OXFORD MEDICAL

Autonomic Failure

Autonomic Failure

A Textbook of Clinical Disorders of the Autonomic Nervous System

THIRD EDITION

Edited by

SIR ROGER BANNISTER

C.B.E., Hon. L.L.D., Hon. D.Sc., M.A.,
M.Sc., D.M. (Oxon), F.R.C.P.
Master, Pembroke College, Oxford;
Hon. Consultant Physician, National Hospital for
Neurology and Neurosurgery, London;
Hon. Consultant Neurologist, St Mary's Hospital, London,
Oxford District Health Authority, and
Oxford Regional Health Authority

and

CHRISTOPHER J. MATHIAS

D.Phil. (Oxon), F.R.C.P.
Professor of Neurovascular Medicine and Consultant Physician
Cardiovascular Medicine Unit, Department of Medicine,
St Mary's Hospital and Medical School/Imperial College of Science,
Technology and Medicine, London;
and Autonomic Unit, National Hospital for Neurology and
Neurosurgery, and University Department of Clinical Neurology,
Institute of Neurology, London

Oxford New York Tokyo
OXFORD UNIVERSITY PRESS

Oxford University Press, Walton Street, Oxford OX2 6DP

Oxford   New York   Toronto
Delhi   Bombay   Calcutta   Madras   Karachi
Kuala Lumpur   Singapore   Hong Kong   Tokyo
Nairobi   Dar es Salaam   Cape Town
Melbourne   Auckland   Madrid
and associated companies in
Berlin   Ibadan

Oxford is a trade mark of Oxford University Press

Published in the United States
by Oxford University Press Inc., New York

First published, 1983 (ed. Sir Roger Bannister)
Second edition, 1988 (ed. Sir Roger Bannister)
Third edition, 1992
First published in paperback, 1993

A catalogue record for this book is
available from the British Library

Library of Congress Cataloging-in-Publication Data

Autonomic failure : a textbook of clinical disorders of the autonomic
nervous system / edited by Sir Roger Bannister and Christopher J. Mathias.
—3rd ed.
(Oxford medical publications)
Includes bibliographical references and index.
1. Autonomic nervous system—Diseases.   I. Bannister, Roger.
II. Mathias, C. J.   III. Series.
[DNLM: 1. Autonomic Nervous System—physiopathology.   2. Autonomic
Nervous System Diseases.   WL 600 A939]
RC407.A95   1992   616.8'8—dc20   91-37457
ISBN 0-19-262218-8 (Pbk)

Printed in Great Britain by
Butler & Tanner Ltd, Frome, Somerset

Preface to the third edition

In this third edition we aim to provide a comprehensive basis for the diagnosis and treatment of the wide range of autonomic disorders which are now being recognized with increasing frequency. It describes these disorders in a range of general diseases, such as diabetes, as well as in various syndromes of acute, subacute, and chronic autonomic failure. Since the second edition there have been many advances in the subject and these have led to the addition of 20 new chapters as well as extensive revision of previous chapters. The international flavour is preserved with authors from the United States of America, different parts of Europe, and Australia.

In the past few years, more autonomic investigation units have been set up around the world and it has become increasingly necessary to describe the scientific basis and the clinical background needed to diagnose and manage a variety of autonomic disturbances. The first two sections deal with the basic aspects of the autonomic nervous system and its function. The third section of the book describes the autonomic tests in detail, their normal values, and the critical interpretation of the abnormalities, which can be quite complex. The fourth section of the book deals with the primary autonomic failure syndromes. The importance of these chronic syndromes has increased in the past few years since it was recognized that some 10 per cent of patients thought to have Parkinson's disease have, in fact, multiple system atrophy, in which there is an important element of autonomic failure requiring detailed investigation and management. There have been advances in the diagnosis of multiple system atrophy (MSA) by the use of refined techniques for catecholamine and neuropeptide measurements, and new techniques such as magnetic resonance imaging (MRI) and *in vivo* neurochemical mapping made possible by positron emission tomography (PET). The pathological examination of ganglia, the counting of autonomic nerve fibres, and the use of microneurography have all increased our understanding of the lesions. The fifth section describes the increasing number of peripheral autonomic neuropathies which are now recognized, including those due to HIV infection, and these have required reclassification since the last edition as a result of the use of more refined techniques for investigation. A new chapter is included on genetically determined autonomic failure syndromes, of which the recently recognized dopamine β-hydroxylase deficiency is of particular interest.

The sixth and last section of the book deals with other autonomic disorders from fainting, through hypertension and cardiac failure, to ageing and the relationship between the sympathetic nervous system and pain.

Better clinical management rests on the attempt to bridge the gap between basic science, which is discussed in the introductory sections of the book, and clinical medicine, thus making diagnosis more precise and treatment more effective. It is hoped that this new edition will continue to provide physicians in different fields, including neurology, diabetology, cardiology, geriatrics, and internal medicine, with a rational guide to the management of autonomic disorders.

Oxford   R.B.
London   C.J.M.
January 1992

Acknowledgements

We wish to acknowledge our gratitude to our clinical colleagues and research associates at the National Hospital for Neurology and Neurosurgery and Institute of Neurology, St Mary's Hospital and Medical School/Imperial College, and the Oxford District Hospitals. We especially wish to thank our staff in the Autonomic Investigation Unit at the National Hospital and the Cardiovascular Medicine Unit at St Mary's Hospital Medical School. We are grateful to various charitable bodies and especially the Wellcome Trust for their sustained support. Finally it is a particular pleasure to thank Miss Alison Blake in Oxford and Mrs Rosalind Mathias for their skilled secretarial assistance and support.

Preface to the first edition

In the past 10 years the clinical syndromes of autonomic failure have been studied by a wide range of new physiological, pharmacological, pathological, and neurochemical techniques, but the information is scattered in papers in many different journals and is not easily available to the clinician. Much is still to be learnt about these syndromes and their management but it is now possible to review these recent advances.

The presenting symptoms of autonomic failure, such as low blood pressure, may overlie unrecognized disturbances of function which are widespread and involve altered control of many different parts of the body including the heart, the kidneys, the pancreas, the bladder, the gut, and the pupils. Symptoms may therefore lead patients to many different specialists who are unfamiliar with these autonomic syndromes. The cardiologist, for example, sees some of the patients with idiopathic orthostatic hypotension and the neurologist, patients with orthostatic hypotension associated with parkinsonism or multiple system atrophy (Shy–Drager syndrome). The general physician encounters many problems of autonomic failure in association with diseases such as diabetes, alcoholism, or amyloidosis. The geriatrician sees the consequences of failure of body-temperature regulation. The genitourinary surgeon is often presented with a difficult problem of the neurogenic bladder. It would be wrong to think of autonomic failure as a single disease entity but progressive autonomic failure in which pathological lesions are to some degree established provides a model for investigation which can be compared with other diseases in which defective autonomic function is part of a wider picture, as in diabetes.

This book aims to provide clinicians in many fields with a guide to useful tests of differing complexity which are now needed to identify autonomic defects of a particular organ in which they have a special interest and should help them to interpret these tests. Interpretation is as important as knowing how to undertake the tests because the autonomic nervous system includes more subtle variations in response than the somatic nervous system and has many compensating mechanisms for impending failure. The practical tests described in the book are set against the more general background of current advances in physiology and pathology of the autonomic nervous system in order to form a basis for rational management in a field which is generally recognized to be exceedingly difficult.

The book also aims to introduce the clinician to new theoretical concepts of the organization of the autonomic nervous system. The old-fashioned notion of a simple duality of a sympathetic–adrenal system causing rather unselective 'fight or flight' responses and a parasympathetic–cholinergic system providing tonic activity, has given way to a new view of a highly selective autonomic nervous system with an integrative action at least as complex as that of the somatic nervous system. New transmitters and modulators abound and receptors, both pre- and postsynaptic, can be blocked, activated, or modified in their numbers and affinities. New general biological principles have emerged with 'up' and 'down' regulation of receptor numbers and affinities and manipulation pharmacologically of pre- and postsynaptic receptors by transmitter depletion or blockade. These fields provide an exciting prospect for future biological as well as medical research. It is appropriate to end with a quotation from my teacher, the late Sir George Pickering, who also concluded a review of autonomic function with the words that it was 'in fact no more than an overture. The main body of the work is to come'.

London   R.B.
September 1982

Contents

Contributors

Anne E. Aber-Bishop, Department of Histochemistry, Royal Postgraduate Medical School, Hammersmith Hospital, DuCane Road, London W12 0NN, UK.

Praveen Anand, Department of Neurology, Royal London Hospital and The London Hospital Medical School, Turner Street, London E1 1BB, UK.

Roger Bannister, Autonomic Investigation Department, National Hospital for Neurology and Neurosurgery, Queen Square, London WC1, UK.

Eduardo E. Benarroch, Department of Neurology, Mayo Clinic and Foundation, Rochester, Minnesota 55905, USA.

Terence Bennett, Department of Physiology and Pharmacology, Medical School, Queen's Medical Centre, Nottingham NG7 2UH, UK.

Christopher D. Betts, Department of Uro-Neurology, National Hospital for Neurology and Neurosurgery, Queen Square, London WC1N 3BG, UK.

David J. Brooks, MRC Cyclotron Unit, Hammersmith Hospital, London W12 0HS, UK.

Geoffrey Burnstock, Department of Anatomy and Developmental Biology, University College London, Gower Street, London WC1E 6BT, UK.

Sudhansu Chokroverty, Division of Clinical Neurophysiology and Department of Neurology, UMDNJ–Robert Wood Johnson Medical School, New Brunswick, New Jersey; and the Neurology Service, Veterans Affairs Medical Center, Lyons, New Jersey 07939, USA.

Jay N. Cohn, Cardiovascular Division, Department of Medicine, University of Minnesota Medical School, Minneapolis, Minnesota 55455, USA.

Kenneth J. Collins, University College and Middlesex School of Medicine, University of London; and Department of Geriatric Medicine, St Pancras Hospital, London NW1 0PE, UK.

Ian Craig, Genetics Laboratory, Department of Biochemistry, Oxford University, Oxford OX1 3QU, UK.

Sally Craig, Genetics Laboratory, Department of Biochemistry, Oxford University, Oxford OX1 3QU, UK.

Susan E. Daniel, Parkinson's Disease Society Brain Bank, Institute of Neurology, 1 Wakefield Street, London WC1N 1PJ, UK.

William C. de Groat, Departments of Pharmacology and Behavioral Science and Center for Neuroscience, University of Pittsburgh, Pittsburgh, Pennsylvania 15261, USA.

Gerald F. DiBona, Department of Internal Medicine, University of Iowa College of Medicine; and Veterans Administration Medical Center, Iowa City, Iowa 52242, USA.

M. E. Edmonds, Diabetic Department, King's College Hospital, Denmark Hill, London SE5 9RS, UK.

Marjorie Ellison, National Hospital for Neurology and Neurosurgery, Queen Square, London WC1 3BG, UK.

David J. Ewing, University Department of Medicine, The Royal Infirmary, Edinburgh EH3 9YW, UK.

R. D. Fealey, Department of Neurology, Mayo Clinic, Rochester, Minnesota 55905, USA.

Nicholas A. Flores, Department of Cardiovascular Medicine, St Mary's Hospital Medical School, Paddington, London W2 1NY, UK.

Clare J. Fowler, Department of Uro-Neurology, National Hospital for Neurology and Neurosurgery, Queen Square, London WC1N 3BG, UK.

Gary S. Francis, Cardiovascular Division, Department of Medicine, University of Minnesota Medical School, Minneapolis, Minnesota 55455, USA.

Hans L. Frankel, National Spinal Injuries Centre, Stoke Mandeville Hospital, Aylesbury, Bucks HP21 8AL, UK.

Sheila M. Gardiner, Department of Physiology and Pharmacology, Medical School, Queen's Medical Centre, Nottingham NG7 2UH, UK.

Roger Hainsworth, Department of Cardiovascular Studies, University of Leeds, Leeds LS2 9JT, UK.

Robert W. Hamill, Department of Neurology, University of Rochester School of Medicine and Dentistry, Rochester, New York, USA.

Wilfrid Jänig, Physiologisches Institut, Christian-Albrechts-Universität, Olshausenstrasse 40, 2300 Kiel, Germany.

Ralph H. Johnson, Medical School Offices, Oxford University Medical School, John Radcliffe Hospital, Headington, Oxford OX3 9DU, UK.

Edmund F. LaGamma, Department of Pediatrics, State University of New York at Stonybrook, Stonybrook, New York, USA.

A. J. Lees, Department of Neurology, National Hospital for Neurology and Neurosurgery, Queen Square, London WC1N 3BG, UK.

Stafford L. Lightman, Neuroendocrinology Unit, Charing Cross and Westminster Medical School, Charing Cross Hospital, London W6 8RF, UK.

Phillip A. Low, Department of Neurology, Mayo Clinic, Rochester, Minnesota 55905, USA.

Ian A. Macdonald, Department of Physiology and Pharmacology, Medical School, Queen's Medical Centre, Nottingham NG7 2UH, UK.

J. G. McLeod, Department of Medicine, University of Sydney, Sydney, New South Wales 2006, Australia.

Allyn L. Mark, Cardiovascular Division, Department of Internal Medicine, University of Iowa College of Medicine, Iowa City, Iowa 52242, USA.

Christopher J. Mathias, Cardiovascular Medicine Unit, Department of Medicine, St Mary's Hospital and Medical School/Imperial College of Science, Technology and Medicine, London W2; and Autonomic Unit, National Hospital for Neurology and Neurosurgery, and University Department of Clinical Neurology, Institute of Neurology, Queen Square, London WC1N 3BG, UK.

Margaret R. Matthews, Department of Human Anatomy, University of Oxford, Oxford OX1 3QX, UK.

Pamela Milner, Department of Anatomy and Developmental Biology, University College London, Gower Street, London WC1E 6BT, UK.

John Morgan-Hughes, National Hospital for Neurology and Neurosurgery, Queen Square, London WC1N 3BG, UK.

H. A. W. Neil, Department of Public Health and Primary Care, University of Oxford, Gibson Laboratories Building, Radcliffe Infirmary, Oxford OX2 6HE, UK.

Julia M. Polak, Department of Histochemistry, Royal Postgraduate Medical School, Hammersmith Hospital, DuCane Road, London W12 0NN, UK.

Ronald J. Polinsky, Clinical Neuropharmacology Section, Clinical Neuroscience Branch, National Institute of Neurological Disorders and Stroke, Bethesda, Maryland 20892, USA.

Christopher Porter, Genetics Laboratory, Department of Biochemistry, University of Oxford, Oxford OX1 3QU, UK.

G. D. Schott, National Hospital for Neurology and Neurosurgery, Queen Square, London WC1N 3BG, UK.

J. T. Shepherd, Mayo Clinic and Foundation, Rochester, Minnesota 55905, USA.

R. F. J. Shepherd, Mayo Clinic and Foundation, Rochester, Minnesota 55905, USA.

Desmond J. Sheridan, Cardiovascular Medicine, St Mary's Hospital Medical School, Paddington, London W2 1NY, UK.

Shirley A. Smith, Diabetes and Endocrine Day Centre, St Thomas' Hospital, London SE1 7EH, UK.

Virend K. Somers, Cardiovascular Division, Department of Internal Medicine, University of Iowa College of Medicine, Iowa City, Iowa 52242, USA.

K. M. Spyer, Department of Physiology, Royal Free Hospital School of Medicine, Rowland Hill Street, London NW3 2PF, UK.

B. Gunnar Wallin, Department of Clinical Neurophysiology, University of Göteborg, Sahlgren's Hospital, S-413 45 Göteborg, Sweden.

P. J. Watkins, Diabetic Department, King's College Hospital, Denmark Hill, London SE5 9RS, UK.

Wouter Wieling, Department of Medicine, Academic Medical Centre, University of Amsterdam, 1105 AZ Amsterdam, The Netherlands.

Christopher S. Wilcox, Departments of Medicine and Pharmacotherapy, University of Florida College of Medicine; and Division of Nephrology and Hypertension, Veterans Administration Medical Center, Gainesville, Florida 32608, USA.

T. D. M. Williams, Neuroendocrinology Unit, Charing Cross and Westminster Medical School, Charing Cross Hospital, London W6 8RF, UK.

David L. Wingate, Gastrointestinal Science Research Unit, The London Hospital Medical College, London E1 2AJ, UK.

P. A. van Zwieten, Departments of Pharmacotherapy and Cardiology, Academic Medical Centre, University of Amsterdam, 1105 AZ Amsterdam, The Netherlands.

Abbreviations

AADC	aromatic L-amino acid decarboxylase deficiency
ACE	angiotensin-converting enzyme
ACh	acetylcholine
AChE	acetylcholinesterase
ACTH	adrenocorticotrophic hormone (corticotrophin)
ADH	antidiuretic hormone (vasopressin)
AF	autonomic failure
AMP	adenosine monophosphate
ANP	atrial natriuretic peptide
ANS	autonomic nervous system
ATP	adenosine triphosphate
AV	atrioventricular
BDNF	brain-derived neurotrophic factor
BMI	body mass index
BP	blood pressure
CAM	cell adhesion molecule
cAMP	cyclic adenosine monophosphate
CAT	computerized axial tomography
CCK	cholecystokinin
CDF	cholinergic differentiation factor
cGMP	cyclic guanosine monophosphate
CGRP	calcitonin gene-related peptide
ChAT	choline acetyltransferase
CHF	congestive heart failure
CI	confidence interval
CNS	central nervous system
CNTF	ciliary neurotrophic factor
CRF	corticotrophin releasing factor
CSF	cerebrospinal fluid
CT	computerized tomography
CV	coefficient of variation
DA	dopamine
DBH	dopamine β-hydroxylase
DBN	down-beat nystagmus
DDAVP	desmopressin
DHPG	dihydroxyphenylglycol
DL-DOPS	DL-threo-dihydroxy-phenylserine (also with prefixes D and L separately)

DM	diabetes mellitus
DMPP	dimethyl phenylpiperazine
dopa	3,4-dihydroxyphenylalanine
EAN	experimental allergic neuritis
ECG	electrocardiogram
EEG	electroencephalogram
EDRF	endothelium-derived relaxing factor
E:I	expiratory : inspiratory ratio
EMG	electromyographic
Enc	encephalin
ENS	enteric nervous system
e.p.s.p.	excitatory postsynaptic potential
ERSNA	efferent renal sympathetic nerve activity
ESR	erythrocyte sedimentation rate
FAP	familial amyloid neuropathy
FD	^{18}F-6-fluorodopa
FDG	^{18}F-2-fluoro-2-deoxy-D-glucose
FFT	fast Fourier transform
FGF	fibroblast growth factor
FSH	follicle-stimulating hormone
GABA	gamma aminobutyric acid
GDH	glutamate dehydrogenase
GFAP	glial fibrillary acidic protein
GFR	glomerular filtration rate
GH	growth hormone
GHRH	growth hormone releasing hormone
GMP	guanosine monophosphate
GRP	gastrin-releasing peptide (bombesin)
HMSN	hereditary motor and sensory neuropathy
HR	heart rate
HRP	horseradish peroxidase
HRV	heart rate variability
HSAN	hereditary sensory and autonomic neuropathy
HVA	homovanillic acid
IAPP	islet-associated polypeptide
IBS	irritable bowel syndrome
i.c.v.	intracerebroventricular
IDDM	insulin-dependent diabetes mellitus
I–E	inspiratory–expiratory difference
i.m.	intramuscular
IML	intermediolateral column
i.p.s.p.	inhibitory postsynaptic potential
i.v.	intravenous

L-Enc	leucine encephalin
LH	luteinizing hormone
LHRH	luteinizing hormone releasing hormone
MANSF	membrane-associated neurotransmitter stimulating factor
mCPP	*m* chlorophenylpiperazine
MHPG	3-methoxy-4-hydroxyphenylglycol
MMC	migrating myoelectric complex
MNSA	muscle nerve sympathetic activity
MPTP	1-methyl-4-phenyl-1,2,3,6 tetrahydropyridine
MRI	magnetic resonance imaging
MSA	multiple system atrophy
NA	noradrenaline
NANC	non-adrenergic, non-cholinergic
NC	neural crest
N-CAM	neural cell adhesion molecule
NGF	nerve growth factor
NIDDM	non-insulin-dependent diabetes mellitus
NMDA	*N*-methyl-D-aspartate
NMF	^{11}C-nomifensine
NNP	nucleated neuronal profile
NPY	neuropeptide Y
NTF	neuronotrophic factors
NTS	nucleus of the tractus solitarius
OH	orthostatic hypotension
OPCA	olivopontocerebellar atrophy
PACAP	pituitary adenylate cyclase activating peptide
PAF	pure autonomic failure
PASP	peripheral autonomic skin potential
PCR	polymerase chain reaction
PCT	pupil cycle time
PD	Parkinson's disease
PET	positron emission tomography
PF	plasma flow
PHI	peptide histidine isoleucine
PHM	peptide histidine methionine
PNMT	phenylethanolamine *N*-methyltransferase
PRA	plasma renin activity
PSP	progressive supranuclear palsy
Q-SART	quantitative sudomotor axon reflex test
RAC	^{11}C-raclopride
RBF	renal blood flow
rCBF	regional cerebral bloodflow

rCMRGlu	regional cerebral glucose metabolism
rCMRO$_2$	regional cerebral O$_2$ metabolism
REM	rapid eye movement (in sleep)
RFLP	restriction fragment length polymorphism
R–R interval	heart rate variability
RSD	reflex sympathetic dystrophy
SAM	substrate adhesion molecule
s.c.	subcutaneous
SCG	superior cervical ganglion
SD	standard deviation
SIF	small intensely fluorescent (of cells)
SHR	spontaneously hypertensive rats
SMP	sympathetically maintained pain
SMS 201-995	somostatin analogue octreotide
SNA	sympathetic nerve activity
SND	striatonigral degeneration
SNSA	skin nerve sympathetic activity
SP	substance P
THC	tetrahydrocannabinol
TOH	tyrosine hydroxylase
TRH	thyrotrophin releasing hormone
TSH	thyroid stimulating hormone
TST	thermoregulatory sweat test
VIP	vasoactive intestinal polypeptide
VLM	ventrolateral medulla
VMA	vanillylmandelic acid
5-HIAA	5-hydroxyindoleacetic acid
5-HT	5-hydroxytryptamine (serotonin)
6-OHDA	6-hydroxydopamine

1. Introduction and classification of autonomic disorders

Roger Bannister and Christopher J. Mathias

The autonomic nervous system innervates every organ in the body, creating, as Galen suggested, 'sympathy' between the various parts of the body. It has as complex a neural organization in the brain, spinal cord, and periphery as the somatic nervous system, but remains largely involuntary or automatic. Claude Bernard wrote 'nature thought it provident to remove these important phenomena from the capriciousness of an ignorant will'. Langley, who in 1898 first proposed the term 'autonomic nervous system', based his experiments on the blocking action of nicotine at synapses in ganglia. In 1921 Loewi discovered 'Vagusstoff' which was released by stimulation of the vagus nerve and proved to be acetylcholine. In the same year Cannon discovered that 'sympathin', later shown to be noradrenaline, was produced by stimulation of the sympathetic trunk. The basis was therefore laid for Dale's distinction between cholinergic and adrenergic transmission in the autonomic nervous system.

Peripheral autonomic function

The peripheral autonomic nervous system, an efferent system, is made up of neurons that lie outside the central nervous system and that are concerned with visceral innervation. Both sympathetic and parasympathetic systems have preganglionic neurons in the brain and spinal cord arranged as shown in Fig. 1.1. The afferent limbs of autonomic reflexes may lie in any afferent nerve. The preganglionic sympathetic fibres are myelinated and leave the spinal roots as white rami communicantes and synapse in the ganglia. Unmyelinated postganglionic fibres rejoin the anterior spinal roots by the arrangement shown in Fig. 1.2, although some sympathetic fibres traverse the ganglia and synapse in more peripheral ganglia, following the arrangement of the parasympathetic fibres.

The transmitter at all preganglionic terminals is acetylcholine, which is not blocked by atropine (the nicotinic effect), whereas the action of acetycholine at the distal end of the cholinergic postganglionic fibres is blocked by atropine (the muscarinic effect). Muscarinic receptors are now subdivided into at least

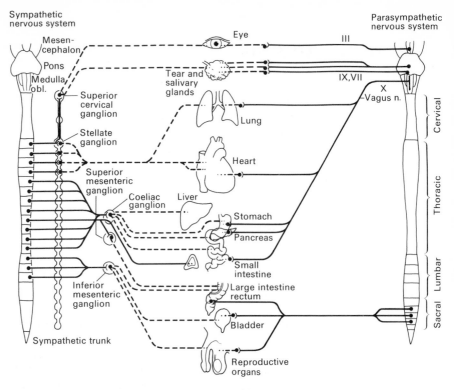

Fig. 1.1. Peripheral autonomic nervous system. The sympathetic innervation of vessels, sweat glands, and piloerector muscles is not shown. Solid lines, preganglionic axons; dashed lines, postganglionic axons. (Taken with permission from Brain (1985).)

three subtypes. Noradrenaline is the principal transmitter for postganglionic sympathetic nerves, but there are a few areas where there is cholinergic transmission. These exceptions include sudomotor nerves, vasodilator fibres to muscle, and the adrenal medulla, which is innervated by preganglionic (cholinergic) fibres and which itself secretes both adrenaline and noradrenaline. Noradrenaline is stored in the terminals and is released by nerve activity or by sympathomimetic drugs, which may act partly indirectly on the ganglia or more centrally, e.g. ephedrine and amphetamine, or on the terminals, e.g. phenylephrine or tyramine. The different actions of noradrenaline and adrenaline are caused by relative effects on different receptors. α-adrenoceptors may be either postsynaptic (α_1) or presynaptic (α_2, which when stimulated decrease the release of the transmitter). α_2-adrenoceptors are also present at the postsynaptic level and they mediate vasoconstriction when stimulated with agonists. β-receptors mediate vasodilatation, especially in muscles, increase the rate and force of the heart

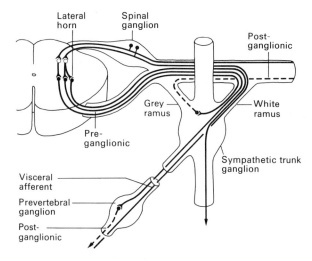

Fig. 1.2.   The autonomic spinal reflex arc. (Taken with permission from Brain (1985).)

with a tendency to arrhythmias, and cause bronchial relaxation. They are further subdivided into β_1-receptors, mediating the chronotropic cardiac action of isoprenaline, and β_2-receptors, which are responsible for most of the peripheral effects of β-adrenergic stimulation (see Chapter 6). Though descriptions of autonomic sensitivity phenomena were first made more than a century ago, the research was summarized by Cannon and Rosenblueth in 1949 under the title, *The supersensitivity of denervated structures: a law of denervation*. Attention since then has concentrated on the 'up' and 'down' regulation of receptor function depending on the availability of the transmitter.

The cells of the autonomic nervous system tend to act in conjunction and this is achieved mainly by specialized intercellular junctions at the ganglion cells which have been demonstrated by electron microscopy and freeze fracture techniques (see Chapter 32). The autonomic ganglia also contain small intensely fluorescent cells ('SIF' cells) which contain many peptides, thought to act as modulators and transmitters at synaptic sites. Substance P, vasoactive intestinal peptide (VIP), encephalins, and somatostatin have all been identified in autonomic ganglia although their precise role in control of nerve transmission is not yet known (see Chapter 32).

The previously held distinction between cholinergic and catecholaminergic cells, underlying the dual hypothesis of antagonism in the autonomic nervous system, is no longer tenable. Immature ganglion cells in culture contain both acetylcholine and catecholamines (see Chapter 2). Sympathetic ganglia have about 45 per cent of acetylcholine-containing neurons in which non-adrenergic, non-cholinergic transmission is now accepted. Within any central pathway there is no simple consistency of a single transmitter and some cells have multiple transmitters: posterior root ganglion cells, for example, have been found to have as many as 10 neuropeptides and putative transmitters. After birth, sweat glands change from adrenergic to cholinergic sympathetic innervation, whereas innervation of some gut structures is switched from sympathetic to cholinergic mechanisms. Presynaptic cholinergic endings may affect noradrenergic sympathetic transmission, and noradrenaline may act not only directly as a transmitter but indirectly by modulating the effect of acetylcholine, as has been shown peripherally where small doses of adrenaline and noradrenaline facilitate transmission but in larger doses inhibit it. The complex interactions of central autonomic control require much further study but, with advances in biochemical typing of cells and in neuroanatomical and neurophysiological techniques, such complex neuronal effects are now being identified.

Central control of the autonomic nervous system

The hypothalamus can be considered the 'highest' level of integration of autonomic function. It remains under the influence of the cortex and the group of structures known as the 'limbic system', which includes the olfactory areas, the hippocampus and amygdaloid complex, the cingulate cortex, and the septal area. These regions of the brain regulate the hypothalamus and are critical for emotional and affective expression. In phylogenetic development the limbic system represents the older or palaeomammalian cortex as opposed to the neomammalian cortex. Its function is thought to be concerned with levels below cognitive behaviour and inductive and deductive reasoning, though it nevertheless is concerned with a feeling of individuality and identity. It analyses the significance of the input of sensation to the organism in relation to the instinctive drives which promote the perpetuation of the individual by satisfying hunger, thirst, and sexual needs.

The hypothalamus is also concerned with maintaining homeostasis against a changing environment and ensures the propagation of the species by sexual and parental drives which can at times override the more selfish self-perpetuating drives of the individual. The essence of its function is choice of patterns of behaviour based on sensory information. As it overlaps both with sensory and motor systems it is essential for many aspects of memory and learning. The autonomic nervous system and many metabolic functions are under the control of the limbic system by means of nerve centres, many of which are situated in the hypothalamus, lying ventrally to the thalamus and constituting the floor of the third ventricle. The hypothalamus contains a large number of scattered ganglion cells, which have been differentiated into a number of nuclei (see Appenzeller 1990). The projections of the hypothalamus are not yet completely known and discussion in detail is beyond the scope of this book.

The hypothalamus controls the autonomic nervous system in two ways, by means of the pituitary and hence other endocrine glands (see Chapter 19) and by direct descending nervous pathways (see Chapter 3). Despite these descending pathways, some regions of the brainstem are to some extent autonomous and function in animals after pontine section of the brainstem. These include cardiac and respiratory function and 'centres' for vomiting and micturition, but under natural circumstances cardiovascular responses never occur in isolation but accompany the processes of exercise, digestion, sexual function, and temperature regulation. The integration of these changes takes place in the hypothalamus. The main course taken by descending sympathetic fibres from the hypothalamus is uncrossed and by way of the lateral tegmentum of the brainstem and lateral medullary formation. Some fibres end directly on the intermediolateral column cells, while others synapse in the reticular formation (see Chapter 4).

Diseases of the autonomic nervous system

The lesions of the nervous system in autonomic failure, with their widespread consequences, are, in Claude Bernard's terms, 'real experiments by which physicians and physiologists profit'. Some may complain that nature is an imprecise experimentalist. The study of individuals with rare disorders can sometimes throw much light on the subtle and complex integration of the autonomic nervous system. A recent example is the newly described disease with a specific enzyme fault, dopamine β-hydroxylase deficiency (Chapter 38). The syndromes of chronic autonomic failure also offer an example of the system degenerations which are so common in neurology and are yet so baffling. We need to find some common biological basis for this curious selective vulnerability. If we can do this, we shall be closer to finding an effective treatment, not only for these particular diseases but possibly also for a wider range of disabling progressive degenerative diseases of the nervous system.

The systematic application of physiological techniques of study to patients with autonomic failure started in the 1960s. Research interest in postural hypotension, the usual presenting symptom of autonomic failure, was stimulated by its occurrence after the weightlessness of space travel. Since then there have been striking advances in the investigation and classification of the syndromes of autonomic failure which were until recently both confused and confusing. Peripheral neuropathies with an autonomic component have long been recognized, particularly in diabetes, alcoholism, and amyloid. Sharpey-Schafer and Taylor (1960) showed that the sympathetic vasoconstrictor pathway to the hands was intact in diabetic autonomic neuropathy, and they therefore attributed the absence of circulatory reflexes and the postural hypotension to an afferent lesion. Though an afferent lesion could not be excluded, their interpretation was probably incorrect because the sympathetic efferent pathway to resistance vessels is often defective in diabetes and the patchiness of lesions on the efferent side is now appreciated.

Much of this book is concerned with the chronic or primary neurological disorders in which the autonomic nervous system is selectively involved by both pre- and postganglionic neuronal degeneration (Shy and Drager 1960; Johnson *et al.* 1966; Bannister *et al.* 1967). Some might doubt the worth of such serious attention given to rare diseases but there are many precedents to show that just such studies of rare disease often lead to the recognition of an entirely new group of disorders of which other examples are then found. It is certain that the detailed study of these diseases by the extensive range of biochemical, physiological, and histochemical techniques now available has yielded a rich harvest of knowledge, much of it unexpected, which can now be applied more widely. In one sense we can classify autonomic disorders as changes of receptor function which are one of the major growing points of medicine, especially the development of autoantibodies against receptors. The detailed studies of autonomic failure are complemented by the sections of the book which are devoted to particular diseases such as diabetes (Chapter 16) in which sooner or later autonomic disturbances occur. Diabetes is overwhelmingly more common than other forms of autonomic dysfunction, and rapid advances have been made now that the methods of testing, most of which were pioneered in relation to autonomic failure, are being applied to the even more complex disturbances in diabetes. There are also large groups of patients with autonomic symptoms: first, patients with parkinsonian symptoms who may have MSA; second, the elderly; and third, patients on drugs which affect autonomic function.

First symptoms of autonomic failure

Most forms of autonomic failure are insidious in their onset, with mild symptoms which are concealed for years because of autonomic or other compensatory mechanisms. As Cannon (1929) pointed out, this system can respond to many and varied stresses from the internal and external environment in ways which conceal its dysfunction. When man first took it upon himself millions of years ago to stand on his two legs he posed great strains on the cardiovascular control needed to protect him against the effect of pooling of blood in the lower extremities. Postural hypotension occurring in emotional syncope raises the intriguing teleological question of whether it has evolutionary significance in avoiding danger by a sudden fall into the horizontal position and the simulation of death. However, a true fainting attack (vasovagal attack) as opposed to other causes of transient loss of consciousness requires an intact autonomic nervous system (see Chapter 39), although persistent postural hypotension is the cardinal feature of autonomic failure. Patients may start with mild symptoms of vague weakness, postural dizziness, or faintness, which can very easily be overlooked or result in erroneous referral to a psychiatrist or cardiologist. The crux of the diagnosis is the measurement of blood pressure when standing rather than lying, still often neglected, which can, like the tip of an iceberg, reveal a much more complex underlying autonomic disturbance. In certain circumstances postural hypotension may be unmasked by food, alcohol, or exercise. The blood pressure control mechanisms at the lower end of the scale are just as elaborate and fascinating as those which cause the more commonly studied problems of hypertension, though the study of these patients has in fact thrown light on the mechanisms of hypertension. Some patients with autonomic failure first have bladder symptoms or impotence, not postural hypotension. In addition to the group of patients with autonomic failure alone, 'pure autonomic failure', a second group of patients may present with symptoms of autonomic failure but within months also develop other neurological symptoms, usually parkinsonism or cerebellar symptoms. However, there may be subtle features which suggest that the parkinsonism is atypical, with a predominance of rigidity and akinesis over tremor or the presence of mild pyramidal signs. Such parkinsonian patients may develop marked postural hypotension when treated with levodopa or may fail to respond to this drug. Some may have additional bulbar involvement. These features raise the possibility of more widespread involvement of the central nervous system and point to the diagnosis of multiple system atrophy.

Classification

Accurate diagnosis is essential for proper management of autonomic failure (AF) but in attempting to classify autonomic disease there is a philosophical point to be borne in mind. As in much of medicine, we use a mixed diagnostic classification. We have a list of diseases of largely known pathology such as diabetes and we make a diagnosis of 'secondary' autonomic failure when abnormal tests in life point to a structural disturbance of autonomic reflexes and pathways in patients or a specific disease. Other patients, without certainly known pathology in common, share certain autonomic symptoms and, from tests in life and observation of similar patients after death, we choose to use the word 'primary' disease. In such patients tests can hardly be said to prove a disease but this is the only way we can place patients in different categories and hope, by research, to improve their treatment.

Autonomic fibres are damaged secondarily in a variety of medical disorders, most commonly in diabetes and alcoholism, but also in a wide range of acute, subacute, and chronic peripheral neuropathies (see Table 1.1). This does not provide a problem of classification but is discussed later (Chapter 35).

Table 1.1.   General classification of autonomic failure

1. Primary

(a) Chronic

  (i) Pure autonomic failure (PAF) formerly called idiopathic orthostatic hypotension (Bradbury and Eggleston 1925)
  (ii) Autonomic failure (AF) with multiple system atrophy (MSA) which includes striatonigral degeneration (SND) and olivopontocerebellar atrophy (OPCA); AF with MSA first described by Shy and Drager (1960)
  (iii) Autonomic failure (AF) with Parkinson's disease (PD), (Fichefet *et al.* 1965)

(b) Acute and subacute

  (i) Pandysautonomia
  (ii) Cholinergic dysautonomia

2. Secondary causes of peripheral autonomic dysfunction (from McLeod, Chapter 35, this volume). Disorders associated with peripheral neuropathy

(a) Autonomic dysfunction clinically important
  (i) Diabetes
  (ii) Primary amyloidosis and familial amyloid neuropathy Type I (Portuguese)
  (iii) Acute inflammatory neuropathy
  (iv) Acute intermittent porphyria
  (v) Hereditary sensory and autonomic neuropathy (HSAN) HSAN type III (Riley–Day syndrome, familial dysautonomia); HSAN type IV

(b) Autonomic dysfunction usually clinically unimportant
  (i) Hereditary neuropathies:
   Hereditary motor and sensory neuropathies
   Fabry's disease
   Hereditary sensory and autonomic neuropathy (HSAN types I & II)
   Amyloid disease (some familial amyloid polyneuropathies, secondary amyloidosis)
  (ii) Chronic inflammatory demyelinating polyradiculoneuropathy
  (iii) Metabolic disorders:
   Chronic renal failure
   Chronic liver disease
   Vitamin B_{12} deficiency
  (iv) Alcoholism and nutritional disorders
  (v) Malignancy
  (vi) Toxic causes (vincristine, acrylamide, heavy metals, perhexiline maleate, organic solvents)

(continued)

Table 1.1. *(continued)*

   (vii) Connective tissue diseases:
       Rheumatoid arthritis
       Systemic lupus erythematosus
       Mixed connective tissue diseases
   (viii) Infection
       Leprosy
       Human immunodeficiency virus (HIV)
       Chagas' disease

3. Ageing (Chapter 44)

4. Genetically determined metabolic disease (Chapter 38)

5. Spinal cord lesions (Chapter 43)

6. Drugs

(a) Central
    (i) Alcohol, Wernicke's encephalopathy
    (ii) Tranquillizers: phenothiazines, barbiturates
    (iii) Antidepressants: tricyclics, monoamine oxidase inhibitors
    (iv) Centrally acting hypotensive drugs: methyldopa, clonidine

(b) Ganglion-blocking drugs: hexamethonium, mecamylamine

(c) Peripherally acting drugs

    (i) Adrenergic neuron-blocking drugs: guanethidine, bethanidine, debrisoquine
    (ii) α–Adrenergic blocking drugs: phenoxybenzamine, labetalol

---

We can now consider the more complex problem of the classification of the group of patients in whom autonomic failure appears to result from a primary or unexplained selective neuronal degeneration. This may occur in a 'pure' form without any other neurological signs. Or it may occur in association with two quite different degenerations of the nervous system, multiple system atrophy and Parkinson's disease.

Historically, the first reported cases of autonomic failure were described by Bradbury and Eggleston (1925) as 'idiopathic orthostatic hypotension' because of their presenting features. This term is misleading because it stresses only one feature of autonomic failure and ignores the more usually associated neurological disturbances of bladder, sexual function, and sweating, and also because the word 'idiopathic' implies that it is a single disease entity, which is not proven. The term 'pure autonomic failure' (PAF) is now accepted generally for this syndrome.

Two cases now recognized as autonomic failure (AF) with multiple system atrophy (MSA) were described by Shy and Drager in 1960 and it is appropriate to quote from their original description.

The full syndrome comprises the following features: orthostatic hypotension, urinary and rectal incontinence, loss of sweating, iris atrophy, external ocular palsies, rigidity, tremor, loss of associated movements, impotence, the findings of an atonic bladder and loss of rectal sphincter tone, fasciculations, wasting of distal muscles, evidence of a neuropathic lesion in the electromyogram that suggests involvement of the anterior horn cells, and the finding of a neuropathic lesion in the muscle biopsy. The date of onset is usually in the 5th to 7th decade of life.

Though they noted degeneration of the intermediolateral column cells in their pathological report, credit for first specifically linking this with the presenting features of postural hypotension rests with Johnson *et al.* (1966). At this stage olivopontocerebellar atrophy had not been linked with autonomic failure.

Autonomic failure may rarely also be associated with otherwise apparently typical Parkinson's disease (PD) (Fichefet *et al.* 1965; Vanderhaegen *et al.* 1970). Such cases pathologically have hyaline eosinophillic cytoplasmic neuronal inclusions known as Lewy bodies, also present in PD (see Chapter 30). It is an important fact that Lewy bodies, some of which may contain catecholamine degeneration products, are usually also found in the brains of patients with PAF, without parkinsonian features, but very rarely in patients with MSA. This evidence, discussed below, tends to separate patients with autonomic failure into two groups pathologically—MSA without Lewy bodies and PAF, and AF with PD with Lewy bodies.

It must be recognized that at an early stage an accurate prognosis of autonomic failure cannot be given. It may remain as PAF for a few years, relatively static, or in time it may also come to be associated either with PD or MSA; with care the earliest features of the other condition may be detected clinically. Conversely, the earliest features of autonomic failure may be detected later in some patients with PD or MSA. For example, Miyazaki (1978) has shown that careful study of cases of non-familial olivo-pontocerebellar atrophy with significant postural hypotension shows a high incidence of urinary, pyramidal, and extrapyramidal symptoms and signs, whereas familial cases, without postural hypotension, very rarely have these additional features.

There is good evidence (see Chapter 30) that virtually all patients with primary autonomic failure as opposed to secondary autonomic failure, studied at post-mortem, have severe loss of intermediolateral column cells, the final common pathway cell for the sympathetic nervous system. It is becoming more probable that the pathological process, whether viral, biochemical, immunological, or of some other kind, that leads to this loss of intermediolateral column cells differs significantly in PAF (and probably in autonomic failure with PD) from that in autonomic failure with MSA. In PAF there appears to be an additional loss of ganglionic neurons (see Chapter 32) which are relatively intact in MSA. This suggests the existence of a more distal process in PAF than in MSA. The hypothesis that at least one of the lesions in PAF is also more distal accords with the evidence that, in general, plasma noradrenaline levels are lower in PAF than in AF with MSA (see Chapter 17). This view now finds support from the magnetic resonance imaging (MRI) and positron emission tomography (PET) scans of patients with PAF which have failed to show evidence of central lesions (see p. 550).

When considering the effects of treatment, so that like is compared with like, it is vital to diagnose patients as precisely as possible on the basis of physiological, pharmacological, biochemical, and scanning findings, even though the ultimate criterion of diagnosis is the post-mortem pathological findings. Moreover, it seems probable that there is a number of different types of sympathetic terminal dysfunction in autonomic failure, which may be the consequence of pathological processes that differ in degree or kind (Nanda *et al.* 1977; Bannister *et al.* 1979; Man in't Veld *et al.* 1987; Mathias *et al.* 1990; see Chapter 38). Just as the defects of nicotinic and muscarinic receptors in human disease have proved to be far more complex than was ever expected (Bannister and Hoyes 1981), disturbances of sympathetic receptors will also prove at least as complex (Fraser *et al.* 1981).

The evaluation and accurate diagnosis of the cause of autonomic symptoms is necessary in order to plan treatment. Even if specific treatment is not available this evaluation will make it easier to manage the patient in such a way that the quality of life can be maintained for as long as possible.

References

Appenzeller, O. (1990). *The autonomic system* (4th edn). Elsevier/North Holland, Amsterdam.

Bannister, R. and Hoyes, A. D. (1981). Generalised smooth-muscle disease with defective muscarinic receptor function. *Br. Med. J.* **282**, 1015–18.

Bannister, R., Ardill, L., and Fentem, P. (1967). Defective autonomic control of blood vessels in idiopathic orthostatic hypotension. *Brain* **90**, 725–46.

Bannister, R., Davies, I. B., Holly, E., Rosenthal, T., and Sever, P. (1979). Defective cardiovascular reflexes and supersensitivity to sympathomimetic drugs in autonomic failure. *Brain* **102**, 163–76.

Bradbury, S. and Eggleston, C. (1925). Postural hypotension: a report of three cases. *Am. Heart J.* **1**, 73–86.

Cannon, W. B. (1929). Organisation for physiological homeostasis. *Physiol. Rev.* **9**, 399–431.

Cannon, W. B. and Rosenblueth, A. (1949). *The supersensitivity of denervated structures: a law of denervation*. MacMillan, New York.

Fichefet, J. P., Sternon, J. E., Franken, L., Demanet, J. C., and Vanderhaegen, J. J. (1965). Etude anatomo-clinique d'un cas d'hypotension orthostatique 'idiopathique'. Considérations pathogénique. *Acta Cardiol.* **20**, 332–48.

Fraser, C. M., Venter, J. C., and Kaliner, M. (1981). Autonomic abnormalities and auto-antibodies to beta-adrenergic receptors. *New Engl. J. Med.* **305**, 1165–70.

Johnson, R. H., Lee, G. de J., Oppenheimer, D. R., and Spalding, J. M. K. (1966). Autonomic failure with orthostatic hypotension due to intermediolateral column degeneration. *Quart. J. Med.* **35**, 276–92.

Man in't Veld, A. J., Boomsa, H., Moleman, P., and Schalekamp, M. A. D. H. (1987). Congenital dopamine-beta-hydroxylase deficiency: a novel orthostatic syndrome. *Lancet* **i**, 183–7.

Mathias, C. J., Bannister, R., Cortelli, P., Heslop, K., Polak, J. M., Raimbach, S., Springall, D. R., and Watson, L. (1990). Clinical, autonomic and therapeutic observations in two siblings with postural hypotension and sympathetic failure due to an inability to synthesize noradrenaline from dopamine because of a deficiency of dopamine beta hydroxylase. *Quart. J. Med.*, New Series **75** (278), 617–33.

Miyazaki, M. (1978). Shy–Drager syndrome—a nosological entity? In *International Symposium on Spinocerebellar Degenerations*. Medical Research Foundation, Tokyo.

Nanda, R. N., Boyle, R. C., Gillespie, J. S., Johnson, R. H., and Keogh, H. J. (1977). Idiopathic orthostatic hypotension from failure of noradrenaline release in a patient with vasomotor innervation. *J. Neurol. Neurosurg. Psychiat.* **40**, 11–19.

Sharpey-Schafer, E. P. and Taylor, P. J. (1960). Absent circulatory reflexes in diabetic neuritis. *Lancet* **i**, 559–62.

Shy, G. M. and Drager, G. A. (1960). A neurological syndrome associated with orthostatic hypotension. *Arch. Neurol., Chicago* **3**, 511–27.

Vanderhaegen, J. J., Perier, O., and Sternon, J. E. (1970). Pathological findings in idiopathic orthostatic hypotension: its relationship with Parkinson's disease. *Arch. Neurol., Chicago* **22**, 207–14.

PART I

Autonomic integration:
scientific aspects of structure and function

2. Autonomic nervous system development

Robert W. Hamill and Edmund F. LaGamma

Introduction

A central theme in developmental neurobiology is the interactions between the forces of 'nature' versus 'nurture' (Bunge *et al.* 1978; Black 1982). More specifically, 'nature' refers to the cell's intrinsic potential, i.e. its genetic make-up which provides the potential for a neuron's eventual repertoire of cellular processes and adult characteristics. 'Nurture' refers to extrinsic forces which influence the developmental cascade of neural maturation and serve to shape ontogenetic processes and determine the neuron's adult state. Although the exact mechanisms of these processes are unknown, the autonomic nervous system (ANS) has served as a model system to examine these developmental issues (for reviews see Black 1978, 1982; Bunge *et al.* 1978; LeDouarin 1982; Patterson 1990). This chapter on autonomic development will briefly review the embryology and maturation of spinal and peripheral components of the ANS, addressing the following areas: developmental stages; regulatory phenomena, interneuronal influences, environmental influences, trophic factors, proto-oncogenes, and plasticity; and clinical issues including normal adaptive autonomic responses and developmental disorders.

Stages of development

Embryonic

Embryologically, ANS ontogeny is related to two main processes: basal plate development within the spinal cord; and neural crest development, migration, and phenotypic expression. In man, neural development begins during the third week when the ectoderm thickens to form the neural plate. Fusion of the neural folds, which form from the elevated lateral edges of the neural plate, results in the formation of the neural tube; neurulation is completed by approximately 26–28 days of gestation (Kissel *et al.* 1981). Upon closure, neuroepithelial cells become neuroblasts, which form the mantle zone surrounding the neuroepithelial layer. As more neuroblasts accrue, dorsal and ventral thickenings appear, and in between the alar and basal plates, progenitors of the dorsal and ventral horns, a smaller collection of neuroblasts form the intermediolateral horn. The preganglionic neurons and ventral nerve rootlets are apparent by the fifth week of maturation.

During the fifth week of human intrauterine development, midthoracic preganglionic fibres (white rami communicans) appear and subsequently exist along the entire length of the sympathetic chain (Kanerva *et al.* 1974). The grey rami communicans develop from the sixth to the eighth week. During the fifth to seventh week vagal parasympathetic preganglionic fibres are present along the trachea, reach the pulmonary parenchyma as well as the proximal intestinal tract (oesophagus and stomach), and form the cardiac plexus (Pappano 1977). Fibres appear in the conduction system of the heart and epithelium of the lung during the tenth week, and, as target organ and enteric ganglion development occurs, preganglionic maturation continues in a craniocaudal fashion (Kissel *et al.* 1981).

Neural crest (NC) cells are initially located dorsomedially between the neural tube and the overlying ectoderm. Before neurulation is complete, crest cells begin to migrate in a rostrocaudal manner along two distinct paths—dorsolaterally and ventrolaterally. The ventral pathways result in the development of autonomic and sensory neurons, paraganglia, chromatophores (non-neuronal support cells), and adrenal chromaffin cells. NC cells are the progenitors of a wide variety of neuronal and neuroendocrine populations which are distinct in phenotypic and functional characteristics. The possible mechanisms by which these crest cells arrive at their terminal differentiated adult character have been reviewed (see Black 1978, 1982; LeDouarin 1982) and it appears that environmental signals exert a major influence on the almost pluripotential nature of crest cells. Table 2.1 summarizes the neural fates and transmitter characteristics of NC.

The timetable of normal human sympathetic development indicates that by the fifth week migrating NC cells coalesce to form primitive sympathetic chains and during the sixth week the chain extends rostrally into the superior cervical ganglion region and caudally with segmentation (Kanerva *et al.* 1974). Postganglionic fibres are also developing: grey rami appear by the sixth week and fluorescent axons are growing toward targets shortly after the appearance of the catecholamine transmitters at approximately 8–9 weeks. Enteric ganglia maturation in human occurs rostrocaudally; ganglion cells appear in the gut early in the first trimester with Auerbach's plexus visible by 9–10 weeks; Meissner's plexus follows at 13–14 weeks. By 24 weeks ganglion cells have reached the rectum.

Noradrenergic fibres innervate the ductus arteriosus very early and by 8–10 weeks of fetal life catecholaminergic fibres are present within the mesentery and gut wall (Kanerva *et al.* 1974). The heart responds to cholinergic stimuli by 4 weeks, adrenergic stimuli by 7 weeks, and the hormones glucagon and

Table 2.1. Neuronal derivatives of neural crest

Primitive cell	Adult cell/structure	Transmitter characteristics (not all inclusive)*
Bipolar neuroblast	**Dorsal root ganglia**	
Multipolar neuroblast	**Sympathetic neurons**	
	Paravertebral ganglia	NA, CCK, somatostatin,
	Prevertebral ganglia	SP, Enc, ACh,
	Terminal ganglia	VIP, 5-HT, NPY
	Parasympathetic ganglia	
	Major parasympathetic ganglia	
	Ciliary	
	Sphenopalatine	ACh, VIP, SP, CA's-SIF,
	Otic	NPY
	Submandibular/sublingual	
	Pelvic ganglia	
	Terminal parasympathetic ganglia (target tissue)	
	Enteric neurons	
	Myenteric plexus (Auerbach's)	GABA, ACh, VIP, 5-HT,
	Submucosal plexus (Meisner's)	SP, Enc, SRIF, motilin-like
	Enteric ganglia	peptide, bombesin-like peptide
	Chromaffin cells of adrenal medulla	A, NA, Enc, NPY, APUD
	Paraganglia–chromaffin	5-HT, DA, A
	Small intensely fluorescent (SIF) cells, ganglia	5-HT, DA, A

*NA, noradrenaline; CCK, cholecystokinin; SP, substance P; Enc, encephalin; ACh, acetylcholine; VIP, vasoactive intestinal polypeptide; 5-HT, 5-hydroxytryptamine; CA's-SIF, catecholamines—small intensity fluorescent; GABA, gamma aminobutyric acid; SRIF, somatostatin; NPY, neuropeptide Y; APUD, amine precursor uptake and decarboxylation; DA, dopamine; A, adrenaline.

triiodothyronine by 11 weeks. Parasympathetic nerves appear by 8 weeks, and sympathetic nerves by 10 weeks, whereas neuroeffector transmission is not present until 11 weeks (cholinergic) and 14 weeks (adrenergic). The heartbeat appears by 1 month, but is generally not auscultated until 18 weeks of intrauterine life. By 20 weeks changes in fetal heart rate may be observed (Walker 1975; Papp 1988). The iris, pineal, and vas deferens are not substantially innervated until after birth (Kanerva *et al.* 1974).

Postnatal

The ANS is at various developmental stages at birth, and, as discussed below, interruption of mechanisms governing neuronal maturation within the first 2–3 weeks of life will produce life-long developmental deficits. Postnatal human development is normally gauged by physiological observations (see 'Clinical issues', p. 30). Blood flow, bowel transit, and bladder emptying depends upon maturation of peripheral neural structures as well as central autonomic control mechanisms. Peripherally, the differentiation of neuroblasts into enteric ganglion cells and mature plexuses is quite delayed; in fact, at birth only approximately one-third of the neuroblasts are differentiated and development continues throughout the first 5 years of life (Kissel *et al.* 1981). Similarly, the development of autonomic ganglia and the innervation of pelvic structures involved in micturition are delayed. Voluntary control over these functions eventually ensues by 2 to 3 years of age.

Two clinical areas, thermoregulation and cardiovascular control, have received considerable attention. Although a newborn human infant can initiate vasodilation and panting in response to hyperthermia and releases catecholamines to vasoconstrict and augment thermogenesis during hypothermia, the neonate and infant adapt poorly to temperature stress. In general, cardiovascular control appears more mature than temperature control. Although incomplete vascular responses to thermal stimuli may be present until about 2 to 3 months of age, cardiovascular responses controlling normal vasomotor tone are present before birth, as early as the end of the second trimester (Gootman and Gootman 1983) and the newborn's cardiovascular response to cold stress is normal, implying intact sympathoadrenal responses and baroreceptor mechanisms (Gootman and Gootman 1983). Studies examining neurotransmitters and their metabolites reveal that all adrenergic compounds are present at birth, but adult levels are not approached until 5 years of age and not reached until adolescence. Laboratory studies in swine and rodent are available which provide a substantial review of the morphological, physiological, and neurochemical development of noradrenergic and baroreceptor systems involved in cardiovascular control (Gootman and Gootman 1983; Slotkin 1985).

Regulatory phenomena

The problem of complexity

In even the simplest analysis, explaining the process of organization of the nervous system's one billion neuronal cells represents a formidable challenge to mechanistic biologists. Decision schema require a remarkable degree of accuracy and precision. To accomplish this feat, an impressive array of biological 'cues' is utilized. In view of the fact that broad categorical mechanisms may contain up to 40 or 50 possible mediators each, the problem of correctly addressing cell location, differentiation, or connectivity and of how developmental disorders appear is perhaps not so surprising after all. The following discussion highlights intrinsic and extrinsic mechanisms while fully recognizing that our knowledge is limited and all important studies cannot be referenced. A schematic diagram illustrating the course of transmitter development is presented in Fig. 2.1.

Intrinsic influences on peripheral
autonomic development ('nature')

Genetic encoding

Defining relationships between environmental stimuli and cell responsiveness at the molecular level is central to an understanding of biological adaptation and phenotypic expression throughout development. Many of these processes require tissue-specific gene control in which factors initiating transcription are critical determinants of function or of choices made during development (Yamamoto 1985). Consequently, during development a dynamic balance must exist between processes intrinsic to the cell (nature) and epigenetic factors (i.e. extrinsic factors) which function as critical determinants of cell outcome (nurture). If true, how do these events transpire; what are the guiding rules? What are the signals, and through which intracellular pathways are signals transduced to guide the developing neuron through a myriad of progressively restricted biochemical choices which define cell lineage? Finally, once committed, to what extent may a cell be modified, that is, how 'plastic' or 'mutable' are neurons in maturity? The following section outlines some of the mechanisms regulating development.

Pattern formation in the nervous system
(Homeobox, PAX, and POU genes)

Hierarchical activation of certain gene families appears responsible for temporal, spatial, and, in all likelihood, phenotypic choices of cell lineage during development. Contemporary strategies have begun to exploit common features among certain genes and then to search for other members of that

Stage:	Embryo	Fetus		Neonate	Adult
Transmitter mutability	++++	++++	+++	++	+

Developmental signals	Embryonic	Microenvironment ?NGF		Afferent transsynaptic signals
				Efferent: target signals
				Trophic factors
				  NGF/CNTF/BDNF/FGF
				Differentiation factors
				  CDF/MANS
				Glucocorticoids
				Gonadal steroids	

Transmitter development	Early expression	Definitive expression	Modulation	Regulation (e.g. inducibility)	

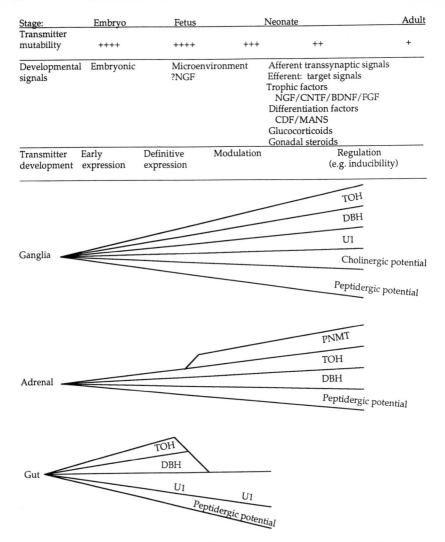

Fig. 2.1. Schematic representation of transmitter development. Developmental age proceeds from left to right in each panel, and vertical alignment among the entries in different panels approximates simultaneous processes or events. Lower segment of schema represents appearance and development of individual transmitter characters for sympathetic ganglia, adrenal chromaffin cells, and the transiently noradrenergic cells of the gut. Phenylethanolamine N-methyltransferase (PNMT) appears during definitive expression in the adrenal and tyrosine hydroxylase (TOH) and dopamine betahydroxylase (DBH) disappear in the gut cells, while a high-affinity uptake system for noradrenaline (U_1) persists. NGF, nerve growth factor; CNTF, ciliary neurotrophic factor; BDNF, brain-derived neurotrophic factor; FGF, fibroblast growth factor; CDF, cholinergic differentiation factor; MANS, membrane-associated neurotransmitter stimulating factor. (Adapted from Black (copyright 1982 by the AAAS).)

gene's family (Kessel and Gruss 1990). In this novel approach, once a gene is identified, experimental evaluation of its protein function follows. Pattern formation gene families are known as homeobox genes (Hox genes), paired-box genes (PAX), and POU genes (Kessel and Gruss 1990). At present, only one example exists that appears to be related to a programme for maturation (*Hox 1.4* discussed later in this section; Wohlgemuth *et al.* 1989).

Homeobox (Hox) proteins number greater than 30 and contain a 61-amino-acid DNA binding domain. These Hox gene protein products are believed to function as transcription factors involved in initiating whole programmes of gene expression, thus evoking broad patterns of phenotypic changes during development. Paired-box gene proteins (PAX 1–8) are similar to Hox proteins, but contain a second DNA binding domain. The third group of proteins, POU proteins (Pit, Oct, and Unc), are also transcription factors. The POU family of proteins contains a carboxy terminal region, homologous to the homeobox binding sites (61 amino acid region), but also has a common 76 amino terminal region. Two other classes of transcription factor proteins in this group include Oct (Oct 1 and Oct 2) and Unc 86. Oct 1 is a ubiquitous human transcription factor protein but Oct 2 and Unc 86 proteins are expressed primarily in neuronal and lymphocytic cell lineages. Whether these protein families serve a role in maturation has yet to be explored.

Considering the organizational importance of pattern formation gene programmes, a fundamental understanding of their regulation is of obvious importance. In addition, one might also anticipate that even their regulation may share common features for the group as well. Indeed, this is the case since one such common transcription factor is the retinoic acid receptor, a protein homologous to the thyroid hormone receptor. The fundamental nature of this molecule's importance is evident by the ubiquitous role of thyroid hormone in ANS development (Slotkin 1985) and the irreversible nature of cretinism (congenital hypothyroidism).

Many investigators are attempting to define the role of pattern formation genes by inserting mutated versions of them into germ lines of mice. Subsequent effects of the mutated protein products during development can then be evaluated (reverse genetics approach; Kessel and Gruss 1990). One successful result from this approach involves overexpressing the *Hox 1.4* gene (Wohlgemuth *et al.* 1989). Excess Hox 1.4 protein resulted in mice with a functional stenosis and improper innervation of the colon, decreased peristaltic activity, and absent enteric ganglia. These phenotypic features are reminiscent of Hirschsprung's disease. Hence, a reverse genetics approach may eventually bring new insights into the basis of Hirschsprung's disease as well as other perplexing ANS disorders through analysis of the role of pattern formation gene programmes.

Genetic mechanisms: intra- and intercellular signalling

Communication between cells results from a plethora of biochemical messages including amines, amino acids, peptides, proteins, etc. This method of organized interaction allows only selected cells to respond to specific signals evoked by changes in the cellular environment, resulting in integrated responses at the level of the whole animal. This specificity of the signals is imparted largely by cell surface (e.g. acetylcholine, adrenergic, etc.) or intracellular (e.g. glucocorticoids) receptors. However, other mechanisms also exist: N-CAM (neural cell adhesion molecule), glycoprotein cell surface molecules, and growth factors. Figure 2.2 schematically presents the complexity of regulatory phenomena for an adrenal chromaffin cell, but similar mechanisms obtain for peripheral autonomic neurons.

Transduction: conversion of extracellular signals to intracellular messages

Neurohormonal messages are detected by cell surface receptors which convert the external biochemical signal into a cellular response (e.g. transmitter release, protein synthesis, etc.). This is often associated with increased

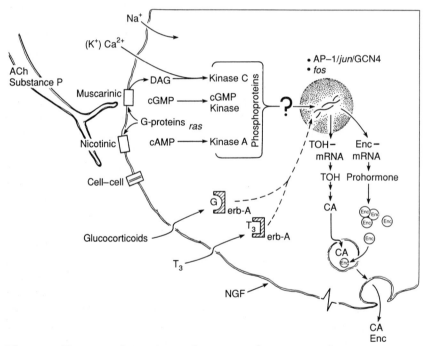

Fig. 2.2. Factors and signal-transduction mechanisms regulating transmitter gene expression in adrenal chromaffin cells. A wide variety of intercellular signals interact to regulate transmitter gene expression in maturity and during development. This includes activation of cell surface receptors, cell–cell interactions, and exposure to growth factors and hormones. ACh, acetylcholine; cAMP, cyclic adenosine monophosphate; cGMP, cyclic guanosine monophosphate; NGF, nerve growth fctor; DAG, 1.2 diacylglycerol; TOH, tyrosine hydroxylase; CA, (catecholamines); Enc (encephalin).

transmembrane flux of sodium, potassium, or calcium ions which in turn activates other intracellular transduction systems. In contrast, transduction for intracellular receptors differs. Activated glucocorticoid receptors cause intracellular responses either directly by activating gene transcription or at epigenetic (i.e. cellular) loci (Yamamoto 1985).

Selective receptor activation is further diversified by intracellular signal-transduction processes providing an additional level of complexity, interaction, and control to expand the cell's functional repertoire. Many of these changes are shown to affect transcriptional events: cell surface receptors linked to membrane-bound G-protein-dependent mechanisms trigger adenylate cyclase-induced increases in cyclic adenosine monophosphate (cAMP) production, activating protein kinase A, which phosphorylates numerous cytosolic proteins. These generalized signal-transduction and second-messenger schemes are central to current thinking in molecular developmental neurobiology, linking biochemical observations with phenotypic expression, neuromodulation, and neuronal function (Fig. 2.2).

Gene regulation: mechanisms for responding to biochemical messages

Control over the levels of individual messenger RNA (mRNA) species is extremely important in generating the diversity and abundance of proteins encoded by the message. Proteins, in turn, define the phenotype and the function of neuronal cells. Moreover, during development, control over expression of certain genes allows differentiation and clonal cell lines to emerge. Molecular mechanisms governing genomic control reside at several levels. Apparently, removal, replacement, or modification of a histone-type DNA-binding protein relaxes the complex chromosomal structure allowing specific regulated gene subunits the opportunity to be transcriptionally activated by biochemical signals. In addition, control is thought to be imparted by changes in the methylation state of nucleotides in the regulatory region of the gene which may also alter DNA conformation.

Once chromatin geometry is rearranged, current evidence indicates gene activation is dependent on binding of various proteins with site-specific DNA affinity to regulate expression (Yamamoto 1985). Thus, protein interactions at enhancer, promoter, or repressor sites enhance or repress gene read-out (i.e. transcription) by altering the 'transcriptional efficiency' of the gene. Regulatory phenomena are likely to reside at the level of biochemical modification of DNA-binding proteins, in proteins required for splicing RNA transcripts (e.g. small nuclear ribonuclearprotein particles) and/or in mechanisms of message RNA stabilization.

Translation and posttranslational control:
extracellular signals result in lasting biochemical responses

Transport of mature mRNA past the nuclear membrane to the cytosolic machinery precedes its binding to ribosomes for translation. After the protein product (prohormones) is generated, it is often biochemically modified (e.g. amidated, glycosylated, etc.) before the mature active molecule exists. The mature protein (or processed peptide product) can now influence other intracellular or extracellular events. Thus, if one of these newly synthesized proteins also serves as a transcriptional control molecule, as is the case with certain oncogenes (e.g. *fos*, *jun*), the additional complexity of interactions that may subsequently arise is enormous.

Regulated neuronal communication and gene expression at the molecular level

At present relevant regulatory phenomena are largely unknown. However, an emerging area of interest will focus on the identification of regulatory proteins which alter expression of neuronal genes (LaGamma *et al.* 1989; LaGamma *et al.* 1991). For inducible genes, does the amount of factor increase or is the factor instead modified to enhance its affinity for the gene? These questions can only be answered by characterizing convenient model systems, such as the ANS. In this way the role of environmental stimuli on nervous system development or function can be further understood at the cellular and molecular level.

Extrinsic influences on peripheral autonomic development ('nurture')

Environmental signals are known to influence autonomic neuron maturation from the earliest stages of neural crest migration to the development and maintenance of the neuron's adult character. Mature neurons apparently are not immutable since alteration of the environmental milieu during adulthood will alter neuronal characteristics.

Adhesion systems—cell migration (CAMs, SAMs, integrins, cadherins)

Peripheral morphogenesis and vector tracking of developing neurons are modified by local 'ques' (factors) including hormones, transmitters, and various growth factors. Directionality also involves cell–cell interactions (cell adhesion molecules: CAMs), and cell–substrate interactions (substrate adhesion molecules: SAMs). Subtypes of adhesion molecules are expressed in a distinct spatial and temporal pattern during neurogenesis.

Putative functions of cell adhesion molecules depend on their transmembrane location, on the local concentration of calcium ions (the cadherins), and on the number of adhesion molecules in the cell membrane. These molecules cause morphological changes and motility by altering features of a cell's cytoskeleton. SAMs and CAMs derive target specificity through an extracellular receptor-linked actin-related mechanism. The cytoplasmic domain of these receptors is linked to actin through a class of molecules known as catenins. At the external surface the transmembrane portion of the SAM family receptors utilizes a class of proteins known as integrins. Integrins interact with extracellular molecules such as fibronectin, collagen, laminin, and proteoglycans to convey information. Growth factors (and, we presume, other regulatory molecules) modify expression of integrins and cadherins on the cell surface. In turn, many extracellular matrix molecules amplify this interaction by affecting growth factors. This synergy contributes to the underlying precision necessary for correct navigation to target structures.

Hormonal regulation

Investigations of the hormonal control of ANS development have focused on thyroid hormone, glucocorticoids, and testosterone. Thyroid ablation prevents normal biochemical and morphological development in the superior cervical ganglion and noradrenergic terminal development in the submaxillary gland (Black 1978) and delays adrenal maturation (Slotkin 1985). Thyroid administration postnatally results in a precocious increase in submandibular gland nerve growth factor and epidermal growth factor; these increases are dependent on noradrenergic nerve terminals (Lakshmanan *et al.* 1986). Glucocorticoids influence the appearance of small, intensely fluorescent (SIF) cells in paravertebral sympathetic ganglia and may alter phenotypic expression in migrating neural crest cells (Black 1982). In addition, glucocorticoids are critical for development of adrenal medullary cells, and influence the transmitter characteristics of SIF cells, as well as co-localized catecholamine and opiate peptides (LaGamma *et al.* 1989).

Gonadal steroids influence a wide variety of neuronal characteristics throughout life and are thought to exert organizational effects during early critical perinatal periods and activational effects during maturity. Both patterns are operant in the ANS. Prenatal and postnatal alterations in the hormonal milieu influence cell number and synaptic input and neuro-transmitter chemistry. During adulthood bilateral castration decreases baseline tyrosine hydroxylase (TOH) activity, noradrenaline (NA) levels, and neuropeptide Y (NPY) in the hypogastric ganglion, and testosterone treatment reverses these effects (Hamill and Schroeder 1990). The potential mechanisms underlying these gonadal regulatory events include the control of TOH mRNA and nerve growth factor mRNA by testosterone.

Interneuronal influences: peripheral and
central regulation of autonomic development

Interneuronal and neuron-target regulatory mechanisms exist during ontogeny and influence neuronal survival and neuronal characteristics. Anterograde transsynaptic influences regulate the development of noradrenergic characteristics of rat sympathetic neurons. Preganglionic neurectomy precludes the development of postsynaptic TOH activity and noradrenaline levels. Similarly, denervation alters adrenal opiate peptide accumulation.

Conversely, retrograde developmental regulatory influences exist between postsynaptic and presynaptic neural components in ganglia. Preganglionic choline acetyltransferase (ChAT) activity fails to develop following ablation of postsynaptic noradrenergic cells, and preganglionic cell bodies within the intermediolateral cell column exhibit reduced survival if adrenergic neurons are destroyed in the periphery (see Black 1978 for review).

There appears to be a critical time during development when central nervous system lesions alter sympathetic maturation. Spinal transection at 10 days of age results in altered cholinergic and adrenergic biochemical maturation, abnormalities which persist throughout the first year of life (Hamill *et al.* 1983). Synapse number within the ganglia is substantially reduced as well and the loss of synapses correlates well with reductions in ChAT activity.

Target organs regulation

Target organs influence the development of the innervating neuron. For instance, removal of the iris or salivary glands prior to any substantial innervation results in failed development of neurotransmitter enzymes in the superior cervical ganglion and a decrease in neuron number within the superior cervical ganglion. The peripheral field of innervation of a neuron may be increased and such studies have demonstrated increased neuronal survival. Salivary glands may be enlarged by pharmacological manipulations which either increase acinar cells (isoproterenol treatment) or tubular portions (testosterone treatment) of the glands. Only the latter treatment results in an increase in enzyme activities and cell number. Since the salivary glands are known to contain nerve growth factor (NGF) and since NGF is synthesized in the gland's tubular portions, it is hypothesized that testosterone treatment increases the availability of NGF which is retrogradely transported to the noradrenergic cell bodies in the superior cervical ganglion. Thus, target organs may influence sympathetic development via NGF (see Black 1978 for review). In turn, sympathetic cells influence target development. Neural crest cells migrating to the embryonic heart contribute to the normal formation of its outlet and influence the intrinsic rate of beating. Removal of these cells prior to migration results in cardiac malformations (Kirby 1987).

Neuronotrophic factors (NTF)

Nerve growth factor (NGF) is the prototype of an ever-expanding group of peptide molecules which regulate neuronal growth and development, influencing either neuronal survival, neuronal growth (neurite outgrowth), or both. Over the last five years a number of new growth factors influencing ANS development have been identified. A brief outline of these neuronotrophic factors is listed in Table 2.2 and several recent reviews address this subject in more detail (Manthorpe *et al.* 1989; Walicke 1989).

NGF is critical for normal prenatal and postnatal sympathetic development (for a review see Levi-Montalcini 1987). Neonatal treatment with antibodies

Table 2.2. Neuronal growth and differentiation factors

Growth/differentiation factor*	Neural-crest-derived target cells†	Source	Molecular weight (kDa)	Effects‡
NGF	Sympathetic nervous system + Dorsal root ganglion + Nodose ganglion 0 Jugular +	Salivary glands Vas deferens Heart Iris Spleen	13.2	↑Survival ↑Neurite growth ↑Transmitter enzyme—TOH
CNTF	Ciliary ganglion +	Sciatic nerve Iris/eye Heart	22.5–24	Superior cervical ganglion: ↑ChAT; ↓NA; ↑VIP Ciliary ganglion: ↑ChAT; ↑cell no.; ↑neurite growth
BDNF	Dorsal root ganglion sensory neurons + Nodose ganglion +/jugular + Dorsomedial trigeminal + Mesencephalic trigeminal + Sympathetic nervous system 0 Ciliary ganglion 0	CNS	12.3	↑Survival ↑Neurite growth
FGF Acidic Basic	Ciliary ganglion + Ciliary ganglion + PC 12 +	Fibroblasts (mitogen for mesenchymal cells)	17–20 (each) (53% homology)	Acidic: Ciliary ganglion: ↑survival; ↑neurites; Basic: Ciliary ganglion: ↑survival; ↑neurites PC 12 neuronal differentiation
CDF	Ciliary neurons 0 Superior cervical ganglion +	Heart	45	Superior cervical ganglion: ↑ChAT; ↓NA; ↑VIP; ↑SP
MANS	Ciliary neurons + Superior cervical ganglion +	Spinal cord	29	Superior cervical ganglion: ↑ChAT; ↓NA; ↑SP

*NGF, nerve growth factor; CNTF, ciliary neurotrophic factor; BDNF, brain-derived neurotrophic factor; FGF, fibroblast growth factors; CDF, cholinergic differentiation factor; MANS, membrane-associated neurotransmitter stimulating factor.

† +, present; 0, absent

‡ ↑, Increased; ↓, decreased; TOH, tyrosine hydroxylase; NA, noradrenaline; VIP, vasoactive intestinal polypeptide; SP, substance P.

directed against NGF will result in sympathectomy, and exposure to anti-NGF prenatally, via maternal transfer of antibody, or postnatally, via cross-fostering experiments with immunized mothers, precludes the normal morphological and biochemical development of peripheral ganglia. The clinical relevance of NGF's role is evident; the immune incompetence associated with the fetal syndrome may be associated with alcohol-induced perturbation of the normal NGF-influenced noradrenergic regulation of the immune system or the interaction between NGF and other hormonal factors such as thyroid and glucocorticoids (Gottesfeld *et al.* 1990). In total, NGF exerts regulatory influences on sympathetic systems throughout life.

The development of cholinergic neurons of the peripheral parasympathetic nervous system is also dependent on neuronotrophic factors for normal maturation. Ciliary ganglion neurons undergo substantial cell death during normal development; 50 per cent die. Death occurs around the time that synaptic contact with the iris, the target organ of the ciliary ganglion, occurs. Ciliary neurotrophic factor (CNTF), a critical neuronotrophic factor produced by ciliary ganglion targets, influences ciliary ganglion neuronal survival. Immunoparasympathectomy may be produced with a monoclonal antibody to CNTF (Hendry *et al.* 1988) suggesting that CNTF is in fact critical for normal maturation of cholinergic components of the ANS. Fibroblast growth factors (FGF) also appear to have an ability to influence neuronal survival in the ciliary ganglion as well. Interestingly, CNTF also influences differentiation of sympathetic neurons; the transmitter phenotype in rodent superior cervical ganglion in culture will change from noradrenergic to cholinergic in the presence of CNTF.

Brain-derived neurotrophic factor (BDNF), originally purified from brain tissue, has been shown to regulate the development of the central processes of neural crest derived peripheral sensory neurons. Additionally, trigeminal mesencephalic neurons and brainstem proprioceptive neurons derived from neural crest also depend on BDNF. BDNF does not increase the survival of sympathetic or parasympathetic neurons. Thus, a scenario appears to exist: the maturation of the peripheral components of a dorsal root ganglion neuron may depend on NGF, and the survival of centrally coursing fibres and central connectivity may depend on BDNF. The extent to which BDNF may influence the maturation of central connections of efferent autonomic pathways is unknown.

Cholinergic differentiation substances have also been identified. These molecules appear to influence the transmitter phenotype of the neuron. For instance, sympathetic neurons in the superior cervical ganglion destined to innervate sweat glands will convert from noradrenergic to cholinergic, and this switch is dependent upon substances derived from the target tissue (Schotzinger and Landis 1988). Factors purified from a number of sources appear to influence transmitter phenotype; cholinergic differentiation factor (CDF), membrane-associated neurotransmitter stimulating factor (MANS), and CNTF all result in a similar transition from catecholaminergic to cholinergic phenotype (Rao *et al.* 1990).

Trophic factors and proto-oncogenes

Oncogenes were discovered in the process of examining retroviral systems of cell transformation to tumours. These viral-incorporated cellular oncogenes have analogues which are part of normal cells: these progenitor constituents were designated proto-oncogenes and approximately 60 have been recognized. Transcription of these genes leads to the production of oncogene-encoded proteins which regulate not only transcriptional activity of genes, including their own, but also interact with second messenger systems within the cell. Thus, nuclear and cytoplasmic proto-oncogene proteins exist and appear to be involved in signal transduction from the cell membrane to the nucleus, as well as gene regulation. Not surprisingly, the natural role for these molecules includes a means by which cells respond to extracellular signals involved in growth and development. Specific proto-oncogenes are activated by NGF. Neoplastic cells from phaeochromocytomas (PC 12 cells) respond to NGF by changing their replicative nature and converting to a neuronal (sympathetic) phenotype which includes sending out processes. Proto-oncogenes are part of the key response mechanisms of these cells. NGF administration to PC 12 cells activates three proto-oncogenes: c-*fos*, c-*myc*, and c-*jun* (Wu *et al.* 1989). The proteins produced regulate the transcription of these, as well as other genes involved in cellular differentiation, and cell growth and development. Other trophic molecules appear to utilize proto-oncogenes in a similar fashion: platelet-derived growth factor induces c-*fos* gene and protein, and the c-*erb*-β gene encodes the epidermal growth factor receptor.

Proto-oncogenes may also be key molecules in the neuron's response to other extracellular signals, namely hormonal factors. Neurons in the central nervous system exhibit induction of fos protein following oestrogen administration (Insel 1990) and oestrogen activation of the ovalbumin gene involves the *fos–jun* proto-oncogene complex. These proto-oncogenes and their protein products are also involved in the regulation of transcriptional activation and inhibition by other steroid hormones such as glucocorticoids. The glucocorticoid receptor will repress AP-1 (*fos:jun* dimer) mediated transcriptional activation. In turn, *jun* inhibits the normal activation of glucocorticoid steroid responsive genes. Although examination of cytoplasmic and nuclear proto-oncogenes and their oncoprotein products in the ANS has not been extensive, these processes will undoubtedly be involved in the aforementioned regulatory phenomena, affecting neuronal growth and survival and phenotypic expression.

The concept of plasticity

Traditional teachings concerning neuronal plasticity maintained a restricted view in which neuronal tissue was believed to be committed, unresponsive, or immutable. Recently, the collective work of many investigators has revealed a remarkable degree of synaptic, transmitter, and receptor plasticity, and, indeed, ongoing neuronal cell division. Most intriguing is the recognition that the fundamental basis of plasticity is the expression of certain proteins. Control of protein synthesis reflects the cell's specificity in control of gene expression. In turn, gene expression results fron *trans*-acting DNA binding proteins functioning in *cis* (LaGamma and Weisinger 1991).

Clinical issues

Developmental disorders

Two ANS developmental disorders which illustrate ontogenetic aberrations of neural crest cells are familial dysautonomia (Riley–Day syndrome) and Hirschsprung's disease. Familial dysautonomia, an autosomal inherited recessive trait, is essentially confined to Ashkenazic Jews, a pattern suggestive of an altered single mutant allele at one gene locus. Patients experience symptom complexes related to underlying disturbances of autonomic and sensory neurons: cardiovascular instability, swallowing and gastrointestinal dysfunction (vomiting crises), tearing and taste bud alterations, and insensitivity to pain and temperature. Since NGF plays a critical role in autonomic development and since anti-NGF (*vide supra*) produces similar pathological changes in animals, a defect in NGF was proposed. Although β-NGF in serum and fibroblast from these patients was believed to be reduced, recombinant DNA techniques have been utilized to establish that the structural gene for β-NGF is not defective. Whether defects in the processing of NGF or in the NGF receptor exist remains unknown.

Hirschsprung's disease results from the absence of enteric ganglia from a segment of bowel and presents clinically as intestinal obstruction. There is substantial dilatation of the bowel proximal to the aganglionic section and megacolon may result. Hirschsprung's disease occurs in approximately one of every 5000 to 8000 births and 80 per cent of the patients are male. Initial hypotheses suggested that, since the pathology is most frequently localized to the distal bowel, rectum, and rectosigmoid colon (70–80 per cent of cases), a defect in neural crest migration must exist. However, since other neurocristopathies such as Waardenburg's syndrome, Marcus Gunn ptosis, and von Recklinghausen's disease may be associated with Hirschsprung's disease, a primary alteration in the differentiation of neural-crest-derived neuroblasts may occur. A similar disease occurs in animals following overexpression of the *Hox 1.4* gene (Wohlgemuth *et al.* 1989). Whether this occurs in humans has yet to be determined. Alternatively, failure of neuroblasts to survive within the bowel because of a defect in the microenvironment may be the underlying pathophysiological mechanism.

Functional development

Maturation of integrated sympathoadrenal function has been an area of interest for fetal, neonatal, and perinatal physiologists and clinicians for many years (Gootman and Gootman 1983; Papp 1988). In the human, catecholamines appear in the adrenal medulla by 8–9 weeks gestation with reflex release by 10 weeks. Reflex control of heart rate and integrated distribution of blood flow begins between 10 and 20 weeks gestation and matures considerably thereafter (Pappano 1977; Papp 1988). Of interest is the slightly earlier appearance of functional parasympathetic reflex responsiveness (Pappano 1977; Papp 1988). For example, well developed baroreflex function exists in nearly all viable preterm neonates (>24 weeks gestation), but is less sensitive and allows for greater blood-pressure and heart-rate variability (Gootman and Gootman 1983; Papp 1988).

At the cellular level, the human fetus will release catecholamines from non-innervated paraganglia to a greater extent than the partially innervated adrenal medulla. These responses mature to become qualitatively similar to adult responses by birth when, for example, hypoxia or head-up tilting results in preferential release of noradrenaline over adrenaline. In contrast, insulin, as in the adult, primarily causes release of adrenaline (Slotkin 1985).

In the broadest sense, the practical issues of neuronal development have achieved a new prominence in perinatal medicine with the survival of increasingly smaller neonates (as early as 24 weeks (400–500 g) gestation). Therefore, the clinical urgency for application of information regarding the neurobiology of neuronal development has become critical. For example, these newborns will undergo a four- to five-fold increase in their birth weight while under the direct care of the clinician in the neonatal intensive care unit, prior to becoming mature enough for discharge from the hospital to parents. Consequently, a failure to comprehend or a lack of appreciation of the ramifications of environmental influences (e.g. drugs, therapy, etc.) on human neonatal development could have disastrous consequences. This is illustrated by the long recognized association of autonomic neuronal dysfunction in infants of drug addicts or in those neonates born to women who abuse ethanol in pregnancy.

Other aspects of sympathoadrenal function are recognized as critical mediators of the successful adaptation into extrauterine life. For example, in the well characterized catecholamine system, catecholamine transmitters serve an important function in temperature regulation, brown fat metabolism, glucose homeostasis, blood pressure, heart rate, and distribution of blood flow regulation, as well as in pulmonary surfactant production and release. As stated earlier, the physiological mechanisms evoked by stress-responsiveness at the cellular level utilize the same biochemical signals (i.e. transmitters, hormones, growth factors, cell–cell interactions, etc.) as those necessary during development or for regulated expression and function in maturity.

Developmental issues and their relationship to
autonomic failure, including the multiple system atrophies

Fundamental to a number of autonomic syndromes is an understanding of
why specific cell populations appear uniquely susceptible to disease processes.
Relevant questions might include: why do certain chemically defined neuronal
populations fail to develop normally; why during adulthood do specific
components of the ANS exhibit dysfunction, degenerate, and die; why do
specific cell groups appear to exhibit functional decline with age?

Since cellular processes are on a continuum and mechanisms existing during
ontogeny probably exist throughout life—from birth through senescence—
the aetiologies of various autonomic syndromes may be viewed in terms of
developmental mechanisms. It seems reasonable to hypothesize that,
throughout life, many of the intrinsic and extrinsic forces described earlier
must continue and provide for normal function as well as survival of
autonomic neurons. As mentioned, such extrinsic factors as interneuronal
mechanisms, hormonal influences, target tissue regulatory influences, and
trophic factors are operative throughout life. Accordingly, interruption of
these processes may underlie disease expression. The developmental
disorders—familial dysautonomia and Hirschsprung's disease—illustrate the
potential interrelationships of altered developmental mechanisms and disease.
Conceivably, autonomic failure during adulthood may result from
interruption of these extrinsic factors. For instance, NGF and insulin are
somewhat structurally related and, as mentioned, anti-NGF will result in an
immunosympathectomy. Thus, high titres of antibodies to insulin might
participate in the autonomic neuropathy in diabetic patients. However, studies
to date do not support a clear relationship between autonomic dysfunction
and insulin antibody titres. Alternatively, if axoplasmic transport fails in
diabetic autonomic neuropathy, an alteration in the availability of NGF from
target tissues may occur. It might be of value to measure NGF levels in
patients with various autonomic syndromes, but the assay systems remain
complex and generally either not sensitive or specific enough for us to be
sure about the validity of the measures in man. Central and peripheral
interneuronal regulatory mechanisms have been examined in pure autonomic
failure. Deficits in catecholamine-transmitter-synthesizing enzymes and
morphological abnormalities in catecholaminergic neurons exist peripherally
and centrally, whereas cholinergic markers in ganglia appear preserved. These
studies suggest that normal regulatory mechanisms are altered in disease
states. Disruption of central and peripheral transsynaptic mechanisms results
in failed interneuronal communication and trophic interactions, and such
alterations might underlie the apparent system degenerations which attend
autonomic failure. However, whether these alterations are part of the
pathogenesis or secondary to the disease state remains unclear.

The recent 'explosion' in molecular neuroscience suggests that we may soon begin to examine the effects of altered intrinsic (genetic control) mechanisms in autonomic systems on the pathophysiology and expression of autonomic failure (e.g. Hox 1.4; Wohlgemuth *et al.* 1989). Recently, the gene locus of the neurofibromatosis 1, Von Recklinghausen's disease (a disorder of neural crest-derived Schwann cells), has been located to the pericentromeric region of chromosome 17 (Barker *et al.* 1987), and for neurofibromatosis 2 (central or bilateral acoustic neurofibromatosis) the gene defect is near the centre of the long arm of chromosome 22 (22q11.1–22q13.1) (Wertelecki *et al.* 1988). Whether these effects result from interference with homeobox proteins or retinoic acid receptors remains to be demonstrated. Certainly in the genetic disorder, Riley–Day syndrome, the chromosomal and gene locus may eventually be explored utilizing similar molecular techniques. It is apparent therefore that molecular biological tools will permit an understanding of the genetic control of normal, as well as abnormal, human autonomic growth and development. In addition, defining molecular mechanisms influencing neuronal ontogeny and neuroplasticity will provide insights into neuronal responses to disease, as well as possibly permit new understandings of how disease processes alter cell function and how neurons thus fail to function, degenerate, and/or die.

Acknowledgements

Investigations in the authors' laboratories are supported by NINCDS Grant NS22103, University of Rochester/Monroe Community Hospital Research Fund, and March of Dimes Basic Research Award, Dysautonomia Foundation, NSF 8719872, SUNY Stonybrook.

References

Barker, D., Wright, E., Nguyen, K., Cannon, L., Fain, P., Goldgar, D., Bishop, D. T., Carey, J., Baty, B., Kivlin, J., Willard, H., Waye, J. S., Greig, G., Leinwant, L., Nakamura, Y., O'Connell, P., Leppert, M., Lalouel, J. M., White, R., and Skolnick, M. (1987). Gene for von Recklinghausen neurofibromatosis is in the pericentromeric region of chromosome 17. *Science* **236**, 1100–2.

Black, I. B. (1978). Regulation of autonomic development. *Ann. Rev. Neurosci.* **1**, 183–214.

Black, I. B. (1982). Stages of neurotransmitter development in autonomic neurons. *Science* **215**, 1198–204.

Bunge, R., Johnson, M., and Ross, C. D. (1978). Nature and nurture in development of the autonomic neuron. *Science* **199**, 1409–16.

Gootman, N. G. and Gootman, P. M. (1983). *Perinatal cardiovascular function.* Marcel Dekker, New York.

Gottesfeld, A., Morgan, B., and Perez-Polo, J. R. (1990). Prenatal alcohol exposure alters the development of sympathetic synaptic components and of nerve growth factor receptor expression selectivity in lymphoid organs. *J. Neurosci. Res.* **26**, 308–16.

Hamill, R. W. and Schroeder, B. A. (1990). Hormonal regulation of adult sympathetic neurons: the effects of castration on neuropeptide Y, norepinephrine, and tyrosine hydroxylase activity. *J. Neurobiol.* **21**, 731–42.

Hamill, R. W., Cochard, P., and Black, I. B. (1983). Long-term effects of spinal transection on the development and function of sympathetic ganglia. *Brain Res.* **266**, 21–7.

Hendry, I. A., Hill, C. E., Belford, D., and Watters, D. J. (1988). A monoclonal antibody to parasympathetic neurotrophic factor causes immunoparasympathectomy in mice. *Brain Res.* **475**, 160–3.

Insel, T. R. (1990). Regional induction of c-fos-like protein in rat brain after estradiol administration. *Endocrinol.* **126**, 1849–53.

Kanerva, L., Hervonen, A., and Hervonen, M. (1974). Morphological characteristics of the ontogenesis of the mammalian peripheral adrenergic nervous system with special remarks on the human fetus. *Med. Biol.* **52**, 144–53.

Kessel, M. and Gruss, P. (1990). Murine developmental control genes. *Science* **249**, 374–9.

Kirby, M. L. (1987). Cardiac morphogenesis - recent research advances. *Pediat. Res.* **21**(3), 219–24.

Kissel, P., Andre, J. M., and Jacquier, A. (1981). *The neurocristopathies*, pp. 1–15, 165–83, 219–21. Year Book Medical Publishers, Chicago.

LaGamma, E. F., DeCristofaro, J. D., and Weisinger, G. (1991). Cholinergic agonist induced binding of adrenal medullary nuclear proteins to the rat preproenkephalin promoter. *Mol. Cell. Neurosci.* **2**, December 1991.

LaGamma E. F., DeCristofaro, J. D., Agarwal, B. L., and Weisinger, G. (1989). Ontogeny of the opiate phenotype: an approach to defining transynaptic mechanisms at the molecular level in the rat adrenal medulla. *Int. J. Dev. Neurosci.* **7**, 499–511.

Lakshmanan, J., Padbury, J., Macaso, T., Wang, D., Berl, U., and Fisher, D. A. (1986). Involvement of developing sympathetic nervous system in thyroxine-mediated submandibular gland nerve growth factor and epidermal growth factor responses. *Pediat. Res.* **20**, 232–6.

LeDouarin, N. (1982). *The neural crest*, pp. 22–53, 144–97. Cambridge University Press, New York.

Levi-Montalcini, R. (1987). The nerve growth factor 35 years later. *Science* **237**, 1154–62.

Manthorpe, M., Ray, J., Pettmann, B., and Varon, S. (1989). Ciliary neurontrophic factors. In *Nerve growth factors* (ed. R. A. Rush), pp. 31–56. John Wiley and Sons, New York.

Papp, J. G. (1988). Autonomic responses and neurohumoral control in the human early antenatal heart. *Basic Res. Cardiol.* **83**(1), 2–9.

Pappano, A. J. (1977). Ontogenetic development of autonomic neuroeffector transmission and transmitter reactivity in embryonic and fetal hearts. *Pharmacol. Rev.* **29**, 3–34.

Patterson, P. H. (1990). Control of cell fate in a vertebrate neurogenic lineage. *Cell* **62**, 1035–8.

Rao, M. S., Landis, S. C., and Patterson, P. H. (1990). The cholinergic neuronal differentiation factor from heart cell conditioned medium is different from the cholinergic factors in sciatic nerve and spinal cord. *Dev. Biol.* **139**, 65–74.

Schotzinger, R. and Landis, S. C. (1988). Cholinergic phenotype developed by noradrenergic sympathetic neurons after innervation of a novel cholinergic target *in vivo*. *Nature* **335**, 637–9.

Slotkin, T. A. (1985). Development of the sympathoadrenal axis. Endocrine control of synaptic development in the sympathetic nervous system: the cardiac-sympathetic axis. In *Developmental neurobiology of the autonomic nervous system* (ed. P. M. Gootman), pp. 69–96. Humana Press, New York.

Walicke, P. A. (1989). Novel neurotrophic factors, receptors, and oncogenes. *Ann. Rev. Neurosci.* **12**, 103–26.

Walker, D. (1975). Functional development of the autonomic innervation of the human fetal heart. *Biol. Neonate* **25**, 31–43.

Wertelecki, W., Rouleau, G. A., Superneau, D. W., Forehand, L. W., Williams, J. P., Haines, J. L., and Gusella, J. F. (1988). Neurofibromatosis 2: clinical and DNA linkage studies of a large kindred. *New Engl. J. Med.* **319**, 278–83.

Wohlgemuth, D. J., Behringer, R. R., Mostoller, M. P., Brinster, R. L., and Palmiter, R. D. (1989). Transgenic mice overexpressing the mouse homeobox-containing gene Hox 1.4 exhibit abnormal gut development. *Nature* **27**, 464–7.

Wu, B., Fodor, E. J. B., Edwards, R. H., and Rutter, W. J. (1989). Nerve growth factor induces the proto-oncogene c-*jun* in PC 12 cells. *J. Biol Chem.* **264**, 9000–3.

Yamamoto, K. R. (1985). Steroid receptor regulated transcription of specific genes and gene networks. *Ann. Rev. Genet.* **19**, 209–52.

3. Central neurotransmitters and neuromodulators in cardiovascular regulation*

Eduardo E. Benarroch

Introduction

In recent years, advances in anatomical, physiological, and pharmacological techniques have provided a wealth of information about the neurochemical and functional organization of central pathways controlling cardiovascular function. This includes: (1) immunocytochemical identification of neurons, fibres, and synaptic terminals containing neuropeptides and specific neurotransmitter-synthesizing enzymes; (2) mapping of neurochemically defined pathways by retrograde, anterograde, and transneuronal transport techniques combined with immunocytochemistry (double-labelling method); (3) localization of neurotransmitter receptors by autoradiography; (4) recording of changes in blood pressure (BP), heart rate (HR), and sympathetic nerve activity after local administration of neurochemicals in restricted areas of the brain; and (5) intracellular or extracellular recording of the activity of central 'cardiovascular neurons' and their responses to microiontophoretic administration of agonists and antagonists.

The central neural circuits controlling autonomic and humoral output to cardiovascular effectors reside at all levels of the neuraxis, have complex neurochemical organization, and are highly interconnected with each other (Loewy 1990). These central structures integrate and co-ordinate central and peripheral commands to: (1) maintain continuous level of activity in cardiovascular effectors; (2) prevent wide fluctuations of BP through compensatory cardiovascular reflexes; and (3) initiate complex adaptive cardiovascular responses (see Chapter 4).

The central autonomic circuits interact in a complex manner via a 'chemical coding' provided by two main types of signals: (1) fast, 'relay type' excitation or inhibition, mediated by amino acid neurotransmitters; and (2) slower-onset and longer-acting 'modulation' of neuronal excitability, mediated by acetylcholine (ACh), monoamines, and neuropeptides. The complexity of this neurochemical coding is the result of the various receptor subtypes for a given neurotransmitter, the coexistence of several neurotransmitters or neuromodulators in a given neuron, and the presence of presynaptic and postsynaptic interactions among various neurochemical pathways.

The central cardiovascular effects of several of these neurochemicals have been reviewed recently (Philippu 1988; Gardiner and Bennett 1989). This chapter provides an overview of the neurochemical organization and pharmacology of some of the central autonomic areas that have been most extensively investigated in recent years. More detailed information can be obtained in several recent excellent reviews (Ciriello *et al.* 1986; Swanson *et al.* 1986; Blessing and Willoughby 1987; Coote 1988; Laskey and Polosa 1988; Guyenet *et al.* 1989). The neurochemistry and neuropharmacology of peripheral autonomic pathways are described in Chapters 6 and 7.

Overview of the functional anatomy of central cardiovascular control

The areas involved in control of circulation comprise: (1) the so-called 'core' of the neuraxis, including the paraventricular nucleus, the nucleus of the tractus solitarius (NTS), and other areas (Loewy 1990); and (2) the autonomic regions of the ventrolateral pons, caudal raphe, ventromedial medulla, and, most importantly, the ventrolateral aspect of the medullary 'intermediate reticular zone' (Tork *et al.* 1990) or ventrolateral medulla (VLM).

The NTS is the first relay station for baroreceptor and other afferents affecting cardiovascular function, and it is the initial site of relay and processing of the baroreceptor reflex (see Chapter 4). The NTS projects to: (1) 'effector' cardiovascular areas of the brainstem for reflex control of sympathetic and cardiovagal outflows; and (2) multiple areas of the central autonomic core involved in integrated cardiovascular responses (Loewy 1990).

The VLM contains two regions involved in tonic and reflex control of cardiovascular function (see Ciriello *et al.* 1986, Guyenet *et al.* 1989 for reviews). The rostral VLM plays a critical role in tonic maintenance of sympathetic activity and blood pressure. Stimulation of rostral VLM neurons produces sympathoexcitation, whereas their inhibition results in a collapse of BP comparable to that obtained by spinal transection. The rostral VLM is also the final common link for most sympathoexcitatory and sympathoinhibitory reflexes. The caudal VLM tonically inhibits the rostral VLM (Blessing and Li 1989) and is involved in the reflex control of vasopressin (antidiuretic hormone; ADH) release (Blessing and Willoughby 1987; Day 1989).

The paraventricular nucleus of the hypothalamus integrates autonomic and neuroendocrine responses to stress such as hypoglycaemia or hypovolaemia. Functionally distinct sets of paraventricular nucleus neurons secrete ADH, activate the pituitary–adrenal axis, or produce widespread autonomic influences via projections to brainstem and spinal autonomic nuclei (Swanson *et al.* 1986). ADH-secreting magnocellular neurons of the paraventricular nucleus form a functional unit with similar neurons in the supraoptic nucleus, and they are the target of multiple humoral and neural influences.

The final output of these central regulatory circuits is mediated by: (1) sympathetic preganglionic neurons of the intermediolateral cell column (IML) of the spinal cord; (2) vagal cardiomotor neurons in the nucleus ambiguus; and (3) ADH-secreting magnocellular neurons of the supraoptic and paraventricular nuclei.

Chemical signalling in central cardiovascular regulatory circuits

The neurochemical signals within the central autonomic nervous system, as well as other areas of the central nervous system (CNS), may be schematically subdivided into two types: (1) 'relay type' or 'classical' fast synaptic excitation or inhibition mediated predominantly by excitatory amino acids and γ-aminobutyric acid (GABA), respectively; and (2) 'modulation' of spontaneous activity and responsiveness of neurons, mediated by ACh, monoamines, and neuropeptides.

Relay-type neurotransmission

Excitatory inputs mediated by L-glutamate (L-glu) or other endogenous excitatory amino acids and inhibitory inputs mediated by GABA control the spontaneous and baroreflex-related activity of cardiovascular neurons in the NTS, the rostral and caudal VLM, nucleus ambiguus, IML, and hypothalamus. All these areas contain neurons and terminals synthesizing L-glu or GABA as well as receptors for these neurotransmitters (see, for example, Morrison *et al.* 1989; Ruggiero *et al.* 1989).

Effects of amino acid receptor agonists on central cardiovascular neurons

Excitatory amino acids such as L-glu produce fast excitatory postsynaptic potentials via activation of both N-methyl-D-aspartate (NMDA) and non-NMDA (kainate/quisqualate) receptors. These receptors are blocked non-selectively by kynurenic acid or by selective NMDA and non-NMDA receptor antagonists. In addition to L-glu, other endogenous excitatory amino acid receptor agonists, such as homocysteic acid, may mediate central excitatory signals. GABA produces synaptic inhibition predominantly via a GABA A receptor-mediated increase in chloride conductance (fast inhibitory post-synaptic potentials). GABA A receptors are stimulated by agents such as muscimol and inhibited by drugs like bicuculline.

Local microinjections of excitatory and inhibitory amino acids have been used as pharmacological 'probes' to identify and characterize central circuits controlling circulation. Unlike electrical stimulation, these agents selectively affect cell bodies but not fibres of passage (McAllen *et al.* 1987).

In the NTS, excitatory amino acids produce baroreflex-like responses, that is, hypotension and bradycardia (Talman 1989), whereas GABA inhibits the response to baroreceptor stimulation (Spyer 1989). In the caudal VLM, excitatory amino acids elicit sympathoinhibition and increase ADH release, whereas GABA agonists produce hypertension and block ADH responses (Blessing and Willoughby 1987; Blessing and Li 1989). In the rostral VLM, excitatory amino acids produce a marked sympathoexcitation, which is topographically organized according to different sympathetic outputs (McAllen *et al.* 1987), whereas GABA agonists or the inhibitory amino acid glycine produce a profound collapse of BP (Ciriello *et al.* 1986).

Amino acid neurotransmitters in central cardiovascular circuits

Recent evidence indicates that amino acid neurotransmitters mediate: (1) tonic inhibitory control of basal neural activity in central cardiovascular circuits; (2) tonic activation of sympathetic preganglionic neurons; (3) relay of information in the baroreflex circuits; (4) supraspinal sympathoexcitatory reflexes; and (5) adaptive changes in baroreflex responses.

1. GABA may play an important role in tonic inhibitory control of central cardiovascular neurons. Bicuculline, a GABA A receptor antagonist, activates neurons in the NTS, the caudal VLM (Blessing and Li 1989), the rostral VLM (Guyenet *et al.* 1989), and the nucleus ambiguus (Spyer 1989).

2. L-glu may mediate the tonic excitatory reticulospinal inputs from 'pacemaker' neurons of the rostral VLM (Guyenet *et al.* 1989), which are critical for maintenance of spontaneous firing of sympathetic preganglionic neurons and thus vasomotor tone. Stimulation of the rostral VLM or the lateral funiculus releases L-glu from terminals contacting sympathetic preganglionic neurons and elicits fast excitation of sympathetic preganglionic neurons possibly via activation of kainate receptors in the IML (Morrison *et al.* 1989).

3. Excitatory and inhibitory amino acid neurotransmission is an essential part of the baroreflex circuit (Fig. 3.1). The evidence for the role of excitatory amino acids and GABA in baroreflex responses has been reviewed (Guyenet *et al.* 1987).

   (a) An excitatory amino acid is likely to be the primary neurotransmitter of baroreceptor inputs to the NTS. Recent studies indicate that baroreceptor activation of NTS neurons may be mediated by an excitatory amino acid other than L-glu (Talman 1989).

   (b) Baroreceptor-induced cardiovagal activation may involve an excitatory amino acid input from the NTS to neurons in the nucleus ambiguus.

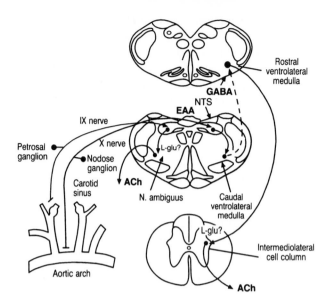

Fig. 3.1. Current view of amino acid neurotransmitter pathways in baroreflex arc. Primary baroreceptor afferents may use an excitatory amino acid (EAA) other than L-glutamate (L-glu) to activate baroreceptive neurons in the nucleus of tractus solitarius. These neurons may send excitatory inputs to cholinergic cardiovagal neurons of the nucleus ambiguus and sympathoinhibitory neurons of the caudal ventrolateral medulla. Inputs from the caudal ventrolateral medulla produce GABA-mediated inhibition of tonic sympathoexcitatory neurons of the rostral ventrolateral medulla. These 'pace-maker' neurons may use L-glu as a neurotransmitter to activate cholinergic sympathetic preganglionic neurons. ACh, acetylcholine; NTS, nucleus tractus solitarius.

(c) Baroreflex-induced sympathetic inhibition involves a GABAergic input to rostral VLM neurons (Guyenet *et al.* 1987). The GABAergic input to the RVLM does not appear to arise directly from the NTS, but it may originate in the caudal VLM. Neurons of the caudal VLM tonically inhibit rostral VLM neurons via GABAergic mechanisms, and they may be activated via NMDA receptor-mediated inputs during sinus nerve stimulation (Blessing and Li 1989).

4. Excitatory amino acid inputs to the rostral VLM are an essential link for many supraspinal sympathoexcitatory reflexes. Administration of kynurenic acid into the rostral VLM does not affect resting sympathetic activity, but it blocks sympathoexcitatory responses elicited by stimulation of somatic afferents (somatosympathetic reflex), fastigial nucleus (fastigial pressor response), and lateral hypothalamus (defence reaction) (Guyenet *et al.* 1987).

5. Amino acids may play a major role in adaptive cardiovascular responses, such as those elicited from the 'hypothalamic defence area'. The sympathoexcitation elicited from hypothalamic stimulation involves an excitatory amino acid at the level of the rostral VLM (Guyenet *et al.* 1987). Local GABAergic mechanisms, probably via interneurons, mediate the resetting of the baroreflex and tachycardia during the defence reaction (Spyer 1989).

Neurochemical modulation of central cardiovascular circuits

The function of central cardiovascular controlling circuits depends on a continuous modulation of neuronal excitability and responsiveness to excitatory amino acid inputs. This is provided by complex chemical coding mediated by ACh, catecholamines, serotonin (5-HT), and neuropeptides.

Functional anatomy of neuromodulatory systems

The areas involved in central autonomic control have abundant cell bodies and terminals containing monoamines and neuropeptides as well as their respective receptors. Many of these cell groups and receptors have been identified in human brain (Tork *et al.* 1990).

Catecholamines and other amines   Catecholaminergic innervation of central autonomic areas arises from the A5, A1, and A2 groups of noradrenaline-synthesizing neurons and from the C1 and C2 groups of adrenaline-synthesizing neurons. The A5 group of the ventrolateral pons innervates the IML and several brainstem autonomic areas. The ventrolateral C1/A1 and the dorsomedial C2/A2 groups occupy the 'intermediate reticular zone' of the medulla (Tork *et al.* 1990) (Fig. 3.2). Both groups, particularly the C1/A1 neurons, relay visceral information to the hypothalamus and may play an important role in the control of ADH and corticotrophin (ACTH) secretion (Swanson *et al.* 1986). The C1 neurons of the rostral VLM may play an important role in integration of autonomic responses (Ruggiero *et al.* 1989). They: (1) project massively to sympathetic preganglionic neurons; (2) have reciprocal connections with the NTS and rostral autonomic areas; (3) provide an important input to the locus ceruleus, an area involved in arousal and attention; and (4) project both to the pial surface and local blood vessels and may have chemosensitive and vasomotor function (Ruggiero *et al.* 1989).

Neurons containing 5-HT are located in the so-called parapyramidal region of the medulla, including the caudal raphe nuclei, and in the adjacent ventromedial medulla (Helke *et al.* 1989), and they innervate the NTS, VLM, and IML. Neurons containing ACh have been identified in the NTS and the VLM by immunocytochemical staining for choline acetyltransferase (ChAT). These may constitute local or short projection neurons.

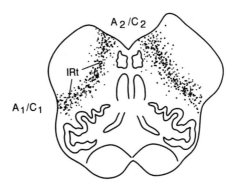

Fig. 3.2. Section of human medulla showing localization of intermediate reticular zone (IRt) (*shaded areas*). IRt contains the ventrolateral A1/C1 group and dorsomedial A2/C2. C1 and C2 synthesize adrenaline and are immunoreactive for PNMT (phenylethanolamine methyltransferase). A1 and A2 neurons are noradrenergic and are immunoreactive for tyrosine hydroxylase (non-selective marker of catecholamine-synthesizing neurons) but not PNMT.

Neuropeptides Central autonomic areas contain a great variety of neuropeptides and their respective receptors. Neuropeptides exert potent cardiovascular effects when administered into the CNS (Gardiner and Bennett 1989). They may act locally at their site of release, or affect distant targets, either by diffusion into the interstitial space (paracrine function) or as circulating hormones. Neuropeptides frequently coexist with other neurotransmitters, are coreleased in a frequency-dependent fashion, and are active at low concentrations, producing a potent, long-latency, and long-duration effect (see Chapter 7).

Substance P is an excitatory neuropeptide located in afferent, intrinsic, and projection neurons of the NTS, VLM, and IML. It may coexist with 5-HT and other neuropeptides in raphe nuclei and ventromedial medullary neurons and with catecholamines in C1 neurons. Enkephalins are inhibitory neuropeptides located in interneurons and in raphe and ventromedial medullary projections to the NTS, VLM, and IML (Helke *et al.* 1989). Neuropeptide Y coexists with catecholamines in the C1/A1 and C2/A2 groups and may modulate catecholaminergic synapses presynaptically or postsynaptically. ADH, angiotensin II (AII), and atrial natriuretic peptide (ANP) affect renal and peripheral autonomic function via several mechanisms. They may act as circulating hormones, humoral signals relayed centrally via the circumventricular organs, or neuromodulators in intrinsic central pathways (Phillips 1987; Share 1988).

Mechanisms of neuromodulation

Monoamines and neuropeptides have complex synaptic effects and this may explain conflicting data about their central cardiovascular effects (Philippu 1988).

A given neurotransmitter may activate different receptor subtypes and, thus, produce various effects depending on its site of action and receptor distribution. For example, catecholamines produce postsynaptic excitation via α_1-receptors and both presynaptic and postsynaptic inhibition via α_2-receptors (see Chapter 5).

In addition, several neurochemical receptor mechanisms may affect the same second messenger or ionic conductance. For example, α_2-adrenergic, 5-HT1 serotonergic, M2 muscarinic, opioid, and GABA B mechanisms produce synaptic inhibition through an increase in K^+ conductances, whereas α_1-adrenergic, M1 muscarinic, and substance P mechanisms produce synaptic excitation via a decrease in K^+ conductances. β-Adrenergic receptors activate, whereas α_2 and opioid receptors inhibit production of cyclic adenosine monophosphate (cAMP).

Neuromodulators may presynaptically affect their own release or the release of other neurotransmitters. Thus, noradrenaline produces postsynaptic effects as well as α_2-autoreceptor-mediated inhibition of its own release.

Neuropeptides coexisting with other neurotransmitters may pre- or postsynaptically modulate the effects of these substances (see Chapter 7).

Neurochemical organization of specific circuits and clinical correlations

Paraventricular and supraoptic nuclei

Functional considerations

The paraventricular nucleus of the hypothalamus integrates neuroendocrine and autonomic responses to stress, such as hypovolaemia and hypoglycaemia. It contains three types of output neurons: (1) magnocellular neurons which, together with similar neurons in the supraoptic nucleus, synthesize ADH (and oxytocin) and release it into the circulation; (2) parvocellular neurons, which synthesize corticotrophin-releasing hormone (CRH), somatostatin, and thyrotrophin-releasing hormone (TRH); and (3) 'autonomic' neurons, which provide direct inputs to several autonomic centres, including the NTS/dorsal vagal complex, the VLM, and the IML of the spinal cord. The functional organization of the paraventricular nucleus and its important role in integrated responses to stress have been reviewed (Swanson *et al.* 1986).

The ADH output of the magnocellular paraventricular and supraoptic nuclei constitutes an important humoral mechanism for cardiovascular control. Circulating ADH may affect cardiovascular function through multiple mechanisms (see Share 1988, for review). Despite its potent vasoconstrictor effects in humans and animals, ADH does not increase BP in normal conditions, due to its concomitant effect in increasing the gain of the baroreflex. ADH levels increase in the upright position, but this peptide does not contribute significantly to maintenance of orthostatic blood pressure in normotensive, normally hydrated individuals with normal sympathetic and renin responses (see Chapter 5).

Neurochemical inputs to the paraventricular and supraoptic nuclei

The magnocellular ADH-secreting paraventricular and supraoptic nuclei, as well as parvocellular CRH neurons of the paraventricular nucleus, receive three main inputs: (1) influences from circulating angiotensin II and ANP, acting via receptors in the circumventricular organs of the anteroventral third ventricle; (2) catecholaminergic projections from the brainstem; and (3) GABAergic inputs from limbic areas (Swanson *et al.* 1986).

Circulating angiotensin II and ANP act via receptors in the subfornical organ and the anteroventral third ventricle. Angiotensin II activates magnocellular neurons and stimulates ADH release, and it also increases thirst, sodium appetite, and BP via receptors in the subfornical organ (Phillips 1987). ANP antagonizes the effects of angiotensin II. There is an overlap between the distribution of intrinsic angiotensin II and ANP neurons and pathways as well as their respective receptors, which suggests that they may constitute physiologically antagonistic systems.

Reflex control of ADH release

Catecholaminergic and GABAergic mechanisms may play an important role in reflex control of ADH release (Fig. 3.3).

The caudal VLM contains the A1 noradrenergic neurons and plays an important role in reflex control of ADH secretion. It receives cardio-pulmonary and other visceral mechanoreceptor and chemoreceptive inputs from NTS and spinoreticular pathways, and its stimulation monosynaptically excites ADH-secreting neurons and increases the plasma level of ADH. Noradrenaline increases the activity of vasopressinergic cells and ADH secretion via activation of α_1-receptors (Day 1989). NPY, a co-transmitter in these pathways, potentiates these effects (Blessing and Willoughby 1987).

The precise role of C1/A1 inputs in the control of ADH secretion by cardiovascular reflexes is still undetermined (Day 1989). Some studies indicate that ascending catecholaminergic inputs to magnocellular neurons may be important in mediating increases in ADH release during haemorrhage or other conditions associated with unloading of arterial baroreceptors or atrial stretch receptors (Blessing and Willoughby 1987). On the other hand, it has also been suggested that baroreflex inhibition of ADH release may involve a polysynaptic pathway that uses GABA as the final neurotransmitter (Renaud and Jhamandas 1987) (Fig 3.3).

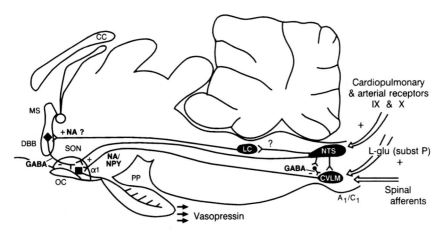

Fig. 3.3. Proposed central networks for reflex control of vasopressin secretion, in this case by magnocellular neurons of the supraoptic nucleus (SON). Ascending catecholaminergic projections from the A1/C1 groups, also containing neuropeptide Y (NPY), excite SON neurons. Baroreflex inhibition of vasopressin release may involve polysynaptic pathway from nucleus of tractus solitarius (NTS), with possible relay in locus ceruleus (LC), which indirectly inhibits SON through GABA interneurons located in the diagonal band of Broca (DBB). Alternatively, baroreflex inputs may inhibit A1/C1 neurons via GABAergic mechanisms in the caudal ventrolateral medulla (CVLM). Cardiopulmonary and arterial receptors may activate NTS and CVLM neurons by using glutamate-like substance (L-glu) and substance P (subst P). The direct excitatory pathway from the CVLM may mediate the chemoreceptors and spinal inputs of vasopressin neurons in the SON. CC, corpus callosum; MS, medial septum; NA, noradrenaline; OC, optic chiasm; PP, posterior pituitary. (Modified from Renaud and Jhamandas (1987).)

Control of ACTH release

Ascending medullary catecholaminergic inputs to the paraventricular nucleus may activate CRH-synthesizing neurons via α_1-mechanisms, and central α_1-agonists stimulate ACTH secretion in humans. CRH stimulates the release of ACTH and β-endorphin in response to stress, such as hypoglycaemia.

Nucleus of the tractus solitarius

Functional considerations

The neurophysiology of the NTS is discussed in Chapter 4. The internal organization and cytoarchitecture of the NTS in humans has been delineated recently (Tork *et al.* 1990). The NTS contains a wide variety of neurotransmitters, identified in its afferents and intrinsic neurons, and these substances may affect the processing of baroreflex signals at the NTS level.

Neurochemical modulation of the baroreflex

Both L-glu and substance P have been postulated as the excitatory neuro-transmitter in primary baroreceptor afferents to the NTS. As discussed above, current evidence indicates that an excitatory amino acid other than L-glu is probably the primary baroreceptor neurotransmitter in the NTS (Talman 1989). Substance P is located not only in baroreceptor afferents but also in local interneurons and in afferents from the raphe nuclei. Substance P may potentiate the effects of excitatory amino acids, but its slow temporal profile of action makes it unlikely as the primary baroreceptor neurotransmitter.

GABAergic neurons may tonically inhibit baroreceptor-sensitive neurons via GABA A and GABA B receptor mechanisms, and they may mediate the resetting of the baroreflex during behavioural adaptive responses (Spyer 1989).

Catecholaminergic inputs may play a complex role in the processing of baroreceptive information at the NTS level. α_2-Adrenergic mechanisms may modulate synaptic activity in the NTS. Local application of adrenaline, noradrenaline, clonidine, or α-methyl-noradrenaline (metabolite of α-methyl-dopa) produces an α_2-receptor-mediated hypotension and bradycardia, and catecholamine denervation of the NTS leads to chronic labile BP and HR. Neuropeptide Y (NPY), a co-transmitter modulator in catecholaminergic synapses, also produces hypotension and bradycardia when administered into the NTS, perhaps via modulation of α_2-receptor mechanisms.

Activation of M2 muscarinic (Sapru 1989) and 5-HT2 serotonergic receptors in the NTS produces hypotension and bradycardia.

Enkephalins are abundant in the NTS and produce a naloxone-sensitive reduction of baroreflex responses. Opioids may exert a modulatory but not tonic inhibition of baroreceptive neurons.

ADH, angiotensin II, and atrial natriuretic factor may modulate baroreflex responses by acting either as circulating hormones via receptors in the area postrema or as neurotransmitters in intrinsic inputs to the NTS. ADH released from paraventricular nucleus projections to the NTS may inhibit baroreflex responses, whereas circulating ADH increases baroreflex gain via receptors in the area postrema (Share 1988). Circulating angiotensin II inhibits baroreflex-induced bradycardia via receptors in the area postrema (Phillips 1987). Atrial natriuretic factor increases activity of baroreceptive neurons, potentiates baroreceptor inputs, and produces hypotension and bradycardia when injected into the NTS.

Rostral ventrolateral medulla

Functional considerations

The anatomical and functional features of the ventral medulla are described in recent reviews (Ciriello *et al.* 1986; Guyenet *et al.* 1989). The rostral VLM occupies the rostroventrolateral aspect of the 'intermediate' reticular zone of the medulla (Ruggiero *et al.* 1989; Tork *et al.*1990). In animals and humans, the VLM is characterized by the presence of C1 adrenaline neurons, which may also contain NPY, substance P, or enkephalins, and by abundant angiotensin II receptors (Ruggiero *et al.* 1989).

The rostral VLM is critical for tonic control of BP and sympathetic activity (see Guyenet *et al.* 1989 for review). Neurons of the rostral VLM provide direct, topographically organized excitatory inputs to functionally different subsets of preganglionic sympathetic neurons (McAllen *et al.* 1987). Recent studies indicated that the rostral VLM may contain two types of baroreceptor-sensitive, spinal projecting neurons: (1) nonadrenergic pace-maker or 'tonic neurons' which may provide the tonic glutamatergic background excitation of sympathetic preganglionic neurons; and (2) C1 adrenergic cells which have a slow spontaneous discharge, project monosynaptically to sympathetic preganglionic neurons as well as rostrally, and are inhibited by clonidine (Guyenet *et al.* 1989).

The rostral VLM is also an integrative reflex centre subserving multiple cardiovascular reflexes and autonomic adjustments to emotional and arousing stimuli. Neurons of the rostral VLM mediate: (1) the baroreceptor reflex; (2) somatosympathetic reflexes provoked by exercise, posture, and nociception; (3) sympathoexcitatory response to cerebral ischaemia; and (4) hypothalamic–mesencephalic defence responses (Guyenet *et al.* 1987, 1989; Ruggiero *et al.* 1989).

Neuropharmacology of the rostral ventrilateral medulla

The rostral VLM contains a great variety of neurotransmitters in neurons and afferent terminals as well as their respective receptors (Ruggiero *et al.* 1989; Fig. 3.4).

Endogenous glutamate receptor mechanisms are the link for most supraspinal sympathoexcitatory reflexes (Guyenet *et al.* 1987, 1989). Tonic GABAergic mechanisms mediate the baroreceptor reflex (Guyenet *et al.* 1987) and tonic sympathoinhibition from the caudal VLM (Blessing and Li 1989).

Local cholinergic neurons synapse on both adrenergic and nonadrenergic neurons in the rostral VLM (Ruggiero *et al.* 1989). Cholinergic stimulation activates rostral VLM neurons and increases sympathetic nerve activity, BP, and HR via M2 receptor mechanisms (Sapru 1989).

The precise role of adrenergic inputs in the modulation of rostral VLM neurons is still undetermined. The rostral VLM may be the central site of action of antihypertensive drugs. Clonidine, a potent α_2-agonist, inhibits C1 adrenergic neurons and decreases BP when applied in the rostral VLM (Guyenet *et al.* 1989). A β-adrenoceptor-mediated accumulation of cAMP increases pace-maker activity of rostral VLM cells, and this may explain the hypotensive effects of propranolol when applied to the rostral VLM (Guyenet *et al.* 1989).

Eduardo E. Benarroch

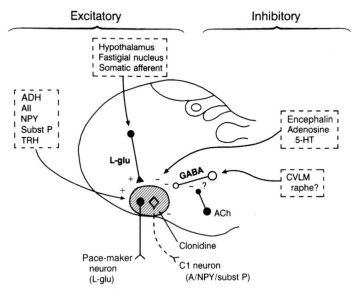

Fig. 3.4. Excitatory and inhibitory neurochemical influences on pace-maker and C1 neurons of the rostral ventrolateral medulla. L-glutamate (L-glu) and GABA may constitute the final link for sympathoexcitatory and sympathoinhibitory reflexes, respectively. Clonidine inhibits C1 adrenergic neurons but not glutaminergic pace-maker neurons. Acetylcholine (ACh) may induce sympathoexcitation via inhibition of local GABAergic neurons. A, adrenaline; AII, angiotensin II; ADH, vasopressin; CVLM, caudal ventrolateral medulla; 5-HT, 5-hydroxytryptamine (serotonin); NPY, neuropeptide Y; subst P, substance P; TRH, thyrotrophin-releasing hormone.

The rostral VLM contains numerous neuropeptides in afferents and intrinsic neurons as well as their respective receptors (Ruggiero *et al.* 1989). Neuropeptides may affect the pace-maker activity of rostral VLM neurons and produce marked changes in BP when microinjected into the rostral VLM. Substance P, NPY, ADH, TRH, and AII may increase pace-maker activity and BP (Guyenet *et al.* 1989). Enkephalins inhibit pace-maker and C1 neurons (Guyenet *et al.* 1989).

Sympathetic preganglionic neurons

Functional considerations

The functional organization and pharmacology of sympathetic preganglionic neurons have been discussed extensively in excellent reviews (Coote 1988; Laskey and Polosa 1988).

The sympathetic preganglionic neurons of the IML are the final site of integration of central influences controlling postganglionic and adreno-medullary sympathetic activity. The sympathetic preganglionic neurons have

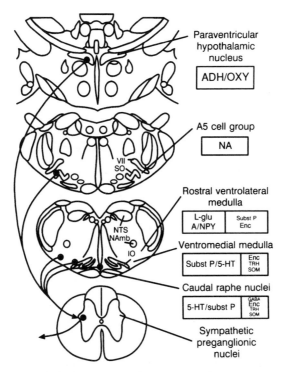

Fig. 3.5.   Supraspinal inputs to sympathetic preganglionic neurons, as identified with transneuronal tracing techniques. A, adrenaline; ADH, vasopressin; Enc, encephalin; 5-HT, 5-hydroxytryptamine (serotonin); IO, inferior olive; N Amb, nucleus ambiguus; NA, noradrenaline; NPY, neuropeptide Y; NTS, nucleus of the tractus solitarius; OXY, oxytocin; SO, superior olive; SOM, somatostatin; subst P, substance P; TRH, thyrotrophin-releasing hormone. (Modified from Strack *et al.* (1989).)

viscerotopic organization and form discrete functional units that innervate specific targets in the periphery (Coote 1988; Laskey and Polosa 1988).

The tonic discharge of sympathetic preganglionic neurons depends on the presence of background synaptic excitation (Laskey and Polosa 1988).

Neurochemical control of sympathetic preganglionic neurons

At least five regions of the autonomic core provide neurochemically defined inputs to the IML (Fig. 3.5): the rostral VLM; the caudal raphe; the ventromedial medulla; the A5 groups; and the paraventricular nucleus (Coote 1988; Strack *et al.* 1989).

The rostral VLM provides: (1) glutamatergic inputs from non-adrenergic pace-maker neurons (Guyenet *et al.* 1989; Morrison *et al.* 1989); and (2) massive C1 projections containing adrenaline, NPY, and, to a lesser extent, substance P and enkephalins (Ruggiero *et al.* 1989).

The caudal raphe and the ventromedial medulla send projections containing 5-HT, substance P, TRH, GABA, encephalin, and somatostatin, alone or in various combinations (Helke *et al.* 1989). The A5 group in the ventro-lateral pons provide the main noradrenergic input to the IML. The paraventricular nucleus provides inputs containing ADH and oxytocin (Swanson *et al.* 1986).

Descending inputs to sympathetic preganglionic neurons maintain the tonic background excitation of sympathetic preganglionic neurons, modulate segmental somatosympathetic and viscerosympathetic reflexes, and selectively activate specific pools of sympathetic preganglionic neurons for co-ordinated simultaneous control of several vascular beds.

As mentioned above, the tonic excitatory input to sympathetic preganglionic neurons originates in pace-maker neurons of the rostral VLM (Guyenet *et al.* 1989). However, the spontaneous activity of sympathetic preganglionic neurons depends not only on the ongoing subthreshold excitation by glutamatergic inputs from the rostral VLM but also on intrinsic properties of the membrane of sympathetic preganglionic neurons (Laskey and Polosa 1988), which may be the target of complex monoaminergic and peptidergic modulation.

Catecholaminergic inputs from adrenaline C1 and noradrenaline A5 cell groups may exert a dual effect on sympathetic preganglionic neurons. α_1-Receptors mediate slow excitation and may induce a 'pace-maker' mode of activity in sympathetic preganglionic neurons (Laskey and Polosa 1988). The more abundant α_2-adrenoceptors mediate slow inhibitory postsynaptic potentials in sympathetic preganglionic neurons (Laskey and Polosa 1988). This inhibition of sympathetic preganglionic neurons is mimicked by local application of clonidine (Coote 1988).

Serotonergic inputs from the caudal raphe and ventromedial medulla may also produce two opposite effects on sympathetic preganglionic neurons, excitation via 5-HT1 and inhibition via 5-HT2 receptors (Coote 1988).

Inputs to sympathetic preganglionic neurons that release substance P originate from bulbospinal pathways and from primary afferents and local interneurons in the spinal cord (Loewy 1987; Helke *et al.* 1989). Substance P produces a long-latency and long-duration excitation of sympathetic preganglionic neurons and interneurons (Loewy 1987; Coote 1988), and it may induce a long-lasting subthreshold depolarization so that cells are more easily excited by other stimuli. NPY, enkephalin, and TRH may also modulate neurotransmission in the IML.

In summary, it is likely that the participation of many neurotransmitter mechanisms (e.g. α_1-adrenergic and substance P) may be necessary to bring sympathetic preganglionic neurons above their firing threshold and to modulate their frequency coding (Guyenet *et al.* 1989).

Another important function of these various chemically coded supraspinal inputs is to provide 'differential innervation' to specific subgroups of sympathetic preganglionic neurons in order to allow differential patterns of sympathetic response (Coote 1988).

In addition to supraspinal influences, local mechanisms may modulate the excitability of sympathetic preganglionic neurons. GABA-containing and glycine-containing neurons in the IML may participate in tonic inhibitory control of sympathetic preganglionic neurons. These inhibitory interneurons are activated by excitatory substance P inputs and may provide negative feedback to limit excessive stimulation of sympathetic preganglionic neurons.

Clinical correlations

Tetraplegia

Patients with chronic tetraplegia have intact supraspinal baroreflex circuits and appropriate release of ADH to cardiovascular stimuli. They show a marked increase of ADH release in response to a profound decrease in their BP during tilt, and they have exaggerated pressor responses to ADH (see Chapters 19 and 43).

Interruption of reticulospinal inputs from pace-maker and clonidine-sensitive C1 neurons of the rostral VLM may explain the abnormalities in control of sympathetic output observed in tetraplegic patients (see Chapter 42). In these patients: (1) supine BP, sympathetic nerve activity, and blood catecholamine levels are lower than in normals; (2) head-up tilt produces an immediate decrease in BP with no compensatory increase in sympathetic nerve activity or catecholamine levels; (3) there is an exaggerated pressor response to ADH; and (4) there is no sympathoactivation in response to mental arithmetic or other adaptive-emotional stimuli.

Clonidine decreases BP and plasma catecholamine levels in normal and hypertensive subjects, but it has no effect on resting blood pressure in tetraplegic patients. In addition, interruption of neurochemical supraspinal mechanisms modulating segmental sympathetic reflexes is responsible for the massive, unpatterned sympathoexcitation observed in autonomic dysreflexia. In those patients clonidine does not affect resting BP, but it prevents these hypertensive responses to segmental stimulation. This underscores the importance of local α_2-mechanisms in controlling the excitability of sympathetic preganglionic neurons.

Multiple system atrophy

Catecholaminergic inputs to hypothalamic neurons may be necessary for reflex stimulation of ADH and CRH release in humans (see Chapter 19). The human brain contains A1/C1 catecholamine neurons (Tork *et al.* 1990) and abundant α_1-receptors in the supraoptic and paraventricular nuclei.

Patients with multiple-system atrophy (MSA) have catecholaminergic denervation of the hypothalamus (see Chapter 30). These patients, unlike those with tetraplegia, show impaired ADH responses despite a profound decrease in BP during tilt but normal ADH response to osmotic stimuli (see Chapter 19).

Patients with MSA, but not those with pure autonomic failure, have impaired ACTH and β-endorphin responses to hypoglycaemia, which has been attributed to central cholinergic dysfunction (see Chapter 17). However, it is also possible that this may reflect dysfunction of adrenergic inputs to the paraventricular nucleus.

Patients with multiple system atrophy have decreased levels of substance P (Loewy 1987) as well as catecholamine, 5-HT, and ACh markers in cerebrospinal fluid (see Chapter 17). It is possible that the lack of excitatory and inhibitory modulation of sympathetic preganglionic neurons may contribute to orthostatic hypotension and supine hypertension, respectively, in these patients.

References

Blessing, W. W. and Li, Y. W. (1989). Inhibitory vasomotor neurons in the caudal ventrolateral region of the medulla oblongata. *Prog. Brain Res.* **81**, 83–97.

Blessing, W. W. and Willoughby, J. O. (1987). Central neural pathways mediating baroreceptor-initiated secretion of vasopressin. In *Cardiogenic reflexes* (ed. R. Hainsworth, P. N. McWilliam, and D. A. S. G. Mary), pp. 301–17. Oxford University Press, Oxford.

Ciriello, J. Caverson, M. M., and Polosa, C. (1986). Function of the ventrolateral medulla in the control of the circulation. *Brain Res. Rev.* **11**, 359–91.

Coote, J. H. (1988). The organisation of cardiovascular neurons in the spinal cord. *Rev. Physiol. Biochem. Pharmacol.* **110**, 147–285.

Day, A. D. (1989). Control of neurosecretory vasopressin cells by noradrenergic projections of the caudal ventrolateral medulla. *Prog. Brain Res.* **81**, 303–17.

Gardiner, S. M. and Bennett, T. (1989). Brain neuropeptides: actions on central cardiovascular control mechanisms. *Brain Res. Rev.* **14**, 19–116.

Guyenet, P. G., Sun, M.-K., and Brown, D. L. (1987). Role of GABA and excitatory aminoacids in medullary baroreflex pathways. In *Organization of the autonomic nervous system: central and peripheral mechanisms* (ed. J. Ciriello, F. R. Calaresu, L. P. Renaud, and C. Polosa), pp. 215–25. Alan R. Liss, New York.

Guyenet, P. G., Haselton, J. R., and Sun, M.-K. (1989). Sympathoexcitatory neurons of the rostroventrolateral medulla and the origin of the sympathetic vasomotor tone. *Prog. Brain Res.* **81**, 105–16.

Helke, C. J., Thor, K. B., and Sasek, C. A. (1989). Chemical neuroanatomy of the parapyramidal region of the ventral medulla in the rat. *Prog. Brain Res.* **81**, 17–28.

Laskey, W. and Polosa, C. (1988). Characteristics of the sympathetic preganglionic neuron and its synaptic input. *Prog. Neurobiol.* **31**, 47–84.

Loewy, A. D. (1987). Substance P neurons of the ventral medulla; their role in the control of vasomotor tone. In *Cardiogenic reflexes* (ed. R. Hainsworth, P. N. McWilliams, and D. A. S. G. Mary), pp. 269–85. Oxford University Press, Oxford.

Loewy, A. D. (1990). Central autonomic pathways. In *Central regulation of autonomic functions* (ed. A. D. Loewy and K. M. Spyer), pp. 88–103. Oxford University Press, New York.

McAllen, R. M., Dampney, R. A. L., and Goodchild, A. K. (1987). The sub-retrofacial nucleus and cardiovascular control. In *Organization of the autonomic nervous system: central and peripheral mechanisms* (ed. J. Ciriello, F. R. Calaresu, L. P. Renaud, and C. Polosa), pp. 251-63. Alan R. Liss, New York.

Morrison, S. F., Ernsberger, P., Milner, T. A., Callaway, J., Gong, A., and Reis, D. J. (1989). A glutamate mechanism in the intermediolateral nucleus mediates sympathoexcitatory responses to stimulation of the rostral ventrolateral medulla. *Prog. Brain Res.* **81**, 159–69.

Philippu, A. (1988). Regulation of blood pressure by central neurotransmitters and neuropeptides. *Rev. Physiol. Biochem. Pharmacol.* **111**, 1–115.

Phillips, M. I. (1987). Functions of angiotensin in the central nervous system. *Ann. Rev. Physiol.* **49**, 413–35.

Renaud, L. P. and Jhamandas, J. (1987). Neurophysiology of central baroreceptor pathway projecting to hypothalamic vasopressin neurons. *Can. J. Neurol. Sci.* **14**, 17–24.

Ruggiero, D. A., Cravo, S. L., Ranago, V., and Reis, D. J. (1989). Central control of the circulation by the rostral ventrolateral reticular nucleus: anatomical substrates. *Prog. Brain Res.* **81**, 49–79.

Sapru, H. N. (1989). Cholinergic mechanisms subserving cardiovascular function in the medulla and spinal cord. *Prog. Brain Res.* **81**, 171–9.

Share, L. (1988). Role of vasopressin in cardiovascular regulation. *Physiol. Rev.* **68**, 1248–84.

Spyer, K. M. (1989). Neural mechanisms involved in cardiovascular control during affective behaviour. *Trends in Neurosciences* **12**, 506–13.

Strack, A. M., Sawyer, W. B., Hughes, J. H., Platt, K. B., and Loewy, A. D. (1989). A general pattern of CNS innervation of the sympathetic outflow demonstrated by transneuronal pseudorabies viral infections. *Brain Res.* **491**, 156–62.

Swanson, L. W., Sawchenko, P. E., and Lind, R. W. (1986). Regulation of multiple peptides in CRF parvocellular neurosecretory neurons: implications for the stress response. *Prog. Brain Res.* **68**, 169–90.

Talman, W. T. (1989). Kynurenic acid microinjected into the nucleus tractus solitarius of rat blocks the arterial baroreflex but not responses to glutamate. *Neurosci. Lett.* **102**, 247–52.

Tork, I., McRitchie, D. A., Rikard-Bell, G. C., and Paxinos, G. (1990). Autonomic regulator centers in the medulla oblongata. In *The human nervous system* (ed. G. Paxinos), pp. 221–59. Academic Press, New York.

4. Central nervous control of the cardiovascular system

K. M. Spyer

Introduction

In my chapter in the previous edition of this volume it was stressed that over the period since 1970 considerable advances had been made in identifying the basic neural processes that regulate the cardiovascular system. These changes have required a reappraisal of many of the accepted notions regarding central processing and represent, in particular, a move away from the proposition that cardiovascular regulation is accomplished largely through a discrete 'vasomotor centre' located in the medulla oblongata. Instead, it appears that control is exerted by a longitudinally arranged series of parallel pathways involving specific regions of the neuraxis extending from cerebral cortex to the spinal cord. The subject of the present review is to identify some of the anatomical features of this integrative network and the interactions that occur within it. This will provide a basis for understanding the role of the central nervous system in homeostatic regulation and in the changes that occur in developing major changes in cardiovascular function that accompany, and support, behavioural activities.

Innervation of autonomic preganglionic neurons

In considering the central nervous regulation of the cardiovascular system it is necessary to note that the preganglionic vagal and sympathetic neurons are the final common pathway within the central nervous system through which this control is exerted. Sympathetic preganglionic neurons are localized within the intermediolateral cell column of the thoracic and upper lumbar spinal cord (for detailed review see Cabot 1990). 'Vasomotor' neurons are distributed throughout the extent of the column, but those sympathetic neurons that influence cardiac activity, both chronotropic and inotropic, are restricted to the upper thoracic segments of the cord (T1–T4). The vagal preganglionic neurons that affect cardiac control are largely located within the nucleus ambiguus of the lateral medulla, with a variable occurrence of similar neurons in the dorsal vagal nucleus: this localization is highly species-selective (see Jordan and Spyer 1987; Loewy and Spyer 1990). It is, as yet, not resolved whether individual vagal preganglionic neurons subserve both inotropic and chronotropic function: considerably more is known of the details of central nervous function in heart rate control than of its influence on cardiac dynamics.

Sympathetic neurons

There is an extensive literature indicating the pattern of innervation of these groups of autonomic neurons from studies using conventional neuroanatomical approaches with various retrograde and anterograde traces (see Loewy 1990 for review). The more recent development of retrograde transsynaptic viral traces has added much to this knowledge (Loewy 1990). With regard to sympathetic neurons innervating the adrenal medulla, a particularly clear picture has been provided using these methods (see Fig. 4.1). Secretions from the adrenal medulla have profound cardiovascular influences. These data are consistent with an earlier report from Loewy and his colleagues, using more conventional approaches (Loewy and Neil 1981), and indicate that a range of descending pathways innervate these sympathetic preganglionic neurons. They arise from hypothalamic, midbrain, pontine, and medullary cell groups. These include cell groups that have been shown, using immunocytochemistry, to contain particular amines and peptides. In this regard, it is notable that some 20 putative neurotransmitter substances have been located within the immediate vicinity of preganglionic sympathetic neurons (Cabot 1990), and include glutamate, GABA, glycine, noradrenaline, adrenaline, dopamine, serotonin, substance P, encephalin, oxytocin, vasopressin, and numerous other neuropeptides, many of which may be localized (see Chalmers and Pilowsky 1991 for review). For the purpose of the current discussion, we will concentrate on the serotonergic innervation of a sympathetic preganglionic neuron that arises from the raphe complex and the adrenaline and noradrenaline innervation that originates in the ventrolateral medulla and A5 pontine noradrenergic neurons. Indeed, physiological significance may reside in the pattern of innervation of individual sympathetic neurons from these various central cell groups but this is, as yet, unproven (see Chalmers and Pilowsky 1991). The belief would be that neurons of a particular class, for example, vasomotor to skeletal muscle, would have a distinctive pattern of innervation, distinguishing them from, say, a sympathetic preganglionic neuron destined to influence other vascular beds or gastrointestinal function. This physiological role of brainstem cell groups innervating the intermediolateral cell column, excitatory or inhibitory, and particularly those arising from the medulla, has been assessed using a range of electrophysiological techniques by Gebber and his colleagues (see Gebber 1990 for review). A major attempt has been made to assess the temporal relationships between the firing of brainstem neurons and

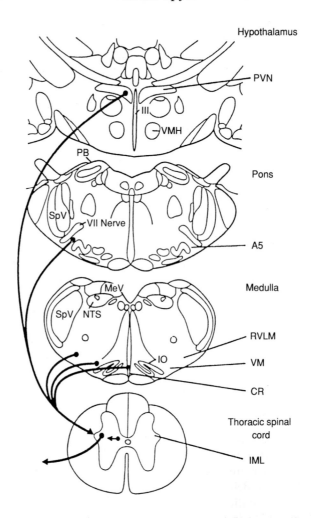

Fig. 4.1. Illustration of the innervation of preganglionic sympathetic neurons. PVN, paraventricular nucleus; A5, A5 group of noradrenergic neurons; RVLM, rostroventrolateral medulla; VM, ventromedial medulla; CR, caudal raphe nuclei; IML, intermediolateral cell column; III, third ventricle; VMH, ventromedial hypothalamus; PB, parabrachial nucleus; SpV, spinal trigeminal nucleus; MeV, medial vestibular nucleus; NTS, nucleus tractus solitarius; IO, inferior olivary nucleus. (Reproduced with permission from Spyer (1989).)

sympathetic pre- or postganglionic activity neurons as a basis for connectivity. To this have been added studies, using antidromic mapping techniques, to determine the specific projections of individual brainstem neurons. Neurons in the rostral ventrolateral medulla (VLM), including those of the C1 group, have been shown to innervate the intermediolateral cell column and the intermediate regions of the spinal cord. Complementary evidence has now been obtained at ultrastructural level for direct monosynaptic connections of rostral VLM neurons with both the soma and dendrites of sympathetic neurons (Milner *et al.* 1988; Bacon *et al.* 1990). Similar evidence exists for connections from the raphe complex, in particular the raphe magnus and pallidus, and these are implicated in the 5-HT innervation of the intermediolateral cell column (Morrison *et al.* 1988; Zagon and Bacon 1991).

With regard to the rostral VLM projection to the spinal cord, Guyenet and others (see Gebber 1990; Guyenet 1990) have indicated that these bulbospinal neurons have properties indicative of a sympathoexcitatory function (see Fig. 4.2). They have a strong cardiac rhythm in their ongoing discharge, and this rhythm appears to involve an inhibitory input from the arterial baroreceptors. In the rat, they fire at around 20 Hz, and the magnitude of their discharge is directly related to the level of arterial blood pressure (see Fig. 4.2). Another dispersed group of medullary neurons, located in the lateral tegmental field, show a temporal relationship to sympathetic discharge that, when compared with the equivalent relationship between rostral VLM neurons and sympathetic discharge, suggests that they feed an excitatory input on to rostral VLM neurons (Gebber 1990). Equally, it appears that many brainstem neurons affect sympathetic discharge in a manner that can be independent of baroreceptor input. Gebber and his colleagues have demonstrated intrinsic rhythms in both medullary and hypothalamic neurons that are also represented in sympathetic discharge in the absence of baroreceptor input. This implies that sympathetic 'tone' is generated by widely distributed neuronal groups distributed throughout the brainstem.

With regard to raphe spinal connections, there are indications that these may mediate both excitatory and inhibitory control of sympathetic neurons (Coote 1988; Gebber 1990). A proportion of raphe spinal neurons have small myelinated axons that are known to contain 5-hydroxytryptamine (serotonin; 5-HT). 5-HT, when delivered by ionophoresis on to lumbar sympathetic neurons, evokes excitation in a majority of cases but inhibition in a small number (Gilbey and Stein 1991). This prevalence of excitation confirms earlier observations in thoracic sympathetic neurons (Coote 1988). The studies of Bacon *et al.* (1990) have now provided convincing evidence for raphe neurons making monosynaptic connections with those sympathetic preganglionic neurons that innervate the adrenal medulla. Gilbey and Stein's observations go further in indicating the potential functional implications of such an innervation. Those lumbar sympathetic neurons that were excited by 5-HT were invariably inhibited by noxious input, whilst those few that were inhibited by 5-HT were excited by the equivalent noxious input. The basis for these actions may be related to the specialization of raphe spinal connections with regard to function (see earlier), and the heterogeneity of 5-HT receptor subtypes located in the intermediolateral column of the spinal cord. Whichever explanation is correct, these connections appear to be

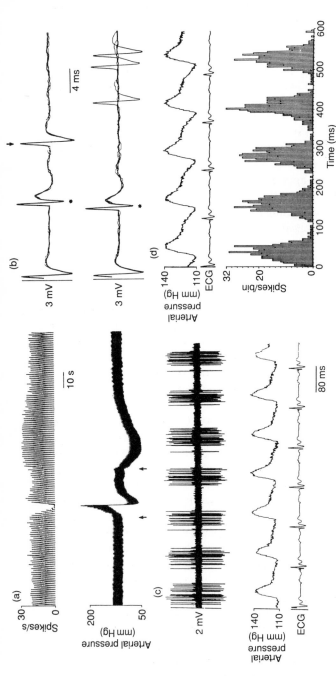

Fig. 4.2. Characteristics of the identified rostral ventrolateral spinal 'vasomotor' neurons. (a) Effect of change in arterial pressure on the neuronal discharge rate. Neuronal activity is represented in the form of integrated rate histogram. Arterial pressure was elevated via descending aortic constriction (started at the first arrow and stopped when the neuron became silent) and reduced by i.v. injection of 0.1–0.2 mg sodium nitroprusside (at the second arrow). (b) Spinal projection of the neuron. The evoked antidromic spikes (arrow) by the spinal cord stimulation (asterisks) collided with spontaneously occurring spikes and failed to occur at recording site when the stimulation was applied within a critical period after spontaneously occurring spikes (bottom trace). (c) Pulse-synchronous discharge of the rostral ventrolateral spinal 'vasomotor' neuron. The arterial pressure trace (middle) and ECG signal (bottom) represent a single sweep, whilst the trace of neuronal discharge represents 12 consecutive sweeps, all triggered on ECG signals. (d) ECG-triggered time histograms of the neuronal activity (300 sweeps, 3 ms/bin). The top and middle traces represent averaged arterial pressure and ECG signals, respectively (50 sweeps each). (Reproduced with permission from Sun and Spyer (1991b).)

important in patterning sympathetic activity in regard to noxious inputs and, presumably, to the cardiovascular adjustments that accompany these inputs.

In an analogous manner, there is evidence for both α_1- and α_2-adrenergic receptors within the intermediolateral column, and evidence that both noradrenergic and adrenergic fibres project from the brainstem to this region (for discussion see Coote 1988). The actions of adrenergic ligands on the activity of sympathetic neurons have been controversial. Both excitatory and inhibitory effects have been seen, and there are considerable differences in the literature between observations made *in vivo* and those made using *in vitro* preparations. From some recent excellent *in vitro* studies initiated by Nishi and his collaborators amongst others (see discussion in Coote 1988). There is now good evidence that α_1-mediated effects are largely excitatory whilst α_2-mediated effects are inhibitory and that, on occasions, both actions can be identified on individual preganglionic neurons. Recent studies by Gilbey and his co-workers have provided a basis for the *in vivo* α_1-mediated excitatory response. These observations could be taken as support for a role of the C1 group of neurons in evoking an excitatory control of sympathetic neurons through the release of adrenaline. However, other studies would seem to indicate that the descending pathway may act through a local release of glutamate in the spinal cord (for discussion see Guyenet 1990), and this may indicate the corelease of glutamate with adrenaline (for discussion see Chalmers and Pilowsky 1991).

Medullary premotor sympathetic or 'vasomotor' neurons

As indicated above, there is convincing evidence that neurons in the rostral VLM provide significant excitatory input to sympathetic preganglionic neurons. These neurons appear to form a relatively discrete group of cells in close proximity to the facial nucleus (Fig. 4.3). Indeed, there is a belief that these neurons, which include a subclass defined as the C1 adrenaline-containing neurons, represent the classical 'vasomotor' centre (Guyenet 1990). This conclusion has resulted, in part, from a demonstration that their destruction, or inhibition, by the topical application of glycine to the ventral medullary surface, results in a fall of blood pressure to a level that is associated with that seen in an acute spinal preparation (Feldberg and Guertzenstein 1976). More recent studies have indicated that the acute effects seen in both cat and rat are not apparent under more chronic situations, and previous data reviewed would seem to add emphasis to the importance of multiple descending pathways in affecting sympathetic activity. These rostral VLM neurons do, however, have a pivotal role since they have properties that indicate that they integrate inputs from several reflex pathways and also from the output of regions of the central nervous system that have been shown to be involved in cardiovascular control. In addition, there are some

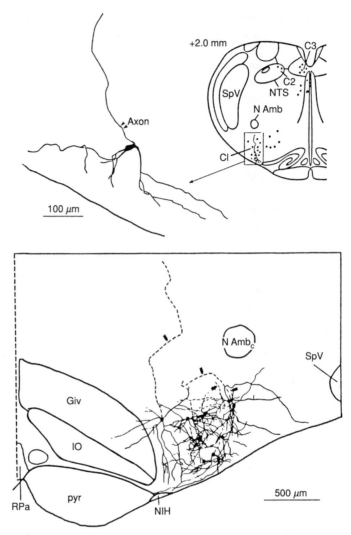

Fig. 4.3. Morphology of pace-maker neuron in the rostral ventrolateral medulla. (Above) An intracellularly labelled pace-maker neuron is shown in relationship to C1 neurons represented as dots. Recordings were made *in vitro* and the staining done by intracellular injection of lucifer yellow. This particular neuron (as shown in higher magnification on the left) exhibits features typical for this cell group, viz. three or four major dendrites that divide a maximum of three times, a limited dendrite span spreading 500–700 μm mediolaterally, and 120–200 μm rostrocaudally, and an axon devoid of local collaterals (n = 14). Pace-maker neurons, like many reticular cells, have dendrites that spread out in a plane perpendicular to the long axis of the brain (unpublished data from Sun and Guyenet). (Below) Nine intracellularly labelled pace-maker neurons are superimposed on a standardized section to show overall dendritic spread. Axons

suggestions that they have intrinsic pace-maker properties, since they are rhythmically active in an *in vitro* slice preparation and this discharge is not silenced in the presence of kynurate, the non-selective antagonist of glutamate (Guyenet 1990). The ongoing discharge of these cells does not appear to be modified by other ionic means of modifying synaptic transmission, and the activity of these cells is reset by applying hyperpolarizing currents. However, these properties are not shown exclusively by rostral VLM neurons, as there are many demonstrations of 'beating' neurons in other areas of the medulla under similar experimental circumstances. However, these neurons receive a powerful inhibitory input from the arterial baroreceptors that is mediated by GABA acting at a $GABA_A$ receptor, an excitatory input from the arterial chemoreceptors, and variable influences from vagal afferents. They often exhibit a respiration-related discharge, largely showing heightened activity during inspiration, and evidence of a pulmonary stretch afferent input. Numerous regions of the CNS which are concerned with different behavioural activities and associated with large changes in the cardiovascular system, such as the hypothalamic defence area, when activated produce marked changes in the discharge of rostral VLM bulbospinal neurons. Equally, variable inputs to these neurons have been described when activating regions of the cerebellum, pons, and midbrain and, more recently, a powerful biphasic influence from the area postrema has been shown (Sun and Spyer 1991*a*). In addition, they are affected powerfully by noxious inputs delivered to the limbs and tail in the anaesthetized rat, and their pattern of response to these inputs is consistent with them playing a major role in the expression of the cardiovascular responses in nociception (Gilbey and Stein 1991; Sun and Spyer 1991*b*).

Other studies have shown that, aside from those rostral VLM neurons with spinally projecting axons, there are numerous cells in the same general area that receive varying patterns of peripheral and central input concerned with cardiovascular regulation. This implies that this area may have a major, yet not exclusive, role in cardiovascular control, since the inputs to this area, both central and peripheral, are distributed to other cell groups located in the lower brainstem which equally well may have powerful connections on to sympathetic neurons of the spinal cord.

Vagal preganglionic cardiomotor neurons

Vagal cardioinhibitory neurons have been shown to be located primarily within the ventrolateral subdivision of the nucleus ambiguus (Loewy and

---

Fig. 4.3 (*continued*)   are indicated by dotted lines. SpV, spinal trigeminal nucleus; NTS, nucleus of the tractus solitarius; N Amb, nucleus ambiguus; Giv, gigantocellular reticular nucleus; IO, inferior olive; pyr, pyramid; RPa, raphe pallidas; NIH, nucleus infrafascicularis hypoglossi; $NAmb_c$, compact rostral end of nucleus ambiguus. (Reproduced with permission from Guyenet, 1990.)

Spyer 1990). This localization places them within close apposition to the premotor sympathetic neurons of the rostral VLM described above. In addition, they share input with these neurons from numerous regions of the forebrain hypothalamus and amygdala as well as lower brainstem. The nucleus ambiguus has been shown to receive afferents from at least 123 different regions of the brain in the rat, which include: (1) the bed nucleus of the stria terminalis; (2) the substantia innominata; (3) the central nucleus of the amygdala; (4) the paraventricular hypothalamic nucleus; (5) the dorsomedial hypothalamic nucleus; (6) the lateral hypothalamic area; (7) the zona inserta; (8) the posterior hypothalamus; (9) the mesencephalic central grey; (10) the mesencephalic reticular formation; (11) the parabrachial nucleus including the Kölliker–Fuse nucleus; (12) the nucleus of the tractus solitarius (NTS); (13) the medullary reticular formation—all of these innervate the rostral VLM. A particularly powerful source of afferent input to the nucleus ambiguus arises from the CNTS, and recent ultrastructural studies (Izzo 1991), using the anterograde transport of biocytin, have shown monosynaptic connections being made from the NTS on to vagal neurons of the nucleus ambiguus. Similarly, evidence has been derived to show that cardiomotor neurons are contacted by synaptic boutons containing 5-HT. As yet, the source of this input is unknown but, interestingly, many vagal neurons, other than cardiomotor neurons of both the nucleus ambiguus and dorsal vagal motonucleus, also show a powerful 5-HT innervation.

Reflex control of cardiovascular control

It is well documented that several groups of peripheral receptors contribute to the reflex control of circulation. These include the arterial baroreceptor and chemoreceptors, receptors within the heart as well as the airways and lungs (Spyer 1981, 1990).

   The primary site of interaction of these afferents within the central nervous system is at the level of the NTS (Spyer 1981, 1982, 1984; Jordan and Spyer 1986 for detailed reviews). Neurophysiological studies have shown that specific areas of the NTS receive innervation from the arterial baroreceptors (see Fig. 4.4), and that these same regions of the nucleus receive a variable innervation from other vagal afferents and the arterial chemoreceptors. In particular, the dorsolateral and dorsomedial regions of the NTS at levels rostral to the obex have been shown using an antidromic mapping technique to receive an input from both myelinated and unmyelinated carotid sinus baroreceptor afferents, and also from aortic baroreceptors (Jordan and Spyer 1986; Spyer 1990). Since the NTS receives a patterned input from afferents arising from receptors which reflexly affect both the cardiovascular and respiratory systems (see Fig. 4.4) and also receives inputs from many regions of the central nervous system (see Fig. 4.10), it is a potential site of integration

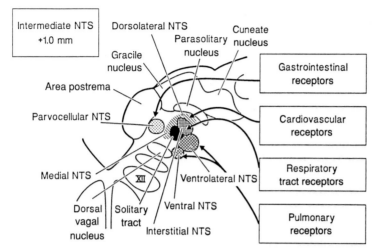

Fig. 4.4. Drawing showing the viscerotropic pattern of innervation of the nucleus of the tractus solitarius (NTS). This drawing illustrates the nucleus of the tractus solitarius of the cat in the transverse plane and the number given indicates the distance from the obex. The nomenclature used follows that presented by Loewy and Burton (1978). (Reproduced with permission from Loewy (1990).)

(see Jordan and Spyer 1986 for discussion). Accordingly, interest has been aroused in determining the synaptic underlying transmission of baroreceptor inputs, in particular at this level. The importance of these considerations resides in the fact that, whilst sinoaortic denervation leads to a lability in arterial blood pressure, destruction of the NTS leads acutely to fulminating hypertension with concomitant pulmonary oedema, and chronically to maintained hypertension (see Spyer 1981 for discussion).

The majority of neurophysiological studies have involved extracellular recordings of unit activity whilst stimulating electrically a number of potential afferent inputs or activating receptors with natural stimuli. An extensive survey indicated a marked convergence of the input on to neurons located in the vicinity of the NTS from the glossopharyngeal, carotid sinus, aortic depressor, and superior laryngeal nerves, although few neurons showing such convergence were actually localized within the NTS. More recently, a more detailed pattern of convergence has been observed. The detailed synaptic organization of the NTS, however, remains unresolved. This will require a combined physiological and neuroanatomical approach and also the use of *in vitro* electrophysiological approaches.

The NTS itself makes extensive connections with regions of the lower brainstem, including the nucleus ambiguus and ventrolateral medulla, and to the various pontine nuclei that are concerned with cardiorespiratory regulations and to forebrain regions (see Fig. 4.5). Details of the connections from the NTS to the nucleus ambiguus and, in particular, on to cardiomotor neurons, have been referred to above. The relationship of the NTS to the rostral VLM neurons that regulate sympathetic activity has yet to be resolved. There are, however, strong indications that the baroreceptor reflex control of these neurons is mediated via a GABAergic interneuron located in an adjacent region of the ventrolateral medulla (see Fig. 4.6; Guyenet 1990 for discussion). This lateralization of the baroreceptor reflex was first identified by Spyer (1981) and has now received general recognition. The ascending pathways from the NTS may well play an additional role in mediating baroreceptor and other reflexes, control of neuroendocrine function (Harris and Loewy 1990), although their relative importance in cardiovascular regulation remains to be fully assessed. The present discussion would seem to indicate that the basic reflex is accomplished within the medulla and involves, not merely the cardiomotor neuron of the nucleus ambiguus and the neurons of the rostroventrolateral medulla, but, presumably, baroreceptor actions at the level of other neurons where baroreceptor-mediated influences have been demonstrated (see Gebber 1990). The relationship between baroreceptor input and raphe spinal control of sympathetic discharge remains to be resolved, and it is, as yet, premature to conclude that baroreceptor control of sympathetic discharge is merely the result of a control of brainstem sympathoexcitatory neurons.

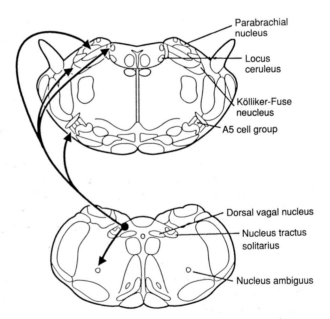

Fig. 4.5. Drawing illustrating the nucleus tractus solitarius projections to the lower brainstem. (Reproduced with permission from Loewy (1990).)

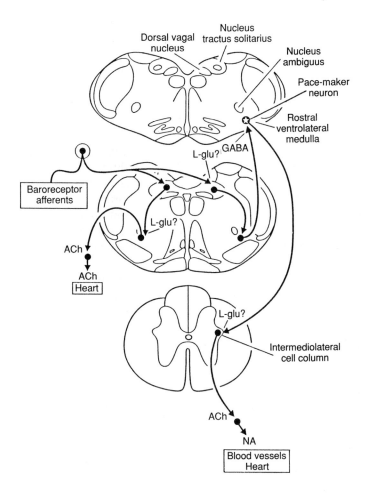

Fig. 4.6. A model of the neural circuitry involved in the baroreflex. Incoming baroreceptor afferents terminate in the nucleus tractus solitarius. These first-order neurons have their cell bodies in the ganglia of the IXth and Xth cranial nerves. The transmitter involved is unknown, but may be L-glutamate (L-glu) or a related chemical. Second-order neurons in the nucleus tractus solitarius project to two sites in the medulla oblongata: cardiac preganglionic neurons (shown on left) and GABA-containing neurons in the region near the nucleus ambiguus (shown on right). The latter are thought to project to pace-maker neurons in the rostral ventrolateral medulla. The pace-maker neurons may project directly to the sympathetic preganglionic neurons and use an L-glutamate or a related chemical as a transmitter. The transmitters used at each central synapse remain speculative because the full requirements needed for proof that a particular chemical is acting as a transmitter have not been fulfilled. ACh, acetylcholine; NA, noradrenaline; GABA, γ-aminobutyric acid. (Reproduced with permission from Guyenet (1990).)

Cardiorespiratory interactions

The role of the cardiovascular system in homeostasis can only be adequately achieved if there is an integration of cardiovascular and respiratory function. This is well evidenced in terms of the parallel changes in cardiac output and respiratory minute volume that occur in relation to changes in the level of activity and metabolic demand. There is also a large body of evidence indicating that extensive interactions occur between those reflexes that provide moment by moment regulation of the cardiovascular and respiratory systems (see Daly 1985). Indeed, the influences exerted by these reflex inputs are not simply explained by algebraic summation of their individual effects, but must involve a complex and as yet unresolved set of interactions at different levels within the central nervous system.

Recently, neurophysiological studies have gone some way to explaining the underlying central mechanisms that are responsible for this integration, at least with regard to cardiac control. As long ago as the 1930s Anrep and his colleagues (for discussion see Daly 1985; Jordan and Spyer 1987) demonstrated that sinus arrhythmia was the consequence of a respiratory control of the vagal outflow to the heart. They identified two distinct factors that were responsible for the generation of this respiratory arrhythmia. The first was central in origin; the second a consequence of reflexes evoked during respiratory movements.

Electrophysiological studies in the cat have now shown that the central mechanism involves a direct synaptic regulation of cardiac vagal motoneurons exerted by a subset of those brainstem neurons that are responsible for generating the respiratory rhythm (Richter and Spyer 1990). The vagal preganglionic motoneurons are actively hypopolarized during inspiration by a wave of chloride-dependent inhibitory postsynaptic potentials (Fig. 4.7). This results in a fall of membrane input resistance, that shunts effectively the excitatory influences of the arterial baroreceptors. Hence, any influence which increases inspiratory drive will lead, by this process, to both a suppression of vagal efferent discharge and a reduced sensitivity of these neurons to other excitatory inputs, whether central or reflex in origin (see Fig. 4.8). The outcome is a tachycardia in inspiration—sinus arrhythmia. The pattern of discharge of vagal motoneurons during the respiratory cycle indicates that they have close similarities to one of the subsets of respiratory neurons, the post-inspiratory neurons that are involved in modulating the discharge and timing of activity in other subsets of the respiratory generator (see Richter 1982; Richter and Spyer 1990). The vagal outflow to the heart and post-inspiratory neurons are most susceptible to reflex inputs during stage 1 of expiration, when there is maintained activity in the phrenic outflow. This respiratory patterning of vagal outflow is also mirrored by similar changes in the excitability of sympathetic preganglionic motoneurons (Richter

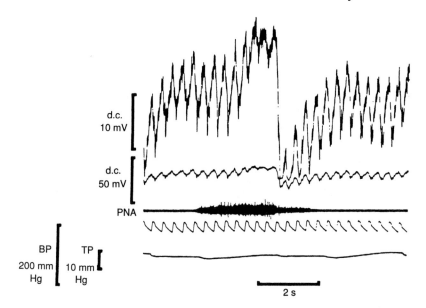

Fig. 4.7. Respiratory modulation of pulse-rhythmic excitatory postsynaptic potentials recording in a cell in which inhibitory postsynaptic potentials have been versed previously by Cl⁻ injection (3 nA for 5 min). Further details in text. Traces from above: high- and low-gain d.c. recordings of membrane potential, phrenic nerve activity (PNA), femoral arterial blood pressure (BP), and tracheal pressure (TP). (Reproduced with permission from Gilbey *et al.* (1984).)

and Spyer 1990). Studies in the rat and cat have shown that sympathetic preganglionic neurons show distinct phases of activity correlating with the central respiratory cycle, as well as being modulated by pulmonary stretch inputs. More recent intracellular studies have gone further to imply that this is imprinted on the discharge of sympathetic neurons, at least as regards inspiration-related activity, by descending excitatory drive. As mentioned earlier, there is evidence that neurons in the rostral VLM that project to the intermediolateral cell column have their activity modulated by respiratory activity, but it remains a possibility that at least a portion of the respiratory discharge of sympathetic neurons is mediated by classical respiratory pathways also (for discussion see Richter and Spyer 1990).

The suppressive action of lung inflation inputs on reflexly evoked bradycardias has been well characterized by Daly (1985), but the central site at which slowly adapting vagal lung stretch afferents act has yet to be discerned. Detailed neurophysiological studies have not revealed an action of this input on baroreceptor or chemoreceptor inputs at the level of the nucleus of the tractus solitarius (Spyer 1990), although there is no doubt that lung inflation modulates the excitability of vagal preganglionic motoneurons

K. M. Spyer

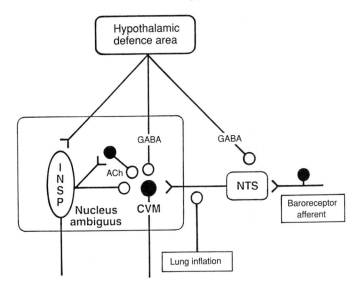

Fig. 4.8. The diagram illustrates the control exerted on vagal cardioinhibitory neurons (CVM) by baroreceptor afferent input, inspiratory neurons (INSP), and the hypothalamic defence area. Excitatory inputs are shown as solid lines with forked endings; inhibitory inputs as lines ending in open circles. NTS, nucleus tractus solitarius; ACh, acetylcholine; GABA, γ-aminobutyric acid. See text for details. (Reproduced with permission from Spyer (1989).)

to these reflex inputs. It is notable that the effects of lung inflation inputs are not of similar magnitude on all reflexes. Reflex activation of those pulmonary receptors excited by phenylbiguanide is much less affected by lung inflation than are either baroreceptor, chemoreceptor, or cardiac afferent inputs (Daly and Kirkman 1989).

Whilst the site of action of lung inflation inputs remains to be resolved, it is clear that changes in respiratory state will exert an enormous direct influence on the sensitivity of both vagal and sympathetic neurons to other inputs. As yet, we have a limited knowledge of the mechanisms by which respiration affects the sympathetic outflow, and this has yet to be correlated directly to the functional role of individual sympathetic preganglionic motoneurons. These influences, however, indicate a potential source of hazard for any input that produces a period of apnoea. At this time, cardiac vagal motoneurons are highly sensitive to other concomitant excitatory inputs, and so can then be viewed as in a state where potentially fatal bradycardia may be induced (see Daly 1985). Aside from providing a plausible explanation for sudden unexplained bradycardias, the apparently tight coupling of cardiac control to respiratory activity ensures a moment by moment matching of cardiac output to respiratory minute volume in diverse physiological situations, such as exercise and breath-hold diving. The underlying neural processes so far considered, will thus provide a framework on which to base further studies into the central nervous basis of cardiorespiratory homeostasis.

Supramedullary control of the cardiovascular system

The cardiovascular system has been shown to be of major importance in homeostasis. It achieves this largely by adjusting the blood supply to different vascular beds in proportion to the level of their activity. Basically, the nervous system achieves this by maintaining arterial pressure within relatively fine limits in consequence of afferent input, whilst regulating cardiac output in the face of different behavioural demands through the interplay of reflex inputs (see above) and central drives. In order to achieve this regulation, the discharge of the autonomic outflows are patterned, and these patterns are highly specific for the different repertoire of responses that can be made by the organism. From studies in man and experimental observations in a range of vertebrates much has now been learned of the cardiovascular response that accompany sleep, exercise, and emotional responses, yet it is only with respect to affective behaviour that we have a detailed description of the central structures and neural pathways that are involved in mediating these changes (see Jordan 1990). The investigations on the defence reaction of the cat by Hilton and his colleagues (see Hilton 1966 for review), and the playing-dead or freezing response of the rabbit (Applegate *et al.* 1983) have shed considerable light on the role of the amygdala and hypothalamus in organizing these responses. These two distinct animal models of behaviour may have provided information of considerable significance in understanding the human adaptations to environmental and emotional stress.

The defence reaction

With regard to the organization of affective behaviour, the hypothalamus has long been seen to play a major role (Hilton 1966). Indeed, the activation of the perifornical region of the hypothalamus, either directly by electrical stimulation through microelectrodes or by activation of other brain areas or general afferent excitation, has been seen to induce patterns of behaviour and autonomic change that is typical of the alerting stage of the defence reaction. The cardiovascular pattern of response accompanying the defence reaction has been shown to involve a rise in heart rate and aortic blood flow (and hence cardiac output), a widespread vasoconstriction, but a characteristic withdrawal of vasoconstrictor tone of the vasculature of skeletal muscle and, in the cat, to an activation of sympathetic cholinergic vasodilator fibres in this particular bed (Hilton 1966; see Fig. 4.9). In all species, vasodilatation in skeletal muscle is enhanced by an increased outpouring of catecholamines

K. M. Spyer

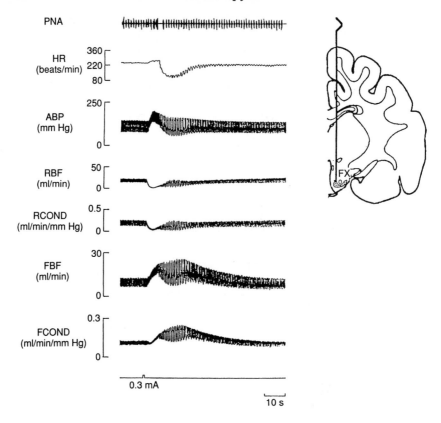

Fig. 4.9. Cardiovascular and respiratory responses to electrical stimulation in the perifornical region of the hypothalamus of the althesin-anaesthetized cat. The diagram on the right illustrates the electrode position on a hemicoronal section (FX, fornix). The stimulus was a 4 s train of 0.5 ms pulses delivered at 100 Hz, initiated at the time shown in the lower trace on the polygraph record shown on the left-hand side. Traces from top to bottom: PNA, phrenic nerve activity; HR, heart rate; ABP, arterial blood pressure; RBF, renal blood flow; RCOND, renal vascular conductance; FBF, femoral blood flow; FCOND, femoral vascular conductance. RBF and FBF were recorded using electromagnetic flow probes. (Reproduced with permission from Spyer (1989).)

from the adrenal medulla. Cutaneous, renal, and mesenteric blood flow is diminished, and arterial pressure and pulse pressure rise dramatically. Further, under appropriate experimental conditions, a similar pattern of response can be elicited on electrical stimulation of the central nucleus of the amygdala in the cat, and there is good evidence that at least a part of the forebrain control of behaviour is mediated via the amygdala which is itself afferent to the hypothalamus (for discussion see Jordan 1990). Recent studies have questioned the importance of the hypothalamus in the integration of this response, since it has proved difficult to elicit the defence reaction by using chemical means to activate neurons in this region of the hypothalamus. However, in the baboon Smith *et al.* (1980) describe how lesions in the perifornical region abolished the cardiovascular component but spared the behavioural component of conditioned adversive responses. The main focus of attention has moved to the amygdala (see above) and to the midbrain periaqueductal grey from where both electrical and chemical stimulation are effective in eliciting the characteristic cardiovascular response (Jordan 1990).

Playing-dead response

Whilst stimulation in the perifornical region of the rabbit hypothalamus may evoke similar cardiovascular responses to those seen in other species, affective behaviour in this species is usually associated with a bradycardia and hypotension and a suppression of motor activity—freezing or playing dead (see Applegate *et al.* 1983). This is accompanied by rapid, shallow breathing. This is the characteristic response that can also be evoked by stimulation of the central nucleus of the amygdala in both anaesthetized and conscious preparations (Cox *et al.* 1987).

Efferent pathways for affective behaviour

The role of the central nucleus of the amygdala and the hypothalamic defence area in patterning the cardiovascular and respiratory responses in affective behaviour has been described. Considerable evidence is now available indicating that the connections of the central nucleus of the amygdala that mediate these affects involve parallel descending pathways influencing several cell groups within the midbrain, including the central grey, the pontine Kölliker–Fuse and parabrachial nuclei, and, within the medulla, the nucleus of the tractus solitarius, dorsal vagal nucleus, nucleus ambiguus, and also the rostroventrolateral medulla (see Fig. 4.10). In many instances reciprocal connections can be shown between these cells groups and the central nucleus. The descending connections of the hypothalamic defence area, which have been mapped electrophysiologically, include many of the same regions of midbrain, pons, and medulla. Indeed, there is now plentiful evidence that activating the hypothalamic defence area and the periaqueductal grey exerts relatively direct control of neurons in the rostral VLM (see Guyenet 1990). These descending pathways are likely to represent the major means by which both sympathetic and vagal neurons are influenced, but other direct connections between the hypothalamus and spinal cord have also been shown (see Loewy 1990 amongst others).

K. M. Spyer

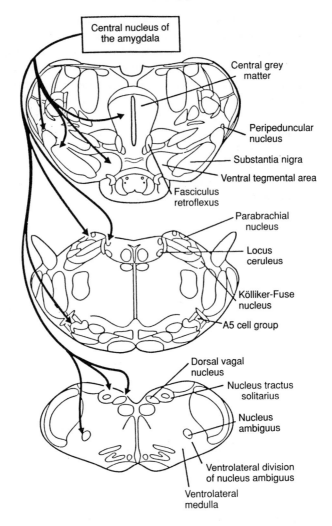

Fig. 4.10. Series of drawings showing the descending projections from the central nucleus of the amygdala that innervate the brainstem. (Reproduced with permission from Loewy (1990).)

Reflex modification

One of the most striking features of the defence reaction elicited on electrical stimulation of either the hypothalamus or the amygdala in the cat, is the concomitant rise in arterial blood pressure and heart rate (see Fig. 4.9). This has been taken to suggest a central suppression of the baroreceptor reflex (Hilton 1966). In part, this resetting could be seen as a consequence of increased inspiratory activity, which, on the basis of our review, would be expected to exert a profound inhibition of cardiac vagal efferent activity. However, both vascular and cardiac components of the reflex appear to be affected (for discussion see Spyer 1981). In contrast, in the rabbit the bradycardia and hypotension resulting from stimulation in the central nucleus of the amygdala appear to involve a facilitatory modulation of the baroreceptor reflex (Cox *et al.* 1986). Since the descending output from both amygdala and hypothalamus appears to have a major target within the NTS (Fig. 4.10), it is probable that this is the site of major interaction between reflex and central drive. In the cat, evidence has now been obtained to show that those NTS neurons that are excited by baroreceptor stimulation receive an inhibitory input on stimulating within the hypothalamic defence area (Fig. 4.11). The

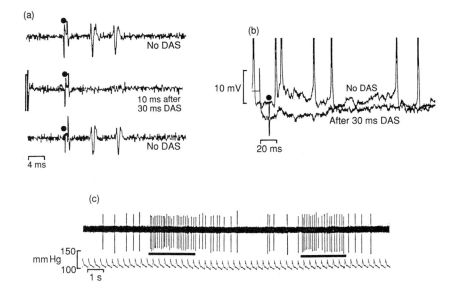

Fig. 4.11. Extracellular and intracellular recording of hypothalamic defence area inhibition of a cell excited by activation of carotid sinus baroreceptors. (a) Extracellular responses to SN (sinus nerve) stimulation (stimulus artefact indicated by ●) in top and bottom traces. Between the two SN stimuli the SN stimulus was preceded by 10 ms by a 30-ms burst of hypothalamic defence area stimulation (DAS; middle trace) that abolished the SN-evoked discharge. (b) Intracellular recording from the same cell. SN stimulation alone (top trace, no defence area stimulation, no hypothalamic defence activator (DAS)) evoked a comparable number of action potentials (truncated) at the same latency as recorded extracellularly. At the end of hypothalamic defence area stimulation (lower trace, after 30 ms DAS) did not evoke discharge. (c) Extracellular recording of response to baroreceptor activation (during period indicated by the bars). Membrane potential, – 53 mV. Potassium citrate-filled electrode. (Reproduced with permission from Mifflin *et al.* (1988*b*).)

inhibitory action is mediated by GABA acting at GABA A receptors and may be antagonized by the iontophoretic application of bicuculline (see Spyer 1989,1990). The descending pathways are likely to converge on intrinsic GABAergic neurons of the NTS, since there is no evidence that descending GABAergic pathways are involved (for discussion see Spyer 1990). These same intrinsic NTS neurons may also be influenced by descending input from the various pontine nuclei involved in cardiorespiratory practice. Interestingly, when the action of this GABAergic descending pathway is antagonized by the application of bicuculline, a hypothalamically mediated excitation often becomes apparent. Conversely, when the central nucleus of the amygdala is activated in the rabbit, NTS neurons receiving baroreceptor input are facilitated. This suggests that two distinct mechanisms may be activated on diencephalic stimulation—the one more prevalent in the cat, involving an inhibition, the other more prevalent in the rabbit exerting facilitation, but both expressed to a degree in each species. The particularly important observation is that these two distinct mechanisms may represent simple operating principles by which the complex forms of behaviour that are associated with stress can express themselves in changes in cardiovascular activity. These powerful actions at the NTS that may be elicited from stimulation in regions of the diencephalon may be enhanced by the action of descending pathways acting at other levels within the brainstem. The powerful inhibition exerted by defence area stimulation in the cat at the level of the NTS, which will remove inhibitory control over medullary premotor sympathetic neurons (i.e. disinhibition) will be reinforced by the more directly distributed excitatory input that rostral VLM neurons receive simultaneously (see Fig. 4.8).

These data provide an insight into the neural substrate through which the effectiveness of the baroreceptor reflex may be modified in relation to emotion. Equally, similar neural interactions may play a role in promoting the parallel changes in the cardiovascular and respiratory systems that accompany other forms of behaviour, such as the response to exercise.

Conclusions

In endeavouring to provide a relatively contemporary analysis of the central nervous control of the cardiovascular system, this review has assessed the neural pathways by which the excitability of both vagal and sympathetic preganglionic motoneurons is regulated. Emphasis has been placed on understanding the reflex and, particularly, the baroreflex control of these two groups of autonomic neurons. Further, attempts have been made to identify the central neural mechanisms by which these reflex inputs are modulated during affective behaviour. It appears that certain simple neural principles dictate the pattern of these interactions, and a fundamental design principle appears to involve a coupling of respiratory and cardiovascular regulation.

These observations indicate that the central nervous system exerts its control over autonomic and specifically cardiovascular function in a manner analagous to the way in which motor activities are controlled. In particular, the modification of reflex action, which can be exerted by rostral brainstem and subcortical areas, may provide an indication of potential mechanisms whereby stress and emotion can cause profound changes in the cardiovascular system. Whether the acute, and clearly reversible, changes of the type reviewed in this discussion may be converted, on repetition, to prolonged and irreversible alterations remain to be investigated.

Acknowledgements

The financial support of the Medical Research Council and British Heart Foundation, and the provision of a Wolfson University Award are gratefully acknowledged.

References

Applegate, C. D., Kapp, B. S., Underwood, M. D., and McNall, C. L. (1983). Autonomic and somatomotor effects of amygdala central nucleus stimulation in awake rabbits. *Physiol. Behav.* **31**, 353–60.

Bacon, S. J., Zagon, A., and Smith, A. D. (1990). Electron microscopic evidence of a monosynaptic pathway between cells in the caudal raphe nuclei and sympathetic preganglionic neurons in the rat spinal cord. *Exp. Brain Res.* **79**, 589–602.

Cabot, J. B. (1990). Sympathetic preganglionic neurons: cytoarchitecture, ultrastructure and biophysical properties. In *Central regulation of autonomic functions* (ed. A. D. Loewy and K. M. Spyer), pp. 44–67. Oxford University Press, New York.

Chalmers, J. P. and Pilowsky, P. M. (1991). Brainstem and bulbospinal neurotransmitter systems in the control of blood pressure. *J. Hypotension* **9**, 675–94.

Coote, J. H. (1988). The organisation of cardiovascular neurons in the spinal cord. *Rev. Physiol. Biochem. Pharmacol.* **110**, 148–285.

Cox, G. E., Jordan, D., Moruzzi, P., Schwaber, J. S., Spyer, K. M., and Turner, S. A. (1986). Amygdaloid influences on brainstem neurones in the rabbit. *J. Physiol., London* **381**, 135–48.

Cox, G. E., Jordan, D., Paton, J. F. R., Spyer, K. M., and Wood, L. M. (1987). Cardiovascular and phrenic nerve responses to stimulation of the amygdala central nucleus in the anaesthetised rabbit. *J. Physiol.* **389**, 541–56.

Daly, M. de B. (1985). Interactions between respiration and circulation. In *Handbook of physiology. The respiratory system II*, pp. 529–94. American Physiological Society, Bethesda, Maryland.

Daly, M. de B. and Kirkman, E. (1989). Differential modulation by pulmonary stretch afferents of some reflex cardioinhibitory responses in the cat. *J. Physiol., London* **417**, 323–41.

Feldberg, W. and Guertzenstein, P. G. (1976). Vasodepressor effects obtained by drugs acting on the ventral surface of the brain stem. *J. Physiol., London* **258**, 337–55.

Gebber, G. L. (1990). Central determinants of sympathetic nerve discharge. In *Central regulation of autonomic functions* (ed. A. D. Loewy and K. M. Spyer), pp. 126–44. Oxford University Press, New York.

Gilbey, M. P. and Stein, R. D. (1991). Characteristics of sympathetic preganglionic neurones in the lumbar spinal cord of the cat. *J. Physiol., London* **432**, 427–43.

Gilbey, M. P., Jordan, D., Richter, D. W., and Spyer, K. M. (1984). Synaptic mechanisms involved in the inspiratory modulation of vagal cardio-inhibitory neurones in the cat. *J. Physiol., London* **356**, 65–78.

Guyenet, P. G. (1990). Role of the ventral medulla oblongata in blood pressure regulation. In *Central regulation of autonomic functions* (ed. A. D. Loewy and K. M. Spyer), pp. 145–67. Oxford University Press, New York.

Harris, M. C. and Loewy, A. D. (1990). Neural regulation of vasopressin-containing hypothalamic neurons and the role of vasopressin in cardiovascular function. In *Central regulation of autonomic functions* (ed. A. D. Loewy and K. M. Spyer), pp. 224–46. Oxford University Press, New York.

Hilton, S. M. (1966). Hypothalamic regulation of the cardiovascular system. *Br. Med. Bull.* **22**, 243–8.

Izzo, P. N. (1991). A note on the use of biocytin in anterograde tracing studies in the central nervous system: application at both light and electron microscopic level. *J. Neurosci. Methods* **36**, 155–66

Jordan, D. (1990). Autonomic changes in affective behaviour. In *Central regulation of autonomic functions* (ed. A. D. Loewy and K. M. Spyer), pp. 349–66. Oxford University Press, New York.

Jordan, D. and Spyer, K. M. (1986). Brainstem integration of cardiovascular and pulmonary afferent activity. In *Progress in brain research*, Vol. 67. *Visceral sensation* (ed. F. Cerevero and F. B. Morrison), pp. 295–314. Elsevier Science Publishers, Amsterdam.

Jordan, D. and Spyer, K. M. (1987). Central neural mechanisms mediating respiratory–cardiovascular interactions. In *Neurobiology of the cardiorespiratory system*, Studies in Neuroscience Series (ed. E. W. Taylor), pp. 342–68. University of Manchester Press, Manchester.

Loewy, A. D. (1990). Central autonomic pathways. In *Central regulation of autonomic functions* (ed. A. D. Loewy and K. M. Spyer), pp. 88–103. Oxford University Press, New York.

Loewy, A. D. and Burton, H. (1978). Nuclei of the solitary tract; efferent projection to the lower brainstem and spinal cord of the cat. *J. comp. Neurol.* **181**, 421–50.

Loewy, A. D. and Neil, J. J. (1981). The role of descending monoaminergic systems in central control of blood pressure. *Fed. Proc.* **40**(13), 56–63.

Loewy, A. D. and Spyer, K. M. (1990). Vagal preganglionic neurons. In *Central regulation of autonomic functions* (ed. A. D. Loewy and K. M. Spyer), pp. 68–87. Oxford University Press, New York.

Mifflin, S. W., Spyer, K. M., and Withington-Wray, D. J. (1988*a*). Baroreceptor inputs to the nucleus tractus solitarius in the cat: postsynaptic actions and the influence of respiration. *J. Physiol.* **399**, 349–67.

Mifflin, S. W., Spyer, K. M., and Withington-Wray, D. J. (1988*b*). Baroreceptor inputs to the nucleus tractus solitarius in the cat: modulation of the hypothalamus. *J. Physiol.* **399**, 369–87.

Milner, T. A., Morrison, S. F., Abate, C., and Reis, D. J. (1988). Phenylethanolamine N-methyltransferase containing terminals synapse directly on sympathetic preganglionic neurones in the rat. *Brain Res.* **448**, 205–22.

Morrison, S. F., Milner, T. A., Pickel, V. M., and Reis, D. J. (1988). Retinospinal vasomotor neurons of the rat rostral ventrolateral medulla (RVLM): relationship to sympathetic nerve activity and the C1 adrenergic cell group. *J. Neurosci.* **8**, 1286–301.

Richter, D. W. (1982). Generation and maintenance of the respiratory rhythm. *J. exp. Biol.* **100**, 93–107.

Richter, D. W. and Spyer, K. M. (1990). In *Central regulation of autonomic functions* (ed. A. D. Loewy and K. M. Spyer), pp. 189–207. Oxford University Press, New York.

Smith, O. A., Asley, C. A., De Vito, J. L., Stein, J. M., and Walsh, K. E. (1980). Functional analysis of the hypothalamic control of the cardiovascular responses accompanying emotional behavior. *Fed. Proc.* **39**, 2487–94.

Spyer, K. M. (1981). Neural organisation and control of the baroreceptor reflex. *Rev. Physiol. Biochem. Pharmacol.* **88**, 23–124.

Spyer, K. M. (1982). Central nervous integration of cardiovascular control. *J. exp. Biol.* **100**, 109–28.

Spyer, K. M. (1984). Central control of the cardiovascular system. In *Recent advances in physiology*, Vol. 10 (ed. P. F. Baker), pp. 163–200. Churchill Livingstone, Edinburgh.

Spyer, K. M. (1989). Neural mechanisms involved in cardiovascular control during affective behavior. *Trends in Neurosciences* **12**, 506–13.

Spyer, K. M. (1990). The central nervous organisation of reflex circulatory control. In *Central regulation of autonomic functions* (ed. A. D. Loewy and K. M. Spyer), pp. 168–88. Oxford University Press, New York.

Sun, M.-K. and Spyer, K. M. (1991*a*). GABA-mediated inhibition of medullary vasomotor neurones by area postrema stimulation in rats. *J. Physiol., London* **436**, 669–84.

Sun, M.-K. and Spyer, K. M. (1991*b*). Nociceptive inputs into rostral ventrolateral medulla-spinal vasomotor neurones in rats. *J. Physiol., London* **436**, 685–700.

Zagon, A. and Bacon, S. J. (1991). Evidence of monosynaptic pathway between cells of the ventromedial medulla and the motoneuron pool of the thoracic spinal cord in rat: electron microscopic analysis of synaptic contacts. *Eur. J. Neurosci.* **3**, 55–65.

5. Control of blood pressure and the circulation in man

R. F. J. Shepherd and J. T. Shepherd

Introduction

The mechanisms that regulate the arterial blood pressure are complex indeed, involving peripheral sensors, centres in the nervous system, autonomic nerves, and humoral and local factors. Continuous measurements over a 24-hour period during which normal activities are pursued have shown that, in healthy individuals, arterial blood pressure varies widely as a consequence of continuous adjustments in autonomic outflow. These adjustments originate directly from centres in the brain and also from the reflexogenic zones in the systemic circulation. They provide the body with the perfusion pressure appropriate to meet, in conjunction with the local regulation of the resistance blood vessels, the changing metabolic requirements of the organs and tissues of the body in response to the many stresses to which the cardiovascular system is subjected.

Circadian pattern

Systolic and diastolic pressures move in the same direction over the 24-hour cycle, so that there is little change in pulse pressure. The arterial baroreflexes exert a buffering influence on the magnitude of the day and night variations in blood pressure. They act to reduce the size of the centrally induced blood-pressure oscillations. They induce short-lived changes in heart rate opposite in direction to the changes in blood pressure, thus increasing heart rate variability. Hence, when the arterial baroreceptors are functioning normally, there occur smaller blood-pressure and larger heart-rate oscillations; if the arterial baroreceptors are ineffective, there are larger blood-pressure and smaller heart-rate oscillations (Mancia and Zanchetti 1986).

Blood pressure variability increases with ageing. In patients with essential hypertension, the arterial pressure variability increases progressively with increasing levels of blood pressure (Mancia and Zanchetti 1986).

Patients with autonomic failure who exhibit postural hypotension retain a circadian variation in pressure; however, this is the inverse of the normal pattern, with the highest pressures being at night and the lowest in the morning. This is consistent with the fact that postural dizziness is most common in the morning. They also have a reduction in heart rate variability (Mann *et al.* 1983).

Studies in animals and man have demonstrated that normal blood pressure control depends on the proper functioning of the sympathetic nervous system to the systemic vessels. While the autonomic nerves to the heart have important roles in regulating heart rate, atrioventricular (AV) conduction, and cardiac contractility, both humans and animals have no problem in blood pressure regulation in the absence of the autonomic nerves to the heart. Some increase in heart rate occurs during exercise due to an intrinsic mechanism and the denervated heart is supersensitive to circulating noradrenaline.

Sympathetic activity

Changes in sympathetic outflow are governed by arterial baroreceptors and chemoreceptors, cardiopulmonary mechanoreceptors, and receptors in skeletal muscles activated by muscular contraction (Fig. 5.1). Changes in sympathetic outflow also occur from primary changes in the activity of brain centres, including the 'central command' originating in the cerebral cortex during exercise and in the hypothalamic centres with emotional stress. It is not surprising, in view of the complexity of these peripheral sensors and of the brain centres that control the cardiovascular system, that the sympathetic outflow is not uniformly altered to meet the various stresses to which the body is subjected. Rather, the sympathetic nerve discharge occurs in a highly differentiated pattern. Thus, in response to reflex or central stimuli, the efferent sympathetic activity varies between the different organs and tissues and, in the same organ or tissue, can vary between resistance and capacitance vessels. In some instances, it may increase in some organs and decrease in others. Multiunit recordings of efferent sympathetic activity in human limb nerves, using tungsten microelectrodes, have shown that, in skin fascicles, the resting activity consists of irregular bursts of impulses, unrelated to the arterial blood pressure. In muscle fascicles, the activity occurs in pulse-synchronous bursts which correlate with variations in diastolic but not systolic blood pressure; the changes in activity are greater when the blood pressure is decreasing than when it is increasing. Thus acute decreases in arterial blood pressure are buffered more efficiently than acute increases, and variations in sympathetic outflow to skeletal muscle vessels are determined mainly by fluctuations in diastolic blood pressure (Wallin 1986).

Plasma levels of noradrenaline are frequently used as an index of sympathetic activity. Such levels are governed by the balance between release of noradrenaline from sympathetic nerve endings, re-uptake into the endings, and catabolism of the amine. Also, the plasma level of noradrenaline gives

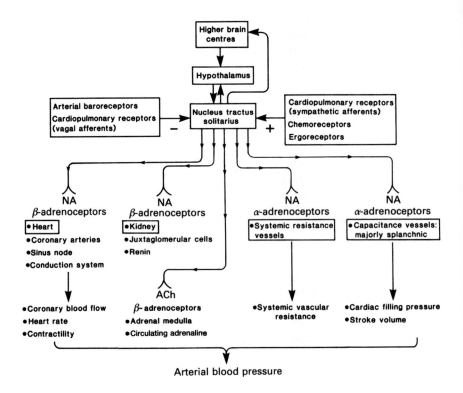

Fig. 5.1. Reflex control of the cardiovascular system. The arterial baroreceptors and the cardiopulmonary receptors with vagal afferents tonically inhibit (–) the vasomotor centres. The cardiopulmonary receptors with sympathetic afferents, the arterial chemoreceptors, and ergoreceptors in the skeletal muscles (when activated by the contraction) stimulate (+) the centres. All these afferent signals are integrated in the central nervous system. As a consequence the sympathetic outflow is modified selectively to adjust appropriately the performance of the cardiovascular system. The noradrenaline (NA) released at the sympathetic terminals acts on beta-adrenoceptors in the heart and the coronary vessels and on the juxtaglomerular cells of the kidney to regulate the release of renin. As a consequence the heart rate and cardiac contractility are augmented, and the main coronary arteries are relaxed. This relaxation is enhanced by a flow-induced release of an endothelium-derived relaxing factor. The sympathetic outflow to the adrenal medulla regulates adrenaline release. The circulating adrenaline also activates the beta-adrenoceptors. The noradrenaline released also activates alpha-adrenoceptors to cause constriction of the resistance vessels and a decrease in the capacitance of the splanchnic vascular bed. As a consequence the systemic vascular resistance and the cardiac filling pressure (and hence the stroke volume and cardiac output) are adjusted to maintain the arterial blood pressure at the appropriate level for the proper perfusion of the organs and tissues of the body.

no indication of the relative changes in sympathetic outflow to the different components of the circulation. The skeletal muscles contribute about one-fifth of the plasma noradrenaline level, whereas the splanchnic bed contributes little since the liver clears catecholamines from the blood (Shepherd and Mancia 1986).

Adrenoceptors

The noradrenaline released from the sympathetic nerves activates α- and β-adrenoceptors in the circulatory system; β_1-adrenoceptors are activated equally by adrenaline and noradrenaline, whereas β_2-adrenoceptors have a greater affinity for adrenaline (see Chapter 6). The former are present on the sinus and atrioventricular nodes, the conducting system and muscle cells of the heart, and conduit coronary arteries. When activated they cause an increase in heart rate and shortening of the refractory period, enhancement of ventricular contractility, and dilatation of the coronary arteries. In the kidneys they are present on the juxtaglomerular cells where they are involved in the control of renin release (Fig. 5.1).

β_2-adrenoceptors, which are not innervated, are present in the resistance vessels of the skeletal muscles. When activated by circulating adrenaline, as in emotional stress, they cause relaxation of these vessels.

The function of the β-adrenoceptors is to adjust the circulation to help meet the stresses imposed by gravitational forces, by muscular exercise, and by emotional stress. Thus, after pharmacological blockade of the β-adrenoceptors, it is only when the cardiovascular system is severely taxed that deficiencies in its performance are apparent.

The α-adrenoceptors are present on the resistance and capacitance vessels of the systemic circulation (Fig. 5.1). These postsynaptic receptors are classified as α_1 and α_2. In general, α_1-adrenoceptors predominate in arterial smooth muscle. In the capacitance vessels, including the human saphenous vein, both types mediate vasoconstriction in response to neuronally released and circulating noradrenaline (Elsner et al. 1986; Steen et al. 1986).

The adrenergic neuroeffector junction

Receptors on sympathetic nerve terminals

Many receptors are present on these terminals. If activated some increase and others decrease the output of the neurotransmitter. In addition, metabolic products and hyperosmolarity can, in addition to causing direct relaxation of the adjacent resistance vessels, depress the outflow of noradrenaline from their sympathetic nerve endings (Shepherd and Vanhoutte 1981; Fig. 5.2).

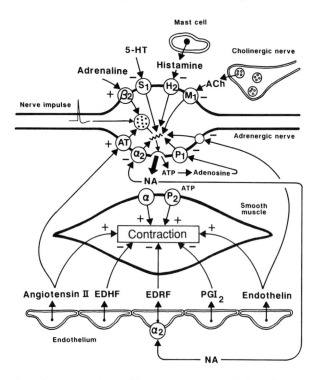

Fig. 5.2. The adrenergic neuroeffector junction. Noradrenaline (NA) released from the adrenergic nerve acts on α-adrenoceptors on the vascular smooth muscle cells (α) to initiate their contraction. Some of the noradrenaline might activate alpha$_2$-adrenoceptors (α_2) on the nerve terminals to reduce its output. Some noradrenaline activates α_2-adrenoceptors (α_2) on the endothelial cells to cause release of endothelium-derived relaxing factor (EDRF). This is likely to be nitric oxide or a labile nitroso compound. Other substances formed in endothelial cells also may modify the smooth muscle response to the noradrenaline. Prostacyclin (PGI$_2$) and endothelium-derived hyperpolarizing factor (EDHF) are vasorelaxant while endothelin would enhance the contraction. Angiotensin II, also formed in endothelial cells, can enhance the contraction by acting on the smooth muscle and also by stimulating an angiotensin II receptor (AT) on the nerve ending to enhance NA release. In some vascular beds in some species, adenosine triphosphate (ATP) is co-released with adrenaline. Thus, activating P$_2$-purinergic receptors on the smooth muscle (P$_2$) can enhance its contraction. However, it is rapidly degraded to adenosine, and the latter, by stimulating P$_1$-purinergic receptors (P$_1$) on the sympathetic nerve endings can inhibit the release of NA and ATP from the nerves. Other receptors on the nerve ending if activated can increase (+) or decrease (–) neurotransmitter release. β_2, β-adrenergic receptor; S$_1$, serotoninergic receptor which can be activated by 5-hydroxytryptamine (5-HT); H$_2$, histaminergic receptor; M$_1$, muscarinic receptor which may be activated by acetylcholine (ACh) released from cholinergic nerves.

Interaction between the sympathetic
nerves and the endothelium

The endothelial cells produce and release a variety of relaxing and contracting substances. These include prostacyclin, nitric oxide (or a labile nitroso compound) and a hyperpolarizing substance which causes relaxation of the underlying smooth muscle, and peptides termed endothelins which depolarize the muscle and cause its contraction. The release of any of these substances can modify the response to sympathetic nerve stimulation. Specifically, noradrenaline not only activates α-receptors on the smooth muscle to initiate contraction, but also activates α_2-receptors on the endothelial cells to release a substance which is not only vasorelaxant (Miller 1991), but also inhibits the calcium-evoked release of noradrenaline from the adrenergic terminals (Tesfamarian et al. 1989; Fig. 5.2).

In addition, the endothelium also can synthesize and secrete angiotensins. This secretion is stimulated by β_2- and inhibited by α-adrenoceptor mechanisms (Tang et al. 1990). Circulating angiotensin II reinforces sympathetic activity by effects on cardiovascular brain centres, on autonomic ganglia, on angiotensin II receptors on the sympathetic nerve endings to increase the noradrenaline output, by inhibition of re-uptake of noradrenaline into sympathetic nerve terminals, and constriction of vascular smooth muscle by activating angiotensin II receptors on the muscle and by enhancing the response of α-adrenoceptors to noradrenaline (Shepherd 1990).

Co-transmitter

In several species and tissues during sympathetic activation adenosine triphosphate (ATP) is coreleased with noradrenaline from perivascular sympathetic nerve terminals. This can modulate sympathetic vasoconstriction through activation of specific receptors. By activating postsynaptic P_2-purinoceptors the vasoconstriction is enhanced. However, adenosine, formed by the rapid breakdown of ATP, stimulates presynaptic P_1-purinoceptors and inhibits noradrenaline release. In humans, from studies of the forearm resistance vessels, there is indirect evidence for a similar role for the purinergic system (Pelleg and Burnstock 1990; Taddei et al. 1990). Thus, when the sympathetic outflow is increased, its final action on a particular vascular bed is the resultant of many complex interactions and feedback mechanisms. These include the degree of nervous activity, the role of co-transmitters, the possibility of activation of prejunctional receptors, and the effect of substances released from the endothelium (Fig. 5.2).

Cardiovascular reflexes

The cardiovascular reflexes initiated from the peripheral sensors can be divided into those which inhibit and those which excite the vasomotor centres in the brain (Fig. 5.1).

The carotid and aortic baroreflexes

A commonly used approach to study the carotid baroreflex in man is to apply negative and positive pressures to the neck to cause increases and decreases, respectively, in carotid sinus transmural pressure. This alters the degree of activation of the carotid sinus baroreceptors. The main limitation of the method is that the alterations of systemic arterial blood pressure induced by changes in the activity of the carotid sinus baroreceptors affect in an opposite manner the aortic baroreceptors and possibly also receptors in the left ventricle.

Other approaches to studying the role of the combined influence of carotid and aortic baroreceptors in the control of heart rate involve using drugs to alter arterial blood pressure and then examining the resultant changes in heart rate. Usually, phenylephrine is used to raise the pressure, and amyl nitrite, nitroglycerin, or nitroprusside to lower it. The same changes in pressure are sensed by the carotid and aortic baroreceptors, but no information, of course, can be obtained by this approach concerning the relationship between baroreceptor activity and arterial blood pressure. Heart rate is only one component of the many complex events which determine the latter.

The primary role of the arterial baroreflexes is the rapid adjustment of arterial blood pressure around the existing mean pressure. This is accomplished by changes in heart rate, stroke volume, cardiac contractility, total systemic vascular resistance, and venous capacitance in response to changes in activity of these stretch receptors in the carotid sinus and ascending aorta.

Carotid baroreflex

The heart rate decreases and increases rapidly in response to increases and decreases, respectively, in the activity of the carotid baroreceptors. This is due to the variations in vagal activity to the sinus node. The speed of the response permits the rate to be regulated on a beat-to-beat basis. An increase in sympathetic outflow to the sinus node, which is slower in onset, contributes to the cardioacceleration during a sustained decrease in carotid sinus pressure. The change in heart rate also depends on the period during the respiratory cycle in which the signal to the baroreceptors is changed; it is less in early- and mid-aspiration and greatest in early expiration. This is explained by modulation of the vagal cardioinhibitory neurons by a central respiratory oscillator.

The arterial pressure decreases when the carotid baroreceptors are activated by the application of negative pressure to the neck and increased when they are deactivated by positive pressure. In normal subjects, the set-point on the curve relating the stimulus to the baroreceptors to the changes in arterial blood pressure is closer to the saturation limit. This makes the reflex more effective in buffering reductions than increases in pressure (Rea and Eckberg 1987).

The changes in arterial blood pressure with activation or deactivation of the carotid baroreceptors result from the balance of changes in cardiac output and in total systemic vascular resistance. However, the buffering action of the carotid sinus baroreceptors is not impaired by combined β-adrenergic and parasympathetic blockade. This implies that adjustments in cardiac output are not essential and that the moment-to-moment control of blood pressure by the arterial baroreceptors depends primarily on changes in total systemic vascular resistance through sympathetically mediated adjustments in vasoconstrictor tone (Shepherd and Mancia 1986).

Studies in dogs have demonstrated that the arterial baroreceptors regulate the overall systemic vascular resistance during and after exercise, while the heart rate and cardiac output are controlled by other mechanisms. If, in dogs with chronic aortic denervation, the influence of the carotid baroreceptors is acutely removed, there is a greater decrease in arterial blood pressure at

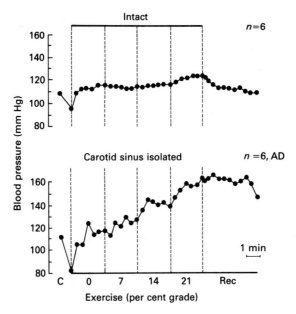

Fig. 5.3. Mean arterial pressure during continuous graded exercise in dogs with aortic-arch denervation before (top) and after (bottom) vascular isolation and pressurization of carotid sinuses. AD, aortic denervation; C, control; Rec, recovery. (Data from Walgenbach and Donald (1983).)

the onset of exercise and, as the severity of the exercise is increased, the blood pressure rises progressively and remains elevated for some time after the exercise ceases (Fig. 5.3). The cardiac output and heart-rate changes are similar with and without the carotid sinuses operative. It seems that the function of the carotid sinus is to oppose the hypotension that develops at the onset of exercise and to limit the elevation in pressure that develops with increasing work load.

Aortic baroreflex

Various studies have been undertaken in normal humans to assess the relative influence of carotid and aortic baroreceptors in circulatory control. These studies suggest that the aortic baroreflex has a greater role than the carotid in the regulation of heart rate responses during elevation of arterial pressure and that, during acute reductions in pressure, it is an important regulator of efferent sympathetic nerve responses (Sanders *et al.* 1989).

Resetting of arterial baroreceptors

The baroreceptor reflex control of the autonomic outflow is governed by the relationship between the arterial blood pressure induced input to the central nervous system and its resultant neural output. An alteration in the efferent autonomic activity in response to a given change in carotid artery and aortic transmural pressure can result from resetting of the baroreceptors. This can occur rapidly in response to different stresses, and permits these baroreflexes to shift their set-point and/or operating range to a higher or lower level. For example, during rhythmic (dynamic) and isometric (static) exercise, the carotid baroreceptors are adjusted quickly to a higher level. This permits the arterial pressure to increase to help meet the metabolic demands of the active muscles. The gain of the reflex is unchanged so that it operates normally around a higher set-point (Shepherd and Mancia 1986). Resetting may result from a change in the coupling, within the central nervous system, of afferent nerve input to efferent nerve activity or, locally, by a change in mechano-electrical transduction in the receptors. Regarding the former, a short-term change in the conditioning pressure of the baroreceptors can reset the central set-point (Tan *et al.* 1989). The latter might result from viscoelastic changes in the wall elements with which the receptors are coupled by alteration of membrane pumps or by a local release of vasoactive factors from the endothelium (Chapleau *et al.* 1989). For example, in normotensive rabbits, a prostanoid released from the endothelium during vascular stretch contributes to baroreceptor activation (McDowell *et al.* 1989).

Cardiopulmonary reflexes

In addition to its key mechanical function, the heart also serves as a sensory and an endocrine organ. Concerning its sensory function, studies in animals have demonstrated that the heart and lungs contain numerous mechano-receptors whose afferent fibres, both myelinated and unmyelinated, course in the vagal nerves to the brainstem. Large unencapsulated endings, confined mainly to the atria and the vein–atrial junctions are subserved by fast-conducting myelinated vagal afferents: one group signals atrial contraction and the other atrial filling. Their different discharge patterns seem to be related to their location rather than to any basic difference in their characteristics. When their activity is increased they cause an increase in heart rate by activating selectively sympathetic fibres to the sinus node. The activity to the myocardium is not increased while that to the kidney is inhibited. This illustrates the reflex selectivity that can occur in the sympathetic outflow (Linden and Kappagoda 1982). These receptors are also involved in the release of vasopressin and hence in the regulation of water reabsorption in renal tubules (Bennett and Gardiner 1985).

Like the arterial baroreceptors, the cardiopulmonary receptors with unmyelinated vagal afferents act continuously to inhibit the vasomotor centre. Studies in dogs demonstrate that receptors in the atria, ventricles, and lungs each contribute to this tonic inhibition. When humans change from the supine to the upright position, there is a gravitational shift of blood from the cardiopulmonary region to the dependent parts. This results in a decrease in the activity of the cardiopulmonary and arterial mechanoreceptors. There follow an increase in heart rate, a decrease in stroke volume, a reflex constriction of muscle, splanchnic, and renal resistance vessels, and an increase in plasma renin activity and in plasma noradrenaline (Shepherd and Mancia 1986). In addition, the capacitance vessels, chiefly the veins, contribute by helping to maintain the mean circulatory filling pressure. This is accomplished by a reflex constriction principally of the splanchnic venous bed, together with passive changes in venous capacity caused by compression of the limb veins by the active muscles and by the reflex constriction of the precapillary vessels (Hainsworth 1990). As a consequence of these neurohumoral responses, the arterial blood pressure is maintained. The mechanisms involved in the fluctuations in heart rate and arterial blood pressure in the first 20–30 seconds of tilting upright (passive change in posture) and standing (active change in posture) are complex. In the latter case, the contraction of the postural muscles contributes to the cardiovascular changes (see Chapter 14).

The application of lower-body negative pressure has been used to study reflexes from the heart and lungs in man. By pulling blood from the central circulation to the periphery, this reduces the cardiac filling pressure and hence the stimulus to mechanoreceptors in the low-pressure side of the central circulation. When small negative pressures are used, the central venous pressure can be reduced without a change in mean arterial pressure or pulse pressure or in arterial dP/dt. Thus, it is assumed that the activity of the arterial baroreceptors is unchanged (Shepherd and Mancia 1986). Using this approach to cause a sustained decrease in central venous pressure, the cardiopulmonary receptors maintain the increase in sympathetic outflow (Joyner *et al.* 1990*a*,*b*). Following orthotopic cardiac transplantation, the reflex constriction of forearm resistance vessels to the application of modest degrees of lower-body negative pressure is reduced. This indicates the importance of mechanoreceptors in the left ventricle in causing the constriction (Mohanty *et al.* 1987).

Since in humans the skeletal muscles constitute about 45 per cent of the body mass, a constriction of their resistance vessels plays a key role in increasing the systemic vascular resistance, particularly in response to gravitational shifts of blood from the central circulation to the periphery. In the calf this constriction can be reinforced by a local sympathetic axon reflex. Both in skin and muscle, this can be triggered by venous congestion. The receptors appear to be in small veins in skin, muscle, and subcutaneous adipose tissue and the effector site in the arterioles supplying these tissues. This axon reflex is an important adjunct to the postural reflexes mediated through the central nervous system so that, on assuming the upright position, the resultant increase in hydrostatic pressure in the veins of the lower limbs causes a local constriction of the resistance vessels (Henriksen 1986). A myogenic response of the smooth muscle of the resistance vessels to the increased transmural pressure also contributes. The relative importance of the cardiopulmonary receptors and of the arterial baroreceptors in the control of renin release in man is not established. However, the evidence suggests that the cardiopulmonary receptors play an important role in the secretion of renin on changing from supine to the upright position (Grassi *et al.* 1985). The increased levels of angiotensin II would reinforce the sympathetic constriction of the systemic vessels by a direct effect on the vascular smooth muscle, its central actions, and the facilitation of noradrenaline release by its effects on the prejunctional sympathetic nerves (Fig. 5.2).

After heart–lung transplantation, which results in afferent and efferent denervation of the transplanted organs, patients are able to maintain their arterial blood pressure during a passive head-up tilt at 45° for 1 hour. Presumably this is due to the contribution of the arterial baroreflex and the local sympathetic axon reflex. However, unlike normal controls, plasma renin activity did not increase. This might be a consequence of cyclosporin treatment, the cardiopulmonary deafferentation, or the high level of atrial natriuretic factor in the transplant group (Banner *et al.* 1990).

Animal studies have demonstrated that some of the cardiopulmonary and aortic mechanoreceptors have afferent fibres which travel in the sympathetic nerves to the spinal cord. One group with myelinated afferents has a spontaneous discharge at normal intracardiac pressures. Another group with unmyelinated afferents discharges irregularly with no apparent relation to cardiac events. Stimulation of the spinal input of these sympathetic afferents causes cardiovascular reflexes that are mainly excitatory although inhibition can also occur. However, it remains to be demonstrated that cardiovascular reflex responses can be induced by natural stimulation of sympathetic mechanoreceptors (Shepherd and Mancia 1986).

In addition to rapid adjustments of the circulation, the sympathetic nervous system via the renal nerves can participate in the longer-term regulation of arterial blood pressure. This is accomplished by promoting or opposing pressure natriuresis (Stella *et al*. 1990).

Ergoreflexes

In humans, as in animals, a strong static contraction of the skeletal muscles or rapid powerful rhythmic contractions cause a marked increase in arterial blood pressure, the so-called blood pressure-raising reflex. This increase helps to oppose the reduction in blood flow to the muscles resulting from the mechanical compression. The evidence indicates that this rise is due to products of muscle metabolism activating chemosensitive endings in the muscles; while the metabolic products have not been identified, it is tempting to suggest that these are the same metabolites which cause the local vasodilatation. The afferent fibres involved are the small myelinated (group III) and unmyelinated (group IV). The pressor response, which is caused by increased sympathetic outflow to the circulation, is proportional to the degree of ischaemia in the exercising muscles and to the mass of the ischaemic muscle. Whether or not the pressor response increases the perfusion of the active muscles has yet to be determined. It is possible that reflex constriction of the resistance vessel in the contracting muscles offsets the increase in arterial blood pressure (Joyner *et al*. 1990*a,b*).

In addition to the reflex from the active muscles, there is a central command from the cerebral cortex to the cardiovascular and respiratory centres in the brainstem. It seems that central command has a key role in increasing the heart rate with isometric or strong dynamic exercise, while the stimulation of the chemosensitive muscle afferents increases the sympathetic outflow to muscle vessels (Mark *et al*. 1986). For unknown reasons, the arterial and the cardiopulmonary mechanoreceptors are rendered unable to prevent the marked pressure increase. The arterial baroreceptors, however, retain their ability to modulate the pressure around the increased level (Shepherd and Mancia 1986).

The afferent projections of the various peripheral sensors that provide information to the brain centres on the functioning of the cardiovascular system terminate in the nucleus of the tractus solitarius (NTS) or closely associated structures. The potential neurotransmitters that have been identified in the NTS include acetylcholine, noradrenaline, oxytocin, vasopressin, and serotonin. It is suggested, however, that glutamate and substance P may have a primary neurotransmitter role in the baroreceptor reflex. There are numerous connections between the NTS and other centres in the brain and spinal cord, and many potential neurotransmitters have been identified (see Chapter 4).

Humoral agents

Vasopressin

Vasopressin (antidiuretic hormone; ADH) is synthesized in the supraoptic and paraventricular nuclei in the hypothalamus. The neurosecretory granules pass along the supraoptic hypophyseal tract to the neurohypothesis. It is released by increases in plasma osmolarity which are detected by osmoreceptors in the hypothalamus. It is also released in response to decreases in blood volume; in dogs this release is governed by cardiopulmonary receptors with vagal afferents, and primarily by large unencapsulated endings at the vein–atrial junctions. These endings, which detect changes in atrial transmural pressure, are subserved by fast-conducting, myelinated vagal afferents (Linden and Kappagoda 1982). The role of the cardiopulmonary receptors versus the arterial baroreceptors in regulating the release of this hormone in man is still uncertain. The plasma vasopressin levels are increased in the upright position; in patients with orthostatic hypotension, tilting upright evokes a greater decrease in arterial blood pressure in those subjects with a subnormal increase in plasma vasopressin. However, if the sympathetic nervous system and the renin–angiotensin system are activated normally by standing, these serve to maintain the arterial pressure in the absence of any increase in circulating vasopressin levels. In studies in which lower-body negative pressure (40 mm Hg for 10 min) was applied to normal subjects, the decrease in mean arterial blood pressure was no greater before and after administration of an angiotensin-converting enzyme inhibitor, indicating again that, when the renin–angiotensin system is inhibited, the sympathetic nervous system and vasopressin can compensate (Bennett and Gardiner 1985).

Studies in dogs have shown that vasopressin acts on the endothelium of the cerebral arteries to cause release of a factor which relaxes the underlying smooth muscle. Since the response is prevented by indomethacin, this indicates that the vasodilator substance is a cyclo-oxygenase derivative. In the coronary arteries vasopressin causes relaxation both by an endothelium-dependent mechanism and by a direct relaxing action on the smooth muscle. In the systemic circulation, it causes constriction which is due to a direct action on the smooth muscle and is not affected by removal of the endothelium (Katusic et al. 1987). Since the major cerebral arteries make a significant contribution to cerebral vascular resistance, these various actions serve to preserve blood flow to the brain and the myocardium while maintaining arterial blood pressure by constriction of systemic resistance vessels. This is of particular importance during hypotensive haemorrhage.

Atriopeptins

The cardiocytes of mammalian atria contain secretory granules that synthesize and, in response to an increase in atrial transmural pressure, release a series of related peptides (cardiac hormones) with diuretic, natriuretic, and vasoactive properties. These are referred to as atriopeptins and are released in response to atrial distension. Together with vasopressin, they have the key role in the regulation of the plasma volume.

When injected into healthy humans, atriopeptins cause, in addition to diuresis and natriuresis, an inhibition of vasopressin and renin release and result in the synthesis of aldosterone and a reduction of systemic arterial blood pressure (Burnett *et al.* 1984). However, in such persons, the sympatho-excitatory responses to unloading of the cardiopulmonary mechanoreceptors are unaltered by circulatory levels of atrial natriuretic factor comparable with those seen in pathophysiological states (Roach *et al.* 1990).

Endothelin

Endothelin circulates in the plasma of normal animals and humans and is increased in experimental heart failure in dogs (Margulies *et al.* 1990). The significance of this remains to be established.

References

Banner, N. R., Williams, M., Patel, N., Chalmer, J., Lightman, S. L., and Yacoub, M. H. (1990). Altered cardiovascular and neurohumoral responses to head-up tilt after the heart–lung transplantation. *Circulation* **82**, 863–71.

Bennett, T. and Gardiner, S. M. (1985). Involvement of vasopressin in cardiovascular regulation. *Cardiovasc. Res.* **19**, 57–68.

Burnett, J. C., Granger, J. P., and Opgenorth, T. J. (1984). Effects of synthetic atrial natriuretic factor on renal function and renin release. *Am. J. Physiol.* **247**, F863–F866.

Chapleau, M. W., Hajduczok, G., and Abboud, F. M. (1989). Peripheral and central mechanisms of baroreflex resetting. *Clin. exp. Pharmacol. Physiol.* (Suppl. 15), 31–43.

Elsner, D., Stewart, D. J., Sommer, O., Holz, J., and Bassenge, E. (1986). Postsynaptic alpha$_1$- and alpha$_2$-adrenergic receptors in adrenergic control of capacitance vessel tone in vivo. *Hypertension* **8**, 1003–14.

Grassi, G., Gavazzi, C., Ramirez, A., Sabadini, E., Turulo, L., and Mancia, G. (1985). Role of cardiopulmonary receptors in reflex control of renin release in man. *J. Hypertens.* (suppl. 3), 263–5.

Hainsworth, R. (1990). The importance of vascular capacitance in cardiovascular control. *News physiol. Sci.* **5**, 250–4.

Henriksen, O. (1986). Circulatory studies: local sympathetic venoarteriolar axon 'reflex'. In *The sympathoadrenal system*, Alfred Benzon Symposium, no. 23 (ed.

N. J. Christensen, O. Hendriksen, and N. A. Lassen), pp. 67–80. Munksgaard, Copenhagen.

Joyner, M. J., Lennon, R. L., Wedel, D. J., Rose, S. H., and Shepherd, J. T. (1990*a*). Blood flow to contracting human muscles: influence of increased sympathetic activity. *J. appl. Physiol.* **68**, 1453–7.

Joyner, M. J., Shepherd, J. T., and Seals, D. R. (1990*b*). Sustained increases in sympathetic outflow during prolonged lower body negative pressure in humans. *J. appl. Physiol.* **68**, 1004–9.

Katusic, Z. S., Shepherd, J. T., and Vanhoutte, P. M. (1987). Endothelium-dependent contraction to stretch in canine basilar arteries. *Am. J. Physiol.* **252** (Heart Circ. Physiol. 21), H671–H673.

Linden, R. J. and Kappagoda, C. T. (1982). *Atrial receptors*, Monographs of the Physiological Soc., no. 39. Cambridge University Press, Cambridge.

Mancia, G. and Zanchetti, A. (1986). Blood pressure variability. In *Handbook of hypertension*, Vol. 7. *Pathophysiology of hypertension—cardiovascular aspects* (ed. A. Zanchetti and R. C. Tarazi), pp. 125–52. Elsevier, Amsterdam.

Mann, S., Altman, D. G., Raftery, E. B., and Bannister, R. (1983). Circadian variation of blood pressure in autonomic failure. *Circulation* **68**, 477–83.

Margulies, K. B., Hildebrand, F. L., Levman, A., Pervella, M. A., and Burnett, J. C. (1990). Increased endothelin in experimental heart failure. *Circulation* **82**, 2226–30.

Mark, A. L., Victor, R. G., Nerhed, C., Seals, D. R., and Wallin, B. G. (1986). Mechanisms of sympathetic nerve responses to static and rhythmic exercise: new insight from direct intraneural recordings in humans. In *The sympathoadrenal system*, Alfred Benzon Symposium, no. 23 (ed. N. J. Christensen, O. Henriksen, and N. A. Lassen), pp. 221–33. Munksgaard, Copenhagen.

McDowell, T. S., Axtelle, T. S., Chapleau, M. W., and Abboud, F. M. (1989). Prostaglandins in carotid sinus enhance baroreflex in rabbits. *Am. J. Physiol.* **257**, R445–R450.

Miller, V. M. (1991). Interactions between neural and endothelial mechanisms in the control of vascular tone. *News Physiol. Sci.* **6**, 60–3.

Mohanty, P. K., Thames, M. D., Arrowood, J. A., Sowers, J. R., McNamara, C., and Szentpeterg, S. (1987). Impairment of cardiopulmonary baroreflexes after cardiac transplantation in humans. *Circulation* **74**, 914–22.

Pelleg, A. and Burnstock, G. (1990). Physiological importance of ATP released from nerve terminals and its degradation to adenosine in humans. *Circulation* **82**, 2269–72.

Rea, R. F. and Eckberg, D. L. (1987). Carotid baroreceptor–muscle sympathetic relation in humans. *Am. J. Physiol.* **253** (Regulatory Integrative Comp. Physiol. 22), R929–R936.

Roach, P. J., Sanders, J. S., Berg, W. J., Mark, A. L., Eberg, T. J., and Ferguson, D. W. (1990). Pathophysiologic levels of atrial natriuretic factor do not alter reflex sympathetic control: direct evidence from microneurographic studies in humans. *J. Am. Coll. Cardiol.* **15**, 1318–30.

Sanders, J. S., Mark, A. L., and Ferguson, D. W. (1989). Importance of aortic baroreflex in regulation of sympathetic responses during hypotension. *Circulation* **79**, 83–92.

Shepherd, J. T. (1990). Volhard Lecture: Increased systemic vascular resistance and primary hypertension: the expanding complexity. *J. Hypertension* **8** (Suppl. 7), S15–S27.

Shepherd, J. T. and Mancia, G. (1986). Reflex control of the human cardiovascular system. *Rev. Physiol. Biochem. Pharmacol.* **105**, 1–99.

Shepherd, J. T. and Vanhoutte, P. M. (1981). Local modulation of adrenergic neurotransmission. *Circulation* **64**, 655–66.

Steen, S., Castenfors, J., Sjöberg, T., Skarby, T., Andersson, K-E., and Norgren, L. (1986). Effects of alpha-adrenoceptor subtype-selective antagonists on the human saphenous veins in vivo. *Acta physiol. scand.* **126**, 15–19.

Stella, A., Golin, R., and Zanchetti, A. (1990). Sympathorenal interactions in the control of cardiovascular functions. *News physiol. Sci.* **5**, 237–41.

Taddei, S., Pedrinelli, R., and Salvetti, A. (1990). Sympathetic nervous system dependent vasoconstriction in humans. *Circulation* **82**, 2061–7.

Tan, W., Panzenbeck, M. J., Hajdu, A., and Zucker, I. H. (1989). A central mechanism of acute baroreflex resetting in the conscious dog. *Circulation Res.* **65**, 63–70.

Tang, S. S., Stevenson, L., and Dzau, V. J. (1990). Endothelial renin–angiotensin pathway. Adrenergic regulation of angiotensin secretion. *Circulation Res.* **66**, 103–8.

Tesfamarian, B., Weisbrod, R. M., and Cohen, R. A. (1989). The endothelium inhibits activation by calcium of vascular neurotransmission. *Am. J. Physiol.* **257**, H1871–H1877.

Walgenbach, S. C. and Donald, D. E. (1983). Inhibition by carotid baroreflex of exercise-induced increases in arterial pressure. *Circulation Res.* **52**, 253–62.

Wallin, B. G. (1986). Functional organization of sympathetic outflow in man. In *The sympathoadrenal system*, Alfred Benzon Symposium, no. 23 (ed. N. J. Christensen, O. Henriksen, and N. A. Lassen), pp. 52–66. Munksgaard, Copenhagen.

6. Adrenergic and cholinergic receptors

P. A. van Zwieten

Introduction

Ever since the discovery of the neurohumoral phenomena associated with the autonomic nervous system there has been a great deal of interest in the receptors that are the targets of the endogenous neurotransmitters, in particular, noradrenaline/adrenaline in the sympathetic and acetylcholine in the parasympathetic system. It goes without saying that this field is of particular interest in physiology and pathophysiology. Much of our present, detailed knowledge of autonomic receptors has been obtained using pharmacological methods and owing to the availability of a large number of experimental compounds, which are more or less selective agonists or antagonists with respect to the numerous receptor subtypes associated with the autonomic nervous system. Conversely, the more detailed knowledge of the various receptor types has also allowed the discovery of new and specific therapeutics for a variety of diseases, predominantly those involving the cardiovascular system. Traditionally, the adrenergic system and its receptors have been studied with great intensity and a wealth of valuable information has been obtained during the past 2–3 decades. More recently, the field of cholinergic receptors has received a new, strong impetus from the discovery that muscarinic receptors are heterogeneous and should therefore be subdivided into different subtypes with different spectra of biological functions and agonists/antagonists. Both the adrenergic and cholinergic receptors deserve our attention and will be discussed in this chapter. The term 'adrenoceptors', officially approved by IUPHAR is preferable to 'adrenergic receptors' and will therefore be used throughout this chapter.

Adrenoceptors (adrenergic receptors)

Subdivision and classification

Adrenoceptors are the primary targets of the endogenous neurotransmitters, noradrenaline and adrenaline, in mediating sympathetic activation to peripheral organs, thus causing well-documented effects like increased cardiac activity (heart rate and contractile force), vasoconstriction, and a rise in plasma glucose levels. In addition, the various adrenoceptors are also important as targets of several synthetic drugs, which can be used to mimic the effects of catecholamines or, conversely, to decrease their actions. Ahlqvist (1948) postulated that the adrenoceptors are different in various organs and he proposed the subdivision into α- and β-subtypes, a classification which is now widely accepted. There has since been further subdivision into β_1/β_2- and α_1/α_2-adrenoceptors (Lands *et al.* 1967). The subdivision and classification into α/β, β_1/β_2 and α_1/α_2 are based upon functional pharmacological data, as reflected by a particular preference for certain agonists and antagonists at postsynaptic (postjunctional) sites with respect to the postganglionic sympathetic neurons and their adjacent synapses. Several of the α- and β-adrenoceptor subtypes have been isolated and their chemical structures (amino acid sequence) have been analysed by molecular biological techniques. The concept of pre- and postsynaptic receptors, which

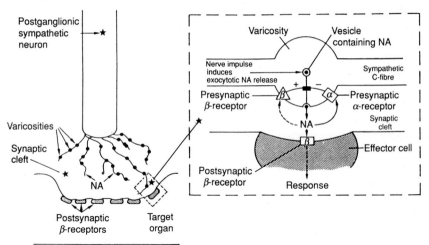

Fig. 6.1. Adrenergic synapse. Nerve activity releases the endogenous neurotransmitter noradrenaline (NA) and also adrenaline from the varicosities. Noradrenaline and adrenaline reach the postsynaptic α- (or β-) adrenoceptors on the cell membrane of the target organ by diffusion. Upon receptor stimulation, a physiological or pharmacological effect is initiated. Presynaptic α_2- adrenoceptors on the membrane (see insertion), when activated by endogenous noradrenaline as well as by exogenous agonists, induce an inhibition and blockade a facilitation of the amount of transmitter noradrenaline released per nerve impulse. Conversely, the stimulation of presynaptic β_2-receptors enhances noradrenaline release from the varicosities. Once noradrenaline has been released, it travels through the synaptic cleft and reaches both α- and β-adrenoceptors at postsynaptic sites thus causing physiological effects such as vasoconstriction or tachycardia.

is not unique for α-adrenoceptors, has been developed and substantiated in the 1970s predominantly by Langer, Starke, and their co-workers (Langer 1981; Starke 1981).

The terminology pre/postsynaptic (or pre/postjunctional) refers to the *anatomical position* of the receptors and does not necessarily coincide with their functional pharmacological profile. Accordingly, presynaptic adrenoceptors belong to the α_2- and β_2-types, whereas in most blood vessels both α_1- and α_2-, but only β_2-adrenoceptors are found at postsynaptic sites. *Postsynaptic* adrenoceptors, located in the end-organs (see Fig. 6.1) are the targets of neurotransmitters and synthetic drugs, and their stimulation or blockade will be translated into a variety of physiological and pharmacological effects. *Presynaptic* receptors are located at the membranes of the presynaptic vesicles which are the stores of noradrenaline. The stimulation (or blockade) of presynaptic adrenoceptors modulates the release of noradrenaline from its vesicular storage sites (Fig. 6.1).

The subdivision into α_1/α_2- or β_1/β_2-adrenoceptors implies that all sympathomimetic and sympatholytic drugs should be defined more precisely

Table 6.1. α-Adrenoceptor agonists and -antagonists: characterization with respect to their selectivity for α_1- and α_2-adrenoceptors.

Agents	Receptor stimulated or blocked
Agonists	
Noradrenaline (neurotransmitter)	$\alpha_1 + \alpha_2 + \beta_1$
Adrenaline (neurotransmitter)	$\alpha_1 + \alpha_2 + \beta_1 + \beta_2$
Phenylephrine (Boralin, Visadron)	$\alpha_1 > \alpha_2$
Clonidine (Catapres, Catapresan)	$\alpha_2 > \alpha_1$
Guanfacine	$\alpha_2 > \alpha_1$
Azepexole (B-HT 933)	α_2
B-HT 920	α_2
UK-14,304	α_2
Antagonists	
Phentolamine (Regitine)	$\alpha_1 + \alpha_2$
Tolazoline	$\alpha_2 > \alpha_1$
Prazosin (Minipress)	α_1
Doxazosin	α_1
Terazosin	α_1
Trimazosin	α_1
Labetalol	$\alpha_1 + \beta_1 + \beta_2$
Corynanthine ⎫ diastereoisomers	α_1
Rauwolscine ⎭	α_2
Yohimbine	α_2
Idazoxan	α_2

Table 6.2. β-Adrenoceptor agonists and antagonists: characterization with respect to their selectivity for β_1- and β_2-adrenoceptors

Agents		Receptors stimulated or blocked
Agonists		
Noradrenaline (neurotransmitter)		$\beta_1 + \alpha_1 + \alpha_2$
Adrenaline (neurotransmitter)		$\beta_1 + \beta_2 + \alpha_1 + \alpha_2$
Dobutamine		$\beta_1 + \alpha_1$
Isoprenaline		$\beta_1 + \beta_2$
Orciprenaline		$\beta_1 + \beta_2$
Fenoterol		$\beta_2 >> \beta_1$
Pirbuterol		$\beta_2 >> \beta_1$
Rimiterol		$\beta_2 >> \beta_1$
Ritodrine		$\beta_2 >> \beta_1$
Salbutamol		$\beta_2 >> \beta_1$
Terbutaline		$\beta_2 >> \beta_1$
Antagonists		
Propranolol Alprenolol Pindolol Oxprenolol Timolol Sotalol	and various other non-selective β-blockers	$\beta_1 + \beta_2$
Practolol		$\beta_1 >> \beta_2$
Atenolol		$\beta_1 >> \beta_2$
Metoprolol		$\beta_1 >> \beta_2$
Acebutolol		$\beta_1 > \beta_2$
Bisoprolol		$\beta_1 >>> \beta_2$
ICI 118,551		$\beta_2 >> \beta_1$

with respect to their receptor profile (see Tables 6.1 and 6.2). The endogenous catecholamines, noradrenaline and adrenaline, are rather unselective since they can stimulate several receptor subtypes simultaneously. Conversely, there are now several synthetic compounds available which are selective stimulants or antagonists with respect to one particular adrenoceptor subtype.

α-Adrenoceptors

α-Adrenoceptors are found in particular in blood vessels and to a less important degree also in the heart as well as in other tissues and organs such as thrombocytes, the vas deferens, the kidneys, and the central nervous system.

In blood vessels the postsynaptic α-adrenoceptors are of both the α_1- and α_2-subtypes. Their stimulation with an appropriate agonist causes vaso-constriction; this is so for both α_1- and α_2-adrenoceptor stimulation. Conversely, the blockade of both α_1- and α_2-adrenoceptors at postsynaptic sites causes vasodilatation. The stimulation of presynaptic α_2-adrenoceptors with an agonist induces the inhibition of noradrenaline from its vesicular stores, whereas α_2-adrenoceptor blockade enhances the release of nor-adrenaline. Since presynaptic α-adrenoceptors are virtually only of the α_2-type, the selective stimulation or inhibition of α_1-adrenoceptors does not interfere with the presynaptic release of noradrenaline. For reviews see Van Zwieten and Timmermans (1984) and Starke (1981).

Stimulation of myocardial α_1-adrenoceptors increases contractility, which is much weaker than that caused by β_1-adrenoceptor excitation. Platelet aggregation is enhanced by stimulation of the α_2-adrenoceptors. Stimulation of α_2-adrenoceptors in certain CNS regions, such as the nucleus tractus solitarii, vagal nucleus, and vasomotor centre, will cause a hypotensive response due to the reduction of peripheral sympathetic nervous activity. This mechanism is the basis of the antihypertensive activity of clonidine and α-methyldopa (via its active metabolite α-methylnoradrenaline), which are α_2-adrenoceptor stimulants. For a review see Van Zwieten et al. 1984. The α_2-adrenoceptors in the brain are similar to, or possibly identical with peripheral vascular α_2-receptors, both in radioligand-binding experiments and with respect to their preference for known selective agonists and antagonists. At the molecular level the α_2-adrenoceptor is known to be coupled to adenylate cyclase. Its structure has been elucidated and also contains the pattern of the seven helices.

α-Adrenoceptor changes associated with disease

Hypertensive disease in an established phase has been reported to be associated with an increased density of α_2-adrenoceptors in thrombocytes. However, other reports indicate that in essential hypertension the α_2-adrenoceptor density is unchanged. This issue remains inconclusive at present. Several authors have established that there exists an exaggerated vasoconstrictor response to α-adrenoceptor agonists in hypertensives, probably for both α_1- and α_2-adrenoceptor stimulants. Congestive heart failure is not associated with important changes in cardiac α-adrenoceptor density.

α-Adrenoceptor agonists and antagonists as therapeutic agents

Vasoconstriction via α_1/α_2-adrenoceptor stimulation is an important physio-logical and pathophysiological principle, although it is of modest therapeutic interest, as in the use of nasal and ophthalmic decongestants or the addition of adrenaline or noradrenaline to local anaesthetic agents. α-Adrenoceptor antagonists (α-blockers) are the major examples of therapeutic agents which owe their efficacy (and most of their side-effects) to their interaction with α-adrenoceptors. Prazosin and related selective α_1-adrenoceptor antagonists (e.g. doxazosin or terazosin) appear to be preferable to non-selective $(\alpha_1 + \alpha_2)$-blockers like phentolamine. The non-selective α-blockers enhance the release of endogenous noradrenaline as a result of presynaptic α_2-receptor blockade, and they cause pronounced reflex tachycardia. These problems are not encountered during the use of selective α_1-blockers, which do not interfere with the α_2-receptor mediated presynaptic mechanisms. Prazosin and related drugs are used as antihypertensives, and occasionally as vasodilators in the treatment of congestive heart failure. Vasodilatation, based on α_1-adrenoceptor blockade, readily explains the therapeutic efficacy of these compounds. Orthostatic hypotension, the major adverse reaction, is also caused by rapid vasodilatation, predominantly in the venous vascular bed. For reviews see Van Zwieten et al. (1984) and Van Zwieten (1990).

Prazosin and possibly the newer related selective α_1-adrenoceptor antagonists have been recently introduced in the treatment of impaired micturition, associated with prostate hypertrophy. We already mentioned the older antihypertensives, clonidine and α-methyldopa, which owe their anti-hypertensive activity to the stimulation of α_2-adrenoceptors in the central nervous system. It has recently been proposed that these compounds would also involve the stimulation of specific imidazoline receptors, closely linked to the α_2-adrenoceptors. The central α_2-adrenoceptors are probably very similar to their peripheral counterparts, although small differences may exist.

β-Adrenoceptors

β-Adrenoceptors are found in various cardiac tissues, in most blood vessels, in the bronchi and intestine, on lymphocytes, and in the central nervous system. Stimulation of postsynaptic β-adrenoceptors will cause a variety of physiological and pharmacological effects as outlined in Table 6.3. β-Receptor blockade by β-adrenoceptor antagonists (β-blockers) suppresses the aforementioned effects and this is the basis of their therapeutic efficacy and also of most of their adverse reactions. β-Adrenoceptors are coupled to adenylate cyclase. The molecular structure of β-receptors in a few tissues and systems has been elucidated. As established for many receptor types the structure of β-adrenoceptors is characterized by the model of the seven helices, with particular areas/regions which are required for the combination with agonists and antagonists (in the extracellular part) or with coupling proteins at intracellular sites.

β-Adrenoceptors at *presynaptic* sites are predominantly of the β_2-type. Their stimulation with an agonist causes enhanced release of endogenous noradrenaline from its vesicular stores. Conversely, the blockade of β_2-adrenoceptors with an appropriate antagonist will reduce the rate of release of endogenous noradrenaline from presynaptic storage sites.

Table 6.3. Effects on the stimulation and blockade by β_1- and β_2-adrenoceptors by means of appropriate agonists and antagonists

Receptor type	Tissue/organ	Stimulation (agonist)	Blockade (antagonist)
β_1	Cardiac pace-maker cells	Heart rate ↑	Heart rate ↓
	AV node	AV conduction ↑	AV conduction ↓
	Myocardium	Contractility ↑	Contractility ↓
	Intestine	Relaxation	—
β_2	Bronchi	Relaxation	Constriction
	Myocardium ($\beta_2 < \beta_1$)	Contractility ↑	Contractility ↓
	Blood vessels	Dilatation	Constriction
	Intestine	Relaxation	—
	Adenylcyclase	Hyperglycaemia	Hypoglycaemia
		Free fatty acids ↑	Free fatty acids ↓

β-Adrenoceptors are present in various structures of the central nervous system, but their functional role and potential basis as a therapeutic target remain uncertain. They are probably similar to their peripheral counterparts, as indicated by radioligand-binding experiments.

β-Receptor changes associated with disease

Radioligand-binding techniques have been used for some years to explore the density and affinity of receptors associated with various diseases. This field is still in the initial stages of development and only recently has it been possible to study the processes of signal transduction subsequent to receptor stimulation with an agonist.

With respect to the influence of disease on the characteristics of β-adrenoceptors the most interesting and convincing results have been obtained in congestive heart failure (CHF). Various types of CHF, caused by severe coronary heart disease and valvular disease, are associated with a significant degree of down-regulation of both β_1- and β_2-adrenoceptors, as reflected by a reduction in the density of both receptor subtypes in the myocardium. In the myocardial tissue of patients with dilated cardiomyopathy the down-regulation remains limited to β_1-adrenoceptors, without changes in the density of β_2-adrenoceptors. The reduced density of β-adrenoceptors is most probably explained by the elevated plasma levels of noradrenaline reported in patients with advanced stages of CHF. The lowered density of cardiac β-receptors in CHF readily explains the well-known tachyphylaxis towards β-adrenoceptor agonists, which may be used in the treatment of CHF. β-Receptor down-regulation may be reversed by treatment with β-blockers in very low doses and this may be the basis of the claim that low-dose β-blocker therapy may be beneficial in CHF, despite the risk of negative inotropic effects. Reports on changes in β-adrenoceptor density (in particular the β_2-receptors on lymphocytes) in hypertension are controversial: increased, decreased, or unchanged β_2-receptor densities on lymphocytes from essential hypertensives, have all been described.

β-Adrenoceptor agonists and antagonists as therapeutic agents

β-Adrenoceptor *agonists* may be used to increase contractile force in patients with CHF, or as bronchodilators in patients with asthma or other types of obstructive airways disease. The use of β-agonists in CHF is associated with various side-effects: these inotropic agents cause a degree of tachycardia, with an increased risk of tachyarrhythmias. None of the β-adrenoceptor agonists so far available can be used orally, making intravenous administration unavoidable. Chronic administration of these compounds leads to down-regulation and desensitization of β-adrenoceptors and hence to tachyphylaxis. Of the drugs available at present, dobutamine is used most frequently.

Salbutamol, terbutaline, and fenoterol are selective β_2-adrenoceptor stimulants. They are well-known bronchodilators, which have replaced non-selective $\beta_1 + \beta_2$-agonists like isoprenaline and orciprenaline. These latter compounds cause a greater degree of tachycardia (as a result of their β_1-component) than observed for the selective β_2-receptor stimulants.

β-Adrenoceptor antagonists (β-blockers) have obtained widespread therapeutic application, especially in the treatment of essential hypertension and angina pectoris. Their therapeutic efficacy is caused by the blockade of β_1-adrenoceptors, and so are most of their adverse reactions. This important subject has been reviewed extensively (Bolli *et al.* 1990).

Cholinergic receptors

Traditionally, cholinergic receptors have been subdivided into nicotinic and muscarinic subtypes, predominantly based on the classical work in this field by Sir Henry Dale and his co-workers in the 1930s. The nicotinic receptors are located in the autonomic ganglia (both sympathetic and parasympathetic) and in the neuromuscular junction. Muscarinic receptors are located in all target organs of the parasympathetic nervous system. More recently, muscarinic receptors have also been demonstrated in certain structures of peripheral sympathetic (adrenergic) neurons. The central nervous system also contains muscarinic receptors, which are involved in cognitive processes, extrapyramidal functions, and probably also in the central regulation of blood pressure and heart rate.

The distinction between nicotinic and muscarinic receptors is based solely upon differential pharmacodynamic effects and preferences for agonists and antagonists. Modern molecular biological techniques have confirmed the different structures and amino acid sequences of both types of cholinergic receptors.

Nicotinic cholinergic receptors

Nicotinic receptors are known to play an important role in the neurohumoral transmission in all autonomic ganglia (parasympathetic and sympathetic) as well as in the neuromuscular junction. It has been proposed that different subtypes of nicotinic receptors may exist but this hypothesis has not been as fully substantiated as for the muscarinic receptors.

For nicotinic receptors both agonists and antagonists have been developed and a few of these are clinically useful. Nicotine (in low doses) and dimethylphenylpiperazine (DMPP) are classical *stimulants* of nicotinic receptors both in the sympathetic and parasympathetic autonomic ganglia. Succinylcholine (suxamethonium) is an agonist particularly with respect to the nicotinic receptors in neuromuscular junction. Its muscle relaxant action, frequently used in anaesthesiology, is based upon the permanent depolarization caused by this compound, thus abolishing the process of neurotransmission.

All inhibitors of the enzyme cholinesterase, such as neostigmine, fysostigmine, pyridostigmine but also the polyalkylphosphates like fluostigmine, parathion, sarin (nerve gas), will cause the accumulation of endogenous acetylcholine, which is a non-specific agonist for both nicotinic and muscarinergic cholinergic receptors. The beneficial effect of neostigmine and related drugs in myasthenia gravis and related disorders of neuromuscular transmission is based upon the stimulation of nicotinic receptors in the neuromuscular junction. Their major side-effects are caused by stimulation of parasympathetic muscarinic receptors. The polyalkylphosphates (some of them nerve gases or insecticides) are only of toxicological interest. Their extremely high toxicity is predominantly based upon a general activation of all cholinergic receptors (including those in the central nervous system) by accumulated endogenous acetylcholine.

Antagonists to nicotinic receptors in the autonomic ganglia are the ganglioplegic agents or ganglion blockers. Examples of these are pentolinium, hexamethonium, or trimetaphan. These compounds were among the first drugs used to treat hypertension. Their antihypertensive activity is based upon the blockade of transmission in sympathetic ganglia. These compounds were effective antihypertensives, but at present are unacceptable because of their severe adverse reactions, which are largely based upon the simultaneous blockade of both sympathetic and parasympathetic ganglia. Trimetaphan is still used occasionally by anaesthetists to lower blood pressure for short periods during surgery.

A second group of nicotinic receptor antagonists are the compounds related to tubocurarine, such as gallamine, pancuronium, and vecuronium. They are muscle relaxants, widely used in anaesthesiology. Their beneficial effect is based upon blockade of transmission in the neuromuscular junction as a result of competitive antagonism at the level of nicotinic receptors.

Muscarinic receptors

Muscarinic receptors are intricately linked to the parasympathetic nervous system as targets of the endogenous neurotransmitter acetylcholine. Recent studies indicate that muscarinic receptors in various organs and tissues are heterogeneous. There are at least three subtypes (M_1, M_2, and M_3) and possibly more. As in the sympathetic system, the existence of presynaptic muscarinic receptors in addition to those at postsynaptic sites has recently been demonstrated.

Furthermore, the classification of muscarinic receptor subtypes requires a more precise designation of receptor agonists/antagonists with respect to their preference for the various classes of muscarinic receptors. As these developments are recent, the receptor classification is less firmly established than that for adrenoceptors. A major problem is the limited availability of highly selective agonists and antagonists, which are suitable as tools in the pharmacological analysis of the muscarinic receptor subtypes.

Subdivision and classification

The subdivision of muscarinic receptors into at least three subtypes is predominantly based upon radioligand-binding studies because of the availability of appropriate ligands and selective M-receptor antagonists. These three subtypes, M_1, M_2, and M_3, and the antagonists used are in Table 6.4, which also shows the tissues where these receptor subtypes can be demonstrated to exist. The introduction of pirenzepine, a selective antagonist to M_1-receptors, has been a major breakthrough in the modern classification

Table 6.4. Various types of muscarinic receptors in different tissues. The effects of receptor stimulation and blockade by appropriate agonists and antagonists are also shown

Receptor type	Organ/tissue	Stimulation (agonist)	Blockade (antagonist)
M_1	Neurons	Excitation	Depression
	Ganglia (sympathetic)	Noradrenaline release ↑	Noradrenaline release ↓
M_2	Heart	Bradycardia Contractility ↓	Tachycardia Contractility ↑
	Smooth muscle	Contraction	Relaxation
M_3	Glands	Secretion ↑	Secretion ↓
	Ileum	Contraction	Relaxation

of M-receptors. The concept of M_1-, M_2-, and M_3-receptors was formulated originally by Doods *et al.* (1987). Apart from these three well-established subtypes a fourth type (M_4) has been proposed, but conclusive evidence for its existence as a separate subtype is currently lacking. The radioligand-binding studies that have been pivotal to the subclassification of M-receptors are being followed up slowly by functional experiments which are globally in line with the findings of the binding data. Table 6.4 shows the functional aspects of the stimulation/blockade of the M-receptor subtypes.

Molecular biological cloning techniques have led to the identification of at least five different muscarinic receptor species, whose amino-acid sequence and structure have been elucidated. Again, the model of the seven helices appears to underlie the structure of these receptor species. These five muscarinic receptor species have been denominated as m_1, m_2, m_3, m_4, and m_5, respectively. The m_1, m_2, and m_3 types broadly coincide with the M_1-, M_2-, and M_3-receptor subtypes established by means of radioligand-binding techniques (Table 6.4). The functional role of the m_4 and m_5 species so far remains unknown (Bonner *et al.* 1987).

Biochemical studies have indicated that muscarinic receptors are coupled to adenylate cyclase. In contrast to β-adrenoceptors the influence of muscarinic receptor stimulation is inhibitory, thus causing a decrease in the cellular concentration of cAMP. Few data are available concerning possible changes of muscarinic receptor density associated with disease and no clear picture has as yet emerged.

Muscarinic receptor agonists and antagonists:
potential therapeutic agents

Acetylcholine, the endogenous neurotransmitter in the parasympathetic nervous system, is a non-selective agent that stimulates muscarinic receptors of the three subtypes, M_1, M_2, and M_3, in addition to nicotinic cholinergic receptors. Most of the classical synthetic muscarinic receptor agonists are non-selective with respect to the various muscarinic receptor subtypes. This lack of selectivity is known for muscarine, aceclidine, pilocarpine, bethanechol, carbachol, and arecoline. Carbachol and arecoline also stimulate ganglionic nicotinic receptors in addition to their agonistic effect on muscarinic receptors.

Methacholine appears to possess some selectivity towards the vascular muscarinic receptors, which may be of the M_2- or the M_3-type, depending on the vascular bed and animal species investigated. The experimental compound McN-A 343 appears to display selectivity towards M_1-receptors, particularly those present in the brain and at the sympathetic ganglia. All other muscarinic receptor agonists available are non-selective with respect to the various M-receptor subtypes. In fundamental pharmacology the development of highly selective agonists for the three (or more) muscarinic receptor subtypes would be most valuable.

Atropine is a non-selective antagonist with a high affinity for the various muscarinic receptor subtypes. Pirenzepine is a selective M_1-receptor antagonist, with a much lower affinity for M_2- or M_3-receptors. AF-DX 116 is a cardioselective antagonist for M_2-receptors as are himbacine and methoctramine. 4-DAMP shows some selectivity for M_3-receptors as do hexahydro-sila-difenidol and related compounds. (For a review see Mutschler *et al.* 1989.)

The present muscarinic receptor classification is predominantly based upon the series of antagonists and agonists mentioned above. Since the number of experimental compounds is rapidly increasing, the receptor classification may well be subject to important future changes.

Therapeutic applications

Muscarinic receptor stimulants have traditionally been used for activation of the smooth muscle of the intestine and/or urinary bladder and for lowering elevated intraocular pressure in glaucoma. Carbachol and bethanechol, which are used to stimulate smooth muscle, are examples of the former. They display a modest selectivity towards intestinal and urinary bladder smooth muscle as compared to that of the cardiovascular system. Adverse reactions are related to stimulation of the peripheral parasympathetic nervous system. Pilocarpine when applied locally to the eye causes miosis and a reduction of intraocular pressure, as in glaucoma. Systemic side-effects usually do not occur.

Therapeutic applications of selective muscarinic receptor agonists are currently a matter of speculation. Highly cardioselective M_2-receptor agonists may be used to reduce heart rate in the treatment of angina pectoris or supraventricular tachycardia. M_1-receptor stimulation in the CNS has been proposed as a potential therapeutic approach to treat Alzheimer's disease. This has been attempted with experimental compounds like RS 86 and with the cholinesterase inhibitor, tetrahydroaminoacridine, but the results so far have been disappointing. Of the muscarinic receptor antagonists, pirenzepine is a selective M_1-agonist which has been introduced in the treatment of peptic ulcer. It appears to have fewer side-effects on the cardiovascular system, the eye, and the exocrine glands.

On theoretical grounds cardioselective M_2-receptor antagonists may benefit patients with impaired atrioventricular (AV) conduction in the period before a pace-maker is implanted and also be useful in conditions such as the sick sinus syndrome, digitalis intoxication, or arrhythmia caused by torsades de pointe (TDP). None of these therapeutic options has been explored clinically on a sufficiently large scale (Goyal 1989). Finally, coronary spasm may involve a cholinergic component in certain patients and the beneficial effects of atropine have been demonstrated. A highly selective antagonist of vascular M_2- (or M_3-) receptors which appear to be involved in this type of spasm may be preferable to a non-selective agent like atropine.

References

Ahlqvist, R. P. (1948). A study of the adrenotropic receptors. *Am. J. Physiol.* **153**, 586–91.

Bolli, P., Fernandez, P. G., and Buehler, F. R. (1990). Beta blockers in the treatment of hypertension. In *Hypertension: pathophysiology, diagnosis and management* (ed. J. H. Laragh and B. M. Brenner), pp. 2181–2208. Raven Press, New York.

Bonner, T. I., Buckley, N. J., Young, A. C., and Brann, M. R. (1987). Identification of a family of muscarinic acetylcholine receptor genes. *Science* **237**, 527–32.

Doods, H. N., Mathy, M-J., Davidesko, D., Van Charldorp, K. J., de Jonge, A., and Van Zwieten, P. A. (1987). Selectivity of muscarinic antagonists in radioligand and in vivo experiments for the putative M_1, M_2 and M_3 receptors. *J. Pharmacol. exp. Ther.* **246**, 929–34.

Goyal, R. K. (1989). Muscarinic receptor subtypes. Physiology and clinical implications. *New Engl. J. Med.* **321**, 1022–8.

Lands, A. M., Arnold, A., McAuliff, J. P., Lunduena, F. P., and Brown, R. G. (1967). Differentiation of receptor systems activated by sympathomimetic amines. *Nature* **214**, 597–8.

Langer, S. Z. (1981). Presynaptic regulation of the release of catecholamines. *Pharmacol. Rev.* **32**, 337–62.

Mutschler, E., Moser, U., Wess, J., and Lambrecht, G. (1989). Muscarinic receptor subtypes: agonists and antagonists. *Prog. Pharmacol.* **7**, 13–31.

Starke, K. (1981). α-Adrenoceptor subclassification. *Rev. Physiol. Biochem. Pharmacol.* **88**, 199–236.

Van Zwieten, P. A. (1990). Alpha-adrenoceptor blocking agents in the treatment of hypertension. In *Hypertension: pathophysiology, diagnosis and management* (ed. J. H. Laragh and B. M. Brenner), pp. 2233–49.

Van Zwieten, P. A. and Timmermans, P. B. M. W. M. (1984). Central and peripheral α-adrenoceptors. Pharmacological aspects and clinical potential. *Adv. Drug Res.* **13**, 209–54.

Van Zwieten, P. A., Timmermans, P. B. M. W. M., and Van Brummelen, P. (1984). Role of alpha-adrenoceptors in hypertension and in antihypertensive treatment. *Am. J. Med.* **77**, 17–25.

7. Structural and chemical organization of the autonomic nervous system with special reference to non-adrenergic, non-cholinergic transmission

Geoffrey Burnstock and Pamela Milner

Introduction

Improvements in the techniques of assessment of autonomic nerve structure and function have revealed the multiplicity of neurotransmitters within these nerves in addition to the classical neurotransmitters, noradrenaline (NA) and acetylcholine (ACh), and have allowed major advances to be made in the description of the roles of these substances. The versatility of the autonomic nervous system has been demonstrated by examination of non-adrenergic, non-cholinergic (NANC) neurotransmission in sympathetic, parasympathetic, and sensory–motor nerves and intrinsic ganglia. Recognition of the concepts of neuromodulation and cotransmission suggests that autonomic failure can operate at many levels. The plasticity of autonomic nerves, even in adult animals, offers the potential for therapy in disease.

The autonomic neuroeffector junction

The autonomic neuroeffector junction between autonomic nerve fibres and smooth muscle cells differs in several ways from the neuromuscular junction in skeletal muscle and from the synapses in the central and peripheral nervous systems (see Burnstock 1986a). The autonomic effector is a muscle bundle rather than a single cell, and low-resistance pathways between individual muscle cells allow electrotonic spread of activity within the effector bundle. Morphologically, the sites of electrotonic coupling are represented by areas of close apposition between the plasma membranes of adjacent cells, which can be identifed under the electron microscope as gap junctions or nexuses. These gap junctions vary in size from punctate junctions to junctional areas of more than $1\mu m$ in diameter. Little is known about the quantity and

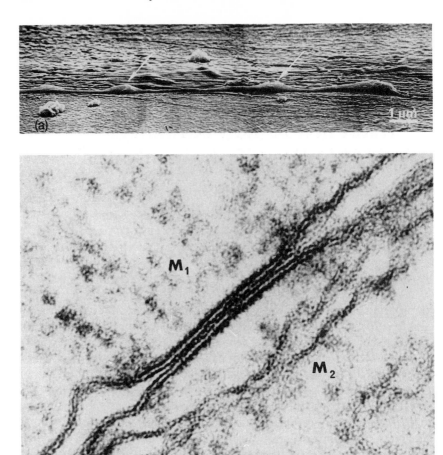

Fig. 7.1. (a) Scanning electron micrograph of varicosities (arrows) in a single nerve fibre growing in a culture of newborn guinea-pig sympathetic ganglia. Photographed at an angle of 70°; scale bar, 1 μm. (From Burnstock (1979).) (b) Gap junction between two cultured smooth muscle cells (M_1, M_2) from embryonic chicken gizzard; scale bar, 0.05 μm. (From Campbell *et al.* (1971).)

arrangement of gap junctions in effector bundles relative to the density of autonomic innervation. Thus, within an effector muscle bundle only a certain percentage of cells are directly innervated, the remainder being coupled to these cells via gap junctions.

Another characteristic of the autonomic neuromuscular junction is that it is not a synapse with a well-defined structure and pre- and postjunctional specializations like the skeletal muscle motor end-plate. Unmyelinated, highly branched, postganglionic autonomic nerve fibres reaching the effector smooth muscle become beaded or varicose (Fig 7.1). These varicosities are not static but are able to move along axons, consistent with the lack of postjunctional specialization. They are 0.5–2 μm in diameter and about 1 μm in length and are packed with vesicles and mitochondria. Neurotransmitters from autonomic nerve fibres are released from these varicosities that occur at intervals of 5–10 μm along axons. The distance of the cleft between the varicosity and smooth muscle varies considerably depending on the tissue, from 20 nm in densely innervated structures such as the vas deferens to 1–2 μm in large elastic arteries. Neurotransmitter is released *en passage* from varicosities during conduction of an impulse along an autonomic axon; however, it is possible that a given impulse will evoke release from only some of the varicosities that it encounters.

Release of neurotransmitter causes a transient change in membrane potential of the postjunctional cell. If the result of a single pulse is a depolarization, the response is called an excitatory junction potential. If an excitatory junction potential reaches sufficient amplitude, the threshold of generation of an action potential may be reached and an all-or-none action potential will propagate through the smooth muscle, resulting in a mechanical contraction. If the result of a single pulse of neurotransmitter release is a hyperpolarization, the response is called an inhibitory junction potential. Inhibitory junction potentials either prevent action potential discharge, thus causing relaxation, or induce relaxation directly. Junction potentials evoked in response to single pulses of nerve stimulation vary in duration from 0.5 to 5 s.

The multiplicity of neurotransmitters in the autonomic nervous system

The classical view of autonomic nervous control as antagonistic actions of NA and ACh causing either constriction or relaxation depending on the tissue was changed in the early 1960s when clear evidence of a NANC system was presented (Burnstock 1986*b*). Inhibitory junction potentials blocked by tetrodotoxin were recorded, using the sucrose-gap technique, in intestinal smooth muscle during stimulation of guinea-pig enteric nerves in the presence of adrenergic and cholinergic blocking agents. At about the same time, other researchers showed that relaxation of the cat stomach following vagal stimulation was resistant to adrenergic and cholinergic blockade. Similar observations were consequently made on a wide variety of tissues, including urinary bladder, lung, oesophagus, seminal vesicles, trachea, and blood vessels.

Purinergic neurotransmission

The first substance that was found to best satisfy the criteria for a neurotransmitter in NANC nerves in the intestine and urinary bladder was the purine nucleotide, adenosine 5′-triphosphate (ATP). Subsequently, the purinergic nerve hypothesis was formulated (Burnstock 1972) which suggested that: (1) ATP synthesized in nerve terminals is stored in large opaque vesicles; (2) after its release and activation of puringergic receptors in the postjunctional membrane, ATP is rapidly broken down by magnesium-activated ATPase and 5′-nucleotidase to adenosine; (3) adenosine is taken up by a high-affinity uptake system, converted to ATP, and reincorporated into physiological stores; (4) any adenosine not taken up this way is broken down by adenosine deaminase to inosine which is inactive and leaks into the circulation.

Based on the relative potencies of purine nucleosides and nucleotides on a variety of tissues, two major types of purinoceptor have been distinguished (see Burnstock 1990a). P_1-purinoceptors are most sensitive to adenosine, are competitively blocked by methylxanthines, and occupation leads to changes in levels of intracellular cyclic adenosine monophosphate (cAMP). P_2-purinoceptors are most sensitive to ATP, are not blocked by methylxanthines nor do they act via an adenylate cyclase system, and their occupation may lead to prostaglandin synthesis. Pharmacological, biochemical, and receptor binding studies have enabled subdivision of these two types of receptor. P_1-purinoceptors are generally of the A_1, A_2, or A_3 type: A_1-receptors are preferentially activated by N^6-substituted adenosine analogues and their occupation leads to decreased cAMP levels, whereas A_2-receptors show preference for 5′-substituted compounds and cAMP levels are increased; occupation of A_3-receptors does not lead to changes in adenylate cyclase. P_2-purinoceptors are generally of the P_{2X} or P_{2Y} type in the autonomic nervous system; however, receptors for ATP have been identified on platelets, mast cells, and lymphocytes that do not respond in the same way and are classified as of the P_{2T} or P_{2Z} type. P_{2X}-purinoceptors are characterized by showing that α,β-methylene ATP is a potent agonist and prolonged exposure to this drug leads to desensitization of the receptor, whilst arylazidoaminoproprionyl-ATP (ANAPP$_3$) is a selective antagonist; 2-methylthio-ATP is a potent agonist of P_{2Y}-receptors, while reactive blue 2, an anthraquinone derivative, is a selective antagonist.

Peptidergic neurotransmission

Hints that there are in fact several different neurotransmitters in the autonomic nervous system came from ultrastructural studies of the enteric nervous system which revealed at least nine distinguishable types of axon profile (Burnstock 1986a). The use of immunohistochemical techniques subsequently led to a rapid expansion in our knowledge of the diversity of the autonomic nervous system since it allowed the identification of several different biologically active peptides and transmitter-synthesizing enzymes in neural elements (Furness and Costa 1987). The following neuropeptides have now been proposed as neurotransmitters in the mammalian autonomic nervous system: enkephalin/endorphin, vasoactive intestinal polypeptide (VIP), and peptide histidine isoleucine (PHI) (methionine in man); substance P (SP) and neurokinins A and B; gastrin-releasing peptide/bombesin, somatostatin, neurotensin, luteinising hormone-releasing hormone (LHRH), cholecystokinin (CCK)/gastrin, neuropeptide Y (NPY) and pancreatic polypeptide; galanin, angiotensin, vasopressin, adrenocorticotrophic hormone, and calcitonin gene-related peptide (CGRP). Recombinant DNA and molecular biological techniques led to the discovery of the previously unknown peptide, CGRP, in neural tissues. It is quite likely that advances in the techniques of molecular cloning and gene expression will lead to the identification of other new bioactive peptides which play a role in autonomic neurotransmission.

By virtue of their structure, the mode and site of synthesis of neuropeptide transmitters differ from those of other neurotransmitters. Neuropeptides are cleaved from larger precursor molecules synthesized in the nerve cell body and transported along the nerve fibre to the site of release, a mechanism quite different from the re-uptake and/or synthesis of other neurotransmitters which occur at the axon terminal. Neuropeptides may thus act in a modulatory capacity and mediate long-term events, rather than functioning as rapidly acting neurotransmitters. As there is no known re-uptake mechanism for removal of neuropeptides from the site of action, it is likely that their action is terminated mainly by metabolism by proteolytic enzymes. A few key ectoenzymes, including endopeptidase 24.11 and angiotensin-converting enzyme, are now thought to account for the degradation of most neuropeptides.

Neuropeptides act on specific receptors which, in turn, activate second messenger systems or G-proteins, a mechanism of action similar to that for the classical neurotransmitters. There are relatively few useful antagonists available to block neuropeptide transmitter actions.

Nitrergic neurotransmission

Evidence is accumulating that nitric oxide (NO) or an NO-related compound has an important role as a primary messenger in transmitting information from nerves to smooth muscles in specific tissues (Bredt *et al.* 1990). NO is formed by oxidation of a terminal nitrogen atom of L-arginine, a reaction catalysed by nitric oxide synthase. Immunohistochemical studies have confirmed, amongst other locations, a neural localization of this enzyme in several tissues, including myenteric neurones of the gut and nerve fibres innervating cerebral arteries. NO is atypical as a neurotransmitter in several ways: it is not stored in vesicles but appears to be synthesized in the cytoplasm on demand; it is released by simple diffusion, not exocytosis; and, rather than acting on membrane receptor proteins, its receptor target is iron in the active centre of the enzyme, guanylyl cyclase, inside the cell. By binding to iron, NO initiates a three-dimensional change in the shape of the enzyme which increases its activity and consequently the production of cyclic GMP (Rand 1992).

Other non-adrenergic, non-cholinergic neurotransmitters

Serotonin (5-hydroxytryptamine, 5-HT), dopamine, and γ-aminobutyric acid have been proposed as autonomic neurotransmitters (Burnstock 1986*a*).

Mechanisms of cotransmission and neuromodulation

The coexistence of more than one neurotransmitter within a single nerve terminal is now well documented (Burnstock 1976, 1990*b*). Peptides or purine nucleotides are often found together with the classic neurotransmitters, NA and ACh. In fact, the majority of nerve fibres in the autonomic nervous system contain a mixture of different neurotransmitter substances that vary in proportion in different tissues and species and probably during development and disease; however, there is usually a preferential association between neurotransmitters which may or may not be stored in the same vesicle within the nerve terminal.

It should be noted that immunohistochemical evidence of coexistence should not necessarily be interpreted as evidence of cotransmission since, in order for substances to be termed cotransmitters, it is essential to show that postjunctional actions to each substance occur via their own specific receptors. Some substances stored and released from nerves do not have direct actions on effector muscle cells but alter the actions of other co-stored transmitters on the pre- and/or postsynaptic membrane; these substances are termed neuromodulators. Many other substances are neuromodulators in that they modify the process of neurotransmission, for example, circulating neurohormones; locally released agents, such as prostanoids, bradykinin, histamine, and endothelin; and neurotransmitters from nearby nerves. Many substances that are cotransmitters are also neuromodulators.

The wide and variable cleft characteristic of autonomic neuroeffector junctions makes them particularly amenable to the mechanisms of neural control mentioned above. There are many different ways in which cotransmitters and neuromodulators interact to effect neurotransmission (Fig. 7.2).

1. *Autoinhibition*. A transmitter, in addition to its postjunctional effects, modifies its own release, often inhibiting it. This, in turn, may effect the release of any cotransmitters.

2. *Cross-talk*. A neuromodulator may act on closely juxtaposed terminals.

3. *Synergism*. Each of two transmitters, either from different nerve terminals or cotransmitters, have the same postjunctional effect so that there is a reinforcement of their individual effects.

4. *Opposite actions*. Rarely, a transmitter may have opposite actions in different effector cells, or the response may depend on the tone of the effector cell.

5. *Prolongation of effect*. A neuromodulator may act on degradative enzymes, for example, peptidases responsible for removal of neuropeptides from the junctional cleft, to prolong the time course of their effect.

6. *Trophic effects*. A neurotransmitter may affect the expression of another transmitter or receptor within a population of neurons (for example, in ganglia) at the level of gene transcription.

All these mechanisms of control of neurotransmission reflect the versatility of the autonomic nervous system.

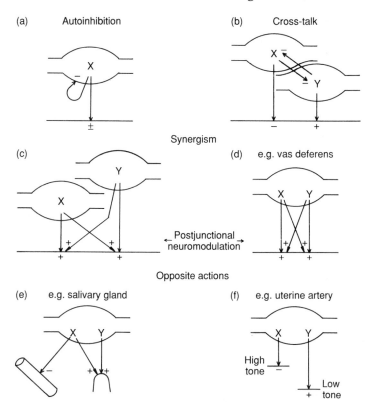

Fig. 7.2. Schematic representation of different types of interactions between two nominal vascular neurotransmitter substances (X and Y). (a) A diagram depicting the process of autoinhibition where, in addition to the neurotransmitter (X) acting postjunctionally to either contract (+) or relax (–) the muscle, it acts on prejunctional receptors (usually of a different subclass) to form a negative feedback system that inhibits release of transmitter. (b) A diagram depicting the process of cross-talk. Transmitters X and Y, contained in separate varicosities, not only act on receptors in the muscle (usually producing opposite actions), but also on prejunctional receptors on each other's nerve terminals to modulate transmitter release. (c) A diagram showing that transmitter X and transmitter Y, contained in separate nerve varicosities, have the same contractile (+) action on the muscle cell. They potentiate each other's actions by the process of post-junctional neuromodulation. This is an example of synergism occurring in another type of cross-talk. (d) A diagram showing where X and Y, released as cotransmitters from a single varicosity, act synergistically on the postjunctional effector cell. (e) A diagram showing how the cotransmitters X and Y can have opposite actions on different effector cell sites, although they again act synergistically on the one effector cell type. (f) A diagram showing how the cotransmitters X and Y express opposite actions depending on the tone of the vessel: in high-tone situations, X produces vasodilatation (–), while in low-tone preparations, transmitter Y dominates producing vasocontraction. (From Burnstock (1987a).)

Neurotransmission at sympathetic neuroeffector junctions: evidence for corelease and roles of NA, ATP, and NPY

There is plenty of evidence to show that NA and ATP are cotransmitters in the sympathetic nervous system in many species (Burnstock 1990c) including man (Taddei *et al.* 1990). There is considerable variation in the proportions of ATP and NA released depending on the tissue and species in question; for example, rabbit saphenous and mesenteric arteries have a substantial purinergic component, whereas in the rabbit ear artery the puringeric component is relatively small. The relative contribution of each compound to neurogenic contractions is dependent on the parameters of stimulation; short bursts (1 s) at low frequency (2–5 Hz) particularly favour the purinergic component, whereas longer periods of nerve stimulation (30 s or more) favour the adrenergic component. NPY is also stored in and is released from most sympathetic nerves, including cardiac and perivascular nerves in many vascular beds in man. NPY release is optimal with high-frequency, intermittent stimulation.

Cotransmission has been investigated extensively in the rodent vas deferens which has a predominantly sympathetic motor innervation. The neurogenic mechanical response of the vas deferens is biphasic, consisting of an initial twitch phase and a slower maintained phase. The rapid twitch phase is resistant to the adrenoceptor antagonist, prazosin, and has been shown to be the purinergic component (it is blocked by the ATP antagonist, $ANAPP_3$, and by the selective desensitizer, α,β-methylene ATP, and the excitatory junction potentials are mimicked by ATP) whilst the second phase is the noradrenergic component. NPY is also stored in sympathetic nerves in the vas deferens and is released concomitantly with ATP and NA upon stimulation of the sympathetic nerves. There is abundant evidence that ATP and NA are stored in the same vesicles; however, differential release of ATP and NA by various agents, such as CGRP, prostaglandin E_2 and angiotensin III, suggests that there may be different subpopulations of sympathetic nerves: some in which ATP and NA are in different storage vesicles; some with different proportions of the cotransmitters in the same vesicle, sometimes even within the same terminal nerve fibre; and possibly some in which the transmitters are not in vesicles at all. Electron microscopic and fractionation studies have shown that NPY is preferentially localized with NA and ATP in large dense-cored vesicles, while no NPY is found in small dense-cored vesicles that are the main storage sites for ATP and NA. This distribution has also been found in human atrial appendage.

In most tissues, including the vas deferens and most blood vessels, NPY does not act as a genuine cotransmitter, having little direct postjunctional effect, but rather acts as a neuromodulator, often by prejunctional reduction of the release of NA and ATP and postjunctional potentiation of the adrenergic and purinergic components of sympathetic nerve responses. Evidence accumulated from the effects of NPY on sympathetic neurotransmission in a variety of tissues has led to the suggestion that the mode of neuromodulation by NPY is related to the width of the junctional cleft: a narrow cleft (20 nm, e.g. vas deferens) favours prejunctional modulation of release of cotransmitters; a medium-sized cleft (100–500 nm, e.g. most blood vessels) favours postjunctional modulation with low concentrations of NPY preceding prejunctional modulation as the concentration of NPY increases: a wide cleft (1000–2000 nm, e.g. large elastic arteries) favours postjunctional modulation.

While the role of NPY is mainly as a neuromodulator in sympathetic nerves, it does have direct vasoconstrictor effects on certain blood vessels, for example of the spleen, kidney, heart, and brain in many species. In man, NPY induces a direct vasoconstrictor response in some vessels which is characteristically slow in onset and long-lasting. A dense plexus of perivascular NPY-containing nerve fibres has been described in many vessels including human omental, mesenteric, skin, spinal, pulmonary, renal, gastric, splenic, coronary, and cerebral vessels (Mione et al. 1990). Because of its distribution and constrictor effects, this component of the sympathetic nervous system has been implicated in the development of hypertension; indeed the innervation of cerebrovascular vessels by NPY-containing nerve fibres is increased in the sponaneously hypertensive rat along with catecholaminergic fibres (Dhital et al. 1988). Abnormalities in purinergic mechanisms have also been reported in hypertension. Perivascular sympathetic hyperinnervation in this condition would explain the increased plasma NA levels found in human essential hypertension. NPY is also a contender as one of the vasospasmic agents responsible for the delayed ischaemic deficit that occurs after subarachnoid haemorrhage. In man the levels of this neuropeptide rise in the cerebrospinal fluid at a time that correlates with the incidence of cerebral vasospasm (Suzuki et al. 1989), a finding which supports previous studies on the experimental induction of subarachnoid haemorrhage in rabbits.

Neurotransmission at parasympathetic neuroeffector junctions: the atropine-resistant components of parasympathetic neurotransmission

The neuropeptide most frequently associated with parasympathetic neurotransmission is VIP. An elegant series of experiments by Lundberg (1981) on the cat exocrine salivary gland with reference to the involvement of VIP and ACh in the control of secretion and blood flow showed that VIP and ACh were stored in separate vesicles in the same nerve terminal and were both released upon transmural nerve stimulation but with different stimulation parameters. ACh was released during low-frequency stimulation to increase salivary secretion from acinar cells and to elicit some minor dilatation of blood vessels in the gland, whereas at high stimulation frequencies, VIP was released to produce marked dilatation of the blood vessels in the gland and to act as a neuromodulator postjunctionally on the acinar gland to enhance the actions of ACh and prejunctionally on the nerve varicosities to enhance the release of ACh. ACh was also found to have an inhibitory action on the release of VIP. VIP has since been shown to have a direct vasodilatory action in the submandibular gland in man.

VIP has been co-localized with the ACh synthesizing enzyme, choline acetyltransferase, in many perivascular nerve fibres where it is localized mainly in large vesicles. Many studies have been carried out on cerebral vessels where VIP-containing nerve fibres innervating the cerebral arteries originate from the cranial parasympathetic ganglia, in particular, from the sphenopalatine ganglion. The anterior vessels of the circle of Willis receive a more dense innervation of VIP-containing nerve fibres than those in the posterior circulation (Mione *et al.* 1990). VIP acts as a direct vasodilator in several blood vessels. A peptide found in human tissue, PHM (peptide with N-terminal histidine and C-terminal methionine), which is derived from the same pre-pro-molecule as VIP (the animal form is PHI, C-terminal isoleucine), has a similar distribution pattern to VIP and also has vasodilator properties, although it is less potent than VIP. Perivascular nerves displaying VIP/PHM immunoreactivity tend to occur more frequently around vessels in regional vascular beds than in association with larger conducting vessels. In addition, small arterioles are generally more sensitive to VIP/PHM than larger vessels.

VIP is thought to play a role in parasympathetic neurotransmission in the urinogenital tract since postganglionic nerves from the pelvic ganglia containing VIP and ACh project to the bladder, colon, and penis (Keast *et al.* 1989). This neuropeptide is implicated in the mechanism of penile erection. Numerous immunohistochemical studies have demonstrated VIP in autonomic nerves in the penile artery and penile tissues from a variety of species including man. Electrical stimulation of pelvic nerves induces vasodilatation of penile blood vessels and increases blood flow to the cavernous tissue. This action may be mediated by VIP since local administration of VIP leads to increased penile volume. VIP *in vitro* induces relaxation of the corpus cavernosum, corpus spongiosum smooth muscle, and blood vessels, and VIP is increased in the venous effluent of the penis during psychogenic-, drug-, or electrically-induced erection. Furthermore, in diabetic impotence in man, there is a dramatic reduction of VIP-immunoreactive nerve fibres in penile vessels. More recently, NO, generated in response to NANC neurotransmission, has been shown to play an important role in the autonomic control of penile erection (Rand 1992). Indeed, several parasympathetic nerves may utilize NO as a cotransmitter.

The human bladder body receives a dense parasympathetic innervation comprising, predominantly, ACh-containing nerves. VIP has been localized

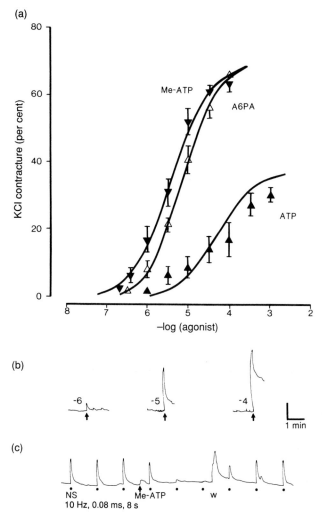

Fig. 7.3. Responses to ATP, α,β-methylene ATP (Me-ATP) and P^1, P^6-diadenosine 5′-hexaphosphate (A6PA) in isolated human urinary bladder detrusor muscle. (a) Concentration–response relationships. The response curve relates contractions due to the agonists to the KCl standard contraction. Points show means $\pm$ SE unless occluded by symbol. Curves are fitted following probit transformation and horizontal averaging. (b) Examples of contractions evoked by A6PA, log molar concentrations applied as indicated at arrows. Scale bar represents 100 mg. (c) Electrical field stimulation of intramural nerves (NS, ●) evoked contractions. α,β-methylene ATP (Me-ATP, 0.3 μM) caused a small contraction which faded and blocked the neurogenic contractions. Following washout of α,β-methylene ATP (W), the neurogenic responses returned. Record obtained in the presence of atropine (0.3 μM). Scale bar repesents 50 mg. (From Hoyle *et al.* 1989).)

in the human bladder wall; however, its role in neuromodulation in this tissue in man is controversial. It is widely accepted that ATP is a cotransmitter utilized by NANC excitatory nerves supplying guinea-pig and rat urinary bladder; however, despite the doubt of the existence of a NANC component of neurotransmission in the human urinary bladder, recent pharmacological studies have demonstrated a small purinergic component in response to electrical field stimulation in man (Fig. 7.3; Hoyle *et al.* 1989). P_{2X}-purinoceptors have also been localized in the human bladder (Bo and Burnstock, personal communication). There are marked regional variations in the distribution of the atropine-resistant component in human bladder and, indeed, ATP responses and receptors are dense in the trigone region but very low or absent in the tip of the bladder dome (see Burnstock 1990*d*). The physiological significance of these responses may be of greater importance in the functionally disturbed bladder.

There are now several reports that some cranial, ciliary, and paracervical parasympathetic ganglia that supply VIP/ACh-containing nerves to cerebral arteries, iris, and uterine artery also contain NPY (Mione *et al.* 1990). Dopamine β-hydroxylase, dynorphin, and somatostatin have also been localized in guinea-pig paracervical ganglia.

Neurotransmission at sensory-motor neuroeffector junctions: the roles of SP, CGRP, and ATP

The phenomenon of antidromic vasodilatation, in which antidromic impulses pass down collateral branches of primary afferent sensory nerves resulting in the release of neurotransmitter thus causing vasodilatation (the axon reflex concept), has been known for some time. More recently, however, interest has been aroused in the dual sensory–efferent functions mediated by sensory neurons, whereby, in addition, these neurons have the ability to release the stored transmitter from the same terminal which is excited by the environmental stimulus. The neurotransmitters essentially involved in sensory–motor neurotransmission are SP, CGRP, and ATP (see Fig. 7.4; Maggi and Meli 1988). The sensory origin of SP- and CGRP-containing nerve fibres has been substantiated by using the selective neurotoxin, capsaicin. Chronic treatment with this drug leads to degeneration of small afferent nerves and a marked loss of SP- and CGRP-containing nerves from most tissues of the cardiovascular system, urinogenital system, and airways. SP and CGRP coexist in large granular vesicles in sensory neurons and perivascular nerves in the guinea-pig; however, in the rat, CGRP immunoreactivity appears to occur in two populations of sensory neurons. In the trigeminal ganglion, small- to medium-sized vesicles contain SP and are sensitive to capsaicin, while larger vesicles contain no SP and are resistant to capsaicin. In addition to its role as a neurotransmitter, CGRP may modulate the action of SP by inhibiting its degradation.

In man SP and other tachykinins have been shown to coexist with CGRP

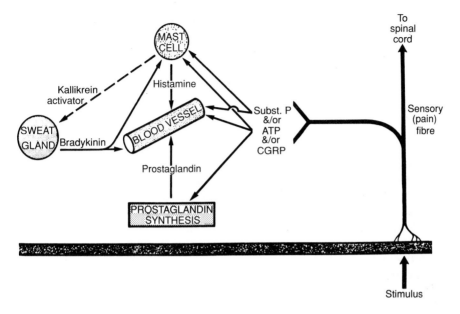

Fig. 7.4. A schematic representation of what might be occurring during an axon reflex in the skin leading to vasodilatation and inflammation. It is suggested that SP, ATP (and possibly CGRP), released during antidromic activation of sensory collaterals, produce dilatation of the blood vessels. In addition, local agents become involved as a secondary consequence of the actions of the transmitters: ATP induces prostaglandin synthesis, while both SP and ATP release histamine from mast cells and also kallikrein activator that leads to production of bradykinin. (From Burnstock (1987*b*).)

in sensory neurons. Activation of the trigeminal cerebrovascular system may be a mechanism involved in cerebrovascular spasm following subarachnoid haemorrhage since the vasoconstriction induced by subarachnoid blood is markedly prolonged following a trigeminovascular pathway lesion but not after trigeminal nerve section. In addition, CGRP levels in middle cerebral arteries are reduced 7–10 days after fatal subarachnoid haemorrhage in man (Edvinsson *et al.* 1991). CGRP and SP levels are also reduced in human cerebrospinal fluid following subarachnoid haemorrhage (Milner, unpublished observations). Indeed, altered functioning of capsaicin-sensitive sensory neurons may be involved in the pathogenesis of several diseases in man, including skin disease, rheumatic disease, asthma and bronchial hyperreactivity, and in the unstable bladder (Maggi and Meli 1988). In the human urinary bladder, VIP, CCK, and dynorphins are present together with SP and CGRP in the afferent projections to the lumbosacral spinal cord. The reduction in innervation by VIP-, SP-, and CGRP-, but not NPY-containing nerve fibres in the unstable bladder with urinary outflow prostatic obstruction indicates possible afferent dysfunction resulting from the prostatic obstruction. VIP has been localized in other sensory neurons, those of the dorsal root and trigeminal ganglion of several species.

Neurotransmission involving intrinsic neurons with special reference to neurotransmitters localized in nerve cell bodies in the heart, bladder, intestine, and lung

Intrinsic neurons are numerous throughout the autonomic nervous system. They have been demonstrated by persistence after extrinsic denervation and by tissue culture techniques in the heart, bladder, lung, and alimentary tract (Hassall *et al.* 1989; Springhall *et al.* 1990). The intrinsic neurons of the myenteric and submucous plexuses of the gastrointestinal tract have been analysed extensively (Furness and Costa 1987). These enteric neurons contain a variety of neuroactive substances, sometimes up to six different neuropeptides existing in a single neuron. It is likely that these substances act as neuromodulators and/or trophic factors rather than neurotransmitters. ATP is still a main contender as a neurotransmitter responsible for the inhibitory junction potentials that predominate from the stomach to the rectum (Hoyle and Burnstock 1989), probably coreleased with NO and VIP, albeit in different proportions in different regions of the gut (Rand 1992). The projections and connections of enteric neurons containing specific neuropeptides have been defined in an elaborate series of surgical manipulations (Furness and Costa 1987). Some enteric neurons project from the intestine to innervate the mesenteric arteries and arterioles of the colon; however, most form a complex network of interconnections between the two major plexuses and the mucosa. With such an integrated system, it is easy to see how an imbalance in the level of just one neuropeptide could lead to disordered intestinal motility; for example, VIP levels are altered in the distal colon in man in two such disorders, being reduced in patients with idiopathic constipation and increased in diverticular disease (Milner *et al.* 1990).

There are many intrinsic neurons in the heart, particularly in the right atrium where guanethidine sympathectomy leads to a depletion of only 46 per cent of NPY (Corr *et al.* 1990). Tissue culture studies on newborn guinea-pig atria have shown immunostaining for NPY and 5-HT (Hassall *et al.* 1989). Projections of these intrinsic neurons form perivascular plexuses in small coronary vessels but do not innervate large coronary arteries (Corr *et al.* 1990).

Intrinsic ganglia in the bladder wall consist of sophisticated circuitry to allow integration of activities in the bladder and urethra. These ganglia have been shown to contain both NPY and somatostatin (Burnstock 1990*d*). Intramural ganglia containing NPY and VIP have been recently identified in the human urethra.

Electrophysiological studies on intramural heart and bladder neurons have revealed significant differences in the electrical properties of these neurons.

Bladder neurons are, in general, highly excitable and frequently exhibit spontaneous activity, whereas only a subpopulation of intracardiac neurons possess these characteristics. In the remainder there are mechanisms which limit the rate and duration of firing, most notably the prominent slow after-hyperpolarization during which the cells are refractory. Bladder neurons, unlike intracardiac neurons, require only small changes in membrane potential or conductance to affect significant alterations in firing rate. These differences in excitability between heart and bladder neurons reflect the different functional roles of these cells: bladder neurons modulate tone, while heart neurons may act to gate information transfer from one area of the heart to another.

Information is unfolding regarding the electrophysiological characteristics of intramural ganglia within the tracheobronchial tree of the airways. Two extreme types of firing behaviour have been identified in intramural paratracheal neurons—short, high-frequency bursts of action potentials at regular intervals in response to prolonged stimulation and no burst firing activity but firing tonically at low frequencies for the duration of the applied stimulus (Fig. 7.5; Allen and Burnstock 1990). The high degree of electrophysiological specialization displayed by these neurons suggests that they may act as sites of integration and/or modulation of the input from extrinsic nerves or permit some local control of aspects of airway function by local reflex mechanisms. The interconnections of intramural ganglia within the respiratory tract and their projections to airway smooth muscle, submucosal glands, and bronchial arteries are only now beginning to be understood.

Plasticity of the autonomic nervous system: some examples of altered expression of neurotransmitters/ neuromodulators in autonomic nerves during development, and ageing, following trauma, surgery, and chronic exposure to drugs, and in disease

Neurons possess the genetic potential to produce many neurotransmitters. The particular combination and quantity that results is partly pre-programmed and partly determined by 'trophic' factors that trigger the expression or suppression of the appropriate genetic machinery. A number of studies have demonstrated the plasticity of the autonomic nervous system in development and ageing; following trauma, surgery, and chronic exposure to drugs; and in disease (Burnstock 1990e).

The pattern of innervation of blood vessels by sympathetic nerves with age is known to vary considerably from one vessel to another. Studies of the development of peptide-containing perivascular nerves show that even peptides that are colocalized within the same nerve fibre do not show the same innervation pattern during development. In cerebral vessels of the ageing

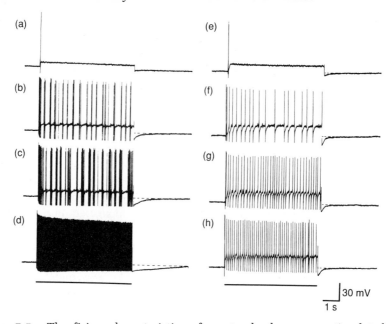

Fig. 7.5. The firing characteristics of paratracheal neurons stimulated by prolonged intrasomal current injection of increasing intensities. The traces in the left-hand column (a–d) were recorded from a burst-firing neuron. (a) Stimulation with low current intensities (150 pA, 5 s) only elicited firing at the onset of current injection. (b) Increasing the current intensity to 300 pA induced the cell to fire short high-frequency bursts of action potentials for the duration of current stimulation. (c) Further increasing the stimulating current to 500 pA increased the duration of these bursts and slightly decreased the interburst interval. (d) At high current intensities (800 pA) the bursts of firing fused and the cell started to fire tonically at high frequencies for the duration of the stimulus. Trains of action potential generated in this way were invariably followed by a prolonged after-hyperpolarization which persisted for up to 3 s and ranged in amplitude between 10 and 20 mV. Records (e)–(h) were obtained under similar conditions from a non-burst-firing cell. (e) At low current intensities the cell again only fired at the start of the stimulus. Note the long spike after-hyperpolarization as compared with the cell in (a). (f) Increasing the stimulus current induced low-frequency multiple firing. (g), (h) Further increases in stimulus intensity produced an increase in this discharge but never to the levels seen in the burst-firing neurons. (From Allen and Burnstock (1990).)

rat there is a decrease in the expression of the vasoconstrictor neurotransmitters, NA and 5-HT, but an increase in the expression of the vasodilator neurotransmitters, VIP and CGRP. In man, a decrease in the levels of NPY, VIP, and SP in cerebral vessels has been reported between the ages of 1 and 46 years, consistent, in terms of relative life span, with the changes reported in rat. During pregnancy, the expression of NPY in perivascular nerves of the uterine artery increases whilst NA levels fall, an event unrelated to systemic progesterone treatment.

In patients with bladder areflexia following lower motor spinal lesion there is increased innervation by VIP-, NPY-, and NA-containing nerve fibres to the striated muscle of the intrinsic external urethral sphincter, which may indicate a regulatory mechanism via the intrinsic ganglia and/or the somatic nervous system to help overcome this type of bladder dysfunction.

Sympathectomy produces remarkable changes in the innervation of tissues: for example, unilateral removal of the superior cervical ganglion results in the reinnervation of the denervated cerebral vessels by sprouting nerves from the contralateral ganglion; surgical ganglionectomy leads to increased SP levels in the iris and ciliary body, increased CGRP in pial vessels, and increased expression of NPY in *parasympathetic* neurons supplying cerebral vessels (Mione *et al.* 1990); and long-term guanethidine sympathectomy results in a drastic increase in the innervation of tissues by the sensory neuropeptide, CGRP, probably due to increased availability to nerve growth factor, for which sensory and sympathetic neurons compete (Aberdeen *et al.* 1990). Following parasympathetic denervation of the cat bladder, there is a reorganization of sympathetic preganglionic connections such that there is a conversion of sympathetic inhibitory pathways to excitatory pathways in the denervated bladder (de Groat and Kawatani 1989). Further, after extrinsic denervation of the human respiratory tract by heart–lung transplantation, the intrinsic parasympathetic neurons that persist express an NA-synthesizing enzyme and NPY, substances normally found in sympathetic nerves (Springhall *et al.* 1990). Chronic stimulation of sympathetic nerves induces structural neuromuscular changes and alters the expression of neurotransmitters in related ganglia.

During the course of experimentally induced diabetes there are marked changes in the expression of neurotransmitters/neuromodulators in nerves supplying the bowel. While there are degenerative changes in VIP- and NA-containing nerves early on in the development of the disease, the expression of 5-HT, SP, and CGRP in nerve fibres changes at different times during the progression of the disease. Patients with autonomic neuropathy, including alcoholic and diabetic neuropathy, have reduced levels of SP in their sural nerves while the change in NA levels is specific to diabetic neuropathy.

These are just a few examples of altered expression of neurotransmitter substances in the autonomic nervous system, some reflecting damage to nerves, some compensatory, and some appearing to lead to an altered neural control of the tissue in question. Knowledge of the factors controlling the expression of these neurotransmitters/neuromodulators may aid manipulation of the autonomic nervous system in disease to encourage beneficial compensatory changes to occur and hence it offers an enormous potential for therapy.

References

Aberdeen, J., Corr, L., Milner, P., Lincoln, J., and Burnstock, G. (1990). Marked increases in calcitonin gene-related peptide-containing nerves in the developing rat following long-term sympathectomy with guanethidine. *Neuroscience* **35**, 175-84.

Allen, T. G. J. and Burnstock, G. (1990). A voltage-clamp study of the electrophysiological characteristics of the intramural neurones of the rat trachea. *J. Physiol., London* **423**, 593-614.

Bredt, D. S., Hwang, P. M., and Snyder, S. H. (1990). Localization of nitric oxide synthase indicating a neural role for nitric oxide. *Nature* **347**, 768-70.

Burnstock, G. (1972). Purinergic nerves. *Pharmacol. Rev.* **24**, 509-81.

Burnstock, G. (1976). Do some nerve cells release more than one transmitter? *Neuroscience* **1**, 239-48.

Burnstock, G. (1979). Non-adrenergic, non-cholinergic nerves in the intestine and their possible involvement in secretion. In *Mechanisms of intestinal secretion*, pp. 147-74. Alan R. Liss, New York.

Burnstock, G. (1986*a*). Autonomic neuromuscular junctions: current developments and future directions. *J. Anat.* **146**, 1-30.

Burnstock, G. (1986*b*). The changing face of autonomic neurotransmission. (The First von Euler Lecture in Physiology.) *Acta physiol. scand.* **126**, 67-91.

Burnstock, G. (1987*a*). Autonomic neuroeffector mechanisms: recent developments. *Funct. Neurol.* **2**, 427-36.

Burnstock, G. (1987*b*). Mechanisms of interaction of peptide and non-peptide vascular neurotransmitter systems. *J cardiovasc. Pharmacol.* **10** (suppl.12) S74-S81.

Burnstock, G. (1990*a*). Classification and characterization of purinoceptors. In *Purines in cellular signalling: targets for new drugs* (ed. K. A. Jacobson, J. W. Daly, and V. Manganiello), pp. 241-53. Springer, New York.

Burnstock, G. (1990*b*). Cotransmission. The Fifth Heymans Lecture—Ghent, February 17, 1990. *Arch. int. Pharmacodyn. Ther.* **304**, 7-33.

Burnstock, G. (1990*c*). Noradrenaline and ATP as cotransmitters in sympathetic nerves. *Neurochem. Int.* **17**, 357-68.

Burnstock, G. (1990*d*). Innervation of bladder and bowel. In *Neurobiology of incontinence*, CIBA Foundation Symposium, no. 151 (ed. G. Bock and J. Whelan), pp. 2-26. John Wiley, Chichester.

Burnstock, G. (1990*e*). Changes in expression of autonomic nerves in ageing and disease. *J. autonom. nerv. Syst.* **30**, 525-34.

Campbell, G. R., Uehara, Y., Mark, G., and Burnstock, G. (1971). *J. Cell Biol.* **49**, 21-34.

Corr, L. A., Aberdeen, J. A., Milner, P., Lincoln, J., and Burnstock, G. (1990). Sympathetic and nonsympathetic neuropeptide Y-containing nerves in the rat myocardium and coronary arteries. *Circulation Res.* **66**, 1602-9.

de Groat, W. C. and Kawatani, M. (1989). Reorganisation of sympathetic preganglionic connections in cat bladder ganglia following parasympathetic denervation. *J. Physiol.* **409**, 431-49.

Dhital, K. K., Gerli, R., Lincoln, J., Milner, P., Tanganelli, P., Weber, G., Fruschelli, C., and Burnstock, G. (1988). Increased density of perivascular nerves to the major cerebral vessels of the spontaneously hypertensive rat: differential changes in noradrenaline and neuropeptide Y during development. *Brain Res.* **444**, 33-45.

Edvinsson, L., Ekman, R., Jansen, I., McCulloch, J., Mortensen, A., and Uddman, R. (1991). Reduced levels of calcitonin-gene-related peptide-like immunoreactivity in human brain vessels after subarachnoid haemorrhage. *Neurosci. Lett.* **121**, 151–4,

Furness, J. B. and Costa, M. (1987). *The enteric nervous system*. Churchill Livingstone, Edinburgh.

Hassall, C. J. S., Allen, T. G. J., Pittam, B. S., and Burnstock, G. (1989). The use of cell and tissue culture techniques in the study of regulatory peptides. In Regulatory peptides, *Experientia* suppl. (ed. J. M. Polak), pp. 113–16. Birkaeuser, Basel.

Hoyle, C. H. V. and Burnstock, G. (1989). Neuromuscular transmission in the gastrointestinal tract. In *Handbook of Physiology, Section 6. The gastrointestinal system,* Vol. I. *Motility and circulation* (ed. J. D. Wood) pp. 435–64. American Physiological Society, Bethesda, Maryland.

Hoyle, C. H. V., Chapple, C., and Burnstock, G. (1989). Isolated human bladder: evidence for an adenine dinucleotide acting on P_{2X}-purinoceptors and for purinergic transmission. *Eur. J. Pharmacol.* **174**, 115–18.

Keast, J. R., Booth, A. M., and de Groat, W. C. (1989). Distribution of neurons in the major pelvic ganglia of the rat which supply the bladder, colon or penis. *Cell Tissue Res.* **256**, 105–12.

Lundberg, J. M. (1981). Evidence for coexistence of vasoactive intestinal polypeptide (VIP) and acetylcholine in neurons of cat exocrine glands. Morphological, biochemical and functional studies. *Acta physiol. scand.* **112** (Suppl. 496), 1–57.

Maggi, C. A. and Meli, A. (1988). The sensory–efferent function of capsaicin-sensitive sensory nerves. *Gen. Pharmacol.* **19**, 1–43.

Milner, P., Crowe, R., Kamm, M., Lennard-Jones, J. E., and Burnstock, G. (1990). Vasoactive intestinal polypeptide levels of the distal sigmoid colon are reduced in idiopathic constipation and increased in diverticular disease. *Gastroenterology* **99**, 666–75.

Mione, M. C., Ralevic, V., and Burnstock, G. (1990). Peptides and vasomotor mechanisms. *Pharmacol. Ther.* **46**, 429–68.

Rand, M. J. (1992). Nitrergic transmission: nitric oxide as a mediator of non-adrenergic, non-cholinergic neuro-effector transmission. *Clin. Exp. Pharmacol. Physiol.* **19**, 147–69.

Springhall, D. R., Polak, J. M., Howard, L., Power, R. F., Krausz, T., Manickam, S., Banner, N. R., Khagani, A., Rose, M., and Yacoub, M. H. (1990). Persistence of intrinsic neurons and possible phenotypic changes after extrinsic denervation of human respiratory tract by heart lung transplantation. *Am. Rev. resp. Dis.* **141**, 1538–46.

Suzuki, Y., Sato, S., Suzuki, H., Namba, J., Ohtake, R., Hashigami, Y., Suga, S., Ishihara, N., and Shimoda, S.-T. (1989). Increased neuropeptide Y concentrations in cerebrospinal fluid from patients with aneurysmal subarachnoid hemorrhage. *Stroke* **20**, 1680–4.

Taddei, S., Pedrinelli, M. D., and Salvetti, M. D. (1990). Sympathetic nervous system-dependent vasoconstriction in humans. Evidence for mechanistic role of endogenous purine compounds. *Circulation* **82**, 2061–7.

PART II

Physiology and pathophysiology of autonomic function

8. Neural control of the urinary bladder and sexual organs

William C. de Groat

Introduction

Various functions of the urogenital tract are controlled by extrinsic nervous pathways which involve neurons in the brain, spinal cord, and peripheral ganglia. Many of these functions are complex, requiring the participation of somatic as well as autonomic efferent mechanisms and the integration of neural and endocrine systems. Due to the complexities of the neurohumoral factors regulating the urogenital organs, the activities of these organs are sensitive to a wide variety of injuries, diseases, and chemicals which affect the nervous system. Thus, neurological mechanisms are an important consideration in the diagnosis and treatment of disorders of the urogenital tract.

This chapter will review experimental studies in animals which have provided insights into the anatomical organization and the transmitters involved in the neural control of urogenital function.

Innervation of the lower urinary tract

The storage and periodic elimination of urine is dependent upon the activity of two functional units in the lower urinary tract: (1) a reservoir (the urinary bladder); and (2) an outlet consisting of bladder neck, urethra, and striated muscles of the urethral sphincter. These structures are, in turn, controlled by three sets of peripheral nerves: sacral parasympathetic (pelvic nerves); thoracolumbar sympathetic (hypogastric nerves and sympathetic chain); and sacral somatic nerves (pudendal nerves) (Fig. 8.1; de Groat and Steers 1990).

Sacral parasympathetic pathways

The sacral parasympathetic outflow provides the major excitatory input to the urinary bladder. Cholinergic preganglionic neurons, located in the intermediolateral region of the sacral spinal cord, send axons via the pelvic nerves to ganglion cells in the pelvic plexus (inferior hypogastric plexus) and

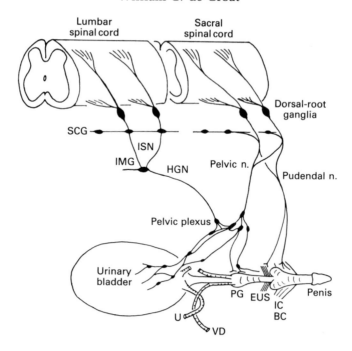

Fig. 8.1. Diagram showing the sympathetic, parasympathetic, and somatic innervation of the urogenital tract of the male cat. Sympathetic preganglionic pathways emerge from the lumbar spinal cord and pass to the sympathetic chain ganglia (SCG) and then via the inferior splanchnic nerves (ISN) to the inferior mesenteric ganglia (IMG). Preganglionic and postganglionic sympathetic axons then travel in the hypogastric nerve (HGN) to the pelvic plexus and the urogenital organs. Parasympathetic preganglionic axons which originate in the sacral spinal cord pass in the pelvic nerve to ganglion cells in the pelvic plexus and to distal ganglia in the organs. Sacral somatic pathways are contained in the pudendal nerve, which provides an innervation to the penis, the ischiocavernosus (IC), bulbocavernosus (BC), and external urethral sphincter (EUS) muscles. The pudendal and pelvic nerves also receive postganglionic axons from the caudal sympathetic chain ganglia. These three sets of nerves contain afferent axons from the lumbosacral dorsal root ganglia. Ureter, U; prostate gland, PG; vas deferens, VD.

in the wall of the bladder. Transmission in bladder ganglia is mediated by a nicotinic cholinergic mechanism, which is sensitive to modulation by various transmitters including muscarinic, adrenergic, purinergic, and peptidergic (Table 8.1; Keast *et al.* 1990). The ganglion cells in turn excite bladder smooth muscle via the release of cholinergic (acetylcholine) and, in some species, non-cholinergic/non-adrenergic transmitters. Cholinergic excitatory transmission is mediated by muscarinic receptors, which are blocked by atropine, whereas non-cholinergic transmission is thought to be mediated by the purinergic

Table 8.1.   Receptors for putative transmitters in the lower urinary tract*

Tissue	Cholinergic	Adrenergic	Other
Bladder body	+ (M_2)	– (β_2)	+ Purinergic (P_2) – VIP + Substance P
Bladder base	+ (M_2)	+ (α_1)	0 Purinergic – VIP
Ganglia	+ (N) + (M_1)	– (α_2) + (α_1) + (β)	– Encephalinergic (δ) – Purinergic (P_1) + Substance P
Urethra	+ (M)	+ (α_1) ± (α_2 – (β_2)	± Purinergic – VIP + NPY
Sphincter striated muscle	+ (N)		

*Letters in parentheses indicate receptor type, e.g. M (muscarinic) and N (nicotinic). + , – , and 0 indicate excitatory, inhibitory, and weak or no effects, respectively.

transmitter, adenosine triphosphate (ATP), acting on P_2 purinergic receptors (Burnstock 1986; Table 8.1). Postganglionic neurons innervating the bladder also contain neuropeptides, such as vasoactive intestinal polypeptide (VIP), neuropeptide Y (NPY), and encephalin (Keast and de Groat 1989). These substances may be coreleased with acetylcholine (ACh) or ATP and function as modulators of neuroeffector transmission.

Thoracolumbar sympathetic pathways

Sympathetic pathways to the lower urinary tract originate in the lumbosacral sympathetic chain ganglia as well as in the prevertebral ganglia (inferior mesenteric ganglia) (de Groat and Steers 1990). Input from the sacral chain ganglia passes to the bladder via the pelvic nerves, whereas fibres from the upper lumbar and inferior mesenteric ganglia travel in the hypogastric nerves. Sympathetic efferent pathways in the hypogastric and pelvic nerves in the cat elicit similar effects in the bladder consisting of: (1) inhibition of detrusor muscle via β-adrenoceptors; (2) excitation of the bladder base and urethra via α_1-receptors; and (3) inhibition and facilitation in bladder parasympathetic ganglia via α_2- and α_1-receptors, respectively (Table 8.1; de Groat and Steers 1990; Keast *et al.* 1990).

Somatic efferent pathways

The efferent innervation of the periurethral and external urethral striated muscles in various species originates from cells in a circumscribed region of the lateral ventral horn, which is termed Onuf's nucleus or the sphincter motor nucleus. These cells send their axons into the pudendal nerve. The sphincter motor nucleus exhibits a number of morphological and histochemical characteristics which distinguish it from other motor nuclei controlling the limb muscles. In regard to dendritic patterns and spectrum of peptidergic inputs, the sphincter motor nucleus closely resembles the sacral autonomic nucleus, with which it has a close functional relationship (Thor *et al.* 1989).

Afferent pathways

Afferent axons innervating the urinary tract are present in the three sets of nerves (de Groat 1986; Jänig and Morrison 1986; de Groat and Steers 1990). The most important afferents for initiating micturition are those passing in the pelvic nerve to the sacral spinal cord. These afferents are small myelinated (Aδ) and unmyelinated (C) fibres which convey impulses from receptors in the bladder wall to neurons in laminae I, V, VII, and X of the spinal cord (Morgan *et al.* 1981). Aδ bladder afferents in the cat respond in a graded manner to passive distension as well as to active contraction of the bladder (Jänig and Morrison 1986) and exhibit pressure thresholds in the range of 5–15 mm Hg, which are similar to those pressures at which humans report the first sensation of bladder filling. These fibres also code for noxious stimuli in the bladder. On the other hand, C-fibre bladder afferents in the cat have very high thresholds and commonly do not respond to even high levels of intravesical pressure (Habler *et al.* 1990). However, activity in some of these afferents is unmasked or enhanced by chemical irritation of the bladder mucosa. These findings indicate that C-fibre afferents in the cat have specialized functions, such as the signalling of inflammatory or noxious events in the lower urinary tract.

The central projections of pelvic, pudendal, and hypogastric nerve afferents have been studied in several species including the cat, rat, and monkey using axonal transport of horseradish peroxidase (HRP) (de Groat 1986). In the cat the general population of visceral afferents in the pelvic nerve (Fig. 8.2), including afferents from the bladder (Fig. 8.3(a)), project to restricted regions of the spinal cord. The afferent axons enter Lissauer's tract and then send collaterals through the marginal zone laterally and medially around the dorsal horn. Afferent terminals are heavily concentrated in lamina I, particularly on the lateral side of the dorsal horn (termed the lateral collateral pathway) and in lateral laminae V–VII in the area of the sacral parasympathetic nucleus as well as in the dorsal commissure (Morgan *et al.* 1981).

Pudendal afferent pathways from internal tissues such as the urethra and urethral sphincters exhibit a similar pattern of termination in the sacral spinal cord (Fig. 8.3(b)), whereas pudendal afferent pathways from cutaneous receptors have a prominent projection to the deeper layers of the dorsal horn and the dorsal commissure (Thor *et al.* 1989). The overlap of bladder and urethral afferents in the lateral collateral pathway and dorsal commissure

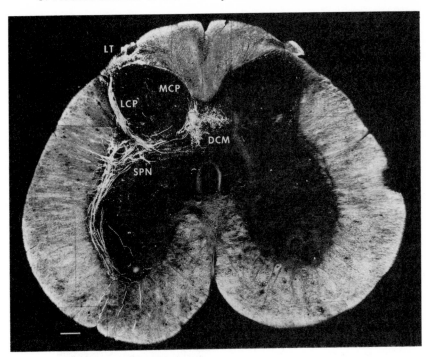

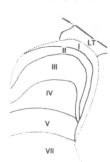

Fig. 8.2. Transverse section of S2 spinal cord showing labelling of primary afferents and preganglionic neurons after application of HRP to the left pelvic nerve in the cat. Pelvic afferents enter Lissauer's tract (LT). Afferent collaterals enter lamina I and extend laterally in a large bundle, the lateral collateral pathway (LCP), into the area of the sacral parasympathetic nucleus (SPN). Collaterals also extend medially in a smaller group, the medial collateral pathway (MCP), into the dorsal grey commissure (DCM), where they expand into a large terminal field ipsilaterally and contralaterally. Small numbers of afferents are also present in contralateral laminae I and V. This photomicrograph was made using darkfield illumination with polarized light. Bar represents 200 μm. Inset shows the laminar organization of the sacral dorsal horn according to Rexed. (From Morgan *et al.* (1981).)

indicates that this region is likely to be an important site of viscerosomatic integration and to be involved in co-ordinating bladder and sphincter activity during micturition.

The central projections of afferents from the lower urinary tract have also been demonstrated by measuring c-*fos* protein in spinal neurons. C-*fos* is a proto-oncogene which is rapidly and transiently induced in neurons by

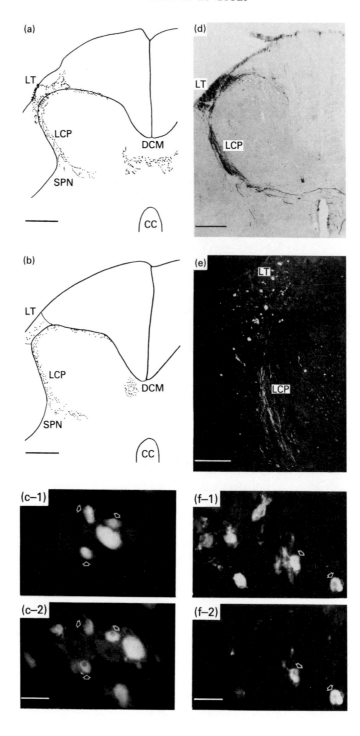

synaptic input. The protein product of the c-*fos* gene is therefore useful in tract-tracing as an indirect marker of neuronal activity. Activation of urethral afferents and distension or chemical irritation of the bladder increases neuronal c-*fos* in those regions of the spinal cord receiving afferent input from the lower urinary tract (Fig. 8.4). Combined axonal tracing and immunocytochemical studies revealed that in lateral laminae, V–VII, 20–25 per cent of the c-*fos* positive neurons activated by bladder afferents are spinal tract cells projecting to the brainstem. A small percentage (<5 per cent) are preganglionic neurons, and the remainder are presumably propriospinal or segmental interneurons.

Immunohistochemical studies have shown that a large percentage of bladder afferent neurons contain peptides including: calcitonin gene-related peptide (CGRP), vasoactive intestinal polypeptide (VIP), substance P, encephalins, and cholecystokinin (CCK) (de Groat 1987). In addition, multiple peptides with both inhibitory (e.g. encephalins) and excitatory actions (VIP) can be co-localized in the same neuron (Fig. 8.3(f)). In the spinal cord, certain peptidergic afferent terminals, e.g. VIP, have a distribution very similar to the distribution of pelvic nerve and bladder afferents labelled with HRP (Fig. 8.3(d), (e)). Nerves containing these peptides are also common in the bladder

---

Fig. 8.3.   Afferent pathways to the sacral spinal cord. (a) Camera lucida drawing of the central projections of bladder afferents in the sacral (S2) dorsal horn (DH) of the cat. Afferent terminals were labelled by transganglionic transport of HRP from nerves on the surface of the bladder. Labelled axons were present in Lissauer's tract (LT), the lateral collateral pathway (LCP), the sacral parasympathetic nucleus (SPN), and the dorsal commissure (DCM). (b) Afferent projections in the S2 dorsal horn of the cat labelled by HRP injected into the external urethral sphincter. (c) Two photomicrographs of the same section through the S2 dorsal root ganglion showing bladder afferent cells (c-1) labelled by fast blue injected into the bladder wall. Several of these labelled cells (arrows in (c-1) and (c-2)) contain VIP-immunoreactivity (VIP–IR). Dye-labelled cells were blue when visualized with UV light at 340–380 nm excitation wavelength and VIP cells were green when visualized with UV light at 430–480 nm wavelength. (d) The distribution of VIP–IR in LT and LCP of the S2 segment of the cat spinal cord. (e) VIP–IR in the sacral dorsal horn of the S3 segment of the human spinal cord. Large bundles of VIP axons are present in LT and smaller numbers of axons are present in lamina I on the lateral edge of the dorsal horn. (f) Co-localization of substance P-IR and VIP–IR in sacral (S2) dorsal root ganglion cells of the cat. Substance P-IR (f-1) stained with TRITC (red colour, at 530–560 nm excitation wavelength) and in (f-2) the same section showing VIP–IR in two of the same ganglion cells (arrows) stained with FITC (green colour at 430–480 nm excitation wavelength). VIP was detected with rabbit polyclonal antisera, whereas substance P was detected by rat monoclonal antisera. Calibration represents 250 μm in (a) and (b), 50 μm in (c), 300 μm in (d), 220 μm in (e), and 60 μm in (f). (From de Groat *et al.* (1986).)

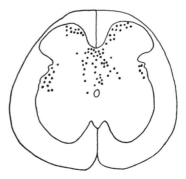

Fig. 8.4. Distribution of neurons on the L_6 spinal cord of the rat exhibiting c-fos immunoreactivity following chemical irritation of the urinary bladder with 1 per cent acetic acid.

wall within the subepithelial and submucosal layers and around blood vessels. Capsaicin, a neurotoxin, which can release peptides from afferent terminals produces inflammatory responses, including plasma extravasation and vasodilatation, when applied locally to the bladder in experimental animals (Maggi and Meli 1986). Large doses of capsaicin, which can deplete peptide stores or destroy peptidergic afferents, can under certain conditions depress the micturition reflex (see next section). These findings suggest that the neuropeptides may be important transmitters in the afferent pathways from the lower urinary tract.

Central reflex pathways to the lower urinary tract

The neural mechanisms regulating micturition seem to be organized as simple on–off switching circuits, which maintain a reciprocal relationship between the bladder and the urethral outlet. During urine storage, a low level of afferent activity in the pelvic nerve and possibly also in proprioceptive afferents in the pudendal nerve initiates reflex efferent firing in sympathetic and somatic pathways to the bladder base and urethra, while the parasympathetic efferent outflow to the bladder body is quiescent (Table 8.2). During micturition a high level of vesical afferent activity reverses the pattern of efferent outflow, producing firing in the parasympathetic pathways and inhibition of the sympathetic and somatic pathways.

These basic reflex mechanisms require the integrative action of neuronal populations at various levels of the neuraxis (Fig. 8.5). Certain reflexes, for example, those mediating the excitatory outflow to the sphincters and the sympathetic inhibitory outflow to the bladder, are organized at the spinal level (Fig. 8.6), whereas the parasympathetic outflow to the detrusor has a

Table 8.2. Reflexes to the lower urinary tract

Afferent pathway	Efferent pathway	Central pathway
Urine storage		
Low-level vesical afferent activity (pelvic nerve)	1. External sphincter contraction (somatic nerves) 2. Internal sphincter contraction (sympathetic nerves) 3. Detrusor inhibition (sympathetic nerves) 4. Ganglionic inhibition (sympathetic nerves) 5. Sacral parasympathetic outflow inactive	Spinal reflexes
Micturition		
High-level vesical afferent activity (pelvic nerve)	1. Inhibition of external sphincter activity 2. Inhibition of sympathetic outflow 3. Activation of parasympathetic outflow	Spinobulbospinal reflexes

more complicated central organization involving spinal and bulbospinal pathways (Fig. 8.5).

Parasympathetic pathways

Electrophysiological and neuroanatomical studies in animals indicate that the spinobulbospinal parasympathetic pathway passes through a centre in the rostral brainstem (the pontine micturition centre) which is located in the region of the locus ceruleus or locus ceruleus alpha in the cat and in the lateral dorsal tegmental nucleus in the rat (Satoh *et al.* 1978; Torrens and Morrison 1987; de Groat and Steers 1990). This centre, in conjunction with neuronal circuitry in adjacent areas of the brain (e.g. the locus subceruleus and lateral parabrachial nucleus), appears to play a major role in co-ordinating the neuronal mechanisms underlying both urine storage and release. Thus, destruction of the pontine micturition centre or interruption of the neuraxis below the pons causes the immediate elimination of the micturition reflex and the slow development of involuntary, uncoordinated, spinal mechanisms which mediate automatic voiding in paraplegic patients and animals (de Groat *et al.* 1990).

The central pathways that are likely to mediate the spinobulbospinal micturition reflex have been demonstrated with axonal tracing techniques.

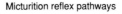

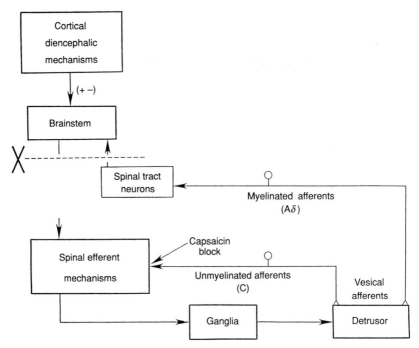

Fig. 8.5. Diagram of the central reflex pathways which regulate micturition in the cat. In animals with intact neuraxis, micturition is initiated by a supraspinal reflex pathway passing through a centre in the brainstem. The pathway is triggered by myelinated afferents (Aδ) connected to tension receptors in the bladder wall. In spinal animals, connections between the brainstem and the sacral spinal cord are interrupted (X) and micturition is initially blocked. However, in chronic spinal animals a spinal reflex mechanism emerges which is triggered by unmyelinated (C-fibre) vesical afferents. The C-fibre reflex pathway is usually weak or undetectable in animals with an intact nervous system. Capsaicin (20–30 mg/kg body weight, s.c.) blocks the C-fibre reflex in chronic spinal cats, but does not block micturition reflexes in intact cats.

For example, it has been shown that the dorsal pontine tegmentum receives inputs from neurons located in lateral laminae I, V, VII, of the sacral spinal cord. Neurons in these areas of the spinal cord receive dense projections from bladder afferent pathways (Figs 8.5 and 8.7) and respond to distension or contraction of the bladder. It is assumed that these neurons represent the spinal ascending limb of the micturition reflex pathway.

Descending projections from the pontine micturition centre to the spinal cord have also been identified in the cat and rat (Holstege *et al.* 1986; Fig. 8.7). In the cat, neurons in the dorsomedial pons send direct projections to the sacral parasympathetic nucleus and to lamina I on the lateral edge

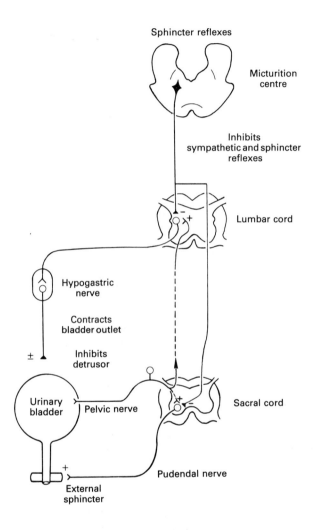

Fig. 8.6.   Diagram showing detrusor–sphincter reflexes. During the storage of urine, distention of the bladder produces low-level vesical afferent firing, which in turn stimulates: (1) the sympathetic outflow to the bladder outlet (base and urethra); and (2) pudendal outflow to the external urethral sphincter. These responses occur by spinal reflex pathways and represent 'guarding reflexes', which promote continence. Sympathetic firing also inhibits detrusor muscle and transmission in bladder ganglia. At the initiation of micturition, intense vesical afferent activity activates the brainstem micturition centre, which inhibits the spinal guarding reflexes.

William C. de Groat

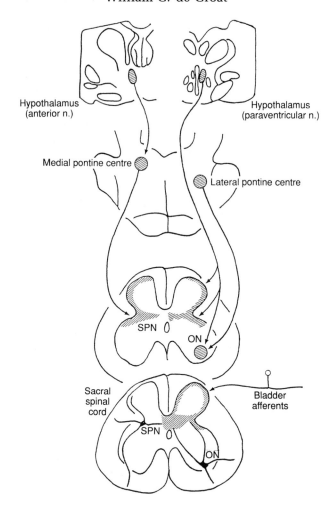

Fig. 8.7. Neural connections between the brain and the sacral spinal cord that may be involved in the regulation of the lower urinary tract in the cat. Lower section of spinal cord shows the location and morphology of a pre-ganglionic neuron in the sacral parasympathetic nucleus (SPN), a sphincter motoneuron in Onuf's nucleus (ON), and the sites of central termination of afferent projections from the urinary bladder. (Based on the studies of Nadelhaft *et al.* 1980; Morgan *et al.* 1981; Thor *et al.* 1989.) Upper section of the spinal cord shows the sites of termination of descending pathways arising in the pontine micturition centre (medial), the pontine sphincter or urine storage centre (lateral), and the paraventricular nuclei of the hypothalamus. Section through the pons shows the projection from the anterior hypothalamic nuclei to the pontine micturition centre. (Based on studies of Holstege 1987; Holstege *et al.* 1986.)

of the sacral dorsal horn, an area that contains dendritic projections from the sacral preganglionic neurons and afferent inputs from the bladder (Morgan *et al.* 1981; de Groat *et al.* 1986). Thus, the sites of termination of descending projections from the pontine micturition centre are optimally located to regulate reflex mechanisms at the spinal level. A second area located somewhat more laterally in the pons sends projections to the sphincter motor nucleus in the sacral spinal cord (Holstege *et al.* 1986; Fig. 8.7). Electrical stimulation of this dorsolateral area elicits sphincter contractions and inhibits bladder activity, whereas stimulation of the more medial pontine micturition centre produces the opposite effects: inhibition of sphincter activity and excitation of the bladder.

Electrical stimulation in the pons also influences the storage function of the bladder. In both rats and cats continuous stimulation in dorsomedial sites reduces bladder capacity, whereas stimulation at ventral sites in the reticular formation increases bladder capacity. These observations suggest that the micturition switching circuit can be modulated by local input within the pons.

Neurophysiological data are consistent with the concept of a spino-bulbspinal micturition reflex pathway. In both cats and rats stimulation of bladder afferents activates neurons in the pons at latencies of 30–40 ms, whereas electrical stimulation in the pons excites sacral preganglionic neurons at latencies of 45–60 ms (de Groat and Steers 1990). The sum of latencies for the spinobulbar and bulbospinal components of the reflex pathway approximate the latency (65–100 ms) for the entire reflex.

Single unit recordings in the pontine micturition centre of cats and rats have identified several populations of cells exhibiting firing correlated with bladder activity. One group of cells fires just prior to and during reflex contractions of the bladder, whereas another group is inhibited during bladder contractions. The all-or-none pattern of activity of these units, coupled with pharmacological data (see below), provides support for the view that this region of the pons contains the neuronal switching circuit responsible for controlling the storage/voiding cycle of the lower urinary tract.

There is also evidence that a switching or gating circuit is present in the spinal cord (de Groat *et al.* 1990). For example, in chronic spinal animals reflex mechanisms within the lumbosacral spinal cord are capable of duplicating many of the functions performed by the reflex pathways in the intact animal. In addition, the firing of sacral preganglionic neurons, elicited by bladder distension in chronic spinal cats following recovery from spinal shock, is similar to that occurring in intact cats.

However, despite these similarities electrophysiological studies in rats and cats have shown that the reflex pathways in intact and chronic animals are markedly different (Mallory *et al.* 1989; de Groat *et al.* 1990). In both species, the central delay for the micturition reflex in chronic spinal animals is considerably shorter (< 5 ms in rats; 15–40 ms in cats) than in intact animals (60–75 ms). In addition, in chronic spinal cats the afferent limb of the micturition reflex consists of unmyelinated (C-fibre) afferents, whereas in intact cats it consists of myelinated (Aδ) afferents (Fig. 8.5). Thus, there seems to be a considerable reorganization of reflex connections in the spinal cord following the interruption of descending pathways from the brain. C-fibre afferent-evoked reflexes, which are weak and occur in only 50 per cent of cats with an intact neuraxis, are facilitated, whereas reflexes evoked by Aδ afferents are completely eliminated in chronic spinal animals.

The role of C-fibre bladder afferents in the initiation of micturition has also been examined using the neurotoxin capsaicin, which is known to disrupt the function of C-fibre afferents. In normal cats capsaicin does not block Aδ-fibre evoked bladder reflexes; however, in chronic spinal cats the toxin (20–30 mg/kg body weight, s.c.) blocks C-fibre-evoked micturition contractions (Fig. 8.5; de Groat et al. 1990).

These data indicate that two distinct central pathways (supraspinal and spinal), utilizing different peripheral afferent limbs (A and C-fibre), can mediate bladder reflexes in the cat (Fig. 8.5). The supraspinal pathway seems to have the major role in the initiation of bladder contractions in animals with an intact neuraxis, while the spinal reflex pathway is essential for the development of automatic micturition in paraplegic animals. It is not known whether the spinal pathway is functional in normal animals or whether this circuit becomes functional as a consequence of synaptic reorganization following spinal cord damage.

Enhancement of the spinal micturition reflex pathway also occurs in another pathological condition: chronic partial urethral obstruction in rats (de Groat et al. 1990). It is also noteworthy that urethral obstruction like spinal cord injury can lead to a hyperactive bladder in both animals and man. This has prompted the speculation that bladder hyperactivity may be linked to changes in spinal reflex pathways.

Axonal tracing studies have also revealed morphological changes in the afferent and efferent pathways to the bladder following partial urethral obstruction (Steers et al. 1990). For example, in obstructed animals bladder afferent neurons in the dorsal root ganglia exhibit an increase in size (45 per cent increase in cross-sectional area) and there is also an increase in density of wheat germ agglutinin (WGA–HRP) labelled bladder afferent terminals in the region of the parasympathetic nucleus in the lumbosacral spinal cord. Bladder post-ganglionic neurons in the pelvic ganglia also exhibit hypertrophy (90 per cent increase in size). It has been speculated that these neuromorphological changes might be due to the action of increased levels of neurotrophic factors released by the hypertrophied bladder (Steers et al. 1990) and that expansion of afferent projections in the spinal cord might underlie the facilitation of the spinal micturition reflex pathway. Expansion of afferent projections in the sacral cord has also been noted in cats following spinal cord injury (de Groat et al. 1990).

The organization of suprapontine pathways controlling micturition is less well defined, despite the fact that there is a large body of literature dealing with the responses of the lower urinary tract to lesions or electrical stimulation of the brain (Torrens and Morrison 1987; de Groat and Steers 1990). In brief, it appears that the voluntary control of micturition in humans is dependent upon: (1) connections between the frontal cortex and the septal and the preoptic regions of the hypothalamus; and (2) connections between the paracentral lobule and the brainstem and spinal cord. Lesions to these areas of cortex resulting from tumours, aneurysms, or cerebrovascular disease appear to remove inhibitory control over the anterior hypothalamic area which normally provides an excitatory input to micturition centres in the brainstem.

Electrical stimulation of anterior and lateral hypothalamic regions in animals induces bladder contractions and voiding, whereas stimulation of posterior and medial hypothalamic areas inhibits bladder activity (Torrens and Morrison 1987; de Groat and Steers 1990). According to results obtained in cats, the inhibitory and excitatory effects of hypothalamic stimulation are believed to be mediated, respectively, by activation of sympathetic inhibitory pathways and activation of parasympathetic excitatory pathways to the bladder (Torrens and Morrison 1987).

Axonal tracing studies in cats have shown that the anterior hypothalamic area sends direct projections through the medial forebrain bundle to the pontine micturition centre (Fig. 8.7; Holstege 1987). On the other hand, medial and posterior hypothalamic areas, including the paraventricular nucleus, send direct projections to the sacral parasympathetic nucleus, the sphincter motor nucleus (Onuf's nucleus), and to certain sites of bladder afferent termination (laminae I and X) in the sacral spinal cord (Holstege 1987). Thus the modulatory effect of hypothalamic centres on the reflex pathways to the lower urinary tract are probably mediated by direct inputs to both pontine and sacral micturition centres.

Sympathetic pathways

The integrity of the sympathetic input to the lower urinary tract is not essential for the performance of micturition. However, physiological experiments in cats and rats indicate that, during bladder-filling, the sympathetic system does provide a tonic inhibitory input to the bladder as well as an excitatory input to the urethra. This sympathetic input is physiologically significant since surgical interruption or pharmacological blockade of the sympathetic innervation can reduce urethral outflow resistance, reduce bladder capacity, and increase the frequency and amplitude of bladder contractions recorded under constant volume conditions.

Sympathetic reflex activity is elicited by a sacrolumbar intersegmental spinal reflex pathway which is triggered by vesical afferent activity in the pelvic nerves (Fig. 8.6). The reflex pathway is inhibited when bladder pressure is raised to the threshold for producing micturition. This inhibitory response is abolished by transection of the spinal cord at the lower thoracic level, indicating that it originates at a supraspinal site, possibly the pontine micturition centre. Thus, the vesicosympathetic reflex represents a negative feedback mechanism whereby an increase in bladder pressure tends to increase inhibitory input to vesical ganglia and smooth muscle thus allowing the bladder to accommodate large volumes (Fig. 8.6). Increased sympathetic excitatory input to the bladder base and urethra would complement these mechanisms by increasing outflow resistance. During micturition these reflexes are suppressed by supraspinal controls thereby facilitating bladder-emptying.

Somatic pathways to the urethral sphincter

Motoneurons innervating the striated muscles of the urethral sphincter exhibit a tonic discharge which increases during bladder-filling. This activity is mediated in part by low level afferent input from the bladder. During micturition the firing of sphincter motoneurons is inhibited. This inhibition is dependent in part on supraspinal mechanisms, since it is not as prominent in chronic spinal animals. Electrical stimulation of the pontine micturition centre induces sphincter relaxation suggesting that bulbospinal pathways from the pons may be responsible for maintaining the normal reciprocal relationship between bladder and sphincter.

Neurotransmitters in micturition reflex pathways

The sacral parasympathetic reflex pathway to the urinary bladder is essentially a positive feedback circuit. In the absence of inhibitory modulation this circuit would trigger voiding at very low bladder volumes and therefore not allow adequate urine storage, a situation that does occur with injuries or diseases of the central nervous system (Torrens and Morrison 1987). Thus, it is clear that the reflex must be under tonic inhibitory control. There has been considerable interest in defining the properties and in particular the neurotransmitters involved in the putative inhibitory mechanisms (Fig. 8.8).

Encephalins

Immunocytochemical and pharmacological experiments have focused attention on the role of encephalinergic inhibitory mechanisms in the regulation of micturition. Encephalinergic varicosities are very prominent in the region of the sacral parasympathetic nucleus and the external urethral sphincter motor nucleus (Onuf's nucleus) in the sacral spinal cord as well as in the region of the pontine micturition centre of various species.

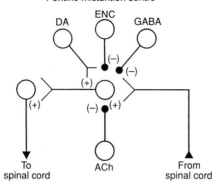

Fig. 8.8.   Diagram showing the variety of neurotransmitters that may regulate transmission in the pontine micturition centre. DA, dopamine; ENC, encephalins; GABA, γ-aminobutyric acid; ACh, acetylcholine; + , excitatory; – , inhibitory.

Administration of exogenous encephalins or opiate drugs to the brain by intracerebroventricular injection, microinjection into the pontine micturition centre, or by intrathecal injection to sacral spinal cord in the cat and rat depresses micturition and sphincter reflexes (de Groat and Steers 1990). Three types of opioid receptors mediate these depressant effects, μ, δ, and K. In the cat spinal cord δ opioid receptors are primarily responsible for inhibition of the micturition reflex, whereas both μ and δ opioid receptors mediate inhibition in the cat brain or the rat and human spinal cord. Sphincter reflexes are resistant to the actions of μ and δ opioid agonists administered to the spinal cord, but are inhibited by the intrathecal administration of K receptor agonists.

A role of endogenous opioids in the control of micturition has been suggested by the effects of the opioid antagonist, naloxone (de Groat *et al.* 1986; Maggi and Meli 1986). The administration of naloxone systemically, intrathecally, intracerebroventricularly, or by microinjection into the pontine micturition centre facilitates the micturition reflex. In low doses, naloxone reduces the bladder volume necessary to evoke micturition. Naloxone also increases the frequency and magnitude of low-amplitude pressure waves on the tonus limb of the cystometrogram in chloralose-anaesthetized cats. These pressure waves are similar to uninhibited contractions seen in patients with hyperactive bladder reflexes. Injection of small doses of naloxone into the pontine micturition centre of decerebrate cats also lowers the micturition threshold. In high doses, the drug produces sustained contractions of the bladder and firing on bladder postganglionic nerves. The effect is noted in anaesthetized animals with an intact neuraxis and in decerebrate unanaesthetized animals. In acute spinal animals where the spinobulbospinal micturition reflex pathway is interrupted, naloxone does not induce reflex bladder contractions, but does unmask the C-fibre afferent evoked spinal reflex (de Groat *et al.* 1990).

However, in chronic paraplegic cats and rats that exhibit automatic micturition, naloxone administered systematically or injected intrathecally induces rhythmic bladder contractions, as well as spontaneous urination, and facilitates somato-bladder reflexes (de Groat *et al.* 1986). These data indicate that the spinal pathways mediating micturition in paraplegic cats are also under a tonic encephalinergic inhibitory control. This is in contrast to normal animals where intrathecal naloxone does not change bladder capacity. Thus, bladder capacity in normal animals appears to be controlled by encephalinergic mechanisms in the brain, whereas in paraplegic animals this function shifts to the spinal cord.

Naloxone also affects bladder function in man. In normal patients, a significant rise in intravesical pressure (i.e. decreased bladder compliance) has been noted during cystometry following naloxone. Naloxone also increases instability during cystometry in patients with incomplete suprasacral spinal cord lesions, reducing by approximately one-third the bladder volume necessary to induce micturition. These data suggest that endogenous encephalinergic mechanisms in the brain and spinal cord have an important role in regulating the storage and release of urine.

Vasoactive intestinal polypeptide (VIP)

In the cat VIP is present in a large percentage (25 per cent) of bladder afferent neurons in the sacral dorsal root ganglia and is contained exclusively in C-fibre afferents (de Groat 1987). These data coupled with the observation that C-fibre afferents initiate micturition reflexes in paraplegic cats prompted an investigation of the effects of VIP on bladder reflex pathways. In normal cats intrathecal injections of VIP (1–10 μg) depressed reflex bladder contractions and firing on bladder postganglionic nerves. On the other hand, in chronic spinal cats small doses of VIP (0.1–1 μg) facilitated bladder activity, whereas large doses (2–10 μg) still depressed activity (de Groat *et al.* 1990). In chronic spinal cats, VIP-ergic afferent fibres also exhibited a significantly broader distribution in lateral lamina I of the spinal dorsal horn. These data are consistent with the concept of afferent axonal sprouting following spinal cord injury and suggest that the actions of a putative C-fibre afferent transmitter change in concert with the emergence of C-fibre evoked micturition reflexes in paraplegic animals.

Gamma aminobutyric acid (GABA)

Injections of GABA agonists intracerebroventricularly into the pontine micturition centre or intrathecally inhibit the micturition reflex. Bicuculline, a GABA-A receptor antagonist, administered into the pontine micturition centre in decerebrate unanaesthetized cats, blocks the inhibitory effects of GABA agonists and also decreases the bladder volume threshold for inducing micturition. The latter data indicates that GABAergic inhibitory mechanisms in the pons are involved in regulating bladder capacity (Fig. 8.8).

GABA also inhibits bladder reflex pathways when applied to the sacral spinal cord. Baclofen, a GABA-B receptor agonist, which mimics the inhibitory effect of GABA has been used clinically via intrathecal administration in patients with hyperactive bladders to suppress bladder activity and to promote urine storage.

5-hydroxytryptamine

5-hydroxytryptamine may also have a transmitter role in central pathways to the lower urinary tract since the lumbosacral sympathetic and parasympathetic autonomic centres receive a dense serotonergic input from the raphe nuclei in the caudal brainstem. In addition, the systemic administration of the serotonergic precursor, 5-hydroxytryptophan, inhibits the parasympathetic micturition reflex and facilitates the vesicosympathetic urine-storage reflex (de Groat *et al.* 1979). In the rat *m*-chlorophenyl-piperazine, a $5-HT_{IC}$ receptor agonist, inhibits bladder reflexes (Steers and de Groat 1989). Since electrical stimulation of the serotonergic neurons in raphe nuclei also inhibits bladder activity (Torrens and Morrison 1987), it is possible that bulbospinal serotonergic pathways are involved in modulating the micturition reflex.

Other putative transmitters

The role of other transmitters in reflex pathways to the lower urinary tract is less clear. For example, exogenous glutamic acid and dopamine injected into the pontine micturition centre facilitate bladder reflexes, whereas injections of cholinergic muscarinic receptor agonists inhibit the reflexes. Further studies are necessary to determine whether endogenously released substances can duplicate these effects. Preliminary experiments focusing on this question have revealed that in cats and rats the systemic administration of MK 801, a substance that blocks glutamate–NMDA channels (NMDA, *N*-methyl-D-aspartate), increases bladder capacity and inhibits reflex bladder contractions. These data implicate glutamic acid as an excitatory transmitter at some point in the micturition reflex pathway, although the specific site is uncertain.

Innervation of sexual organs

In man the physiological changes initiated by erotic stimuli are divided into four distinct phases (excitement, plateau, orgasm, and resolution) which

William C. de Groat

Table 8.3. Male sexual reflexes

Response	Afferent nerves	Efferent nerves	Central pathway	Effector organ
Penile erection				
Reflexogenic	Pudendal nerve	Sacral parasympathetic	Sacral spinal reflex	Dilatation of arterial supply to corpus cavernosum and corpus spongiosum
Psychogenic	Auditory, imaginative, visual,	Sacral parasympathetic, lumbar sympathetic	Supraspinal origin	
Glandular secretion	Pudendal nerve	Sacral parasympathetic, lumbar sympathetic	Sacral spinal reflex	Seminal vesicles and prostate
Seminal emission	Pudendal nerve	Lumbar sympathetic	Intersegmental spinal reflex (sacrolumbar)	Contraction of vas deferens, ampulla, seminal vesicles, prostate, and closure of bladder neck
Ejaculation	Pudendal nerve	Somatic efferents in pudendal nerve	Sacral spinal reflex	Rhythmic contractions of bulbocavernosus and ischiocavernosus muscles

are designated collectively the sexual response cycle. Although anatomical differences obviously preclude identical responses in male and female during each phase of the cycle it is clear that similar secretory responses (vaginal lubrication, prostatic and bulbourethral gland secretion), vascular responses (penile and clitoral erection), and responses of smooth and striated muscles occur in both sexes (Table 8.3). This section will review experimental studies in animals which examined the neural mechanisms regulating these physiological responses.

Innervation

The sex organs like the lower urinary tract receive an innervation from three sets of nerves: sacral parasympathetic (pelvic); thoracolumbar sympathetic (hypogastric and lumbar sympathetic chain); and somatic (pudendal) nerves (Fig. 8.1; Elbadawi and Goodman 1980; de Groat and Steers 1988, 1990; Sachs and Meisel 1988).

Parasympathetic pathways

Preganglionic axons arising from neurons in the sacral spinal cord provide an excitatory input to parasympathetic ganglion cells (Fig. 8.9) in the pelvic plexus which in turn innervate: (1) erectile tissue in the penis and clitoris; (2) smooth muscle and glandular tissue in the prostate, urethra, seminal vesicles, vagina, and uterus; and (3) blood vessels and possibly secretory epithelia in various structures. Among the numerous sexual functions controlled by the sacral parasympathetic pathway, the one which has attracted the most research interest and for which there is the most detailed information is penile erection.

Since the initial observation by Eckhard in 1863 that electrical stimulation of the pelvic nerves in the dog produced penile erection, the mechanisms involved in erection have been investigated in various species. It is clear that parasympathetic neural activity induces vasodilatation in penile blood vessels and increases blood flow to the cavernous tissue (de Groat and Steers 1988; Lue and Tanagho 1988). However, the mechanisms underlying the vasodilatation and the transmitters mediating the response are still being investigated. Two putative transmitter mechanisms, cholinergic and peptidergic, are currently receiving the most attention.

Cholinergic mechanisms

Although acetylcholine (ACh) has been identified as a transmitter at many parasympathetic postganglionic neuroeffector junctions and acetylcholinesterase-containing nerves (presumably cholinergic) are present in the penis, the role of ACh in the penile erection has been questioned. This is based on the lack of convincing and consistent pharmacological data.

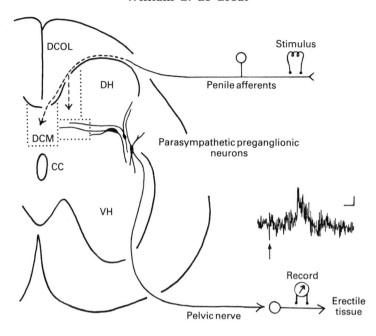

Fig. 8.9. Diagram showing the reflex pathway for inducing penile erection. Horseradish peroxidase axonal tracing studies in the cat have shown the relationship between sacral parasympathetic preganglionic neurons and afferent projections from the penis. Penile afferents in the pudendal nerve project to the medial side of the dorsal horn (DH) and the dorsal commissure (DCM) in the S2 segment of the spinal cord. Preganglionic neurons send dendrites into regions of afferent termination. Dorsal column (DCOL), ventral horn (VH), and central canal (CC). In the rat electrical stimulation of the penile afferents in the dorsal nerve of the penis elicits reflex firing in efferent pathways to the penis. Inset is an example of a reflex discharge in parasympathetic postganglionic axons in penile nerves. The reflexes which occur at a long latency (mean 75 ms) are present in normal and chronic spinal rats and are blocked by section of the pelvic nerve. Stimulus marked by arrow. Horizontal calibration 20 ms, vertical calibration 10 μV.

For example, in some species atropine, a muscarinic cholinergic antagonist, reduces but does not completely block penile erections, whereas in other species, including man, it has no effect on erections (de Groat and Steers 1988). Furthermore, the local administration of exogenous ACh increases penile volume in some species but has never been shown to induce complete erections.

In vitro studies on isolated cavernosal smooth muscle also provide some support for a cholinergic mechanism in erection. Studies in the rabbit reveal that ACh relaxes cavernosal muscle strips first contracted by noradrenaline.

The relaxation is blocked by atropine, indicating that muscarinic receptors can mediate a relaxation of penile smooth muscle. ACh-induced relaxation also occurs *in vitro* in human corpus cavernosal tissue. In addition, electrical field stimulation of the tissue elicits a relaxation which is potentiated by physostigmine, an anticholinesterase drug, and which is partially blocked by atropine. These studies suggest that cholinergic neurotransmission plays an important though not exclusive role in the relaxation of corpus cavernosal smooth muscle.

The relaxant actions of exogenous ACh on penile smooth muscle may be indirect via the release of endogenous substances which in turn activate second messenger systems in the smooth muscle cells (Burnstock 1986; de Groat and Steers 1988). It is known that the actions of exogenous ACh on large arteries are dependent upon the release of endothelial-derived relaxing factor (EDRF) from endothelial cells. EDRF stimulates guanylate cyclase which increases the intracellular levels of cyclic guanosine monophosphate (cGMP) leading to relaxation of the smooth muscle. cGMP has been implicated in neurally evoked relaxation of bovine and canine penile arteries as well as bovine penile smooth muscle.

Peptidergic mechanisms

The identification of neuropeptides as mediators of non-cholinergic, non-adrenergic transmission at various sites in the mammalian peripheral nervous system (Burnstock 1986) has focused attention on the possible role of these agents in the vasodilator pathways to the penis. Several substances, including VIP, substance P, and neuropeptide Y, have been identified in nerves supplying the penile vasculature (Burnstock 1986). Among these peptides VIP is the most promising transmitter candidate. VIP immunoreactivity in penile nerves in human, monkey, and dog is associated with large, dense, core vesicles which are located in varicosities containing small clear, presumably cholinergic vesicles (Burnstock 1986; de Groat and Steers 1988). These findings are consistent with immunocytochemical results in the rat demonstrating that cholinergic pelvic ganglion cells projecting to the penis contain VIP. Additional evidence for a role of VIP in penile erection includes experiments in which local administration of VIP to man, monkey, or dog increased penile volume. VIP also induces relaxation of *in vitro* preparations of corpus cavernosum, corpus spongiosum smooth muscle, and penile blood vessels from many species. Finally, an increase in VIP concentration occurs in the venous effluent of the penis of man and dog during psychogenically, drug, or electrically induced erections.

The effect of VIP in penile erectile tissue may involve several mechanisms. Direct relaxation of smooth muscle may be mediated by increased levels of cAMP. In addition, VIP could facilitate muscarinic cholinergic transmission in the penis as it does in other organs such as the salivary gland and autonomic ganglia. Since VIP and ACh are co-localized in the penile nerves it is possible that a synergistic interaction between these two transmitters occurs during erection.

Sympathetic pathways

Sympathetic pathways to the reproductive organs follow three routes: (1) the hypogastric nerves; (2) the pelvic nerves; and (3) the pudendal nerves (Fig. 8.1). The sympathetic nerves provide an input to penile and clitoral erectile tissue and to blood vessels throughout the reproductive organs as well as to smooth muscle of the ductus deferens, seminal vesicles, prostate, vagina, and uterus (Elbadawi and Goodman 1980; Sachs and Meisel 1988).

Sympathetic postganglionic neurons are thought to release primarily noradrenaline; however, other substances, such as ACh, ATP, and neuropeptides, have also been identified as transmitters in these neurons (Burnstock 1986).

Sympathetic inputs to the erectile tissue can initiate tumescence as well as detumescence by release of different transmitters (de Groat and Steers 1988). Inputs from the caudal sympathetic chain ganglia, which contain noradrenaline and possibly neuropeptide Y, produce vasoconstriction of penile blood vessels and detumescence via actions on α-adrenergic and peptidergic receptors. On the other hand, inputs from the hypogastric nerve which pass through ganglionic relay stations in the pelvic plexus can produce vasodilatation and penile erection as well as detumescence. Pharmacological experiments indicate that ACh and non-cholinergic transmitters, such as VIP, mediate the erectile response.

Sympathetic nerves provide excitatory inputs to the ductus deferens, seminal vesicles, prostate, vaginal, and uterine smooth muscle (Elbadawi and Goodman 1980). These excitatory responses are mediated by an action of noradrenaline on α-adrenoceptors. In the ductus deferens and seminal vesicles a second excitatory transmitter, ATP, is coreleased with noradrenaline and acts on non-adrenergic, purinergic receptors (Burnstock 1986).

Somatic pathways

The pudendal nerves arising from the lumbosacral segments of the spinal cord provide efferent excitatory input to the bulbocavernosus and ischiocavernosus muscles (Fig. 8.1). These muscles are responsible for ejaculation in the male and contribute to the rhythmic perineal contractions during orgasm in the female (Levin 1980). In many species, including cat, monkey, and man, the motoneurons innervating these muscles are located in Onuf's nucleus, whereas in the rat they are located in a separate nucleus in the medial part of the ventral horn.

In rat, dog, and man the bulbocavernosus nucleus is sexually dimorphic, males having a considerably larger number of motoneurons than females (de Groat and Steers 1988). This sexual dimorphism has been attributed to the trophic influence of androgens during neonatal development. Androgens also have an influence in adult animals. For example, castration in the adult rat and dog produces a dramatic decrease in somal size and dendritic length of bulbocavernosus motoneurons. The changes are reversed by the administration of testosterone. These data are consistent with behavioural studies in the rat which show that sexual reflexes in rats are influenced by the actions of androgen on neural elements in the spinal cord.

Afferent pathways

Afferent pathways to the penis, clitoris, and vagina are present in the pudendal nerves (Levin 1980). Afferent pathways to deeper structures such as the uterine cervix and uterine horns are present in the pelvic and hypogastric nerves, respectively. Cervical afferent neurons are located primarily in the sacral dorsal root ganglia, whereas uterine horn afferent neurons are located primarily in the upper lumbar dorsal root ganglia. Electrophysiological studies have shown that afferents from the penis respond to tactile stimuli, whereas the great majority of afferents from the uterus are of the polymodal type which respond to non-noxious and noxious mechanical and chemical stimuli.

Substance P and CGRP are present in a considerable proportion of the afferent neurons innervating the genital organs (de Groat 1987). For example, it has been estimated that 45–80 per cent of the lumbosacral dorsal root ganglia cells innervating the female genital tract contain CGRP. VIP is present in a large percentage (70 per cent) of the sacral afferent neurons innervating the uterine cervix of the cat. At many sites the two peptides are co-localized in the same neuron and, therefore, may function as cotransmitters in afferent pathways to the genital organs.

Peptidergic axons are associated with blood vessels, non-vascular smooth muscle, and squamous and glandular epithelium. In the female the most prominent substance P–CGRP innervation occurs in the vagina. In the male, where substance P and CGRP fibres are less dense, they are located in the glans penis, ductus deferens, seminal vesicles, and epididymides (de Groat 1987).

Central reflex mechanisms controlling the sexual organs

Erection

Penile erection is primarily an involuntary or reflex phenomenon that can be elicited by a variety of reflexogenic and psychogenic stimuli and by at least two distinct central mechanisms (i.e spinal and supraspinal) (Table 8.3) which probably act synergistically (de Groat and Steers 1988). The central control of clitoral erection is likely to be mediated by similar mechanisms but has not been studied in detail (Levin 1980).

Reflexogenic erections

Reflexogenic penile erections, which are elicited by exteroceptive stimulation of the genital regions, are mediated by a sacral spinal reflex pathway having an afferent limb in the pudendal nerve and an efferent limb in the sacral parasympathetic nerves (Table 8.3; Fig. 8.9; de Groat and Steers 1988). The central organization of the reflex pathway has been studied in several species of animals. Axonal tracing techniques have revealed that pudendal afferent pathways from the penis of the cat and rat terminate in the medial dorsal horn and dorsal commissure (Fig. 8.9). Interneurons in these regions are activated by tactile stimulation of the penis and presumably are involved in transmitting sensations to the brain in addition to activating parasympathetic preganglionic neurons which induce erection. The preganglionic neurons are located in the intermediolateral nucleus of the sacral spinal cord and send dendritic projections into areas of laminae V–VII and the dorsal commissure which receive afferent input from the penis (Fig. 8.9). Thus the afferent and efferent components of the reflex pathway are in close proximity.

In the rat electrical stimulation of the dorsal nerve of the penis evokes several long latency (mean 75 ms) reflex discharges in postganglionic axons passing from the major pelvic ganglion into the penile nerves (Steers *et al.* 1988; Steers and de Groat 1989; Fig. 8.9). Since some of these reflexes are obtained in both normal and chronic spinal rats and are eliminated by transection of the pelvic nerves, it is clear that they are mediated by a polysynaptic spinal reflex pathway involving efferent neurons in the sacral autonomic outflow.

In the rat penile afferents also project into the ventral horn and appear to make contacts with the soma and dendrites of motoneurons. These connections could be involved in the somatic reflex mechanisms involved in copulation.

Psychogenic erections

Psychogenic erections are initiated by supraspinal centres in response to auditory, visual, olfactory, and imaginative stimuli. The efferent limb of the reflex pathway traverses both the thoracolumbar and the sacral autonomic outflow (Table 8.3). Studies conducted in monkeys and rats indicate that hypothalamic and limbic pathways play a key role in erection and that the medial preoptic–anterior hypothalamic area is an important integrating centre (de Groat and Steers 1988). Electrical stimulation at this site produces full erections in anaesthetized and unanaesthetized animals, whereas lesions at the same site generally suppress sexual behaviour.

Efferent pathways from the medial preoptic area enter the medial forebrain bundle and then pass caudally into the midbrain tegmental region near the lateral part of the substantia nigra. Caudal to the midbrain the efferent pathway for erection travels in the ventrolateral pons and medulla and then in the lateral funiculus of the spinal cord. Descending projections from the hypothalamic nuclei terminate in lumbosacral spinal autonomic and somatic centres involved in erection (Fig. 8.7).

Secretion

During the first and second phases of the sexual response cycle, activity in parasympathetic and sympathetic pathways in the male stimulates mucus secretion from the bulbourethral and Littre's glands and secretion from the seminal vesicles and prostate gland (Table 8.3). ACh has been implicated as an efferent transmitter since cholinomimetic agents mimic neurally evoked secretion from some glands.

In the female, erotic stimuli elicit vaginal lubrication and mucus secretion from Bartholin's glands (Levin 1980). Vaginal lubrication is thought to be secondary to increased vaginal blood flow and possibly changes in capillary permeability leading to increased formation of plasma transudate which passes through the epithelium to the vaginal surface. An active secretory mechanism is unlikely since the vaginal epithelium is devoid of glands. VIP has been implicated as the efferent transmitter in vaginal lubrication and increased vaginal blood flow.

Emission–ejaculation

The third phase of the sexual act (orgasm) in the male, which is accompanied by emission and ejaculation of semen, involves the co-ordination of autonomic and somatic reflex mechanisms at different levels of the lumbo-sacral spinal cord. During the first step in the process (emission) reflex activity in the thoracolumbar sympathetic outflow elicits rhythmic con-tractions of the smooth muscle of the seminal vesicles, prostate, ductus deferens, and ampulla resulting in the ejection of sperm and glandular secretions into the urethra and at the same time closure of the vesical neck to prevent backflow of semen into the bladder. Pharmacological studies have shown that these responses are mediated by the adrenergic transmitter noradrenaline acting on α-adrenoceptors and by the purinergic transmitter, ATP. Seminal emission may be modulated also by cholinergic nerves which can block the release of adrenergic transmitters (Burnstock 1986).

After emission of semen into the proximal urethra, rhythmic contractions of the bulbocavernosus, ischiocavernosus, and periurethral striated muscles result in ejaculation. The afferent and efferent limbs of the ejaculatory reflex are contained in the pudendal nerve. The sensations accompanying ejaculation, or rhythmic vaginal contractions in the female, represent a major component of the orgasmic response (Levin 1980).

Neurotransmitters in sexual reflex pathways

Pharmacological studies in animals have implicated many neurotransmitter systems in the central control of sexual function. The literature relevant to this topic is extensive (Bitran and Hull 1987; Sachs and Meisel 1988; de Groat and Steers 1988, 1990; Hemmie *et al.* 1990) and will be summarized very briefly in this section.

Monoamines

The monoaminergic transmitters (5-hydroxytryptamine, dopamine, and noradrenaline) appear to have varied roles in the central mechanisms underlying sexual behaviour. For example, pharmacological blockade or destruction of the 5-hydroxytryptamine (5-HT) containing pathways in the brain facilitates sexual activity in male rats and rabbits, whereas the administration of a 5-HT precursor decreases sexual activity. These data indicate that 5-HT pathways in the brain exert a general depressant effect on sexual motivation. However, other studies imply that, at the level of the spinal cord, 5-HT mechanisms facilitate seminal emission, but have mixed effects on penile erection in the rat.

The effects of 5-HT in the CNS are due to an action on a variety of 5-HT receptors broadly classified as either 5-HT_1 or 5-HT_2. The 5-HT_1 receptors are further subdivided into 5-HT_{1A}, 5-HT_{1B}, 5-HT_{1C}, and 5-HT_{1D}. Systemically administered 5-HT_{1A} or 5-HT_2 agonists or 5-HT releasing agents inhibit penile erection (see Bitran and Hull 1987; de Groat and Steers 1988; Steers and de Groat 1989 for reviews) but stimulate emission and ejaculation in rats. However, the 5-HT_{1C} agonists, *m*-chlorophenylpiperazine (mCPP) and MK212, induce penile erections in rats and primates (Hemmie *et al.* 1990; Berensen and Broekkamp 1987; Steers and de Groat 1989) but do not affect emission or ejaculation. Electrophysiological analysis of the effect of mCPP on penile erections in the rat has revealed that this agent elicits efferent discharges on the penile nerve accompanied by a rise in intracavernous pressure (Steers and de Groat 1988). This firing is abolished by pelvic nerve transection and 5-HT antagonists, but remains after acute and chronic thoracic spinal cord transection indicating an action at the level of the spinal cord.

Noradrenergic pathways exert an inhibitory influence on sexual function. Clonidine, a centrally acting α_2-adrenoceptor agonist, inhibits erections and copulatory activity in rats. The inhibitory effects of clonidine are reversed by yohimbine, an α_2-adrenoceptor antagonist. The administration of yohimbine alone increases sexual motivation suggesting that sexual activity is tonically inhibited by a noradrenergic pathway.

Dopaminergic pathways have a facilitatory effect on male copulatory behaviour in the rat. Administration of L-dopa, a precursor of dopamine, or the administration of dopamine receptor agonists increases mounting, intromissions, and ejaculations in male rats. On the other hand, lesions of the dopamine system in rats depress copulatory behaviour. In rhesus monkeys, apomorphine, a dopamine receptor agonist, and quinelorane, a D_2 dopamine receptor agonist, facilitate penile erections.

Neuropeptides and GABA

Oxytocin, a neuropeptide which is present in efferent pathways from the hypothalamus to spinal autonomic centres facilitates penile erectile mechanisms in the rat when administered in nanogram quantities into the cerebral ventricles. On the other hand, the opioid peptides and GABA inhibit copulatory behaviour when administered into the brain of male rats, whereas the administration of receptor antagonists for either type of transmitter facilitate copulatory behaviour.

Thus a broad spectrum of neurotransmitters seem to be involved in the control of sexual behaviour in the rodent. It is uncertain whether these findings are generally applicable to man. However, the susceptibility of human sexual function to a broad range of drugs suggests that sexual behaviour in humans, as in rodents, depends on a variety of neurochemical mechanisms.

References

Berendsen, H. H. G. and Broekkamp, C. L. E. (1987). Drug-induced erections in male rats: indications of serotonin$_{1B}$ receptor mediation. *Eur. J. Pharmacol.* **135**, 279–87.

Berendsen, H. H. G., Jenck, F., and Brockkamp, C. L. E. (1990). Involvement of 5-HT$_{1C}$-receptors in drug-induced penile erections in rats. *Psychopharmacology* **101**, 57–61.

Bitran, D. and Hull, E. M. (1987). Pharmacological analysis of male rat sexual behavior. *Neurosci. biochem. Rev.* **11**, 365–89.

Burnstock G. (1986). The changing face of autonomic neurotransmission. *Acta physiol. scand.* **126**, 67–91.

de Groat, W. C. (1986). Spinal cord projections and neuropeptides in visceral afferent neurons. In *Visceral sensation. Progress in brain research*, Vol. 67 (ed. F. Cervero and J. F. B. Morrison), pp. 165–87. Elsevier, Holland.

de Groat, W. C. (1987) Neuropeptides in pelvic afferent pathways. *Experientia* **43**, 801–12.

de Groat, W. C. and Steers, W. D. (1988). The neuroanatomy and neurophysiology of penile erection. In *Impotence and infertility* (ed. E. A. Tanagho, T. F. Lue, and D. D. McClure), pp. 3–27. Williams & Wilkins, Blatimore, Maryland.

de Groat, W. C. and Steers, W. D. (1990). Autonomic regulation of the urinary bladder and sex organs. In *Central regulation of autonomic functions* (ed A. D. Loewy and K. M. Spyer), pp. 310–33. Oxford University Press, Oxford.

de Groat, W. C., Booth, A. M., Krier, J., Milne, R. J., Morgan, C., and Nadelhaft, I. (1979). Neural control of the urinary bladder and large intestine. In *Integrative functions of the autonomic nervous system*, Vol. 4 (ed. C. M. Brooks, K. Koizumi, and A. Sato), pp. 50–67. University of Tokyo Press, Japan.

de Groat, W. C., Kawatani, M., Hisamitsu, T., Booth, A. M., Roppolo, J. R., Thor, K., Tuttle, P., and Nagel, J. (1986). Neural control of micturition: the role of neuropeptides. *J. autonom. nerve. Syst.* suppl. 369–87.

de Groat, W. C., Kawatani, M., Hisamitsu, T., Cheng, C.-L, Ma, C.-P., Thor, K., Steers, W., and Roppolo, J. R. (1990). Mechanisms underlying the recovery of urinary bladder function following spinal cord injury. *J. autonom. nerv. Syst.* **30**, 571–8.

Elbadawi, A. and Goodman, D. C. (1980). Autonomic innervation of accessory male genital glands. In *Male accessory sex glands* (ed E. Spring-Mills and E. S. E. Hafez), pp. 101–28. Elsevier, Holland.

Habler, H. J., Jänig, W., and Koltzenburg, M. (1990). Activation of unmyelinated afferent fibres by mechanical stimuli and inflammation of the urinary bladder in the cat. *J. Physiol., London* **425**, 545–62.

Holstege, G. (1987). Some anatomical observations on the projections from the hypothalamus to brainstem and spinal cord: an HRP and autoradiographic tracing study in the cat. *J comp. Neurol.* **260**, 98–126.

Holstege, G., Griffiths, D., DeWall, H., and Dalm, E. (1986). Anatomical and physiological observations in supraspinal control of bladder and urethral sphincter muscles in the cat. *J. comp. Neurol.* **250**, 449–61.

Jänig, W. and Morrison, J. F. B. (1986). Functional properties of spinal visceral afferents supplying abdominal and pelvic organs, with special emphasis on visceral nociception. In *Visceral sensation, Progress in Brain Research*, Vol. 67 (ed. F. Cervero and J. F. B. Morrison), pp. 87–114, Elsevier, Holland.

Keast, J. R. and de Groat, W. C. (1989). Immunohistochemical characterization of pelvic neurons which project to the bladder, colon or penis in rats. *J. comp. Neurol.* **288**, 387–400.

Keast, J., Kawatani, M., and de Groat, W. C. (1990) Sympathetic modulation of cholinergic transmission in cat vesical ganglia is mediated by $\alpha 1$ and $\alpha 2$ adrenoceptors. *Am. J. Physiol.* **258**, R44–R50.

Levin, R. J. (1980). The physiology of sexual function in women. *Clin. Obstet. Gynecol.* **7**, 213–52.

Lue, T. F. and Tanagho, E. A. (1988). Functional anatomy and mechanism of penile erection. In *Contemporary management of impotence and infertility* (ed. E. A. Tanagho, T. F. Lue, and R. D. McClure), pp. 39–50. Williams & Wilkins, Baltimore, Maryland.

Maggi, C. A. and Meli, A. (1986). The role of neuropeptides in the regulation of the micturition reflex. *J. auton. Pharmacol.* **6**, 133–62.

Mallory, B., Steers, W. D., and de Groat, W. C. (1989). Electrophysiological study of micturition reflexes in the rat. *Am. J. Physiol.* **257**, R410–R421.

Morgan, C., Nadelhaft, I., and de Groat, W. C. (1981). The distribution of visceral primary afferents from the pelvic nerve within Lissauer's tract and the spinal gray matter and its relationship to the sacral parasympathetic nucleus. *J. comp. Neurol.* **201**, 415–40.

Nadelhaft, I., Morgan, C., and de Groat, W. C. (1980). Localization of the sacral autonomic nucleus in the spinal cord of the cat by the horseradish peroxidase technique. *J. Comp. Neurol.* **193**, 265–81.

Satoh, K., Shimizu, M., Tohyama, M., and Maeda, T. (1978). Localization of the micturition reflex center at dorsolateral pontine tegmentum of the rat. *Neurosci. Lett.* **8**, 27–33.

Sachs, B. D. and Meisel, R. L. (1988). The physiology of male sexual behavior. In *The physiology of reproduction* (ed. E. Knobil and J. Neill), pp. 1393–482, Raven Press, New York.

Steers, W. D. and de Groat, W. C. (1989). Effects of *m*-chlorophenylpiperazine on penile and bladder function in rats. *Am. J. Physiol.* **257**, R1441–R1449.

Steers, W. D., Mallory, B., and de Groat, W. C. (1988). Electrophysiological study of neural activity in the penile nerve of the rat. *Am. J. Physiol.* **254**, R989–R1000.

Steers, W. D., Ciambotti, J., Erdman, S., and de Groat, W. C. (1990). Morphological plasticity in efferent pathways to the urinary bladder of the rat following urethral obstruction. *J. Neurosci.* **10**, 1943–51.

Thor, K., Morgan, C., Nadelhaft, I., Houston, M., and de Groat, W. C. (1989). Organization of afferent and efferent pathways in the pudendal nerve of the cat. *J. comp. Neurol.* **288**, 263–79.

Torrens, M. and Morrison, J. F. B. (1987). *The physiology of the lower urinary tract.* Springer-Verlag, Berlin.

9. The gut and the autonomic nervous system

Anne E. Aber-Bishop and Julia M. Polak

Introduction

Although under the overriding control of the central nervous system, the gastrointestinal tract is capable of carrying out its functions of food passage, storage, digestion, and absorption after all central connections are severed. Thus, sympathetic denervation has only a transient effect on gut function; denervation of the parasympathetic nervous sytem usually reduces the tone and degree of peristaltic activity but this is eventually compensated for by increased intrinsic excitability of the enteric plexuses. This autonomy of the gastrointestinal tract has been the subject of much interest and speculation in recent years and terms such as 'minibrain' have been used to describe the gut's intrinsic innervation; some indication of the size and importance of the intramural innervation can be gained from the observation that the number of neurons in the human gut is similar to that in the spinal cord (Furness and Costa 1987). Increased interest has centred largely on the recognition that, far from using only the classical autonomic neuro-transmitters, acetylcholine and noradrenaline, the nervous system of the gut employs a myriad of substances, including amines, γ-aminobutyric acid, adenosine triphosphate, and a variety of peptides, to relay information. In fact, neuropeptides are probably the most abundant neurotransmitter type in the gut and are found singly or in combinations with each other and/or acetylcholine and noradrenaline.

This chapter describes the general anatomy of the autonomic nervous system of the gut with particular reference to the peptidergic innervation in normal and disease states and during development.

General anatomy

Sympathetic innervation

Preganglionic fibres from T8 to L3 of the spinal cord pass through the sympathetic chains to synapse with postganglionic neurons in the coeliac and superior and inferior mesenteric ganglia. The postganglionic fibres spread from these ganglia to innervate all parts of the gut. The fibres either innervate their effector organ (i.e. muscle layers, blood vessels, or epithelium) directly or synapse with neurons of the main ganglionated (myenteric or submucous) plexuses.

Parasympathetic innervation

The parasympathetic innervation of the gut is either cranial or sacral in origin. Cranial parasympathetic fibres run mostly in the vagus nerves, whereas sacral nerves originate from S2–S4 of the spinal cord and pass through the nervi erigentes to innervate the lower bowel. The fibres synapse in the intramural plexuses and postganglionic fibres radiate to effector organs including other cells in the plexuses.

Intramural plexuses

Most of the fibres which innervate the gut arise from the intramural plexuses. These plexuses form a complex, heterogeneous part of the autonomic nervous system, as was recognized very early in the work of Langley (1898). There are two main ganglionated plexuses—the myenteric (or Auerbach's), which lies between the longitudinal and circular muscle coats, and the submucous (or Meissner's), lying between the circular muscle and the muscularis mucosae. The myenteric plexus contains most of the intrinsic nerve cell bodies of the gut. It can be subdivided into three parts: the primary, secondary, and tertiary plexuses. The primary plexus is composed of the neuronal cells and bundles of fibres running between them, i.e. the core of the plexus. The secondary component is formed by fibres running from ganglia or connecting branches of the primary plexus, which pass to the muscle, whereas the fine fibres that run between the ganglia and branches of the primary plexus are known as the tertiary plexus. The submucous plexus has sometimes been described as having two components, one by the muscularis mucosae, known as Meissner's plexus, and the other against the circular muscle, called Henle's plexus. However, the lack of apparent functional and structural differentiation between the two means that they are unified in most of the relevant literature. The intramural ganglia supply fibres that either synapse with cells in the same or other ganglia, or innervate a range of effector organs in the gut as well as sending afferents to the central nervous system.

Neurochemistry

A number of functionally different neuronal types have been identified in the intramural plexuses of the gut, mainly on the basis of electrophysiology, and attempts have been made to relate the function and morphology of the cells. The work of Dogiel (1899) describing three morphologically and, he hypothesized, functionally distinct types of gut neurons subsequently has been shown by the investigation of morphofunctional correlations to be remarkably prescient. In particular, this has been achieved by injection of dye into cells previously characterized electrophysiologically (for review see Furness and Costa 1987). Table 9.1 summarizes the current knowledge of the neurons of Dogiel's classification, as studied in the guinea-pig small intestine. There has been much controversy over the value of Dogiel's work but this classification remains a useful basis for neuronal identification. However, it must be noted that not all gut neurons have been found to fit into the classification.

A large number of different substances have been identified, by pharmacological, physiological, or morphological means, in the autonomic nervous system of the mammalian gut. Not all of these substances have been shown as yet to satisfy all the criteria used to identify neurotransmitters. However, what is clear is that a highly complex, heterogeneous transmitter system exists with subtypes of neurons chemically coded by the presence of a specific substance or combination of substances. Different combinations of the same substances can be found in functionally and morphologically distinct neurons (see Table 9.1, for example). For brevity Table 9.2 provides a list of the main established and candidate transmitters that have been identified in enteric nerves.

Acetylcholine and noradrenaline have long been known to be neurotransmitters in the gut and their excitatory and inhibitory influences on gut function are well described. What has emerged in recent years is the realization that these 'classical' neurotransmitters often coexist with other substances in the gut innervation. For example, in the guinea-pig the peptides, cholecystokinin, somatostatin, neuropeptide Y, and substance P, have been localized to cholinergic neurons, identified by immunostaining of the acetylcholine-synthesizing enzyme choline acetyltransferase (Furness and Costa 1987). Similarly, neuropeptide Y has been demonstrated in postganglionic sympathetic neurons supplying the stomach and colon of several species (Ekblad *et al.* 1984; Su *et al.* 1987).

Although adenosine triphosphate (ATP) has been put forward as the main transmitter in inhibitory gastrointestinal neurons it seems, at present, that it is more widely accepted as also being present in other types of neurons and acting as some kind of cotransmitter (Burnstock 1981). Dopamine, a precursor to noradrenaline, has been found in gastrointestinal nerves, but is likely to be related to the sympathetic nerves rather than existing as a separate neurotransmitter (Furness and Costa 1987). Gamma aminobutyric acid (GABA) appears to cause differential modulation of gastrointestinal motility by stimulating cholinergic neurons via GABA-A receptors or reducing cholinergic contractions via the GABA-B subtype (Ong and Kerr 1983). The

Table 9.1. Dogiel's classification

Type	Dogiel's classification*		Function	Electrophysiology (neuron type)‡	Neuropeptides†,§
	Axons	Dendrites			
I	Project through other ganglia to muscle	4–20; short, end within ganglia	Motor	S	Substance P, dynorphin, encephalin, VIP, NPY, GRP, CCK
II	Project to other ganglia	3–10, long	Sensory	AH	Somatostatin, substance P, CCK
III	Termination not traced	2–10; short, end within ganglia	?	S	Somatostatin, dynorphin, VIP, CGRP, NPY, CCK

*Dogiel (1899).
†Furness and Costa (1987).
‡S, fast excitatory postsynaptic potentials (cholinergic); AH, prolonged after-hyperpolarizations.
§CCK, cholecystokinin; VIP, vasoactive intestinal peptide; NPY, neuropeptide Y; GRP, gastrin-releasing peptide; CGRP, calcitonin gene-related peptide.

Table 9.2. Neurochemicals identified in the innervation of the human gut

Acetylcholine (ACh)
Adenosine triphosphate (ATP)
Dopamine
γ-aminobutyric acid (GABA)
Noradrenaline
Peptides
Serotonin (5-hydroxytryptamine (5-HT))

amine has been identified in the myenteric plexus in neurons which seems to innervate other ganglion cells (Jessen *et al.* 1979).

Serotonin (5-hydroxytryptamine) has long been known to act as a transmitter in the central nervous system but its presence in gastrointestinal nerves was a matter of debate prior to the advent of specific antibodies to the amine. A major problem with evaluation of serotonin as a neuro-transmitter is its relatively high concentration in endocrine cells in all areas of the gastrointestinal mucosa. Serotonin has been localized to the intramural plexuses (Furness and Costa 1987) where it has been suggested to contribute to slow potentials in prolonged after-hyperpolarization neurons.

The most widespread and abundant transmitters in the mammalian gut are the neuropeptides. As yet, not all of them satisfy the classical criteria for neurotransmitters, but they do represent a relatively new discovery in the peripheral nervous system; their numbers are continuously expanding and our understanding of them increasing. The rest of this chapter describes current knowledge of this heterogeneous group of substances, with emphasis on the contribution of morphological investigations.

For brevity, a list of the major peptides currently identifiable in the innervation of the mammalian gut is given in Table 9.3, together with information on their origins, known actions, and number of amino acids. The information in the table is based on data derived from human and experimental animal (rat and guinea-pig) tissues.

Morphological studies of gut neuropeptides

Techniques

Localization of neuropeptides: immunocytochemistry

Most of the literature on the localization of neuropeptides in the gut concerns the application of immunocytochemistry at light or electron microscopical levels. Several immunocytochemical techniques exist and those for light microscopy can be divided broadly into transmitted light methods or

Table 9.3. Major gut neuropeptides

Peptides*	No. of amino acids	Main actions	Main origin(s)
Bombesin (GRP)	27	Multiple stimulatory effects, e.g. gastrin release	Local
CGRP	37	Gastric acid secretion, muscle constriction	Local and sensory
CCK8	8	Not known	Local
Dynorphin	17	Opiate effects	Local
Endothelin-1	21	Vasoconstriction	Local
Galanin	29	Muscle constriction	Local
Leu-encephalin	5	Opiate effects	Local
Met-encephalin	5	Opiate effects	Local
Neuromedin U	8 or 25	Muscle constriction, vasoconstriction	Local
NPY	36	Vasoconstriction	Local and sympathetic
PACAP	38	Adenylate cyclase activation	Local
PHM	27	Muscle relaxation, secretion	Local
Somatostatin	28	Multiple inhibitory effects e.g. gastrin inhibition	Local
Substance P	11	Vasodilatation, muscle constriction	Local and sensory
VIP	28	Vasodilatation, muscle relaxation, secretion	Local

*CGRP, calcitonin gene-related peptide; GRP, gastrin-releasing peptide; NPY, neuropeptide Y; PACAP, pituitary adenylate cyclase activating peptide; PHM, peptide histidine methionine; VIP, vasoactive intestinal polypeptide.

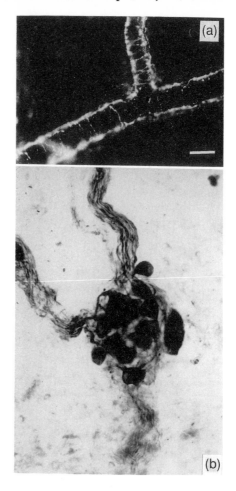

Fig. 9.1. Immunostained peptide-containing nerves in whole mount preparations of the human large bowel. (a) Neuropeptide Y-immunoreactive fibres around a blood vessel in the submucous layer (indirect immunofluorescence). (b) Vasoactive intestinal peptide-immunoreactive ganglion cells and nerve fibres in the submucous plexus (peroxidase antiperoxidase). Scale bar, 50 μm.

fluorescent labelling (for review see Polak and Van Noorden 1986). Of the former, the unlabelled antibody enzyme (peroxidase antiperoxidase) or avidin–biotin complex methods are the most widely used. Fluorescence labelling usually employs an indirect method with fluorescein, rhodamine, or some other fluorescent compound coupled to the secondary antibody. The method of choice is often a matter of personal preference but immunostains visible on transmitted light are permanent and therefore more widely used where

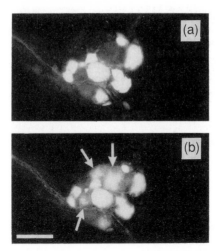

Fig. 9.2. (a) Fluorogold-labelled neurons in a whole mount preparation of the submucous plexus of the human colon after injection of the dye into the submucous layer. (b) Vasoactive-intestinal peptide immunoreactivity in the same specimen. Cells marked with arrows are positive only for immunoreactivity (indirect immunofluorescence). Differential visualization of the dye and immunostain in the same cells was achieved by altering the wavelength of observation light. Scale bar, 50 μm.

quantitative image analysis is required. Immunostains of neuropeptides can be made on tissue sections or on whole mount preparations of intact layers of the gut, e.g. intramural plexuses (Fig. 9.1) or muscle layers. Co-localization of neuropeptides is achieved using serial sectioning through ganglion cells or by administering antibodies to separate neuropeptides, labelled with different colours, to the same section.

Similarly, for electron microscopy a number of methods exist for immunostaining of vesicles containing neuropeptides (and other antigens), the most popular of which are those which employ gold-labelled antibodies. Colloidal gold adsorbs on to the Fc portion of the IgG molecule and is electron-dense. The immunogold staining technique is a straightforward indirect method (De Mey *et al.* 1981; Fig. 9.3) which has been adapted to allow immunostaining of multiple antigens in a single tissue section by the use of antibodies labelled with gold particles of different sizes.

Localization of neuropeptide gene expression: in situ *hybridization*

Immunocytochemistry localizes the final products of gut nerves but information on the sites, rates, and control of neuropeptide gene expression can now be derived from histological preparations using *in situ* hybridization of DNA or RNA species directing neuropeptide synthesis (for review see Polak and McGee 1990). This technique utilizes the capacity of labelled complementary nucleic acid sequences to form stable hybrids with endogenous DNA or mRNA. The complementary sequences, in the form of single-stranded DNA or RNA, double-stranded DNA, or synthetic oligodeoxyribonucleotides, can be labelled with isotopes (e.g. ^{32}P, ^{35}S, ^{3}H, etc.) and localized by autoradiography or with substances subsequently localized by immunocytochemistry (e.g. biotin, digoxigenin).

Morphological studies of gut neuropeptides

Applications

Neural origins

The nature and projections of neuropeptide-containing gut nerves have been studied extensively in experimental animals. Chemical manipulations in combination with immunocytochemistry can help to identify particular nerve types containing neuropeptides. For example, immunostaining of neuropeptide Y (NPY) in rats treated with 6-hydroxydopamine shows a loss of NPY-immunoreactive fibres from around gut blood vessels, suggesting that these are noradrenergic sympathetic nerves (Su *et al.* 1987). Similarly, destruction of primary sensory afferents by administration of capsaicin (8-methyl-*N*-vanillyl-5-nonenamide) removes a proportion of calcitonin gene-related peptide (CGRP)- and substance P-immunoreactive fibres from the rat gut, indicating their sensory nature (Su *et al.* 1987).

Analysis of the origin and projection fields of neuropeptide-containing innervation of the gut requires further manipulations, in the form of surgical interruption of nerve pathways or retrograde tracing using dyes. Interruption of pathways has been a useful way of establishing nerve origins. To continue with the example of NPY-containing nerves, sympathectomy by removal of the coeliac ganglion and plexus and the superior mesenteric ganglion reduces the population of nerves in the rat gut in a similar way to administration of 6-hydroxydopamine (Su *et al.* 1987). Lesioning of pathways can also be used to study neural projections within the gut wall. Myotomy, myectomy, and homotopic autotransplants, with immunocytochemical identification of nerve types, have been used successfully to provide detailed information on the projections of neuropeptide-immunoreactive nerves in certain species and the most complete analysis of neuronal circuitry of the mammalian gut has been achieved by application of these methods in the guinea-pig small intestine (for review see Furness and Costa 1987). However, a less invasive method is retrograde tracing of neuronal pathways, which has the major advantage of being applicable in specimens of human gut, thereby yielding information with direct relevance to clinical gastroenterology. Retrograde tracing uses the ability of nerves to transport dyes retrogradely to their perikarya and consists of injection of a suitable chemical (e.g. horseradish peroxidase,

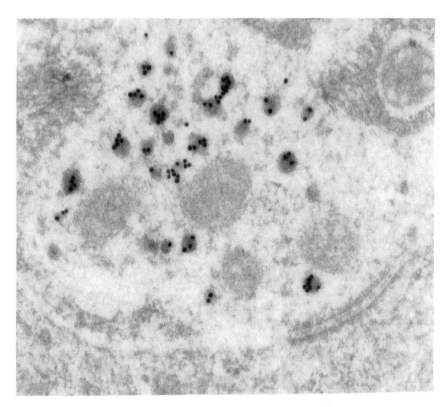

Fig. 9.3. Immunoreactivity for substance P demonstrated in granules in a nerve terminal in guinea-pig colon using the indirect immunogold method. Magnification, 10 000 ×.

radiolabelled amino acids, fluorescent dyes) *in vivo* to the terminal region of interest which is taken up and labels the cell of origin (for review see Su and Polak 1987). This is then identified by neuropeptide immunocytochemistry. In this way, sympathetic, NPY-immunoreactive nerves supplying, for example, the rat stomach have been shown to arise from perikarya in the coeliac and inferior mesenteric ganglia whereas sensory CGRP-immunoreactive fibres are supplied by bilateral dorsal root ganglia at levels T8–T11 (Su *et al.* 1987).

A recent refinement of this technology has been to apply it *in vitro* to study human enteric neural pathways. Injection of a new fluorescent dye, Fluorogold, into human colon maintained *in vitro*, combined with fluorescein immunofluorescence on whole mount preparations, was used to study the projection field of vasoactive intestinal polypeptide (VIP)-containing nerves in three dimensions (Domoto *et al.* 1990) and, thus, provide an entirely new means to study human gut neuroanatomy (Fig. 9.2).

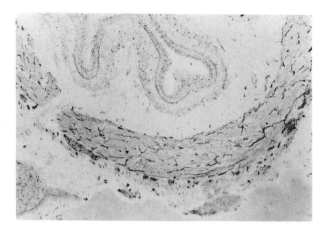

Fig. 9.4. Vasoactive intestinal polypeptide-immunoreactive fibres in the oesophagus of a human fetus (17 weeks gestation). Avidin–biotin complex method; magnification, 100×.

Neuropeptides in the developing human gut

Few studies have been made of neuropeptides in human fetal gut. A recent, comprehensive immunocytochemical study of the ontogeny of major neuropeptides in the human oesophagus revealed their appearance in fibres at 11 (VIP, NPY, gastrin-releasing peptide (GRP)) (Fig. 9.4), 13 (galanin, substance P), 15.5 (somatostatin, met-encephalin), and 18 weeks (CGRP) (Hitchcock *et al.* 1992). Some investigation has been made of the way in which the peptide-containing nerves infiltrate the developing human gut. Traditionally, colonization of the human gut by nerves is considered to occur in a craniocaudal direction, with subsequent passage of neuronal precursors through the muscle to form the major ganglionated plexuses although, in other species, bidirectional migration of neuronal precursors has been detected. Using immunocytochemistry and *in situ* hybridization in combination, the appearance of VIP-containing nerves has been examined in developing human gut (Facer *et al.* 1992). At the earliest stage examined (8 weeks gestation) nerve cells, demonstrated by immunostaining of the general nerve marker protein gene product 9.5, were found throughout the length of the gut, but not transversely. Ganglion cells were first found in both myenteric and submucous plexuses at 9 weeks gestation. VIP immunoreactivity was seen in fibres from 9 weeks gestation but could not be found in perikarya until 18 weeks gestation. With *in situ* hybridization, VIP gene expression in cells was detected much earlier, from 9 weeks gestation, and its temporal appearance was consistent with craniocaudal, transmural neuronal colonization and/or migration (Fig. 9.5).

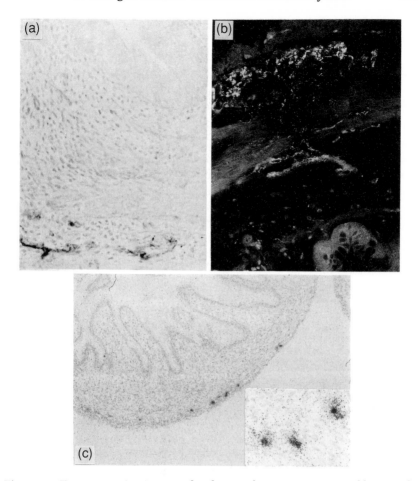

Fig. 9.5. Few vasoactive intestinal polypeptide-immunoreactive fibres in the human fetal colon (9 weeks gestation). Few fibres can be seen in the region of the myenteric plexus. Avidin–biotin complex method; magnification, 250 × . (b) Vasoactive intestinal polypeptide fibres infiltrating the wall of the human fetal small intestine (15 weeks gestation). Indirect immunofluorescence; magnification, 250 × . (c) Groups of silver grains indicating the presence of vasoactive intestinal peptide mRNA detected by *in situ* hybridization in human fetal small intestine (9 weeks gestation). Magnification, 120 × (inset 180 ×).

Neuropeptides in gastrointestinal diseases

Marked abnormalities of the neuropeptide-containing innervation of the gut have been observed in a number of diseases. In view of the rapid breakdown of most neuropeptides, alterations in circulating levels are rare and most changes have been observed on the basis of morphological investigations sometimes coupled with radioimmunological measurement of peptide concentrations in affected tissues.

Constipation

Chagas' disease

Severe disturbance of the normal pattern of neuropeptide-containing nerves has been reported in Chagas' disease, an example of acquired aganglionosis. This disease is a common result of long-standing infection with the flagellate protozoan, *Trypanasoma cruzi*. Ganglionitis occurs in the intramural plexuses with subsequent destruction of cells leading to denervation and distension of gut segments, most commonly manifesting as megaoesophagus and/or megacolon. Comparison with both normal controls and patients with multiple system atrophy (Shy–Drager syndrome) has revealed a reduction in both VIP- and substance P-immunoreactive nerves and tissue content of these neuropeptides only in Chagas' disease (Long *et al.* 1980). Thus the neuropeptides appear to be affected by intrinsic but not extrinsic autonomic neuropathy, indicating that VIP and substance P have mainly intrinsic origins in the human bowel.

A similar reduction in neuropeptides was found in an equine disease, grass sickness, which is in many ways analogous to human Chagas' disease in being acquired aganglionosis, although the pathogenic agent has yet to be identified (Bishop *et al.* 1984).

Idiopathic constipation

The pathogenesis of idiopathic, slow-transit constipation has yet to be clearly defined and, at present, colectomy is often used to treat the condition. Some changes in the morphology of intramural neurons have been noted and a recent study has examined the morphology and concentrations of the three major gut neuropeptides, VIP, substance P, and NPY, in affected bowel (Milner *et al.* 1990). It seems that substance P- and NPY-containing nerves are not altered in the colon of individuals with severe chronic idiopathic constipation, in comparison with normal control bowel. However, VIP content was reduced in the intramural plexuses of the colon, although no consistent alteration of VIP-immunoreactive nerves was seen on immunocytochemistry.

Hirschsprung's disease

In Hirschsprung's disease, or congenital aganglionosis, the neuronal lesions do not appear to be confined to an absence of intramural ganglion cells. Hypertrophied nerve bundles can be observed, often in the serosa or between the longitudinal and circular muscle layers. In addition, alterations of specific nerve types have been noted including increased adrenergic and

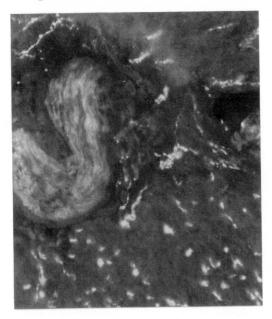

Fig. 9.6. Hyperplastic, numerous neuropeptide Y-immunoreactive fibres in large bowel from a child with Hirschsprung's disease. Indirect immuno-fluorescence; magnification, 350 × .

cholinesterase-positive nerves and loss of intrinsic serotonin-containing nerves. For the neuropeptides, a mixed pattern of changes are seen in aganglionic bowel. VIP- (and its related molecule, peptide histidine methionine), substance P-, met-encephalin-, somatostatin-, and CGRP-immunoreactive nerves are reduced in aganglionic segments, possibly reflecting their mainly intrinsic origin in the human large bowel (Ehrenpreis and Pernow 1953; Tafuri *et al.* 1974; Bishop *et al.* 1981; Hamada *et al.* 1987). In contrast, fibres containing NPY immunoreactivity show a marked increase in aganglionic bowel, particularly in the circular muscle where few such fibres are normally found (Hamada *et al.* 1987; Fig 9.6). As described earlier, NPY-immunoreactive fibres in the gut have a dual origin from intramural ganglion cells and extrinsic noradrenergic nerves and the latter innervate mainly the vasculature and myenteric plexus (Ekblad *et al.* 1984; Su *et al.* 1987). This change in NPY nerves may thus reflect the reported hyperplasia of aminergic fibres in Hirschsprung's disease.

Diabetic neuropathy

Specific alterations of peptide-containing nerves are seen in the enteric neuropathy associated with streptozotocin-induced diabetes mellitus in rats. It has been reported that VIP nerve immunoreactivity increases, whereas

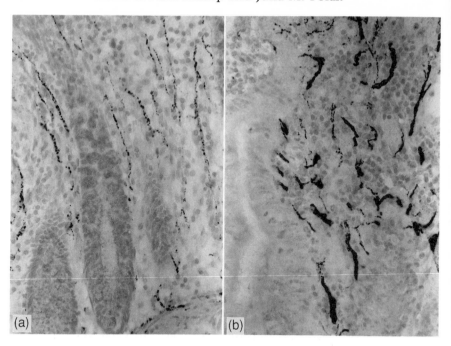

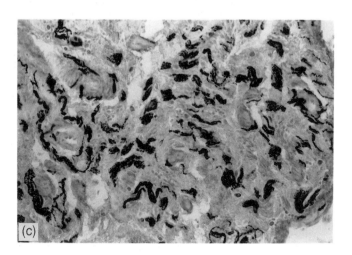

Fig. 9.7. Mucosa from normal human colon with vasoactive intestinal peptide-immunoreactive fibres. Magnification, 380 ×. (b) The same area in colon from a patient with Crohn's disease. The vasoactive intestinal peptide-immunoreactive fibres appear thickened and distorted. Magnification, 380 ×. (c) Fibrosed submucosa from the same patient showing abnormal vasoactive intestinal peptide-immunoreactive nerves Avidin–biotin complex method; magnification, 300 ×.

that of CGRP nerves decreases, whilst substance P- and NPY-immunoreactive nerves remain unchanged (Belai and Burnstock 1990).

Inflammatory bowel disease

Neuronal abnormalities have long been known to occur in Crohn's disease (regional enteritis) and take the form of general nerve proliferation, sometimes termed neuromatous hyperplasia, but their significance remains unknown. Such changes are not characteristic of ulcerative colitis, and it is possible that the transmural inflammatory process that occurs in Crohn's disease stimulates the neural proliferation, as such a stimulus would be absent from all but the most severe cases of ulcerative colitis. No agreement has been reached on the pathology of peptide-containing nerves in inflammatory bowel disease and a variety of different findings has been published (for review see Bishop and Polak 1990). The first study reported that VIP-immunoreactive fibres and the tissue content of VIP is increased in Crohn's disease (ileitis and colitis), in comparison with both ulcerative colitis and normal controls (Fig. 9.7) (Bishop et al. 1980; O'Morain et al. 1984). No evidence has been obtained that these hyperplastic VIP nerves are functional, but it is tempting to speculate that the peptide's potent stimulation of gut secretion and inhibition of motility may contribute to the symptoms of the disease. In contrast, a separate group of researchers reported a reduction of both VIP and substance P nerves in Crohn's disease (Sjolund et al. 1983), whilst the most recent study describes loss of VIP from the mucosa/submucosa in Crohn's and ulcerative colitis and an increase in substance P nerves in ulcerative colitis (Koch et al. 1987). Detailed comparison of the neural changes with histopathology, which was not provided in any of these publications, and investigation of neuropeptide gene expression, using in situ hybridization and/or Northern blotting, may settle this controversy.

Conclusions

The intramural plexuses of the mammalian gut have long been known to form a major part of the autonomic nervous system but their importance has only been recognized comparatively recently with the discovery of their complex neurochemistry and wide range of actions. The application of new techniques for the investigation of gut nerves allows delineation of the neuroanatomy of the gut and is revealing pathological alterations which may provide the basis for future therapeutic measures.

References

Belai, A. and Burnstock, G. (1990). Changes in adrenergic and peptidergic nerves in the submucous plexus of streptozotocin–diabetic rat ileum. *Gastroenterology* **98**, 1427–36.

Bishop, A. E. and Polak, J. M. (1990). Gut endocrine and neural peptides. *Endocrinol. Pathol.* **1**, 4–24.

Bishop, A. E., Polak, J. M., Bryant, M. G., Bloom, S. R., Hamilton, S. (1980). Abnormalities of vasoactive intestinal polypeptide-containing nerves in Crohn's disease. *Gastroenterology* **79**, 853–60.

Bishop, A. E., Polak, J. M., Lake, B. D., Bryant, M. G. and Bloom, S. R. (1981). Abnormalities of the colonic regulatory peptides in Hirschsprung's disease. *Histopathology* **5**, 679–88.

Bishop, A. E., Hodson, N. P., Major, J. H., Probert, L., Yeats, J., Edwards, G. B., Wright, J. A., Bloom, S. R. and Polak, J. M. (1984). The regulatory peptide system of the large bowel in equine grass sickness. *Experientia* **40**, 801–6.

Burnstock, G. (1981). Neurotransmitters and trophic factors in the autonomic nervous system. *J. Physiol.* **313**, 1–35.

De Mey, J., Moeremans, M., Geuens, G., Nuydens, R. and De Brabander, M. (1981). High resolution light and electron microscopic localization of tubulin with the IGS (immunogold staining) method. *Cell Biol. Int. Rep.* **5**, 889–99.

Dogiel, A. S. (1899). Ueber den bau der Ganglien in den Geflechten des Darmes und der Gallenblase des Menschen und der Säugetiere. *Arch. Anat. Physiol. Leipzeig, Anat. Abt.* 130–58.

Domoto, T., Bishop, A. E., Oki, M. and Polak, J. M. (1990). An *in vitro* study of the projections of enteric VIP-immunoreactive neurones in the human colon. *Gastroenterology* **98**, 819–27.

Ehrenpreis, T. and Pernow, B. (1953). On the occurrence of substance P in the rectosigmoid in Hirschsprung's disease. *Acta physiol. scand.* **27**, 380–8

Ekblad, E., Wahlstedt, C., Ekelund, M., Hakanson, R. and Sundler, F. (1984). Neuropeptide Y in the gut and pancreas. Distribution and possible vasomotor function. *Frontiers Horm. Res.* **12**, 85–90.

Facer, P., Bishop, A. E., Moscoso, G., Terenghi, G., Liu, Y. F., Goodman, R. H., Legon, S. and Polak J. M. (1992). Vasoactive intestinal peptide gene expression in the developing human gastrointestinal tract. *Gastroenterology* **102**, 47–55.

Furness, J. B. and Costa, M. (ed.) (1987). *The enteric nervous system.* Churchill Livingstone, Edinburgh.

Hamada, Y., Bishop, A. E., Federici, G., Rivosecchi, M., Talbot, I. C. and Polak, J. M. (1987). Increased neuropeptide Y-immunoreactive innervation of aganglionic bowel in Hirschsprung's disease. *Virchow's Arch.* **A411**, 369–77.

Hitchcock, R. J. I., Pemble, M. J., Bishop, A. E., Spitz, L. and Polak, J. M. (1992). The ontogeny and distribution of neuropeptides in the human fetal and infant oesophagus. *Gastroenterology* **102**, 840–8.

Jessen, K. R., Mirsky, R., Dennison, M. E. and Burnstock, G. (1979). GABA may be a neurotransmitter in the vertebrate peripheral nervous system. *Nature* **281**, 71–4.

Koch, T. R., Carney, J. A., Go, V. L. W. (1987). Distribution and quantification of gut neuropeptides in normal intestine and inflammatory bowel disease. *Digest. Diseases Sci.* **32**, 369–76.

Langley, J. N. (1898) On the union of cranial autonomic (visceral) fibres with the nerve cells of the superior cervical ganglion. *J. Physiol.* **23**, 240–70.

Long, R. G., Bishop, A.E., Barnes, A. J., Albuquerque, R. H., O'Shaughnessey, D. J., McGregor, G. P., Bannister, R., Polak, J. M. and Bloom, S. R. (1980). Neural and hormonal peptides in rectal biopsy specimens from patients with Chagas' disease and chronic autonomic failure. *Lancet* **i**, 559–62.

Milner, P., Crowe, R., Kamm, M. A., Lennard-Jones, J. E. and Burnstock, G. (1990). Vasoactive intestinal polypeptide levels in sigmoid colon in idiopathic constipation and diverticular disease. *Gastroenterology* **99**, 666–75.

O'Morain, C., Bishop, A. E., McGregor, G. P., Levi, A. J., Bloom, S. R., Polak, J. M., and Peters, T. J. (1984). Vasoactive intestinal peptide concentrations and immunocytochemical studies in rectal biopsies from patients with inflammatory bowel disease. *Gut* **25**, 57–61.

Ong, J. and Kerr, D. I. B. (1983). GABA$_A$- and GABA$_B$-receptor-mediated modification of intestinal motility. *Eur. J. Pharmacol.* **86**, 9–17.

Polak, J. M. and McGee, J. O'D. (ed.) (1990). *In situ hybridization.* Oxford University Press, Oxford.

Polak, J. M. and Van Noorden, S. (ed.) (1986). *Immunocytochemistry: modern methods and applications* (2nd edn). John Wright & Sons, Bristol.

Sjolund, K., Schaffalitzky De Muckadell, O. B., Fahrenkrug, J., Hakanson, R., Peterson, B. G., and Sundler, F. (1983). Peptide-containing nerve fibres in the gut wall in Crohn's disease. *Gut* **24**, 724–33.

Su, H. C. and Polak, J. M. (1987). Combined axonal transport tracing and immunocytochemistry for mapping pathways of peptide-containing nerves in the peripheral nervous system. *Experientia* **43**, 761–7.

Su, H. C., Bishop, A. E., Power, R. F., Hamada, Y., and Polak, J. M. (1987). Dual intrinsic and extrinsic origins of CGRP- and NPY-immunoreactive nerves of rat gut and pancreas. *J. Neurosci.* **7**, 2674–87.

Tafuri, W. L., Maria, T. A., Pittella, J. E. and Bogliolo, L. (1974). An electron microscopic study of the Auerbach's plexus and determination of substance P of the colon in Hirschsprung's disease. *Virchow's Arch.* **A362**, 41–50.

10. The kidney and the sympathetic nervous system

Gerald F. DiBona and Christopher S. Wilcox

Introduction

Since the chapter on body fluids and renal function in autonomic failure (AF) in the first edition of this book, there have been major advances in the understanding of the neural control of the kidney. It is the purpose of this chapter to review the physiology and pharmacology of the renal sympathetic nervous system in the regulation of renal function (Kopp and DiBona 1991) and to integrate this information into a clearer understanding of the abnormalities in body fluid regulation which are observed in AF, a condition thought to be characterized by partial or complete renal sympathetic denervation.

Neural control of renal function: physiology and pharmacology

Control of the renal circulation

Alterations in renal nerve activity

It is generally agreed that under physiological conditions basal efferent renal sympathetic nerve activity (ERSNA) is too low to influence renal haemodynamics. In the conscious state, surgical or pharmacological renal denervation does not affect renal blood flow (RBF) or renal vascular resistance. When ERSNA is elevated above its baseline, its effect on renal haemodynamics can be profound. Studies in anaesthetized rats and conscious dogs have shown a frequency-dependent reduction in RBF in response to graded increases in the frequency of electrical renal nerve stimulation with a threshold frequency of about 1 Hz. Current available evidence supports the concept that renal nerves do not play a role in the mechanisms involved in autoregulation of RBF.

Effector loci of renal nerves

The effector loci for renal nerves within the cortical microcirculation have been localized by micropuncture techniques to both the afferent and efferent glomerular arteriole. Renal nerve stimulation decreases single-nephron glomerular filtration rate (GFR) and single-nephron plasma flow. The decreases are due to the increases in afferent and efferent glomerular arteriolar resistances with a resultant decrease in the glomerular hydrostatic pressure gradient and a decrease in the glomerular capillary ultrafiltration coefficient (K_f). Renal nerve stimulation at lower intensities produces similar but quantitatively smaller effects. When ERSNA is low, as is the case in euvolaemic rats, the renal nerves play a minimal role in the control of single nephron GFR. However, acute renal denervation of euvolaemic rats increases urinary sodium excretion in the absence of a change in single-nephron GFR. When ERSNA is elevated, e.g. by sodium depletion (DiBona 1982), single-nephron GFR is reduced due to a reduction in single-nephron plasma flow and K_f. Single-nephron GFR is restored towards control levels by either volume repletion or renal denervation via reductions in afferent and efferent glomerular arteriolar resistances and increases in single-nephron plasma flow and K_f. Further studies (Kon 1989) suggest that the marked fall in K_f caused by renal nerve stimulation is at least partly related to decreased glomerular capillary surface area since morphological studies show that glomeruli (as well as afferent and efferent glomerular arterioles) from the stimulated kidney are markedly smaller than glomeruli (and arterioles) from the contralateral non-stimulated kidney.

Adrenergic receptors

The ratio between α_1- and α_2-adrenoceptor mediated renal vasoconstriction seems to vary between species. In the rat, α_1-adrenoceptors dominate with little evidence for a significant contribution of α_2-adrenoceptors. In the dog, although α_1-adrenoceptors seem to be most important, it is clear that α_2-adrenoceptor agonists can also cause smaller but definite renal vaso-constriction. In the intact rabbit kidney, a combination of α_1- and α_2-adreno-ceptor antagonists produces a greater attenuation of the renal vasoconstrictor reponses to renal nerve stimulation or renal arterial administration of noradrenaline than that produced by α_1-adrenoceptor antagonist alone, suggesting that renal α_1- and α_2-adrenoceptors both participate in the renal vasoconstrictor response. However, *in vitro* studies on isolated rabbit superficial afferent and efferent glomerular arterioles show that α-adrenoceptor mediated vasoconstriction is exclusively mediated by the α_1-adrenoceptor subtype. It has been suggested that the failure to demonstrate the presence of α_2-adrenoceptor mediated vasoconstriction in *in vitro* preparations is related to the absence of endogenous factors necessary for the functional expression of α_2-adrenoceptors and/or that the α_2-adrenoceptors are confined to deeper juxtamedullary arterioles.

Whether the renal circulation can be affected by activation of presynaptic α- and/or β-adrenoceptors has been examined. The intrarenal administration of the α_2-adrenoceptor antagonist, yohimbine, enhances the renal venous overflow of noradrenaline and the renal vasoconstrictor response to renal nerve stimulation. A role for presynaptic β-adrenoceptors in the neural control of the renal circulation has been suggested from studies in isolated perfused rat kidneys. The β-adrenoceptor agonist, isoproterenol, enhances the renal venous overflow of noradrenaline as well as the renal vasoconstrictor response to renal nerve stimulation. Similarly, adrenaline in physiologically relevant doses causes an enhancement of the renal vasoconstrictor response to renal nerve stimulation which was blocked by the β_2-adrenoceptor antagonist, ICI 118, 551. Thus it is possible that neurogenic renal vasoconstriction can be enhanced by increased circulating adrenaline concentration, i.e. during stress.

Recent studies comparing the effects of catecholamines on renal haemodynamics in innervated and denervated kidneys show that chronically denervated kidneys (7–10 days) exhibit supersensitivity to noradrenaline. The denervation supersensitivity is not due to a loss of neuronal uptake of noradrenaline and is not restricted to noradrenaline, since denervated kidneys also showed enhanced renal vasoconstrictor responses to vasopressin (ADH), serotonin, and prostaglandin $F_{2\alpha}$.

Although there is considerable evidence for the existence of nerves in the kidney which contain dopamine (DA) and for renal vasodilator effects of exogenous dopamine (Felder *et al.* 1989), the physiological significance of neurally released dopamine is still controversial. Albeit electrical and reflex renal nerve stimulation result in an increase in renal venous output of dopamine, there is no functional evidence for the existence of renal vasodilator nerves (DiBona 1990). While the kidney contains acetylcholinesterase, this is located in the adrenergic nerve terminals and there is no functional evidence for the existence of renal parasympathetic cholinergic innervation. Direct electrical renal nerve stimulation fails to produce a renal vasodilator response in prazosin (α_1-adrenoceptor antagonist)-treated canine kidneys. On the other hand, studies using electrical stimulation of the midbrain or intracerebroventricular administration of ouabain provide pharmacological evidence for the existence of renal dopaminergic vasodilator fibres that can be activated by central nervous system mechanisms. The renal vasodilatation produced by exogenous dopamine is mediated by activation of postsynaptic DA-1 receptors. *In vitro* and micropuncture studies suggest a role for dopamine in the control of glomerular haemodynamics. Dopamine produces equal relaxation of rabbit afferent and efferent glomerular arterioles by activation of DA-1 receptors but has very little effect on interlobular arteries. Dopamine produces an increase in cyclic adenosine monophosphate (cAMP) production in isolated canine afferent glomerular arterioles which is blocked by a DA-1 antagonist suggesting that increased cAMP production may be the means by which dopamine causes afferent glomerular arteriolar dilatation.

Control of renal tubular solute and water transport

Renal denervation

Renal denervation results in decreased proximal tubular reabsorption of sodium, chloride, bicarbonate, phosphate and water in association with an increased urinary excretion of these ions and water. These changes occur in the absence of alterations in single-nephron or whole-kidney GFR or RBF and interstitial, peritubular capillary oncotic or hydrostatic pressure. Renal denervation also decreases water, sodium, and potassium reabsorption in the loop of Henle and decreases water, Na, and bicarbonate reabsorption in the distal convoluted tubule.

The occurrence of denervation diuresis and natriuresis in conscious rats with chronic renal denervation clearly indicates that the renal response to renal denervation is not due to the removal of an artefactually increased level of ERSNA as is present in anaesthetized surgically stressed animals. The effects of renal denervation are not transient and have been observed for up to 35 weeks after renal denervation.

In consideration of the effect of renal denervation on urinary water and Na excretion, the potentially confounding issue of supersensitivity of the vasculature and tubules of the acutely or chronically denervated kidney to circulating noradrenaline is important. There is evidence of both renal vascular and tubular supersensitivity to noradrenaline in the chronically but not the acutely denervated kidney; however, the plasma noradrenaline concentrations required to demonstrate this are high, producing vaso-constriction with resultant increases in mean arterial pressure and/or decreases in GFR and RBF which could independently influence urinary water and Na excretion. Thus, it seems unlikely that, at prevailing basal plasma noradrenaline concentrations, supersensitivity of the renal vasculature or tubules of the chronically denervated kidney masks the effect of renal denervation to increase urinary flow rate and Na excretion. It is known, however, that infusions of noradrenaline that produce physiological increments ($< 50–100$ per cent increase) in plasma noradrenaline concentration decrease urinary Na excretion without affecting mean arterial pressure, GFR, or RBF in both dogs and humans with innervated kidneys.

Direct and reflex activation of the renal nerves (Table 10.1)

Using a frequency of renal nerve stimulation that was subthreshold for renal vasoconstriction, it was demonstrated in dogs that direct low-frequency electrical stimulation of the renal nerves produced a reversible decrease in urinary Na excretion without a change in renal perfusion pressure, GFR, RBF, or intrarenal distribution of blood flow. Similar observations have been made in the rabbit and the monkey. This antinatriuretic response is abolished by renal α-adrenoceptor blockade with phenoxybenzamine, selective renal

Table 10.1. Renal responses to graded renal nerve stimulation

Renal nerve stimulation frequency (Hz)	Renin secretion rate	$U_{Na}V$	GFR	RBF
0.25	No effect on basal RSR; augments RSR mediated by non-neural stimuli	0	0	0
0.50	Increased without changing $U_{Na}V$, GFR, or RBF	0	0	0
1.0	Increased with decreased $U_{Na}V$ without changing GFR or RBF	↓	0	0
2.50	Increased with decreased $U_{Na}V$, GFR, and RBF	↓	↓	↓

RSR, renin secretion rate; $U_{Na}V$, urinary sodium excretion; GFR, glomerular filtration rate; RBF, renal blood flow.

α_1-adrenoceptor blockade with prazosin, or renal adrenergic blockade with guanethidine. The antinatriuretic response is unaffected by renal blockade to angiotensin II or by prostaglandin synthesis inhibition. These studies demonstrate that low-frequency renal nerve stimulation directly increases renal tubular Na reabsorption via activation of renal tubular α_1 adrenoceptors. The response is not mediated by either angiotensin II or prostaglandins, which are known to be released in response to renal nerve stimulation. It has been demonstrated that both the antinatriuretic and the decreased urinary bicarbonate excretion responses to low-frequency renal nerve stimulation are decreased by inhibition of renal tubular bicarbonate reabsorption with either acetazolamide or intrarenal bicarbonate infusion. These results suggest that the neurogenic antinatriuresis is partly mediated by a tubular mechanism that is dependent on intact renal tubular bicarbonate reabsorption.

A similar direct electrical splanchnic nerve stimulation protocol in rats produces a decrease in ipsilateral urinary flow rate and Na excretion without a change in whole-kidney GFR, single-neuron GFR, or RBF. Simultaneous micropuncture analysis demonstrated an increased fractional and absolute Na and water reabsorption in the proximal tubule and increased sodium chloride but not water reabsorption in the thick ascending loop of Henle.

Reflex increases in ERSNA produce changes in renal Na and water handling similar to those seen after direct electrical stimulation of the renal nerves. Stimulation of carotid baroreceptors with increased ERSNA decreases urinary Na and water excretion without changes in GFR, RBF, or intrarenal distribution of blood flow. In these various studies, the antidiuretic and antinatriuretic responses were shown to be prevented by renal arterial administration of phenoxybenzamine, phentolamine, or guanethidine as well as by renal denervation or carotid sinus nerve section.

Recently, the ERSNA and renal functional responses during head-up tilt have been studied in conscious chronically instrumented dogs. A 1 hour period of 40° head-up tilt resulted in a sustained increase in ERSNA of approximately 50 per cent. Despite a rise in mean arterial pressure that would favour diuresis and natriuresis, there were significant decreases in urinary flow rate and Na excretion without changes in GFR. The antidiuretic and antinatriuretic responses were completely abolished in dogs with chronic bilateral renal denervation indicating their total dependence on the increase in ERSNA. In the absence of the confounding issues of anaesthesia and surgery, these studies indicate that sustained reflex increases in ERSNA directly increase renal tubular Na and water reabsorption resulting in antidiuresis and antinatriuresis.

Activation of left atrial mechanoreceptors ('cardiopulmonary receptors', 'volume receptors') is known to decrease ERSNA (Kopp and DiBona 1991). Distension of the left atrium by inflating a balloon in the left atrium or left atrial appendage produced a reversible decrease in ERSNA, which was accompanied by a diuresis and a natriuresis in the absence of changes in renal perfusion pressure, GFR, RBF, or intrarenal distribution of blood flow. The reduction in ERSNA during left atrial receptor stimulation and the accompanying diuresis and natriuresis are mediated by the Paintal-type atrial receptors with myelinated vagal afferent fibres. Left atrial receptor stimulation produces a reflex whose afferent limb is in the vagus nerves and whose efferent limb for the diuretic response is suppression of ADH release and for the natriuretic response is suppression of ERSNA.

The responses to head-out water immersion, a manoeuvre which translocates fluid from dependent portions of the body to the intrathoracic circulation thus increasing intrathoracic blood volume and left atrial pressure, have been studied in conscious dogs. This produces an abrupt decrease of 50 per cent in ERSNA which is sustained for 120 min during which time there is an increase in urinary flow rate and Na excretion without a change in GFR. When the experiments are repeated following chronic bilateral renal denervation, the diuretic and natriuretic responses are completely abolished indicating that the diuretic and natriuretic responses are totally dependent on the withdrawal of ERSNA.

Studies in conscious rats, dogs, monkeys, and sheep demonstrate that prior bilateral renal denervation attenuates the diuretic and natriuretic response to acute intravascular volume expansion. These findings indicate that the withdrawal of ERSNA that occurs during the volume expansion is a significant contributor to the diuretic and natriuretic responses observed.

Central nervous system lesions

Although a variety of central nervous system lesions have been associated with alterations in the renal handling of water and solutes, the most extensively characterized lesion is that involving the anteroventral portion of the third ventricle (Johnson 1990). Acutely, there is adipsia, hypernatraemia, and marked extracellular fluid volume depletion. Chronically, there is impaired drinking response to thirst challenges, hypernatraemia, impaired natriuretic response to volume expansion, increased plasma renin activity, and increased blood volume.

Adrenergic receptors

The accumulated evidence from studies in dogs, rabbits, and rats indicates that the antidiuretic, antinatriuretic, and antibicarbonaturic responses to increases in renal nerve activity are mediated by postsynaptic α_1-adrenoceptors located at neuroeffector junctions on the basolateral aspect of the tubule throughout the extent of the nephron.

With respect to dopamine, available evidence argues against a role for DA-1 receptors in the antinatriuresis produced by low-frequency renal nerve stimulation. However, renal dopamine may play a role in denervation natriuresis. Whether dopamine antagonists influence the diuretic and natriuretic responses to intravenous volume loading is controversial as both positive and negative results have been reported in rats and dogs. In man, dopamine antagonists attenuate the natriuretic response to both lower-body positive pressure and head-out water immersion. The blunted natriuresis may be related to dopamine-mediated inhibition of proximal tubular Na^+-K^+-ATPase activity. It would appear that non-neuronal dopamine produced locally within the kidney acts as an autocrine or paracrine substance producing a decrease in renal tubular Na reabsorption. Aromatic L-amino acid decarboxylase, which converts L-dopa to dopamine, is present in the proximal convoluted tubule. The dopamine produced in the proximal convoluted tubule may decrease tubular Na reabsorption by binding to DA-1 receptors in the proximal convoluted tubule, the proximal straight tubule, and the cortical collecting duct (Felder *et al.* 1989).

Role of renal nerves in sodium and water homeostasis

As discussed above, denervation diuresis and natriuresis is observed in the conscious animal in the absence of anaesthesia and traumatic operative procedures. Furthermore, the studies in unanaesthetized dogs provide compelling evidence for a significant role for ERSNA in the acute regulation of Na and water homeostasis in the conscious animal. Also, chronic renal denervation attenuates the diuretic and natriuretic response to acute intravascular volume expansion.

As another approach to understanding the role of the renal nerves in Na homeostasis, investigators have used experimental designs which would test the requirement for intact renal innervation under conditions where there existed a requirement for maximum renal Na conservation in conscious animals. The general paradigm was to examine the ability of the denervated kidneys to conserve sodium during dietary Na restriction in the conscious state. A synthesis of the several observations (DiBona 1989; Herman *et al.* 1989) is that severe dietary Na restriction represents a sufficient challenge to maximally engage all mechanisms required for a normal renal adaptive response in order to avoid negative Na balance. Under such conditions, the absence or malfunction of any one of these redundant mechanisms cannot be made up for by another, and a negative Na balance results. Thus, under these circumstances, renal denervation eliminates an essential mechanism, which is revealed by the development of a negative Na balance. A lesser degree of dietary Na restriction would not maximally activate this complex multicomponent homeostatic system, and elimination of one component (e.g. renal denervation) would not result in a defect in renal Na conservation. The overall results lend further support to the argument that the dependence of normal renal Na conservation on intact renal innervation is related to the magnitude of the dietary Na restriction with a severe degree of restriction requiring intact renal innervation and lesser degrees of restriction not requiring intact renal innervation. The studies of Gill and Bartter (1966) and Wilcox *et al.* (1977) (see Fig. 10.3 and below) support the view that intact renal innervation is also essential for the kidney to express its full ability to maximally reabsorb Na in response to a reduction in dietary Na intake in man.

There is general agreement that intact renal innervation is not required for the renal regulation of external Na balance during normal or modest reductions in dietary Na intake. However, it appears likely that more severe degrees of dietary Na restriction maximally engage the many mechanisms known to enable the kidney to appropriately conserve Na and that, under these more stressful conditions, intact renal innervation is essential for normal renal Na conservation.

Control of renin secretion

Alterations in renal nerve activity

Renal nerve stimulation at a frequency of 0.3–0.5 Hz results in an increase in renin secretion rate in the absence of changes in renal haemodynamics and urinary Na excretion; thus the resultant increase in renin secretion rate occurs in the absence of stimulatory input to the vascular baroreceptor and tubular macula densa receptor mechanisms. The increases in renin secretion rate observed with renal nerve stimulation are frequency-dependent.

The increase in renal secretion rate that occurs with dietary Na restriction in human subjects is associated with increased renal noradrenaline spillover as an index of increased ERSNA.

Adrenergic receptors

It is well established that the renin secretion rate response to increases in ERSNA at intensities causing no or minimal changes in renal haemodynamics (low-level renal nerve stimulation) is mediated by activation of renal β_1-adrenoceptors; β_2-adrenoceptors are not involved.

There has been substantial debate concerning the role of α-adrenoceptors in the control of neurally mediated renin secretion. Whereas there is little doubt that the increase in renin secretion rate produced by renal nerve stimulation at intensities causing marked decreases in urinary Na excretion and renal blood flow is partly related to activation of vascular and/or tubular α-adrenoceptors, the role of α-adrenoceptors in the increase in renin secretion rate produced by renal nerve stimulation at intensities causing minimal renal haemodynamic changes is minimal (Osborn and Johns 1989).

The effects of dopamine on renin secretion rate have been extensively studied. *In vitro* studies using kidney slices or juxtaglomerular cells have shown that the increase in renin secretion rate produced by dopamine is mediated by activation of DA-1 receptors and not related to conversion of dopamine to noradrenaline. Similarly, studies in dogs and pithed rats have shown that the renin secretion rate response to dopamine is related to a direct activation of renal DA-1 receptors and is not mediated by the renal nerves. The increase in renin secretion rate produced by dopamine is attenuated by DA-1 antagonists and not reduced by α- or β-adrenoceptor antagonists or ganglionic blockade.

Interaction between neural and non-neural mechanisms

In evaluating the role of each of the mechanisms involved in the control of renin secretion rate, early studies examined each mechanism in a fashion that allowed it to be evaluated independently of the influence of the other two mechanisms. More recent evidence indicates, however, that in many physiological conditions there is an interaction between the neural and non-neural mechanisms in the control of renin secretion rate (Gibbons *et al.* 1984).

Some of the earliest studies suggesting an interaction between the renal nerves and the baroreceptor/macula densa mechanisms showed that furosemide administration or suprarenal aortic constriction elicited a greater renin secretion rate response in the innervated than in the denervated kidney. Since subsequent studies in dogs showed that the greater increase in renin secretion rate from the innervated kidney was not due to an increase in ERNSA, these studies suggested that the increase in renin secretion rate mediated by non-neural mechanisms could be influenced by the prevailing level of ERSNA. This hypothesis was subsequently confirmed by experiments showing that electrical renal nerve stimulation at a frequency that did not affect renin secretion rate at spontaneous renal perfusion pressure enhanced the renin secretion rate response to suprarenal aortic constriction or furosemide. Subsequent studies showed that the interaction between non-neural and neural mechanisms in the control of renin secretion rate is dependent on the level of renal arterial pressure and on the intensity of the renal nerve stimulation. Similarly, studies in humans show that reflex renal nerve stimulation produced by cold pressor stress enhanced the increase in renal venous plasma renin activity produced by renal arterial pressure reduction.

The evidence for an interaction between the renal nerves and the baroreceptor and macula densa mechanisms in the control of renin secretion rate is substantial. Since ERSNA is quite variable, there are times when increases in ERSNA are sufficient to cause a direct neural release of renin. At other times, changes in ERSNA may be more modest but still sufficient to modulate the renin secretion rate responses initiated by other mechanisms. The degree of interaction between the neural and non-neural mechanisms is dependent on the level of activation of the non-neural mechanisms and the intensity of renal nerve activity and requires an intact macula densa receptor mechanism.

Body fluid homeostasis and renal function in patients with autonomic failure

This section contains a concise review of studies of body fluid homeostasis, renal function, and relevant hormones in patients with autonomic failure (AF). These studies are of practical interest since they provide a rational basis for management of orthostatic hypertension.

Studies in patients with AF first established the importance of the autonomic nervous system for body fluid homeostasis. In their original description of pure autonomic failure in 1925, Bradbury and Eggleston described the nocturnal polyuria from which these patients often suffer. Thirty years later, Wagner and Shear demonstrated abnormal patterns of fluid and sodium (Na) excretion, which Gill and Bartter (1966) related to failure of the sympathetic nervous system since they reproduced these defects in normal human subjects by administration of guanethidine. More recently, important differences in key hormones and in body fluid homeostasis have been found between patients whose AF is due to tetraplegia and those with pure autonomic failure (PAF) or multiple system atrophy (MSA).

Body fluid volumes

The median value for plasma volume derived from a survey of published studies of 53 patients with AF due to PAF or MSA is 99.2 per cent of normal (Wilcox *et al.* 1984). However, the regulation of plasma volume during changes in Na intake or posture is clearly abnormal in such patients.

When healthy subjects stand or are tilted upright, their blood pressure (BP) does not change substantially yet plasma volume is reduced by an average of 10 per cent. This orthostatic fall in plasma volume is normally accompanied by a corresponding increase in interstitial volume of the lower limbs due to an increase in the hydraulic pressure in the capillaries of the skin and muscle vessels. In contrast, when patients with AF stand or are tilted upright, there is a sharp fall in BP yet plasma volume is maintained. The absence of a postural contraction of plasma volume in patients with AF suggests that the orthostatic fall in BP is sufficient to counter any increase in capillary hydraulic pressure (Wilcox et al. 1984).

During dietary Na restriction, one study showed that the plasma volume fell by a similar degree in normal subjects and patients with AF, yet the patients lost three times as much body weight due to defective renal Na conservation (see below). Thus, the excessive loss of body fluid derived exclusively from the interstitial (or intracellular) compartment(s). As with head-up tilt, the sharp fall in BP of patients with AF during dietary Na restriction may have reduced the hydraulic pressure in the capillary bed sufficiently to redistribute interstitial fluid into the intravascular compartment (Wilcox et al. 1984).

Preservation of the plasma volume during standing or dietary Na restriction is a vital last line of defence against catastrophic hypotension. In the absence of effective cardiovascular control mechanisms, the BP of patients with AF is closely dependent on cardiac output and venous return (Fig. 10.1). Therefore, the initial fall in BP during standing or Na depletion may prevent a loss of plasma volume and thereby limit the fall in venous return and progressive hypotension.

Hormonal control of renal function

Renin–angiotensin–aldosterone system

The median value of plasma renin activity (PRA) from a survey of 33 reports in 127 patients with AF due to PAF, MSA, or diabetes mellitus (DM) is only 53 per cent of normal while the patients are recumbent and only 48 per cent of normal while they are upright. The reduced levels of PRA in patients while upright indicates a profound blunting of renin release since orthostatic hypotension should be a potent stimulus to renin release. Moreover, cardiac output is sharply reduced on standing and this may reduce hepatic blood flow and prolong the circulatory half-life of renin. These blunted renin levels have been ascribed to a defect in renal renin release, probably due to defective ERSNA or subnormal plasma catecholamine concentrations, rather than to defect in renal renin stores since PRA rises normally in patients with PAF or MSA during severe hypotension produced by a combination of standing and dietary Na restriction (Wilcox et al. 1977) or in response to infusions of dopamine, isoproterenol (isoprenaline), or furosemide (frusemide).

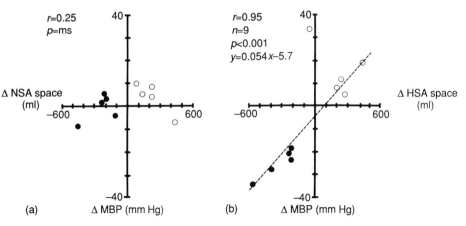

Fig. 10.1. Individual values for changes in mean blood pressure (ΔMBP) and plasma volume (human serum albumin, ΔHSA space) measured while sitting during alteration in sodium intake in (a) control subjects and (b) patients with autonomic failure (AF) due to pure AF or multiple system atrophy (MSA). The data calculation in (b) refer to nine observations; inclusion of the aberrant point reduced the correlation coefficient r to 0.80. Changes in dietary sodium intake: solid circles, from unrestricted to 17 mmol/24 h; open circles, from 17 to 189 mmol/24 h. Note the close correlation between changes in MBP and plasma volume in (a) the subjects with AF in contrast to the stable MBP despite similar changes in plasma volume in (b) the control subjects. (Taken with permission from Wilcox *et al.* (1984).)

In striking contrast are the reports of patients with the Riley–Day syndrome or tetraplegia complicating high cervical spinal cord lesions where a survey of the values for PRA show that the median values are increased by 688 and 277 per cent, respectively. Children have rather higher values of PRA than adults. Therefore, this figure may overestimate the degree of PRA elevation in the subjects with the Riley–Day syndrome who were mostly children. Nevertheless, the difference between the normal or elevated values of PRA in these two categories of AF, compared to the low values seen in patients with PAF, MSA, or DM, despite similar degrees of blockade of sympathetic reflexes has not been adequately explained. One theory ascribes the subnormal PRA values in patients with PAF, MSA, or DM to defective ERSNA. However, an anatomical explanation is unsatisfactory since the dominant lesion in the sympathetic nervous system in patients with MSA is a degeneration of intermediolateral column cells throughout the cervicolumbar spinal cord, yet their subnormal values of PRA differ radically from the supranormal values seen in tetraplegic patients who also have damage at this site. Tetraplegic patients can have overactive autonomic reflexes which might increase ERSNA and hence renin release. However, Mathias *et al.* (1980) found that activation of such reflexes in tetraplegics by bladder stimulation, although provoking a rise in BP and plasma noradrenaline levels indicative of widespread spinal reflex activation, did not increase PRA. Whereas blockade of β-adrenoceptors with propranolol prevented the rise in PRA that normally occurs during upright tilting, it failed to block the rise in PRA in those with tetraplegia. Since the PRA of these patients increased normally during infusion of isoproterenol (isoprenaline), which indicated that β-receptor mediated stimulation of renin release was intact, these authors concluded that the rise in PRA on tilting was not due to residual reflex activity mediated by β-adrenoceptors. They postulated a renal baroreceptor-mediated stimulus to renin release caused by the fall in renal perfusion pressure. However, there remain the problems of explaining, first, the high basal values of PRA in tetraplegic patients while they are recumbent with relatively normal levels of BP and, second, the subnormal PRA responses to tilt in patients with PAF and MSA despite equally impressive orthostatic falls in BP.

As anticipated from the values of PRA, a survey of measurements of the rate of secretion of excretion of aldosterone in 30 patients with PAF or MSA shows that the median values are only 43 per cent of normal while plasma aldosterone levels in patients with the Riley–Day syndrome or tetraplegia are normal or raised. Slaton and Biglieri found that the subnormal aldosterone secretion that they documented in patients with AF due to PAF or amyloidosis was accompanied by a blunted response to short-term stimulation by angiotensin or adrenocortitrophic hormone (ACTH). Since more prolonged stimulation, provided either by dietary Na restriction or by prolonged infusions of angiotensin, increased aldosterone secretion into the normal range, they concluded that the low basal values and subnormal short-term responses represented the effects of a prolonged reduction in angiotensin stimulation of the zona glomerulosa of the adrenal gland due to defective renin release.

The regulation of the renin–angiotensin–aldosterone system in patients with DM has attracted considerable interest. PRA is reduced in diabetics with AF when compared to those with normal autonomic function. However, the interpretation is complicated because patients with advanced DM, but without AF, can have sufficiently low values of PRA and aldosterone to lead to overt hypoaldosteronism with hyperkalaemia and metabolic acidosis (type IV renal tubular acidosis). The suppressed renin–aldosterone axis in these diabetic patients has variously been related to hyalinosis of the renin-containing cells in the afferent arteriole, to a reduced renin release due to prolonged volume expansion, or to a specific defect in renin synthesis. Nevertheless, it is clear that the cause for hyporeninaemic hypoaldosteronism in diabetic patients is usually not AF.

Antidiuretic hormone (ADH)

ADH release is triggered either by a rise in plasma osmolality or by a reduction in blood volume or venous return leading to reduced stretch of low-pressure receptors in the atria and pulmonary vascular circuit. On standing, there is normally a reduction in central venous pressure and plasma volume which can account for the observed increase in ADH release. Although the osmotic regulation of ADH release appears intact in patients with PAF or MSA, postural regulation is often abnormal. Thus, some patients with MSA cannot dilute their urine normally in response to a water load while standing which implies an exaggerated postural release of, or response to, ADH (Wilcox *et al.* 1975). However, other studies have disclosed that patients with MSA can have a blunted postural release of ADH due to abnormal central control via dopaminergic and encephalinergic systems in the brainstem (Puritz *et al.* 1983). Further studies are required to resolve these issues.

Renal haemodynamics

Measurements of RBF and GFR in patients with AF while they are recumbent are usually normal. Moreover, these patients retain a normal renal vasoconstrictor response to infused angiotensin or ADH. During step-wise head-up tilt to reduce the BP progressively, the RBF and GFR are maintained until the lower limits of the autoregulatory response at 65–70 mm Hg are exceeded.

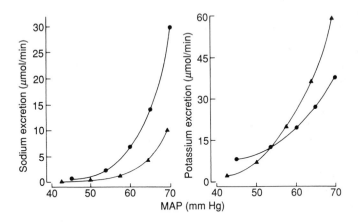

Fig. 10.2.   Data from a single subject with AF showing rates of renal sodium and potassium excretion during a maintained water diuresis in response to graded changes in mean arterial pressure (MAP) induced by tilting. The data depicted by solid triangles were obtained while the subject received aldosterone (2 ng/min) which raised the plasma aldosterone concentration to 250 ng/dl. Note the close dependence of renal sodium and potassium excretion on MAP and the shift of the sodium excretion curve to the right and the potassium excretion curve to the left at higher levels of MAP by aldosterone. (With permission after Schalekamp *et al.* (1985).)

Renal sodium conservation

Schalekamp *et al.* (1985) varied the mean arterial pressure of patients with PAF by grading tilting. They showed a steep increase in renal Na and K excretion with rise in mean arterial pressure above 55 to 60 mm Hg. As shown in Fig. 10.2, a concurrent infusion of aldosterone reduced the Na excretion and increased the K excretion. This study illustrates the predominant importance of renal perfusion pressure and mineralocorticosteroids in regulating Na excretion in patients with PAF.

Normal subjects given a low dietary Na intake reduce their renal Na excretion rapidly over 2–5 days to achieve Na balance at the lower level of intake. A survey of published reports of 23 patients with PAF or MSA studied during dietary Na restriction, revealed that renal Na conservation was impaired in two-thirds; some manifested a remarkable inability to conserve Na. Wilcox *et al.* (1977) contrasted renal Na conservation in a group of five patients with PAF or MSA with five age-matched controls. As shown in Fig. 10.3, while renal Na excretion fell rapidly over 3–5 days in the normal subjects, it was not significantly altered over a week of dietary Na restriction

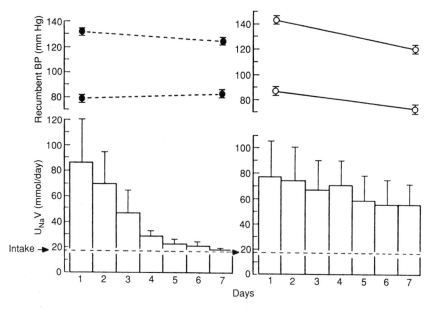

Fig. 10.3. Mean ± SEM values for systolic and diastolic blood pressure (BP) while recumbent and urinary sodium excretion ($U_{Na}V$) in five patients with AF due to pure AF and MSA (right panel, open circles) and five age-matched control subjects (left panel, closed circles) during 7 days of reduced dietary sodium intake (17 mmol/24 h). Note the failure of the patients with AF to achieve Na balance and their fall in BP. (Taken with permission from Wilcox *et al.* (1977).)

in those with AF. This excessive Na loss in the patients with AF was accompanied by a greater loss of body weight, a worsening of orthostatic hypotension, and a deterioration in their clinical state. The worsening orthostatic hypotension was directly related to the fall in plasma volume in these patients (Fig. 10.1). Failure of Na conservation in patients with AF may be ascribed to defective renal sympathetic nerve traffic and catecholamine release since Gill and Bartter (1966) showed that administration of the adrenergic neuron-blocking drug guanethidine to normal human subjects blunted their ability to attain Na balance during dietary Na restriction. The Na wasting in these subjects given guanethidine could not be ascribed to changes in renal haemodynamics or aldosterone excretion since neither were altered. However, the situation is more complicated in patients with PAF or MSA where some of the Na wasting may be ascribed to subnormal aldosterone secretion. Indeed, administration of a mineralocorticoid improves Na homeostasis in these subjects (Wilcox et al. 1977). However, these patients display an inappropriate renal Na excretion while they are recumbent even while they receive supramaximal doses of mineralocorticosteroid replacement. This implies additional mineralocorticosteroid-independent defects which may include a loss of the effects of angiotensin and catecholamines to enhance renal tubular Na and fluid reabsorption. Interestingly, patients with tetraplegia lack the exaggerated natriuresis seen in those with PAF or MSA while recumbent although they do have an exaggerated diuresis. Kooner et al. (1987) ascribed this difference in natriuresis to the higher levels of PRA and aldosterone in tetraplegic subjects. However, one subject with AF due to dopamine β-hydroxylase deficiency studied by Mathias et al. (1990) had a nocturnal diuresis and natriuresis that was not reversed by repletion of catecholamines with treatment with DL-DOPS. Further studies are required to define the precise role of catecholamines in renal Na and fluid homeostasis in patients with AF.

Renal Na wasting in patients with PAF or MSA provides a rational basis for provision of a liberal Na intake supplemented, during periods of intercurrent illness or anorexia, with NaCl capsules or intravenous fluids. Moreover, subnormal aldosterone levels in these patients can be addressed by administration of a mineralocorticosteroid drug. Indeed, 9-α-fludrocortisone (Fluorinef) can alleviate orthostatic hypotension due to prolonged bed-rest, DM, PAF, MSA, and a variety of other categories of AF. Whereas about one-third of patients show a striking benefit, a similar fraction show little or no response and eventually most patients become refractory. Soon after starting treatment with 9-α-fludrocortisone, patients usually retain Na and fluid, there is an expansion of the plasma volume, and the body weight increases by 1–3 kg. However, after some weeks or months of therapy, the plasma volume and body weight return to baseline yet some improvement in orthostatic hypotension persists (Schalekamp et al. 1985). This apparent improvement in autonomic control of the circulation has been ascribed to an enhanced vascular responsiveness to noradrenaline since 9-α-fludrocortisone can increase the pressor sensitivity to infused noradrenaline in patients with PAF or MSA independent of fluid retention.

Overzealous treatment with 9-α-fludrocortisone and Na can lead to excessive fluid retention, recumbent hypertension, K depletion, and alkalosis. This requires a temporary discontinuation of therapy which can later be restarted at a reduced dosage.

Effects of posture on Na and water excretion

Some patients with PAF or MSA are troubled with nocturnal polyuria which can reduce extracellular fluid volume in the morning sufficiently to worsen orthostatic hypotension. Patients with MSA have a normal capacity to eliminate a water load while recumbent, yet a subnormal diuretic response while standing due to an inability to dilute the urine maximally (Wilcox *et al*. 1975). Conversely, during prolonged fluid deprivation, urine flow and Na excretion decrease, and urine osmolality increases normally during standing, yet these changes in the patients with AF are reversed during standing. Two mechanisms have been identified which could account for these striking effects of posture. First, Schalekamp *et al*. (1985) demonstrated a steep relationship between arterial pressure and Na excretion in patients with PAF (Fig. 10.2). Therefore, the greater diuresis and natriuresis while recumbent may relate to higher BP. Second, patients with AF may have exaggerated postural changes in central blood volume due to excessive pooling of blood in the periphery on standing and excessive return of blood to the central compartment on lying. These excessive postural changes could generate exaggerated responses by the low-pressure volume receptors which would be complemented by exaggerated responses by the high-pressure baroreceptor systems due to the orthostatic changes in BP. Therefore, any intact volume-sensitive mechanisms may generate abnormal signals which could dictate excessive postural changes in renal function. One such mechanism could be the release of atrial natriuretic peptide but this requires study. A second may be release of ADH which is regulated by low-pressure receptors. Indeed, measurements in one subject with MSA demonstrated excessive postural changes in ADH excretion (Wilcox *et al*. 1975), although this was not confirmed in a later study of plasma ADH concentration during tilting (Puritz *et al*. 1983). Thus, a role for ADH in the abnormal diuresis of recumbency in patients with AF has yet to be clearly defined. As described above, tetraplegic patients also show an excessive diuresis when recumbent, but, unlike those with PAF or MSA, they do not have major posture-induced changes in Na excretion (Kooner *et al*. 1987).

The demonstration of an inappropriate diuresis and natriuresis in patients with PAF or MSA while recumbent provides a rational basis for postural therapy whereby the patient is kept in the semi-sitting position at night. Such a change in posture can diminish the recumbency-induced natriuresis and diuresis of patients with PAF or MSA and thereby prevent the ensuing worsening of orthostatic hypotension during the following morning. Where such postural therapy is effective, patients often gain 1–3 kg in weight and have a diminished orthostatic fall in BP. Postural therapy may be combined with 9-α-fludrocortisone. In contrast, the normal or elevated values for renin and aldosterone in tetraplegic patients, together with the absence of a recumbency-induced natriuresis or clear evidence of Na wasting in the group of patients, indicate that postural therapy or supplementary fludrocortisone may not be of major benefit for them.

Acknowledgements

Work from the laboratory of GFD was supported by National Institutes of Health grants, DK-15843, HL-35163, HL-40222, HL-14388, and HL 44546, and by the Veterans Administration. Work from the laboratory of CSW was supported by National Institutes of Health grant DK 36079.

References

Bradbury, S. and Eggleston, C. (1925). Postural hypotension: a report of three cases. *Am. Heart J.* **1**, 78–86.

DiBona, G. F. (1982). The functions of the renal nerves. *Rev. Physiol. Biochem. Pharmacol.* **94**, 75–181.

DiBona, G. F. (1989). Renal nerves. *Min. Electrolyte Metab.* **15**, 1–96.

DiBona, G. F. (1990). Renal dopamine containing nerves: ? functional significance. *Am. J. Hypertension* **3**, 64S–67S.

Felder, R. A., Felder, C. G., Eisner, G. M., and Jose, P. A. (1989). The dopamine receptor in adult and maturing kidney. *Am. J. Physiol.* **257**, F315–F327.

Gibbons, G. H., Dzau, V. J., Farhi, E. R., and Barger, A. C. (1984). Interaction of signals influencing renin release. *Ann. Rev. Physiol.* **46**, 291–308.

Gill, J. R. and Bartter, F. C. (1966). Adrenergic nervous system in sodium metabolism. II. Effects of guanethidine on the renal response to sodium deprivation in normal man. *New Engl. J. Med.* **275**, 1466–1471.

Herman, P. J., Sawin, L. L., and DiBona, G. F. (1989). Role of renal nerves in renal sodium retention of nephrotic syndrome. *Am. J. Physiol.* **256**, F823–F829.

Johnson, A. K. (1990). Brain mechanisms in the control of body fluid homeostasis. In *Perspectives in exercise science and sports medicine*, Vol. 3. *Fluid homeostasis during exercise* (ed. C. V. Gisolfi and D. R. Lamb), pp. 347–424. Benchmark, Carmel, Indiana.

Kon, V. (1989). Neural control of circulation. *Mineral Electrolyte Metab.* **15**, 33–44.

Kooner, J. S., da Costa, D. F., Frankel, H. L., Bannister, R., Peart, W. S., and Mathias, C. J. (1987). Recumbency induces hypertension, diuresis and natriuresis in autonomic failure, but diuresis alone in tetraplegia. *J. Hypertension* **5** (suppl. 5), S327–S329.

Kopp, U. C. and DiBona, G. F. (1991). The neural control of renal function. In *The *kidney: physiology and pathophysiology* (ed. D. W. Seldin and G. Giebisch), pp. 1157–1204. Raven, New York.

Mathias, C. J., Bannister, R. R., Cortelli, P., Heslop, K., Polak, J. M., Raimbach, S., Springall, D. R., and Watson, L. (1990). Clinical, autonomic and therapeutic observations in two siblings with postural hypotension due to an inability to synthesize noradrenalin from dopamine because of a deficiency of dopamine beta hydroxylase. *Quart. J. Med.* **75**, 617–33.

Mathias, C. J., Christensen, N. J., Frankel, H. L., and Peart, W. S. (1980). Renin release during head-up tilt occurs independently of sympathetic nervous activity in tetraplegic man. *Clin. Sci.* **59**, 251–6.

Osborn, J. L. and Johns, E. J. (1989). Control of renin and prostaglandin release. *Mineral Electrolyte Metab.* **15**, 51–8.

Puritz, R., Lightman, S. L., Wilcox, C. S., Forsling, M., and Bannister, R. (1983). Blood pressure and vasopressin in progressive autonomic failure: response to postural stimulation, l-dopa and naloxone. *Brain* **106**, 503–11.

Schalekamp, M. A. D. H., Man in't Veld, A. J., and Wenting, G. J. (1985). The second Sir George Pickering Memorial Lecture: what regulates whole body autoregulation? Clinical observations. *J. Hypertension* **3**, 97–107.

Slaton, P. E. and Biglieri, E. G. (1967). Reduced aldosterone excretion in patients with autonomic insufficiency. *J. Clin. Endocrinol. Metab.* **27**, 37–45.

Wilcox, C. S., Aminoff, M. J., and Penn, W. (1975). The basis of the nocturnal polyuria in patients with autonomic failure. *J. Neurol. Neurosurg. Psychiat.* **37**, 677–84.

Wilcox, C. S., Aminoff, M. J., and Slater, J. D. H. (1977). Sodium homeostasis in patients with autonomic failure. *Clin. Sci.* **53**, 321–8.

Wilcox, C. S., Puritz, R., Lightman, S. L., Bannister, R., and Aminoff, M. J. (1984). Plasma volume regulation in patients with progressive autonomic failure during changes in salt intake or posture. *J. Lab. Clin. Med.* **104**, 331–9.

11. The sympathetic nervous system and its influence on metabolic function

Ian A. Macdonald

Introduction

In many of the topics considered in this book, the sympathetic nervous system effects are mediated mainly through the postganglionic noradrenergic and cholinergic innervation of the peripheral tissues. Such innervation is important in the regulation of metabolism, but there is also a key role for catecholamines released from the adrenal medulla. This chapter will deal with the influences of both sympathetic postganglionic nerves and plasma catecholamines on metabolism. These effects can occur either through direct actions of catecholamines within metabolically active tissue, or as a consequence of alterations in the major hormones which regulate metabolism. There is now substantial evidence that changes in metabolic or nutritional status can affect the sympathoadrenal system, and these effects will be considered in the second part of this chapter. The mechanisms by which diabetes mellitus has profound effects on the autonomic and sensory nervous systems are not fully understood. However, it is well established that the pathological consequences of this neuropathy for sympathetic function are extremely serious with regard to the postural control of blood pressure and the regulation of sweating. The implications of such diabetic neuropathy on the control of metabolism are also considered in the section on 'Metabolic and nutritional effects on the sympathoadrenal system'.

Control of metabolism

It is beyond the scope of this book to provide a comprehensive account of the intracellular biochemical processes that may be under sympathoadrenal regulation. This chapter will focus on the metabolism of the three main components of the diet, carbohydrate, fat, and protein, concentrating on effects which have been established through *in vivo* studies (mainly in humans). Consideration will also be given to overall energy metabolism—

197

assessing the effects of the sympathoadrenal system on resting energy expenditure (thermogenesis). Only a few specific references will be given in the text; more detailed accounts of these topics can be found in the reviews by Clutter *et al.* (1988), Niijima (1989), Macdonald *et al.* (1985) and Young and Landsberg (1977).

Direct sympathoadrenal control of metabolism

Carbohydrate metabolism (Fig. 11.1)

The maintenance of an adequate supply of glucose to neural tissue is a fundamental component of homeostasis. The carbohydrate component of food is stored in the liver and skeletal muscle as glycogen, under the influence of insulin released from the B cells of the islets of Langerhans in the pancreas. During the intervals between meals, or in periods of prolonged starvation, the stored glycogen is used to produce free glucose which maintains an adequate blood glucose concentration, thus sustaining neural function. During short periods of starvation (less than 24 h), the breakdown of the liver glycogen store (the process of glycogenolysis) produces free glucose which maintains blood glucose. This hepatic glycogenolysis is regulated in part by glucagon released from the A cells of the pancreatic islets, but it is now clear that adrenaline stimulation of glycogenolysis is also important.

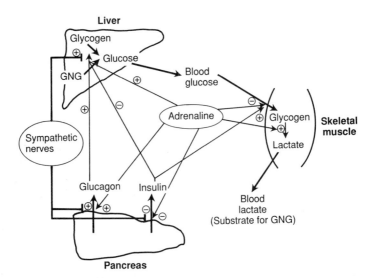

Fig. 11.1. Effects of sympathetic nerves and plasma adrenaline on carbohydrate metabolism. Both direct effects on liver and muscle metabolism and indirect effects via alterations in insulin and glucagon release are illustrated. GNG, gluconeogenesis; +, stimulated; –, inhibited.

In humans, adrenaline stimulates glycogenolysis mainly via activation of β-adrenoceptors. There is evidence that a small component of hepatic glycogenolysis after an overnight fast is due to stimulation of α-adrenoceptors, probably through the sympathetic innervation of the liver. After more prolonged fasting, adrenaline contributes to the maintenance of glucose homeostasis in the first few days, although glucagon has the primary role at this time (Boyle *et al.* 1989).

With more prolonged periods of starvation, the synthesis of glucose (gluconeogenesis) from precursors such as lactate, alanine, and glycerol is of major importance as the glycogen store is not unlimited. This gluconeogenesis occurs mainly in the liver (although the kidneys do contribute) and is stimulated by glucagon and adrenaline. In addition to this direct effect on hepatic gluconeogenesis, adrenaline is one of the main stimuli for increasing muscle glycogenolysis in the resting state. By contrast to the liver, muscle glycogen cannot be broken down to free glucose, but instead lactate is produced and passes into the blood. This lactate is a substrate for hepatic gluconeogenesis and thus muscle glycogen can indirectly contribute to the maintenance of blood glucose (the Cori cycle).

The liver has a sympathetic innervation which has been studied extensively by Lautt (1980). Stimulation of the hepatic sympathetic supply leads to increased glycogenolysis and glucose release. There is no direct evidence that these nerves are involved in the regulation of carbohydrate metabolism under normal conditions, and there do not appear to be any gross abnormalities after liver transplantation. In the latter case it would be rather difficult to identify more subtle alterations, given the previous metabolic disease and posttransplant immunosuppression. It is more likely that hepatic sympathetic nerves are of importance in severe hypoglycaemia or when the other mechanisms are defective.

Fat metabolism (Fig. 11.2)

The major direct metabolic effects of the sympathoadrenal system are in the control of fat metabolism. The storage of fatty acids as triacylglycerols in adipose tissue is regulated by insulin, which stimulates the storage process and inhibits the breakdown of triacylglycerol to non-esterified fatty acids (NEFA or FFA). This breakdown process (lipolysis) increases if plasma insulin levels fall, but the major stimulation is achieved by several hormones, including adrenaline, and by the sympathetic innervation of the adipose tissue. The sympathoadrenal stimulation of lipolysis occurs via β-adrenoceptor mediated processes. By contrast the stimulation of α-adrenoceptors in adipose tissue inhibits lipolysis. This may prevent excessive rates of lipolysis occurring during periods of starvation, as there is evidence that such a state is accompanied by a fall in β-adrenoceptor density and a rise in α-adrenoceptor density in adipose tissue.

Ian A. Macdonald

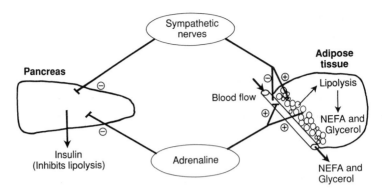

Fig. 11.2. Effects of sympathetic nerves and plasma adrenaline on fat metabolism. Both direct effects on adipose tissue blood flow and metabolism and indirect effects through inhibition of insulin release are illustrated. NEFA, non-esterified fatty acids; +, stimulated; –, inhibited.

The sympathetic innervation of white adipose tissue mainly supplies the vasculature, but in some depots there is a direct innervation of the adipose tissue cells. There is histological evidence that neurotransmitters released from the sympathetic nerves may also stimulate non-innervated adipose tissue cells, thus providing a key role for the sympathetic nervous system in the regulation of adipose tissue blood flow and metabolism (Fredholm 1985). During conditions such as orthostasis, there are transient reductions in human adipose tissue blood flow, mediated by sympathetic nervous innervation of vascular smooth muscle. However, these blood vessels also contain β-adrenoceptors which mediate vasodilatation in response to an increase in plasma adrenaline, or possibly due to diffusion of noradrenaline from the sympathetic neuroeffector junctions. Thus, prolonged sympathetic nervous stimulation to white adipose tissue is accompanied by a type of vasoconstrictor escape, whilst a rise in plasma adrenaline levels produces active vasodilatation (Hjemdahl and Linde 1983). Furthermore, the stimulation of lipolysis by the sympathetic nerves, or plasma adrenaline, leads to a rise in adipose tissue blood flow through metabolic effects—facilitating the transport of fatty acids to other tissues in the body.

Brown adipose tissue has a more dense vascular supply and innervation than white adipose tissue. Furthermore, many more brown adipose tissue cells are sympathetically innervated directly. The vascular innervation appears to be predominantly vasoconstrictor, with the released noradrenaline acting on α-adrenoceptors. However, the stimulation of lipolysis in brown adipose tissue leads to a secondary vasodilation accompanied by a marked increase in the oxygen consumption of the tissue (brown adipose tissue thermogenesis). This metabolic event is mediated by β-adrenoceptors that appear to be somewhat atypical and have been designated β_3 (Arch *et al.* 1984). In humans brown adipose tissue is important as a site of thermogenesis in the newborn, but is of limited significance in the adult (see below).

Protein metabolism

There is no evidence of a direct effect of the sympathetic nervous system on protein metabolism. However, it appears that adrenaline is able to decrease the rate of breakdown of body protein. This is based on observations of the effects of adrenaline infusion (Miles *et al.* 1984), and the physiological and clinical significance are not established.

Indirect effects of the sympathoadrenal system on metabolism

The main indirect effect on metabolism is through the modulation of insulin and glucagon release from the pancreas. Stimulation of the sympathetic innervation of the B cell leads to α-adrenoceptor mediated inhibition of insulin release. Evidence from *in vitro* studies suggests plasma catecholamines inhibit insulin release through activation of α_2-adrenoceptors, but it is not known if these also mediate the sympathetic nervous effects. The pancreatic B cells also contain β_2-adrenoceptors, although it is uncommon for these to be stimulated by plasma adrenaline under physiological conditions—the stimulation of α-adrenoceptors seems to predominate. However, β_2-adrenoceptor agonists such as salbutamol will stimulate insulin release.

The pancreatic A cells are stimulated by both their sympathetic innervation and by plasma catecholamines. Glucagon release results from activation of β-adrenoceptors, although such release has not been demonstrated in all studies of the effects of the infusion of adrenaline.

One of the consequences of pancreatic transplantation would be to produce a denervated pancreas. However, this cannot readily be used to judge the overall importance of the innervation, as the transplant recipients are patients with insulin-dependent diabetes mellitus (IDDM) who also have severe diabetic complications such as end-stage renal failure. Such pancreatic transplantation is judged to be successful if the patient no longer needs to inject insulin (although this is only achieved with continued immunosuppression). The transplanted pancreas is capable of controlling postprandial blood glucose satisfactorily and releases glucagon in response to hypoglycaemia. However, it is not known whether the effectiveness of the pancreas in regulating metabolism is compromised by its lack of a sympathetic (and parasympathetic) innervation.

One of the most important indirect effects of the sympathoadrenal system on metabolism is to reduce the sensitivity of the peripheral tissues to insulin. Thus, in conditions of sympathetic activation or increased adrenal medullary secretion (such as in trauma or after a myocardial infarction) there is a reduction in the effectiveness of insulin to stimulate glucose uptake and utilization in adipose tissue and skeletal muscle. These peripheral effects of the catecholamines seem to be mediated through activation of β_2-adrenoceptors and thus are also produced by drugs such as salbutamol, ritodrine, and terbutaline. Such drugs are commonly used to prevent premature labour. If used in pregnant women with IDDM, these drugs lead to a marked increase in the insulin requirements for achieving adequate control of blood glucose. (The latter is of major importance in preventing the occurrence of macrosomia in the fetus.) Large doses of these β_2-agonists can stimulate adipose tissue lipolysis and pancreatic glucagon secretion, leading to increased ketone production which may develop into diabetic ketoacidosis. In such conditions of possible premature labour, steroids are sometimes given intravenously to the woman to stimulate the fetal lung maturation process, and in patients with IDDM these high doses of steroids will increase the likelihood of diabetic ketoacidosis occurring.

Summary

Physiologically the predominant effects of the sympathoadrenal system are to raise blood glucose concentration through direct effects on glycogenolysis and gluconeogenesis and, indirectly, through reducing insulin release, decreasing insulin sensitivity, and possibly stimulating glucagon release. Of equal, if not greater, importance is the effect of the sympathoadrenal system on the regulation of lipolysis. The sympathetic innervation to adipose tissue and plasma catecholamines both stimulate lipolysis, an effect which is enhanced if there is also a catecholamine-mediated suppression of insulin release.

Thermogenesis

Given the profound effects of the catecholamines on metabolism that were described in the previous section, it would be surprising if there were not also an effect on energy metabolism. It was demonstrated over 60 years ago that the infusion of adrenaline (in amounts which we now know produce plasma adrenaline levels in the physiological range) into humans caused an increase in whole body energy metabolism, as well as stimulating heart rate and respiration (Cori and Buchwald 1930). This effect is now known as adrenaline (catecholamine)-induced thermogenesis (the stimulation of energy metabolism above resting baseline levels) and does not involve an increase in physical activity, although adrenaline will of course increase skeletal muscle tremor. The existence of this catecholamine-induced thermogenesis has been confirmed many times and may be of physiological importance in the control of energy balance and of body temperature.

   The infusion of noradrenaline also stimulates thermogenesis, mainly through an increase in lipolysis and oxidation of free fatty acids (as is the case with adrenaline), although the amounts which have to be used are somewhat larger than for adrenaline. In fact, the plasma adrenaline threshold for increasing thermogenesis is towards the lower end of the physiological range. Higher plasma levels of noradrenaline are needed to stimulate thermogenesis, indicating that under physiological conditions it is more likely that direct stimulation of thermogenesis by noradrenaline occurs due to activation of the sympathetic nerves rather than through an effect of plasma noradrenaline.

When the human neonate is exposed to a cool environment, its total heat production increases (cold-induced thermogenesis) to maintain body temperature. It seems most probable that this cold-induced thermogenesis is mediated through the sympathetic nervous system activating thermogenesis in brown adipose tissue—as seen also in cold adapted rodents and hibernating mammals. Thus, catecholamine-induced thermogenesis is of major importance in neonatal thermoregulation. Studies in adult humans also indicate that cold-induced thermogenesis occurs in the absence of muscle contraction (Jessen et al. 1980), and it has been suggested that this is also stimulated by catecholamines. However, the normal human adult has insufficient brown adipose tissue to contribute significantly to heat production in the cold, and it seems more probable that the splanchnic region and skeletal muscle are the major sites of such thermogenesis. Nevertheless, such non-shivering thermogenesis would be of minor importance in the regulation of body temperature in most situations (this is considered further in Chapter 12).

There is an increasing volume of evidence that sympathoadrenal effects on thermogenesis may be of importance in the overall regulation of energy metabolism. It has been apparent for many years that experimental animals (e.g. rats, pigs) and in some cases humans can regulate overall thermogenesis to maintain energy balance over a wide range of energy intake. Studies in the rat by Rothwell and Stock (1981) indicated that the consumption of excessive amounts of a varied, palatable diet did not produce the expected degree of weight gain, because of a profound increase in energy expenditure. This increased energy expenditure was not due to physical activity, but was a result of increased sympathetic nervous stimulation of brown adipose tissue and of an increased mass of this tissue. Attempts to make similar observations in adult humans foundered because of the small amounts of this tissue present. However, there have now been several demonstrations of marked sympatho-adrenal effects on overall energy metabolism.

The first of these demonstrations relates to the effects of insulin and glucose in normal man. If one raises plasma insulin levels by exogenous infusion, but then infuses glucose to maintain a constant blood glucose, the amount of glucose infused matches the glucose taken up by the tissues and is a measure of the sensitivity of the individual to insulin (the glucose clamp method). In healthy subjects, the glucose taken up by the tissues is either oxidized or stored as glycogen. Acheson and colleagues demonstrated that this combined infusion of insulin and glucose stimulated thermogenesis (increasing resting energy expenditure by 10–20 per cent) and that the observed increase was substantially greater than the expected increase required to provide the necessary energy for the amount of glycogen being synthesized. The demonstration that this extra energy expenditure could be suppressed by administration of a β-adrenoceptor antagonist led to the proposition that part of the observed glucose-induced thermogenesis was due to sympatho-adrenal activation (Acheson 1988).

Further support for a link between glucose metabolism, the sympatho-adrenal system, and thermogenesis comes from the studies of Astrup and colleagues. They demonstrated an increase in thermogenesis in resting skeletal muscle, approximately 4 h after ingestion of a glucose load, coincident with an increase in plasma adrenaline levels. Subsequent studies by this group showed that the ingestion of a mixed meal has a similar effect and that, in both cases, this delayed stimulation of thermogenesis can be prevented by β-adrenoceptor blockade (Astrup *et al.* 1990). In the same review, these authors provided a useful analysis of previous studies which indicated that β-blockade only reduced meal-induced thermogenesis in the later stages and when there was a high carbohydrate content of the ingested food.

Recent work by Schwartz and colleagues has shown a positive correlation between the increase in thermogenesis seen after consuming a mixed meal and the stimulation of the sympathetic nervous system (assessed by measuring plasma noradrenaline turnover). Furthermore, the administration of clonidine to suppress central sympathetic outflow reduced both the sympathetic stimulation and the thermogenic response to the meals (Schwartz *et al.* 1988).

Summary

The sympathoadrenal system can stimulate thermogenesis, and there are a number of physiological conditions in which this effect may operate. The final part of this chapter will consider whether disorders of such effects are involved in the aetiology of obesity or in disturbances of thermoregulation.

Metabolic and nutritional effects on the sympathoadrenal system

In addition to the sympathoadrenal system being important in the regulation of metabolism, it is apparent that alterations in metabolic or nutritional status can affect the activity of the sympathoadrenal system. Some of these effects would be entirely predictable on the basis of the regulation of metabolism discussed above. The best example of this is the effect of an acute reduction in blood glucose concentration producing hypoglycaemia, which leads to adrenaline release from the adrenal medulla and altered sympathetic nervous system activity. However, there are a variety of other metabolic and nutritional effects on the sympathoadrenal system which will now be considered.

Dietary effects on the sympathetic nervous system

Animal studies

The possibility that the amount and composition of the diet may affect the sympathetic nervous system has been addressed by the studies of Landsberg, Young, and colleagues over the past 15 years (Landsberg and Young 1985). They have assessed the activity of the sympathetic nervous system by measuring the rate of turnover of the neurotransmitter noradrenaline in specific organs and tissues of rats and mice. These studies have shown that starvation suppresses and overfeeding enhances sympathetic activity, with an increased dietary carbohydrate content being a particularly potent stimulus. This effect of carbohydrate in stimulating the sympathetic nervous system appears to involve an action of insulin in the hypothalamus. This has led to a series of studies on the effects of insulin on the sympathetic nervous system in humans which will be discussed below and in Chapters 36 and 37.

There are impressive correlations between increased noradrenaline turnover and thermogenesis in brown adipose tissue during both excess dietary intake and cold adaptation in rodents. Thus, it would appear that there is an important functional role for diet-induced changes in sympathetic activity. This is supported by the demonstration that a reduced energy intake leads to a fall in sympathetic activity and in blood pressure in spontaneously hypertensive rats.

Human studies

Assessing the activity of the sympathetic nervous system in humans is restricted to intraneural recording in superficial nerves (Chapter 18), measuring plasma noradrenaline turnover (Esler *et al.* 1990), or measuring plasma or urinary catecholamine concentrations (Chapter 17). Each of these techniques has some limitations, and caution must be exercised when interpreting any results obtained, especially if there are no associated functional measurements. Alterations in dietary intake in humans are accompanied by changes in sympathetic activity (assessed with plasma noradrenaline turnover and plasma and urinary levels) which are qualitatively similar to the effects seen in animals. A reduced energy intake is accompanied by evidence of reduced sympathetic activity and decreased supine blood pressure, with increased energy intake being associated with opposite changes. Although these effects are modest, they may be of some functional significance and are considered further in the section entitled 'Changes in sympathoadrenally regulated processes during metabolic/nutritional disturbances'.

Metabolic effects on the sympathoadrenal system

The most potent metabolic disturbances which affect the sympathoadrenal system relate to alterations in glucose metabolism, or in plasma insulin

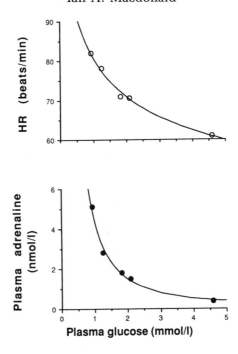

Fig. 11.3. Heart rate (HR) and plasma adrenaline responses to insulin-induced hypoglycaemia. In both cases there is a curvilinear relationship with more profound hypoglycaemia having a progressively greater effect.

concentrations. In healthy adult humans an overnight fast produces blood glucose concentrations of 4–5 mmol/l. Acute reduction of blood glucose to approximately 3.5 mmol/l (with insulin) is followed within 10 min by the secretion of adrenaline from the adrenal medulla. More severe hypoglycaemia is associated with progressively increasing adrenaline responses (Fig. 11.3). This release of adrenaline at a relatively high blood glucose level is part of the early endocrine response which opposes the effect of insulin and occurs before any detectable impairment in cerebral function caused by the fall in blood glucose.

More profound hypoglycaemia (blood glucose 2–3 mmol/l) is accompanied by increases in plasma noradrenaline concentrations, and the rate of appearance of noradrenaline in plasma, and by an increase in muscle and skin nerve sympathetic activity as measured by microneurography (reviewed by Heller and Macdonald 1991). The effect on muscle sympathetic activity is interesting as this appears to be occurring in vasoconstrictor fibres, yet muscle vasodilatation occurs in hypoglycaemia. The latter is not due to the effects of insulin (see below) as it occurs when hypoglycaemia is induced with relatively low plasma insulin levels (below 120 mU/l) whilst the effect of insulin in producing vasodilatation in skeletal muscle does not occur until insulin levels exceed 140 mU/l. It is far more likely that the muscle vasodilatation in hypoglycaemia is due to the increased plasma adrenaline levels as it can be prevented by β-adrenoceptor antagonism. The muscle blood flow response to hypoglycaemia illustrates the need to assess sympathetically mediated function as well as sympathetic nervous system activity.

Such hypoglycaemia occurs most commonly in patients with IDDM. When these patients first develop diabetes, their responses to hypoglycaemia are the same as in non-diabetic subjects. However, within 5 years of the onset of IDDM, most patients lose the ability to release glucagon in response to hypoglycaemia (although not in response to other stimuli). Such patients are then dependent on an adequate adrenaline response, and on the disappearance of the injected insulin, for blood glucose recovery after hypoglycaemia (unless they eat). When such diabetic patients develop autonomic neuropathy of such a severity that they fail to release adrenaline from the adrenal medulla, they will then be at risk of developing prolonged, severe hypoglycaemia if their insulin dose and food intake are poorly matched.

A rise in blood glucose concentration is often accompanied by an increase in plasma noradrenaline, heart rate, and blood pressure consistent with stimulation of the sympathetic nervous system. This is confirmed by the demonstration of increased muscle sympathetic nerve activity after glucose ingestion (Berne *et al.* 1989). The effect of glucose can be explained at least partly by an action of insulin on the sympathetic nervous system. The technique of insulin and glucose infusion (glucose clamping) described above leads to a rise in plasma noradrenaline, heart rate, and systolic blood pressure in normal humans. Studies with microneurography have shown increased muscle sympathetic (vasoconstrictor) nerve activity, but again it is interesting to note that forearm (predominantly muscle) blood flow increases in these circumstances (Scott *et al.* 1988*a*). This raises the possibility that insulin may have direct effects on the vascular smooth muscle (or the sympathetic nerve terminals) to produce vasodilatation which leads to reflex activation of the sympathetic nervous system.

Changes in sympathoadrenally regulated processes during metabolic/nutritional disturbances

Acute (48 h) starvation in healthy humans is accompanied by functional changes consistent with altered sympathoadrenal activity. The regulation of body temperature during cold exposure is impaired with inadequate increases in thermogenesis and reductions in limb blood flow contributing to a fall in core temperature (Macdonald *et al.* 1984). In addition, there is no increase in thermogenesis during insulin and glucose infusion in starvation. As the latter response is normally mediated by the sympathetic nervous system this is consistent with reduced sympathetic activity in starvation. Further evidence of functional impairment of sympathetic control during starvation is provided by the falls in arterial blood pressure on standing seen after 48 h starvation in young men with normal orthostatic responses in the fed state (Bennett *et al.* 1984). These functional impairments seen in acute starvation are not due to the inability to respond to catecholamines, as the cardiac and thermogenic responses to infused adrenaline are actually enhanced after 48 h starvation.

These demonstrations of functional impairments consistent with reduced sympathetic activity are not restricted to acute starvation. Severe weight loss in human babies (due to inadequate food intake) and adults (with Crohn's disease, coeliac disease, or postoperative fistulae) is accompanied by impaired thermoregulation, particularly with reduced or absent thermogenic responses, which is reversed by weight gain. Impaired thermoregulation also occurs in anorexia nervosa, although it is not clear whether these changes are also reversible. It seems most unlikely that weight loss in anorexia nervosa is contributed to by enhanced thermogenic responses to food or to catecholamines, which would increase overall energy expenditure producing the opposite effect to that which may occur in obesity (see below). However, the weight loss associated with chronic respiratory disease is accompanied by increases in resting energy expenditure and urinary catecholamine excretion, providing further evidence of an effect of the sympathoadrenal system on energy metabolism.

Many studies have also shown poor orthostatic tolerance during chronic undernutrition, although this may of course be due to disturbances of fluid and electrolyte balance rather than to nutritional effects on the sympathetic nervous system.

Obesity

The role of the sympathoadrenal system in controlling substrate mobilization and thermogenesis, and the links between nutritional factors and the sympathetic nervous system have led to the proposition that reduced sympathetic activity contributes to the development or maintenance of obesity. Some investigators have shown reduced catecholamine-induced thermogenesis in the obese, and others have observed altered plasma catecholamine kinetics. However, there have been many conflicting reports, and it seems most probable that human obesity is not due to a single metabolic defect, but has varied aetiologies. However, there is no doubt that if an individual fails to respond to increased carbohydrate intake by activating thermogenesis (possibly through the sympathetic nervous system) then they will have a greater tendency to develop obesity than someone who does increase thermogenesis.

There have now been several studies of patients already obese which revealed minor impairments of autonomic function associated with obesity (Peterson *et al.* 1988). Most of these changes were in the parasympathetic nervous system (analagous to the early stages of autonomic neuropathy in diabetes mellitus). There is also evidence of abnormal regulation of platelet α-adrenoceptors in obesity although there is little disturbance of β-adreno-ceptor sensitivity unless such patients are underfed (Berlin *et al.* 1990).

Sympathoadrenal dysfunction

The main consequences of sympathoadrenal dysfunction are considered in other sections of this book, but it is worth noting here that patients with autonomic failure are frequently insulin-resistant and can have impaired glucose tolerance. However, this is likely to result mainly from their low levels of physical activity, and possibly reduced carbohydrate intake, rather than from defects in the autonomic nervous system. The other two clinical situations in which one might expect altered control of metabolism are in adrenal insufficiency (either Addison's disease or post-adrenalectomy) or in diabetic autonomic neuropathy.

Addison's disease is characterized by adrenocortical degeneration and loss of corticosteroids, but the adrenal medulla is usually preserved. However, the enzyme phenyl *N*-ethanolamine methyl transferase (PNMT) involved in the conversion of noradrenaline to adrenaline is only produced in the presence of cortisol. Thus, in untreated Addison's disease there would be a deficiency of adrenaline which would contribute to the problems of hypoglycaemia and intolerance of other stresses which characterize this condition. Once the patients are given glucocorticoid replacement therapy there should be normal production of adrenaline, provided the adrenal medulla is preserved.

There is little evidence of impaired thermoregulation or other aspects of metabolism in adrenalectomized patients, although there have been few studies of such patients using the more sensitive methods now available. The fact that adrenalectomy does not produce serious metabolic disturbances (provided that corticosteroid replacement therapy is adequate) is not too surprising as the sympathetic innervation of blood vessels (to regulate heat loss in thermoregulation) and of the metabolically active tissues and endocrine glands, are probably more important than the effects of circulating adrenaline. The major exception is the prevention of hypoglycaemia during exercise, starvation, or in the presence of an excess of insulin. The primary factor acting to raise blood glucose under these conditions is glucagon, with adrenaline providing a secondary role. Obviously, the absence of a glucagon response in an adrenalectomized patient would then lead to serious problems in the defence of blood glucose concentration. Such an occurrence is likely to be rare, as (apart from the failure to release glucagon in IDDM as mentioned above) the only circumstances likely to affect glucagon release are the infusion of somatostatin or its analogues and, of course, pancreatectomy.

The problems of impaired responses to hypoglycaemia in diabetic autonomic neuropathy were considered above. However, diabetic autonomic neuropathy has other implications for metabolism, as these patients have impaired thermoregulatory responses to cold exposure. Such patients have less vasoconstriction in the feet and legs when exposed to the cold, and are more likely to shiver than diabetic patients without such complications. Furthermore, the rate of resting energy expenditure under thermoneutral conditions of the neuropathic patients who shivered was higher than in non-neuropathic patients who did not shiver when cooled (Scott *et al.* 1988*b*). This indicates that inadequate control of the peripheral circulation through impaired sympathetic function is likely to lead to increased heat loss which requires an elevated resting metabolic rate to maintain thermal balance.

Conclusions

The sympathoadrenal system is an important regulator of metabolism, and an essential feature of homeostasis is the activation of the sympathoadrenal system when the tissue fuel supplies are compromised (e.g. the adrenaline response to hypoglycaemia). However, there does appear to be a more fundamental link between nutritional status and the sympathetic nervous system which may have important implications for the development/maintenance of obesity.

References

Acheson, K. J. (1988). Nutrient induced thermogenesis. In *Clinical progress in nutrition research* (ed. A. Sitges-Serra, A. Sitges-Creus, and S. Schwartz-Riera), pp. 255–64. Karger, Basel.

Arch, J. R. S., Ainsworth, A. T., and Cawthorne, M. A. (1984). Atypical β-adrenoceptor on brown adipocytes as target for antiobesity drugs. *Nature* **309** 163–5.

Astrup, A., Christensen, N. J., Simonsen, L., and Bulow, J. (1990). Effects of nutrient intake on sympathoadrenal activity and thermogenic mechanisms. *J. Neurosci. Methods* **34**, 187–92.

Bennett, T., Macdonald, I. A., and Sainsbury, R. (1984). The influence of starvation on the cardiovascular responses to lower body subatmospheric pressure or to standing in man. *Clin. Sci.* **66**, 141–6.

Berlin, I., Berlan, M., Crespo-Laumonier, B., Landault, C., Payan, C., Puech, A. J., and Turpin, G. (1990). Alterations in β-adrenergic sensitivity and platelet α_2-adrenoceptors in obese women: effect of exercise and calorie restriction. *Clin. Sci.* **78**, 81–7.

Berne, C., Fagius, J., and Niklasson, F. (1989). Sympathetic response to oral carbohydrate administration. Evidence from micro-electrode recordings. *J. clin. Invest.* **84**, 1403–9.

Boyle, P. J., Shah, S. D., and Cryer, P. E. (1989). Insulin, glucagon and catecholamines in prevention of hypoglycemia during fasting. *Am. J. Physiol.* **256**, E651–E661.

Clutter, W. E., Rizza, R. A., Gerich, J. E., and Cryer, P. E. (1988). Regulation of glucose metabolism by sympathochromaffin catecholamines. *Diabetes/Metab. Rev.* **4**, 1–15.

Cori, C. F. and Buchwald, K. W. (1930). Effect of continuous injection of epinephrine on the carbohydrate metabolism, basal metabolism and vascular system of normal man. *Am. J. Physiol.* **95**, 71–8.

Esler, M., Jennings, G., Lambert, G., Meredith, I., Horne, M., and Eisenhofer, G. (1990). Overflow of catecholamine neurotransmitter to the circulation: source, fate and function. *Physiol. Rev.* **70**, 963–85.

Fredholm, B. B. (1985). Nervous control of circulation and metabolism in white adipose tissue. In *New perspectives in adipose tissue: structure, function and development* (ed. A. Cryer and R. L. R. Van), pp. 45–64. Butterworth, London.

Heller, S. R. and Macdonald, I. A. (1991). Physiological disturbances in hypoglycaemia: effect on subjective awareness. *Clin. Sci.* **81**, 1–9.

Hjemdahl, P. and Linde, B. (1983). Influence of circulating NE and Epi on adipose tissue vascular resistance and lipolysis in humans. *Am. J. Physiol.* **245**, H447–H452.

Jessen, K., Rabol, A., and Winkles, K. (1980). Total body and splanchnic thermogenesis in curarized man during a short exposure to cold. *Acta anaesthesiol. scand.* **24**, 339–44.

Landsberg, L. and Young, J. B. (1985). The influence of diet on the sympathetic nervous system. In *Neuroendocrine perspectives* (ed. E. E. Muller, R. M. MacLeod, and L. A. Frohman), pp. 191–218. Elsevier, Amsterdam.

Lautt, W. W. (1980). Hepatic nerves. A review of their functions and effects. *Can. J. Physiol. Pharmacol.* **58**, 105–23.

Macdonald, I. A., Bennett, T., and Sainsbury, R. (1984). The effect of a 48 h fast on the thermoregulatory responses to graded cooling in man. *Clin. Sci.* **67**, 445–52.

Madonald, I. A., Bennett, T., and Fellows, I. W. (1985). Catecholamines and the control of metabolism in man. *Clin. Sci.* **68**, 613–19.

Miles, J. M., Nissen, S. L., Gerich, J. E., and Haymond, M. W. (1984). Effect of epinephrine infusion on leucine and alanine kinetics in humans. *Am. J. Physiol.* **247**, E166–E172.

Niijima, A. (1989). Nervous regulation of metabolism. *Progress Neurobiol.* **33**, 135–47.

Peterson, H. R., Rothschild, M., Weinberg, C. R., Fell, R. D., McLeish, K. R., and Pfeiffer, M. A. (1988). Body fat and the activity of the autonomic nervous system. *New Engl. J. Med.* **318**, 1077–83.

Rothwell, N. J. and Stock, M. J. (1981). Regulation of energy balance. *Ann. Rev. Nutr.* **1**, 235–56.

Schwartz, R. S., Jaeger, L. F., and Veith, R. C. (1988). Effect of clonidine on the thermic effect of feeding in humans. *Am. J. Physiol.* **254**, R90–R94.

Scott, A. R., Bennett, T., and Macdonald, I. A. (1988a). Effects of hyperinsulinaemia on the cardiovascular responses to graded hypovolaemia in normal and diabetic subjects. *Clin. Sci.* **75**, 85–92.

Scott, A. R., Macdonald, I. A., Bennett, T., and Tattersall, R. B. (1988b). Abnormal thermoregulation in diabetic autonomic neuropathy. *Diabetes* **37**, 961–8.

Young, J. B. and Landsberg, L. (1977). Catecholamines and intermediary metabolism. *Clinics Endocrinol. Metab.* **6**, 599–631.

12. The autonomic nervous system and the regulation of body temperature

Kenneth J. Collins

Introduction

Body temperature regulation in mammals depends on the integrated activity of higher central nervous, autonomic, and neuroendocrine systems, with the hypothalamus as the dominant central controller. In analysing reactions to different levels of heat energy a distinction is often made between autonomic and behavioural temperature regulation. Autonomic thermoregulation in the sense of involuntary, self-governing processes, involves control of shivering, non-shivering thermogenesis, cutaneous blood flow, sweat secretion, pilo-erection, and the endocrine responses. Panting and salivation are important mechanisms of body temperature control in many animals but are insignificant in human responses to heat. Thermoregulatory behaviour on the other hand is associated with conscious temperature sensations as well as emotional feelings of thermal comfort or discomfort, which result in complex behavioural adjust-ments in seeking shelter, postural changes, and the use of clothing. Behavioural reactions to heat and cold modify the relationship between the organism and its environment and thereby alter the need for autonomic thermoregulation, though this does not necessarily imply central nervous co-ordination between the two. Autonomic thermoregulation does not always depend on autonomic nervous activity, however. Shivering, for example, is an involuntary response to cold which is controlled via somatic motor pathways through descending tracts leaving the posterior hypothalamus and eventually by the cerebrospinal and reticulospinal pathways to skeletal muscle motoneurones.

The role of the autonomic nervous system in temperature regulation involves two basic elements: first, organization in the central control structures of the hypothalamus and connecting centres and, second, the functions of the efferent autonomic pathways regulating heat loss and heat production. Regulation of heat loss is autonomically dependent on the sympathetic nervous control of vasomotor activity and sweat secretion. Heat production is at least partly dependent on the sympathetic and sympathoadrenal-medullary control of metabolism and, particularly in the human newborn, on sympathetic stimulation of non-shivering thermogenesis.

Central autonomic control of thermoregulation

There are numerous observations showing good correlations between the activity of thermosensitive neurons in the hypothalamus and thermoregulatory responses (reviewed by Hori *et al.* 1989). A principal role in thermoregulation is proposed for thermosensitive neurons responding to small changes in local temperature particularly in the preoptic/anterior hypothalamic area. *In vitro* studies using brain tissue slices have suggested the existence of 'primary' warm-sensitive and cold-sensitive neurons which have inherent thermosensitivity in the preoptic/anterior hypothalamus and other brain areas. The high degree of convergence of thermal signals from local and remote sites on to these neurons further suggests that thermosensitive neurons in one site of the central nervous system are connected to those in other sites and form neuronal control networks within the brain and spinal cord. Many earlier studies had pointed to two linked centres, one concerned with heat loss in the anterior hypothalamus and the other with heat production in a more posterior hypothalamic centre. Bazett (1968) proposed that body temperature regulation depended on a balance between the opposing activity of these two centres with crossed inhibitory control. It is now apparent that there is not just one central control centre in the hypothalamus but a hierarchy of neural integration and control for each thermoregulatory response (Simon *et al.* 1986). In this respect, our understanding of central nervous thermoregulatory control has developed along similar lines to that of the 'vasomotor centre'. The widely held view of a 'vasomotor centre' comprising two mutually antagonistic half-centres located in the medulla oblongata has been superseded by that of a series of multilevel integrating circuits, encompassing the medulla, pons, midbrain, hypothalamus, limbic, and forebrain structures, which allows for greater functional plasticity.

Hypothalamic 'set-point'

Ideas on the theoretical need for a hypothalamic 'set-point' were originally developed by Vendrik (1959) who postulated thermoreceptors in the hypothalamus with temperature–activity characteristics similar to those of peripheral warm and cold receptors (Fig. 12.1). The activity–response curves were depicted as overlapping, and at only one temperature, the 'set-point', did they both have the same activity. Deviation from this temperature would result in the frequency of one sensor increasing and the other decreasing. Indeed, with the use of micro-electrode recordings from the preoptic/anterior hypothalamic region in subsequent mammalian experiments various types of single-unit thermosensitive neurons have been identified that respond with positive or negative temperature coefficients to local temperature changes (Hensel 1981). The notion of a central thermostat control system acting as a

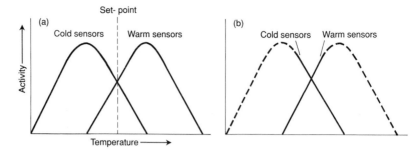

Fig. 12.1. (a) Activity–temperature characteristics of hypothalamic cold sensors and warm sensors. (After Vendrik (1959).) (b) The positive and negative linear activity–temperature relationships of primary cold sensors and warm sensors shown as segments of Vendrik's bell-shaped curves. (After Bligh (1983).)

proportional control between the feedback signal and the set-point (Benzinger *et al.* 1963) was clearly insufficient to account for the thermoregulatory capability of the hypothalamic centres.

Hammel and his colleagues (1963) introduced the idea that temperature regulation depended on a hypothalamic proportional control with an 'adjustable set-point'. A neuronal scheme was proposed involving two populations of neurons in the hypothalamus—primary 'warm' (high Q_{10}) and primary 'cold' (low Q_{10}) with high and low positive responses to temperature, respectively. The 'set-point' was considered to be that hypothalamic temperature at which the activities of the two neuron populations were the same (Fig. 12.2). Thus, in a cold environment, the change in activity characteristics of the neurons results in an upward shift in the 'set-point' temperature and, in a hot environment, in a downward shift.

Others have questioned the 'set-point' hypothesis and proposed that, instead of a 'set-point' shift, thermosensitive cells in the hypothalamus may be subject to a change in 'gain' or sensitivity (Mitchell *et al.* 1970). Thus, in fever, a pyrogen-induced change in sensitivity of the neurons could occur with a change in slope of the thermal responses of single units. In a control system with a single feedback loop, the loop may be 'opened' in order to measure the gain, for example,

$$\text{Gain} = \frac{\Delta T_{co}}{\Delta T_{se}}$$

where ΔT_{co} is the change in core temperature and ΔT_{se} is the temperature change at the sensor. However, in thermoregulation, an open loop gain may

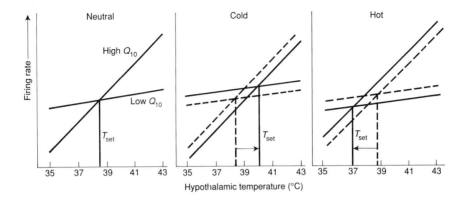

Fig. 12.2. A 'set-point' theory based on firing rate–temperature characteristics of hypothalamic neurons with small (low Q_{10}) or large (high Q_{10}) positive responses to temperature. The 'set-point' of temperature regulation (T_{set}) is considered to be that hypothalamic temperature at which the activities of the two neuron populations are equal. (From Hammel *et al.* (1963).)

be difficult to measure because of an unknown number of other closed loops counteracting the displacement of temperature by setting up feedback signals. A method of direct determination of the gain of the hypothalamic temperature sensors has been devised in animal studies using independent control of hypothalamic, extrahypothalamic (brain), and trunk core temperature with implanted local thermodes and intravascular heat exchangers (Heath and Jessen 1988).

According to Bligh (1983), a workable basis for temperature regulation proposes that the crossed inhibition in hypothalamic centres does not create a 'set-point' but a 'null-point' or 'zone' at or between the temperature thresholds for thermoregulatory heat loss and heat gain effector activities. The converging excitatory and inhibitory influences, including those from peripheral temperature sensors, modify the relation between the activities of core temperature sensors and the thermoregulatory effectors, thereby causing temporary changes in the 'null point' of the regulated body temperature. How the central nervous system interprets the information received from sensors is poorly understood generally and remains a controversial issue. 'Set-point' is variously thought to be based on temperature-insensitive continuously firing neurons, a biochemical gating influence on the thermosensors, or an ionic gating influence on these pathways (see Bligh 1983). A central 'set-point' or 'gain' determinant remains a plausible model but the biological correlates of these functions remain enigmatic.

Thermogenesis and sympathetic nervous activity

While shivering thermogenesis is under the control of somatic nerves, metabolic heat production is also dependent on the sympathetic and sympathoadrenal systems. As discussed in Chapter 11, the sympathoadrenal system stimulates hepatic glycogenolysis and gluconeogenesis and modulates pancreatic insulin and glucagon release. Sympathetic nerves can also directly affect metabolic activity by increasing hepatic glycogenolysis in some circumstances, e.g. severe hypoglycaemia, and by regulating blood flow and metabolism in both white and brown adipose tissues. Thermogenesis produced by sympathetic nervous activity can be distinguished from that produced by the sympathoadrenal system. For example, during fasting when hypoglycaemia is sufficiently severe there may arise a situation where increasing adrenal medullary activity is associated with a relative suppression of sympathetic nervous activity (Young *et al.* 1984). The same combination of changes can occur during acute hypoxia or trauma. The result is a reduction in oxygen consumption, and this is seen as evidence of the greater contribution made by sympathetic innervation than by the adrenal medulla in the control of thermogenesis.

Early classical experiments on the effects of changes in the temperature of blood supplying the brain showed that, if carotid blood was warmed, blood glucose levels fell together with a fall in rectal temperature. Conversely, blood glucose and rectal temperature increased when carotid blood was cooled. The close link between body temperature regulation and energy metabolism suggests a reciprocal process involving hypothalamic and sympathetic nervous control. It has been suggested that the nervous system responds to changes in energy intake such that energy restriction decreases and energy administration increases sympathetic nervous activity (Appenzeller 1983). Insulin appears to be another important link between changes in dietary intake and central sympathetic activity. Diet-induced thermogenesis may be decreased in obese animals and man, though there is no consensus that this results from abnormal dietary regulation of sympathetic responses. However, the connection between dietary intake (mostly carbohydrate) and sympathetic nervous system activity may have important implications for heat and exercise training as well as for obesity and hypertension (Young and Landsberg 1982).

The calorigenic action of catecholamines released by sympathetic stimulation during cold exposure is likely to be of some importance in the control of body temperature (Fig. 12.3). Non-shivering thermogenesis through the sympathetic nervous stimulation of brown adipose tissue is thought to be involved in maintaining heat balance in the neonate. The newborn increase their heat production in the cold without obvious shivering, and intravenous infusion of noradrenaline increases their heat production in the warm. Thermogenesis in the cold may, however, be caused by an increase in muscular

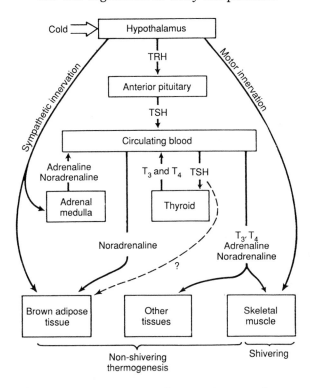

Fig. 12.3. Schematic representation of sympathetic and sympathoadrenal pathways in thermogenesis. TRH, thyrotrophin releasing hormone; TSH, thyroid stimulating hormone. (Reproduced with permission from Maclean and Emslie-Smith (1977) p. 49.)

tone without obvious shivering, and noradrenaline infusion is often accompanied by arousal and crying which increase heat production. Present evidence suggests that there is little brown adipose tissue in the human adult. In subjects exposed to air at 12 °C for 8 hours daily, electromyographic activity and oxygen consumption both decline with successive exposures. The oxygen consumption, however, declines less than muscle electrical activity which could be interpreted as evidence for the development of non-shivering thermogenesis. Outdoor workers such as lumberjacks and timbermen in northern Finland are reported to develop deposits of brown adipose tissue around the carotid arteries (seen at autopsy) while indoor workers of the same age do not. The inference is that people who spend much time out of doors in winter may develop non-shivering thermogenesis as a cold defence mechanism. Thus, there remains some indication that humans may develop the capacity for brown fat non-shivering thermogenesis following acclimatization to cold, though this is small compared to rodents. Non-shivering thermogenesis may arise from other sources (Fig. 12.3). For example, patients with pathological elevations of circulating thyroid hormones show manifestations typical of adrenergic activation including tachycardia, increased non-shivering thermogenesis, and sweating.

Thermoregulatory vasomotor responses

In most areas of the body vascular insulation in skin tissues is regulated by a balance between neurogenic vasoconstriction and local vasodilatation by metabolites, vasoactive substances, and the direct effects of temperature. Sympathetic vasoconstrictor tone is marked in the limbs and generalized vasodilatation can be brought about by inhibition of this tone. Vasodilatiation may, however, also be produced by the release of co-localized transmitters such as vasoactive intestinal polypeptide (VIP) from cholinergic sudomotor nerves (Lundberg *et al.* 1979) during sweating and possibly also by putative active vasodilator neurons.

The possibility that specific vasodilator nerves exist in the skin remains controversial. Indirect evidence from experiments on cats and dogs tends to support their existence. For example, spinal cord heating and electrical stimulation of the preganglionic axons in the lumbar sympathetic trunk evoke an atropine-resistant vasodilatation in the hind paw even after noradrenergic vasoconstrictor block, while the dilator fibre population is distinct from that mediating eccrine sweat secretion (Bell *et al.* 1985). During graded spinal cord warming, it has been shown that, in recordings from single unmyelinated fibres in the cat hind paw, some units can be vigorously activated. It was not proved, however, that these fibres were truly postganglionic. Experiments on humans and animals indicate that the skin may be innervated by a set of functionally distinct sympathetic vasodilator neurons. The transmitter of these neurons is not known. The strict coincidence between sweating and cutaneous vasodilatation could well be explained, however, by the reciprocal organization of the cutaneous sudomotor and vasoconstrictor pathways in the neuraxis, and does not require an active neural vasodilator system.

Sympathetic sudomotor innervation

The sympathetic cholinergic innervation of the eccrine sweat glands was demonstrated originally by Dale and Feldberg in the cat's paw and subsequent experiments have confirmed the dominant response of human glands to acetylcholine and allied substances (Collins 1989). Intravenous administration of 0.5 mg atropine sulphate in humans is sufficient to inhibit sweating within 2 or 3 min. However, human eccrine sweat glands also respond to intradermally administered catecholamines and to intraarterial infusion of adrenaline. Although α-blockers such as phentolamine and guanethidine inhibit adrenaline-induced sweating, these substances possess anticholinergic properties. The existence of both adrenergic and cholinergic periglandular nerves of the eccrine sweat glands of macaques (Uno and Montagna 1975) revived discussion of dual autonomic innervation. The possible role of the adrenergic component may be in the metabolic control of glandular growth and its plasticity (Collins 1989).

The sudomotor nerve terminals are acetylcholinesterase and choline acetyltransferase-rich, and these neurons contain VIP and other peptides such as calcitonin gene-related peptide (CGRP) involved in neurotransmission. The properties of the young adult human sudomotor nerves appear to be similar to those described in the foot pad of the young mature rat (Landis 1990) where the acetylcholinesterase content is high, with intense VIP, some CGRP, and very faint tyrosine hydroxylase (TOH) immunoreactivity. There is marked involution of the neuroeffector sudomotor system in aged humans with a virtual absence of acetylcholinesterase in sudomotor nerve endings (Abdel-Rahman et al. 1992). Connections between neurons and their target organs are subject to continuous adjustment by means of intercellular signals, e.g. by nerve growth factor (NGF). Treatment of newborn rats with antiserum to NGF for example, produces a loss of sympathetic neurons that normally project to eccrine sweat glands in the rat's paw (Hill et al. 1988). NGF is required postnatally for the survival of cholinergic sympathetic neurons and continuity of nerve supply and nervous activity in neuroeffector relationships appears to be important also in adult life. In maturity, decreased levels of postsynaptic nervous activity may increase the trophic stimulus provided by target cells to their innervation while increased postganglionic activity decreases it (Gallego and Geijo 1987). On the other hand, in the aged organism, a minor reduction in the production of NGF by a target organ may lead to impairment of transmitter synthesis within the nerve, and a large reduction might produce degeneration of nerve fibres or even nerve cell bodies (Cowen and Burnstock 1986).

Hypothermia

Hypothermia is sometimes a feature of syndromes arising from autonomic dysfunction and is manifest particularly in old people in cold conditions (see also Chapter 44). Recent experience suggests that the prevalence in the UK is much less than predicted in the 1960s and with a mortality in the population of about 1 per cent of the total excess winter deaths (Collins 1992). The registration of deaths from hypothermia presents difficulties because of the uncertainty as to whether hypothermia is a primary or secondary event. The condition can occur when there is a marked deterioration in vital functions often associated with severe malnutrition and intercurrent illness. It is therefore not exclusively cold-induced and many cases are encountered in marginally nourished tropical populations. A spontaneous fall in deep body temperature may present in the course of infectious diseases (Maclean and Emslie-Smith 1977, p. 283) as has recently been confirmed in a study of elderly patients admitted to hospital with acute illnesses complicated by chest infections (Darowski *et al.* 1991). Hypothalamic dysfunction in temperature control may be a common link between various infective disorders and hypothermia. Recognition of both extrinsic and intrinsic factors in the aetiology of hypothermia is important in the management of the disorder (Wollner and Collins 1992).

Hypothermia can be usefully categorized as follows: (1) primary hypothermia in which there is an inherent failure of the neural control system due to congenital central nervous abnormalities, e.g. corpus callosum agenesis, or to the effects of hypothalamic trauma; (2) secondary hypothermia associated with existing pathological conditions such as diabetes mellitus, or to the effects of drugs (Wollner and Collins 1992); (3) accidental hypothermia resulting from unintentional exposure to overwhelming cold stress; and (4) controlled or therapeutic hypothermia for the purposes of surgery. Any of the first three types are likely to occur in elderly people and sometimes in coexistence. Although old people may be admitted to hospital with accidental hypothermia due to cold exposure superimposed on a failing thermoregulatory system, pathological conditions leading to secondary hypothermia are present in the majority.

While many abnormalities conducive to the occurrence of hypothermia result in impairment of heat production, autonomic control of the rate of heat loss through peripheral vasomotor tone plays a crucial role in the maintenance of body temperature within the zone of thermoneutrality. Persistent peripheral vasolidatation in the cold, by keeping the skin temperature abnormally high, would be expected to lower the threshold of shivering. Indeed it has been found that many of the individual differences in shivering thermogenesis in the cold may be related to the degree of dysfunction of the vasoconstrictor mechanism (Collins *et al.* 1981). In young adults, transient vasoconstrictor responses at rest in a neutral temperature environment may be demonstrated by microelectrode recording of sympathetic activity from human cutaneous nerves (Bini *et al.* 1980). Bursts of vasoconstriction occur rhythmically with a frequency that increases from 2–3 bursts/min to about 10 bursts/min in a cold environment. The responses indicate volleys of vasoconstrictor impulses entrained by central vasomotor rhythm-generating mechanisms. In many elderly people these rhythmic vasoconstrictor bursts are absent in neutral temperature conditions, though by itself this does not necessarily demonstrate diminished autonomic control since target organ responses may change with age.

The physiological mechanisms that dictate survival or non-survival after hypothermic stress are poorly understood. Very little information is available, for example, on the cerebral circulation and oxidative metabolism during hypothermia. The few studies conducted so far (e.g. Hernandez 1983) indicate only that cerebral blood flow and cerebral metabolic rate for oxygen decrease with body temperature.

Hyperthermia

Thermoregulatory impairment due to diminished or absent sweating is one of the factors responsible for the development of heat illness and heat stroke in hot conditions. Heat stroke is characterized by extreme hyperthermia with a core temperature of 41 °C or more, central nervous disturbances leading to convulsions, delirium, and coma, and anhidrosis which is often present but is not pathognomonic. At autopsy, destructive lesions in the hypothalamus have been described which represent severe disorganization of thermoregulation at a high level of autonomic control (Weiner et al. 1984). The high mortality from heat stroke, particularly in persons aged over 65 years, suggests that reduced ability to sweat and to vasodilate might be important precipitating causes of the thermoregulatory failure. Deaths in the elderly during heat waves, however, can usually be ascribed to existing ischaemic heart and cerebrovascular disease (see also Chapter 44). Only a small number of deaths appear to be caused directly by primary thermoregulatory failure in old people during heat waves.

The manifestations of heat stroke in the elderly are usually not typical of those in young adults (Collins 1992). In old people, heat stroke often occurs in epidemic form and in the presence of predisposing disorders such as arteriosclerotic heart disease, congestive cardiac failure, diabetes mellitus, parkinsonism, and recent or old stroke. In young adults, heat stroke is commonly exertional, arising in isolated cases, and less frequently related to an underlying chronic disorder. There is often uncertainty as to whether deficient sweat and vasomotor responses reflect deterioration of effector function rather than autonomic control. Eighty-year olds show striking changes in both neural and target organ morphology in the peripheral sudomotor system (Abdel-Rahman et al. 1992).

A number of problems complicate the circulatory vasomotor adjustments with exercise during hyperthermia. Reduced sympathetic venomotor tone leads to filling of the highly compliant capacitance vessels of the skin and eventually cardiac filling pressure is reduced and stroke volume declines, requiring a compensatory increase in heart rate. The high skin blood flow with exercise in the heat becomes attenuated at a critical skin blood flow which suggests that some degree of vasoconstriction occurs concurrently on achieving maximum heart rate, presumably to prevent a further decrease in stroke volume. It is not known if the heat-induced vasoconstriction is the result of closure of the arteriovenous anastomoses or arteriolar vasoconstriction, or both. But, as a consequence, heat transfer from the core to the periphery is reduced and core temperature will rise. An increase in circulating levels of catecholamines during hyperthermia may contribute towards the cutaneous vasoconstriction. A full discussion of circulatory and other problems in the aetiology and management of heat stroke is given in Khogali and Hales (1983).

Thermoregulation in autonomic failure

Autonomic pathways in the central nervous system are damaged secondarily in a wide range of disorders including central brain lesions and give rise to gross disturbances in thermoregulatory function. This may be manifest as thermal lability, intolerance to heat or cold, and, in more extreme environmental conditions, to an increased risk of developing hypo- or hyperthermia. Some lesions in the hypothalamus lead to recurrent bouts of hypothermia or to anhidrosis and heat intolerance. Episodic hypothermia may progress to chronic hypothermia and this has been observed following traumatic damage in the preoptic/anterior hypothalamic region. Another type of hypothermia has been described in cases of diencephalic epilepsy when intermittent episodes of hypothermia may last for only a few hours and there are inappropriate thermoregulatory responses in cool conditions (Maclean and Emslie-Smith 1977, pp. 312–20).

Abnormal sweating responses in autonomic failure have been well documented (see Chapter 28). Transection of the spinal cord produces anhidrosis below the level of interruption of sympathetic efferent pathways though sweating on the contralateral side can occur through spinal reflexes (see Chapter 43). Degeneration of sympathetic neurons, especially in the intermediolateral spinal columns, leads to segmental or unilateral loss of thermoregulatory sweating. This is often found in autonomic failure associated with other primary neuronal degenerative diseases such as one of the forms of autonomic failure with multiple system atrophy or Parkinson's disease. Anhidrosis may also occur in alcoholic polyneuritis and Wernicke's encephalopathy. It may occur in alcoholic patients without postural hypotension and is evidence of the involvement of postganglionic sympathetic fibres of the limbs though insufficient to induce loss of baroreflex control. Impairment of sweating and vasodilatation has often been described in tetraplegics who may become vulnerable to the effects of environmental heat and to hyperpyrexia in infections. Involvement of the peripheral nerves in leprosy and in remote malignancies similarly results in anhidrotic areas. Impaired sweating is a consequence of autonomic involvement in the Guillain–Barré syndrome and the Holmes–Aidie syndrome.

In peripheral nerve lesions, anhidrosis usually occurs in the area of sensory loss because postganglionic sympathetic fibres are present in the peripheral nerve trunks. In acute and chronic polyneuropathies, sweating is usually impaired predominantly over the distal parts of the extremities, but also on the trunk. Local hyperhidrosis may be seen in partial nerve injuries such as causalgia and when there is pressure on nerve roots such as occurs in malignancy or by pressure on the lower brachial plexus by a cervical rib. Excess sweating can also occur in tetanus due to sympathetic overactivity.

Autonomic dysfunction in the Guillain–Barré syndrome includes various forms of paroxysmal autonomic disturbances with episodes of sweating and peripheral vasoconstriction. Autopsy studies have shown demyelination lesions in the glossopharyngeal and vagus nerves, and in the sympathetic chain and white rami. Paroxysmal disturbances appear to be due to loss of damping of autonomic reflexes by damage to myelinated fibres in the afferent limb of autonomic reflex arcs, to denervation hypersensitivity of receptors in blood vessel walls, or to paroxysmal increases in the firing rate of sympathetic neurons due to inflammatory lesions. In the hereditary sensory and motor neuropathies (formerly known as a group by the name Charcot–Marie–Tooth disease) sweating and vasomotor responses to body heating and cooling are often impaired and there is evidence of denervation hypersensitivity of receptors. Reduction of thermoregulatory sweating in diabetes mellitus is due to a postganglionic lesion affecting the sudomotor nerve fibres. It is commonly associated with absence of piloerection. There is often evidence of anhidrosis over the lower extremities or trunk in patients with diabetic neuropathy and in hot surroundings there is increased susceptibility to heat disorders and heat stroke. The disorder of glucose metabolism may be so severe as to decrease significantly metabolic heat production. Diabetic hyperglycaemic ketoacidotic coma is sometimes associated with hypothermia. Abnormalities of vasomotor function may also contribute to failure of thermoregulatory reflexes in diabetes.

Thermoregulatory tests of autonomic function

Clinical thermoregulatory tests used for investigating the integrity of autonomic control are based mainly on assessments of vasomotor and sudomotor function. They may be part of general thermal tests involving whole body heating or cooling in which autonomic disorders may be a factor in deficient control of thermal balance and result in changes in deep body temperature. Peripheral reflex pathways can be usefully tested by local application of thermal stimuli, i.e. by indirect heating or cooling. Local sudomotor or vasomotor tests usually take the form of local injections or iontophoresis of sympathomimetics, parasympathomimetics, or blocking agents in order to examine the integrity of the peripheral autonomic neuroeffector system. An important part of these studies should be to incorporate direct tests of target organ function. Investigation of human blood vessel compliance under different ambient temperature conditions indicates

Table 12.1. Thermoregulatory tests of autonomic function

Clinical thermal tests

Climatic chamber: tests of heat/cold tolerance for 1–2 h in controlled ambient temperature conditions, with or without physical exercise; usually involves displacement of deep body temperature

Conductive heating/cooling: head-out immersion in warm or cold water for 0.5–1 h; involves displacement of deep body temperature

Convective heating/cooling: by moving air in an enclosed insulated system (e.g. Fox bed) enclosing the whole body, or by forced convection (e.g. Body Cooling Unit); convenient for tests in the vasomotor zone of thermoregulation with constant deep body temperature

Indirect heating/cooling*:

(1) Radiant heat cradle over the trunk for 2–3 min;

(2) Hand or limb immersed in hot/cold water for 15–20 min. Cold pressor test requires the hand to be immersed in water at 4 °C for up to 10 min;

(3) Facial cooling by face immersion in cold water (10–15 °C) for 30 s (diving response), in a cold airstream (0–5 °C), or cold gel packs applied to the face.

Measurement of vasomotor responses

Peripheral blood flow in the finger, hand, forearm, toe, foot, or leg by:

(1) venous occlusion volume plethysmography (quantitative);

(2) mercury-in-rubber or gallium/indium alloy strain-gauge plethysmography (quantitative);

(3) photoelectric plethysmography/pulsimetry (qualitative);

(4) laser Doppler velocimetry (qualitative).

Skin conductance

$$\frac{\text{Metabolic rate (W/m}^2)}{T_{\text{core}} - T_{\text{skin}}(°\text{C})}$$

Heat flux: heat flux transducer (e.g. Hatfield disc)

Measurement of sudomotor responses

Gravimetric. Total sensible body water loss. Continuous weighing balances may also be used to measure partitional sweat losses from different regions. Armbag methods suffer disadvantage of hidromeiosis (sweat suppression)

Local and regional

Qualitative: colorimetric methods using indicators, e.g. bromphenol blue, quinizarine, rhodamine; iodine/starch papers; sweat gland enumeration techniques, e.g. polyvinyl formal, silicone rubber impression; electrical impedance, e.g. palmar galvanic skin response

(continued)

Table 12.1. *(continued)*

Quantitative: ventilated or non-ventilated capsule systems; sudorimeter or evaporimeter methods. (Quantitative measurements are based on micro-gravimetric, hygrometric or infra-red water-vapour analysis.)

Pharmacological tests:

Local intradermal/subcutaneous injections or iontophoresis of:
Nicotine (optimum concentration 1 μg/0.1 ml) stimulates local intra-sympathetic axon reflex.

Methacholine or pilocarpine stimulate glands directly.

Acetylcholine stimulates directly and by axon reflex.

*Thermal reflex tests do not involve displacement of deep body temperature.

a reduced compliance and blood flow in cold conditions which is decreased even further in patients with arteriosclerosis and peripheral vascular disease (Collins 1990). A 'non-constrictor' response may not therefore necessarily signify autonomic nervous failure but may be explained at least partly by structural changes in the walls of peripheral blood vessels. Vascular medial wall calcification, which is shown to be more frequent in diabetes mellitus with autonomic neuropathy compared to diabetes without neuropathy, is therefore an important factor to consider when undertaking tests of vasomotor control.

Thermal tests may also be valuable in investigations of autonomic reflexes involved in cardiorespiratory responses such as the 'diving' response evoked by immersion of the face in cold water or facial cooling in air. A summary of clinical tests employed in examining the autonomic components of thermoregulation is given in Table 12.1. The majority of these tests are non-specific and give information about the total thermal reflex pathways including the function of target organs and do not necessarily delineate the site of autonomic dysfunction.

Drugs affecting autonomic control of thermoregulation

There are many agonist and antagonist autonomic drugs and central nervous transmitter substances that have effects on central and peripheral control of thermoregulation and on 'set-point' adjustments. Body temperature can be affected indirectly through induced toxicity or drug interactions. Some drugs may be regarded as having an effect on thermoregulation in neutral environmental conditions, e.g. the antipyretic action of salicylates, while others cause severe clinical disturbances during thermal stress, e.g. atropine-like substances administered during exposure to hot environments. Little attention has been paid to the question of altered drug reaction as the result of ambient temperature change, and there may be seasonal effects on drug requirements. In the treatment of hypertension, for example, a winter increment in systolic blood pressure as the result of a colder environment could affect therapeutic requirements (Collins 1990).

The effects of autonomic and other drugs on temperature regulation have been studied extensively in animals and much less so in man (Lomax and Schonbaum 1979). The better-known examples of temperature–drug responses in humans are illustrated in the following subsections and it is noticeable that many of these drugs have a dual effect and are capable of inducing either hypothermia or hyperthermia depending on the dose and ambient temperature conditions. Due caution should be observed in interpreting the effects listed here. Reactions to the various classes of drugs or even individual compounds within a group can be variable and will depend on age, environmental conditions, exercise, stress, route of administration, and many other factors.

Alcohol

Alcoholism is commonly considered to be a risk factor in the aetiology of heat stroke, though in fact ethanol causes a downward setting of central nervous control and is more usually associated with cases of secondary and accidental hypothermia. There is central nervous inhibition, hypoglycaemia, peripheral vasodilatation, impairment of behavioural thermoregulation and judgement in low temperatures, and possibly a 'set-point' effect. Moderate amounts of alcohol are found to have only a small effect on heat loss in cold water immersion which may be due to the fact that intense cold stimulation of the skin can override the alcohol-induced vasodilatation. In air, with a less intense cold stimulus, alcohol may be more effective in increasing cutaneous heat loss through vasodilatation. Another important action is on thermogenesis. Severe hypoglycaemia is frequently a feature of acute alcoholism, especially in fasting subjects. In high ambient temperatures alcohol may interfere with normal judgements to the extent that behavioural protective measures are not taken when necessary. In hot conditions, alcohol can help to increase the degree of body dehydration by its diuretic effect but at the same time improve heat loss by vasodilatation.

Phenothiazines

Phenothiazines have a powerful hypothermic action in the cold with a long-term central action on body temperature control and possibly also a peripheral effect through interaction with adrenaline. Both hypothermia or hyperthermia may occur, with ambient temperature being an important determinant of the outcome. Deep body temperatures as high as 42 °C have been observed in adults treated with phenothiazines during exposure to high environmental temperatures and/or severe physical exercise, in some cases with normal therapeutic doses. The risk of hyperthermia or hypothermia is greater with the longer-acting compounds such as fluphenazine enanthate. Phenothiazines have a particularly marked effect in reducing body temperature in conditions when patients are vulnerable to cold such as in the elderly or with hypothyroidism. In cool conditions 0.3–2.0 mg/kg chlorpromazine intravenously can reduce core temperature by 1–2 °C.

Antidepressants

Tricyclic antidepressants can cause rapid reduction of deep body temperature, reduced awareness of cold, and potentiation of the effects of barbiturates or alcohol in inducing hypothermia. These compounds may also cause hyperthermia in high doses, especially in combination with other agents such as amphetamines. Generally, hypothermia is the more common side-effect, the magnitude of the effectiveness of individual compounds being a function of their phenothiazine-like pharmacological activity. There are important interreactions between tricyclics and sympathetic or parasympathomimetics. Hyperpyrexia and heat stroke have been reported after overdose and in combination with monoamine oxidase inhibitors, β-adrenergic blockers, and benzodiazepines.

Barbiturates

In high doses, barbiturates induce coma and depress all thermoregulatory systems including appropriate behaviour so that the individual is virtually poikilothermic and body temperature will fall or rise depending on the external environment. A potentially dangerous combination arises from using alcohol and barbiturates in the presence of heat or cold stress, since the two drugs augment each other in suppressing thermoregulation.

Cannabinoids

At ambient temperatures within or below the thermoneutral range, tetrahydrocannabinol (THC) causes a fall in body temperature, and at high temperatures hyperthermia can develop. With doses in the range of cannabis smoking (about 15–20 mg THC) there is no change or sometimes a slight 0.1–0.2 °C decrease in body temperature in a normal or cool environment. Hallucinogens have been reported to cause hypothermia in cold environments and a raised temperature in a 47 °C ambient temperature which was not found in control subjects in the same environments.

Opiates

Opiate alkaloids, especially morphine, have profound effects on body temperature but the response varies considerably with the dose and the animal model used. In some species the predominant response is a fall in temperature and in others a rise. With therapeutic doses there is no significant effect on core temperature in man although skin vasodilatation occurs, partly due to histamine release. More marked effects are seen during withdrawal in drug-dependent individuals. Profuse sweating and piloerection occur within 8–16 h of withdrawal and by 36 h there is muscle fasciculation, cramps, and a rise in body temperature.

Anaesthetics

General anaesthetics usually depress the central nervous system including the thermoregulatory centres. A number of cases of hypothermia have been reported in which the patient entered a state of hypothermia while anaesthetized. The degree of change of body temperature depends on the depth of anaesthesia and on ambient temperature. Below 24 °C body temperature often falls, whereas at higher ambient temperatures hyperthermia may result. Malignant hyperthermia is a rare and often fatal complication of general anaesthesia found to occur in those who suffer from myopathies. Halothane anaesthesia typically produces muscle contracture in susceptible subjects resulting in a rapid rise in body temperature, generalized muscle rigidity, and a severe metabolic acidosis. The biochemical basis appears to involve an abnormally large release of calcium ions into the myoplasm.

Other drugs affecting thermoregulation

Body temperature elevation has been reported to occur during the first few weeks of treatment of hypertensive patients with methyldopa. Decarboxylation of methyldopa increases levels of sympathomimetic amines and produces cutaneous vasoconstriction. Similarly, amphetamines which affect the release or metabolism of catecholamines have thermoregulatory effects. Hyperthermia is sometimes associated with amphetamine poisoning. The action of amphetamine is not confined to the central nervous system and may include increased skeletal muscle heat production similar to that associated with malignant hyperthermia.

There are now several reported fatalities due to cocaine overdose in which hyperpyrexia, rhabdomyolysis, disseminated intravascular coagulation, and hepatic and renal failure were found. These cases present a picture of classical stress-related heat stroke.

Antimuscarinic drugs such as atropine diminish sweating in hot climates. In infants even moderate doses may induce 'atropine fever'. The effects appear to be at the thermoregulatory centres as well as at postganglionic sudomotor nerve endings.

Deep body temperature can be lowered by hypoglycaemic or antithyroid agents which reduce internal heat production or vasodilators which accelerate peripheral heat loss.

References

Abdel-Rahman, T. A., Collins, K. J., Cowen, T., and Rustin, M. (1992). Immunohistochemical, morphological and functional changes in the peripheral sudomotor neuro-effector system in elderly people. *J. autonom. nerv. Syst.* (In press.)

Appenzeller, O. (1983). Influences of physical training, heat acclimation and diet on temperature regulation in man. In *Heat stroke and temperature regulation* (ed. M. Khogali and J. R. S. Hales), pp. 283–92. Academic Press, New York.

Bazett, H. C. (1968). The regulation of body temperature. In *Physiology of heat regulation and the science of clothing* (ed. L. H. Newburgh), pp. 109–92. Saunders, Philadelphia.

Bell, C., Jänig, W., Kümmel, H., and Xu, H. (1985). Differentiation of vasodilator and sudomotor responses in the cat paw pad to preganglionic sympathetic stimulation. *J. Physiol., London* **364**, 93–104.

Benzinger, T. H., Kitzinger, C., and Pratt, A. W. (1963). The human thermostat. In *Temperature: its measurement and control in science and industry*, Vol. 3 (ed. J. D. Hardy), pp. 637–65. Reinhold, New York.

Bini, G., Hagbarth, K.-E., Hynninen, P., and Wallin, B. G. (1980). Thermoregulatory and rhythm-generating mechanisms governing the sudomotor and vasoconstrictor outflow in human cutaneous nerves. *J. Physiol., London* **306**, 537–52.

Bligh, J. (1983). Basic concepts and applied aspects of body temperature regulation. In *Heat stroke and temperature regulation* (ed. M. Khogali and J. R. S. Hales), pp. 41–52. Academic Press, New York.

Collins, K. J. (1989). Sweat glands: eccrine and apocrine. In *Handbook of experimental pharmacology*, Vol. 87/1 (ed. M. W. Greaves and S. Shuster), pp. 193–212. Springer–Verlag, Berlin.

Collins, K. J. (1990). Age-related changes in autonomic control: the use of β-blockers in the treatment of hypertension *Cardiovasc. Drugs Ther.* **4**, 1257–62.

Collins, K. J. (1992). Temperature homeostasis and thermal stress. In *Oxford textbook of geriatric medicine* (ed. J. Grimley-Evans and T. F. Williams), pp. 93–100. Oxford University Press, Oxford.

Collins, K. J., Easton, J. C., and Exton-Smith, A. N. (1981). Shivering thermogenesis and vasomotor responses with convective cooling in the elderly. *J. Physiol., London* **320**, 76P.

Cowen, T. and Burnstock, G. (1986). Development, aging and plasticity of perivascular autonomic nerves. In *Neurobiology of the autonomic nervous system* (ed. P. M. Gootman), pp. 211–32. The Humana Press, New Jersey.

Darowski, A., Najim, Z., Weinberg, J. R., and Guz, A. (1991). Hypothermia and infection in elderly patients admitted to hospital. *Age Ageing* **20**, 100–6.

Gallego, R. and Geijo, E. (1987). Chronic block of the cervical trunk increases synaptic efficiency in the superior and stellate ganglion of the guinea pig. *J. Physiol., London* **382**, 449–62.

Hammel, H. T., Jackson, D. C., Stolwijk, J. A., Hardy, J. D., and Stromme, S. B. (1963). Temperature regulation by hypothalamic proportional control with an adjustable set point. *J. appl. Physiol.* **18**, 1146–54.

Heath, M. E. and Jessen, C. (1988). Thermosensitivity of the goat's brain. *J. Physiol., London* **400**, 61–74.

Hensel, H. (1981). *Thermoreception and temperature regulation*, Monographs of the Physiology Society, no. 38. Academic Press, New York.

Hernandez, M. J. (1983). Cerebral circulation during hypothermia. In *The nature and treatment of hypothermia* (ed. R. S. Pozos and L. E. Wittmers), pp. 61–8. University of Minnesota Press, Minneapolis.

Hill, C. E., Jelinek, H., Hendry, I. A., McLennan, I. S., and Rush, R. A. (1988). Destruction by anti-NGF of autonomic sudomotor neurones and subsequent hyperinnervation of foot pad by sensory fibres. *J. Neurosci. Res.* **19**, 474–82.

Hori, T., Kiyohara, T., and Nakashima, T. (1989). Thermosensitive neurones in the brain: role in homeostatic functions. In *Thermal physiology 1989.* (ed. J. B. Mercer), pp. 3–12. Excerpta Medica, Amsterdam.

Khogali, M. and Hales, J. R. S. (ed.) (1983). *Heat stroke and temperature regulation.* Academic Press, New York.

Landis, S. C. (1990). Target regulation of neurotransmitter phenotype. *Trends Neurosci.* **13**, 344–50.

Lomax, P. and Schonbaum, E. (1979). *Body temperature regulation: drug effects and therapeutic implications.* Marcel Dekker, New York.

Lundberg, J. M., Hökfelt, T., Schultzberg, M., Uvnäs-Wallensten, K., Köhler, C., and Said, S. I. (1979). Occurrence of vasomotor intestinal polypeptide (VIP)-like immunoreactivity in certain cholinergic neurones of the cat: evidence from combined immunochemistry and acetylcholinesterase staining. *Neuroscience* **4**, 1539–59.

Maclean, D. and Emslie-Smith, D. (1977). Accidental hypothermia. Blackwell Scientific Publications, Oxford.

Mitchell, D., Snellen, J. W., and Atkins, A. R. (1970). Thermoregulation during fever: change of set-point or change of gain. *Pflüger's Arch.* **321**, 293–302.

Simon, E., Picrau, F.-K., and Taylor, D. C. M. (1986). Central and peripheral thermal control of effectors in homeothermic temperature regulation. *Physiol. Rev.* **66**, 235–300.

Uno, H. and Montagna, W. (1975). Catecholamine-containing nerve terminals of the eccrine sweat glands of macaques. *Cell Tissue Res.* **158**, 1–13.

Vendrik, A. J. H. (1959). The regulation of body temperature in man. *Ned. Tijdschr. Geneesk* **103**, 240–4.

Weiner, J. S., Collins, K. J., and Rubel, L. R. (1984). Heat-associated illnesses. In *Hunter's tropical medicine* (6th edn) (ed. G. T. Strickland), pp. 873–9. Saunders, Philadelphia.

Wollner, L. and Collins, K. J. (1992). Disorders of the autonomic nervous system. In *Textbook of geriatric medicine and gerontology* (4th edn) (ed. J. C. Brocklehurst, R. C. Tallis and H. Fillit), pp. 389–410. Churchill-Livingstone, London.

Young, J. B. and Landsberg, L. (1982). Diet induced changes in sympathetic nervous system activity: possible implications for obesity and hypertension. *J. chron. Dis.* **35**, 879–86.

Young, J. B., Rosa, R. M., and Landsberg, L. (1984). Dissociation of sympathetic nervous system and adrenal medullary response. *Am. J. Physiol.* **247**, E35–40.

13. Pain and the sympathetic nervous system: pathophysiological mechanisms

Wilfrid Jänig

Introduction

The sympathetic nervous system is organized in a target-organ-specific way. Its peripheral part is efferent and consists of preganglionic and postganglionic neurons which constitute several functionally separate pathways to the different target organs. This is illustrated schematically in Fig. 13.1. The activity of the postganglionic neurons is transmitted by neuroeffector pathways to the effector organs (e.g. blood vessels, glands, non-vascular smooth musculature, enteric neurons). The activity of the preganglionic neurons is transmitted in the sympathetic ganglia to the postganglionic neurons; each functional set of preganglionic neurons synapses only with a particular set of postganglionic neurons. Thus, many 'private lines' exist between the thoracolumbar spinal cord and the autonomic target organs establishing final common sympathetic motor paths (Jänig 1989). The paravertebral ganglia can be viewed as pure relay stations; the prevertebral ganglia also have relay function, but additionally integrate afferent input from the viscera. Each final common sympathetic motor path, which is defined according to its target organ, is associated with a distinct organization in the spinal cord and in the brainstem, the details of which are still almost unknown. The peripheral and central organization of the sympathetic nervous system is the basis of the smooth co-ordinated regulation of general and specific autonomic functions in the adaptation of the body during different behavioural responses (Jänig 1985a; Jänig and McLachlan 1987).

This remarkably organized system exhibits distinct adaptive reactions when the organism is in pain, yet it is, as far as we know, not involved in the generation of pain under healthy conditions (Jänig 1990). How can it be involved in the generation of pain under pathophysiological conditions, e.g. after peripheral trauma with nerve injury? This chapter will concentrate on this question.

Spinal afferent neurons that project through the corresponding splanchnic nerves to the viscera are 'visceral afferent neurons'. These afferent neurons

231

do not belong to the sympathetic or parasympathetic nervous system in the strict sense and will therefore not be labelled 'sympathetic' or 'parasympathetic'. Neuronal mechanisms of visceral pain that are associated with the excitation of these afferent neurons will not be discussed.

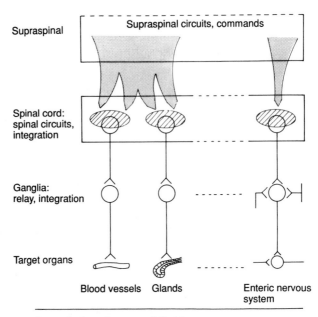

Fig. 13.1. Organization of the sympathetic nervous system. Each target organ (different types of blood vessels, glands, non-vascular smooth musculature, enteric nervous system and others) is supplied by a specific sympathetic pathway which consists of pre- and postganglionic neurons and is called 'final common sympathetic motor path'. The activity of the postganglionic neurons is transmitted to the target organs by way of specific neuroeffector apparatuses. Preganglionic axons synapse in the ganglia with postganglionic neurons according to the target organs, the paravertebral ganglia having largely relay function and the prevertebral ones (left) relay and integrative functions. Each final common sympathetic motor path is associated with a distinct organization in the spinal cord, brainstem and hypothalamus (see Jänig 1985; Jänig and McLachlan 1987).

Some clinical background and problems

Reflex sympathetic dystrophy and related disorders

That the sympathetic nervous system may be involved in the generation and maintenance of pain states has been particularly documented for a disorder that is generically called reflex sympathetic dystrophy (RDS) and for related disorders that follow trauma, particularly affecting deep tissues with and without obvious nerve lesions, sometimes visceral disease, and sometimes even central lesions (for literature see Bonica 1990; Jänig 1990; Chapter 45). The syndrome consists of pain, abnormal regulation of blood flow through skin and possibly deep tissues, abnormal regulation of sweating, trophic changes of skin, appendages of skin and deep tissues (including bone), and motor disturbances. At present we may tentatively distinguish between 'sympathetic maintained pain' (SMP), 'sympathetic algodystrophy' (so-to-speak 'reflex sympathetic dystrophy' *sui generis*), and 'sympathetic dystrophy' (see table 13.1). The first, SMP, is characterized by localized spontaneous pain and touch-evoked allodynia, but allodynia may also be absent (Campbell *et al.* 1988; Price *et al.* 1989); the other symptoms are absent or not very prominent. In the second, sympathetic algodystrophy, all symptoms are present. In the third, sympathetic dystophy, the spontaneous pain is absent or not a dominant symptom.

The classification as proposed in Table 13.1 is tentative. It may undergo changes and further differentiation in future. For example, the SMP patients may be considered as a separate group which is independent of the other RSD patients. The SMP patients may be subclassified into those with touch-evoked allodynia and those without (Price *et al.* 1989). Both groups of SMP patients may be separated from another group of patients with almost the same neuropathic pain which is independent of the sympathetic activity (so-called 'sympathetically independent pain'; see Frost *et al.* 1988). Finally, it is advisable to discriminate between patients in the early stage of RSD (e.g. within 20 days after the initiating event) and those in a later stage who have RSD for months or longer (Blumberg, 1991). This division may not only have considerable diagnostic and therapeutic consequences, but both stages may be characterized by different though related pathophysiological mechanisms. Thus a more reliable and accepted classification and distinction between different types or stages of RSD in future will depend on more reliable and reproducible minimal criteria for its clinical diagnosis and better knowledge of its pathophysiology (Jänig *et al.* 1991).

It is commonly, yet not universally, recommended that RSD be treated by sympathetic blocks and physiotherapy (Bonica 1990). It is irrelevant in the present context (albeit important from the practical point of view) whether the sympathetic blocks are successful in all cases or not and whether

Table 13.1. Tentative classification of reflex sympathetic dystrophy by the leading clinical symptoms*

Symptoms	Reflex sympathetic dystrophy[†]		
	Sympathetically maintained pain	Sympathetic algodystrophy	Sympathetic dystrophy
Abnormal pain (spontaneous, evoked)	+ (allodynia)	+	Absent
Abnormal regulation of blood flow (cutaneous, deep) and sweating	Absent, (+)	+	+
Motor disorders	(+)	+	+
Trophic changes	Absent, (+)	+	+
Territory	Territory of lesioned nerve	Distal (rarely proximal) extremity	Distal (rarely proximal) extremity
Recommended therapies	Sympathetic block	Sympathetic block, physiotherapy	Sympathetic block (?), physiotherapy
Frequency	≤ 5%	~ 90%	≤ 5%

*Based on data from Blumberg and modified from Jänig (1990).
[†] + , present.

temporary blocks may not lead in some cases to permanent relief of pain. It is important to note that intravenous injection of guanethidine into the affected and cuffed extremity distal to the occlusion (Hannington-Kiff 1989) and intravenous injection of an α-adrenoreceptor antagonist (used as diagnostic tool; Arnér 1991) may abolish the pain. Both procedures correlate quite well with the effects of sympathetic blocks by local anaesthetics and strongly support the view that the sympathetic noradrenergic neurons are involved. However, it is poorly understood why temporary sympathetic blocks mostly produce long lasting if not permanent relief of pain.

This and the clinical phenomenology of RSD favour the notion that the (efferent) sympathetic nervous system is an important component in the generation of RSD. A general hypothesis is sketched in Fig. 13.2. It consists of the following components. First, the noradrenergic postganglionic axons are coupled in some abnormal way to the afferent axons in the periphery leading to an abnormal afferent impulse traffic to the spinal cord. Second, the sensory receptors of small-diameter fibres in the affected territory may be changed (sensitized) as a consequence of the lesion. Third, the processing of nociceptive and non-nociceptive afferent information, including its control by supraspinal systems in the spinal cord (particularly the dorsal horn), is changed. Fourth, as a consequence of the latter the discharge pattern in the

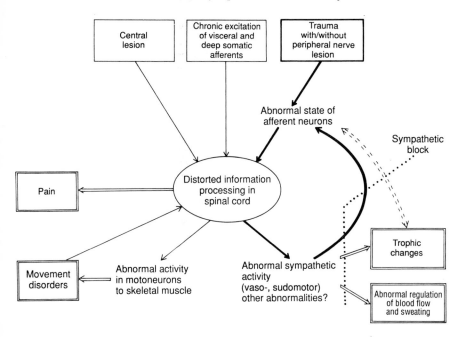

Fig. 13.2. General hypothesis about the neural mechanisms of generation of reflex sympathetic dystrophy (RDS) following peripheral injury with and without nerve lesions, and, rarely, with central lesions and chronic stimulation of visceral afferents. Note the vicious circle (arrows in bold black). An important component of this circle is the excitatory influence of postganglionic sympathetic axons on primary afferent fibres in the periphery. This influence leads to orthodromic afferent impulse activity. But it may also induce antidromically conducted impulses in unmyelinated afferents to the periphery which may contribute to the trophic changes (i.e. by release of substances due to antidromic invasion of axon terminals which leads to vasodilation and plasmaextravasation). These trophic changes may in turn influence the coupling between postganglionic axons and afferent axons (see interrupted double arrow). Another important component that is not emphasized in this diagram may be that the neurovascular transmission is impaired and that the blood vessels develop adaptive supersensitivity to changes in the local micromilieu (e.g. to released vasoactive substances), to circulating substances, to external influences (e.g. increase and decrease of environmental temperatures), and to nerve impulses (Modified from Jänig (1990).)

sympathetic outflow is changed. Fifth, the regulation of small blood vessels by noradrenergic fibres and other components may be changed. This complex concerto of events may establish a vicious circle that is interrupted by blocking the sympathetic impulse traffic to the affected territory (Jänig 1985*b*, 1990).

Table 13.2. Peripheral and central pathobiological mechanisms that are possibly associated with the sympathetic nervous system and may contribute to the generation of RSD after peripheral injury with nerve lesions. Some mechanisms are supported experimentally; some are hypothetical (see Devor *et al.* 1991; Jänig 1985*b*, 1990; Jänig and Koltzenburg 1991*a*; Otten 1991)

1. Retrograde cell reactions: interruption of transport of neurotrophic factors from periphery to sympathetic ganglia; shrinkage of axons and cell bodies; death of postganglionic neurons

2. Anterograde cell reactions; sprouting of postganglionic axons and postganglionic–target organ mismatch

3. Change and failure of synaptic transmission from preganglionic to postganglionic neurons in sympathetic ganglia

4. Development of influence of postganglionic sympathetic fibres on afferent fibres; chemical (by release of noradrenaline); ephaptic (unlikely); indirect via influence on vascular and via influence on other non-neural cells; indirect by change of micromilieu

5. Development of adaptive supersensitivity and subsensitivity of autonomic effector organs after degeneration and regeneration of their postganglionic noradrenergic innervation; abnormal vascular responses to neural impulses, substances released locally, circulating substances, and external influences (e.g. changes in environmental temperature)

6. Abnormal regulation of blood flow through skin and subcutaneous tissues due to mismatch of vasoconstrictor activity to different sections of vascular beds

7. Increase of filtration pressure in capillary beds with subsequent chronic formation of oedema due to imbalance of pre- to postcapillary constriction; increase in vascular permeability due to release of vasoactive substances (e.g. from primary afferents or local cells) or due to other processes

8. Activation of local immune-competent and related cells (macrophages, T and B lymphocytes, polymorphonuclear leucocytes, mast cells) in the microenvironment of primary afferent and noradrenergic fibres. Neuroimmune interaction in sustaining nociceptive impulse activity and inflammatory reactions. Participation of histamine, arachidonic acid derivatives (prostaglandins, leukotrienes), cytokines (e.g. interleukins 1 and 2, tumour necrosis factor), growth factors (e.g. nerve growth factor)

9. Development of abnormal discharge properties and abnormal reflexes in sympathetic neurons supplying the affected extremity (skin, deep somatic tissues, etc) as a consequence of central changes

Other painful disorders in which the sympathetic nervous system may be involved

There exist other painful disorders in which the sympathetic nervous system may be actively involved, though the evidence is more indirect and less well established. This may apply to acute herpes zoster and the development of postherpetic neuralgia and to pain and associated reactions in inflammatory rheumatoid arthritis (see Jänig and Koltzenburg 1991*a*). In both diseases the sympathetic nervous system may act in a more indirect way. It is reported that sympathetic blocks or interventions that reduce the putative influence of the sympathetic nervous system on the inflammatory processes may reduce the peripheral tissue reactions and the pain.

Problems

In this chapter neurobiological processes are discussed through which the sympathetic nervous system may be involved in the generation of pain states after trauma with and without obvious nerve lesions and during chronic inflammations. Particular reference will be made to the RSD syndrome; it is, however, clear that these mechanisms also operate in a generation of other neuropathic pains (see Devor *et al.* 1991). Table 13.2 lists possible pathobiological mechanisms in which the sympathetic nervous system may be involved. The following mechanisms may be particularly important (see Fig. 13.2).

1. The noradrenergic postganglionic fibres are coupled to the afferent fibres or the afferent receptors in the periphery in several ways.

2. Activity in noradrenergic postganglionic fibres influences non-neural cells and leads in this way to sensitization of nociceptive and other afferents.

3. The neurovascular transmission changes after peripheral nerve lesions with degeneration and regeneration of postganglionic and afferent axons. Blood vessels develop adaptive supersensitivity to nerve impulses and to circulating or locally released substances.

4. The pattern of activity in the sympathetic vasoconstrictor neurons supplying blood vessels changes as a consequence of central changes (central sensitization processes) after trauma.

   Changes of primary afferent neurons and the central consequences of these changes following peripheral trauma, though closely related to the present subject, will not be discussed (see Jänig 1988; Cervero *et al.* 1989; Bond *et al.* 1991).

Effects of sympathetic activity on afferent neurons

Physiological conditions

Under physiological conditions there exists almost no influence of sympathetic activity on sensory receptors in skin and deep somatic tissues in mammals. The effects that have been measured under experimental conditions on receptors with myelinated and unmyelinated axons were weak, required synchronous high-frequency stimulation of 5–10 Hz or more of the sympathetic supply, and can in part be explained by changes of the effector organs induced by the activation of sympathetic neurons. These rather negative results do not rule out that noradrenaline or co-localized substances released by the postganglionic terminals have secondary long-term effects on the excitability of sensory receptors (for details see Jänig 1990).

Pathophysiological conditions

Direct chemical coupling

The presence of chemical coupling between sympathetic postganglionic fibres and afferent fibres has mainly been documented following transection of peripheral nerves with and without subsequent regeneration of axons in animal models (Fig. 13.3(a)). Postganglionic fibres can excite myelinated and unmyelinated afferent fibres by release of noradrenaline following nerve lesion. Some myelinated afferent fibres ending in stump neuromas of the sciatic nerve in rat and mice can be excited by systemically administered noradrenaline and during high-frequency electrical stimulation of the lumbar sympathetic trunk 1 to about 3 weeks after the nerve lesion. The responses can be blocked by α-adrenergic antagonists and occur almost exclusively in afferents with ongoing activity. Qualitatively similar results were obtained in the cat, yet the excitation of myelinated and unmyelinated afferent fibres projecting into a stump neuroma were rather small. The α-adrenoceptor which mediates this sensitivity has not been subclassified further (see Jänig 1988).

Little attention has been given to the efficiency of chemical coupling between postganglionic fibres and afferent fibres with respect to the time which has elapsed after the nerve lesion, the type of nerve lesion, and substances that are co-localized with noradrenaline in the postganglionic noradrenergic neurons.

First, it has recently been shown that some 20 to 40 per cent of C-fibre polymodal nociceptors of the rabbit ear can be excited by stimulation of the sympathetic supply of the ear and by noradrenaline given systemically about 10–24 days after a partial nerve lesion has been applied to the auricular nerve (constriction lesion as described by Bennett 1991). The responses of the afferents to sympathetic stimulation, to noradrenaline, and to heat stimuli

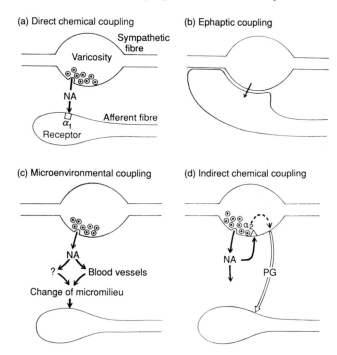

Fig. 13.3. Possible modes of coupling between postganglionic sympathetic and primary afferent fibres under pathophysiological conditions. (a) Direct chemical coupling. Noradrenaline (NA) is released from the varicosity and acts directly on the postsynaptic membrane of the afferent fibre, probably on α_1-receptors. (b) Ephaptic coupling. Electrical cross-talk between sympathetic and afferent fibres, when close membrane appositions are present between axons. This type of coupling has so far never been found between postganglionic and afferent axons. (c) Microenvironmental coupling. Sympathetic neurons affect the micromilieu of primary afferents by changing local blood flow and potentially by further unknown mechanisms. (d) Indirect chemical coupling. Noradrenaline is released from the varicosity and acts back on to presynaptic α_2-receptors, thereby leading to release of other compounds such as prostaglandins (PG), either from the varicosities or from non-neural cells. Only these secondary substances act on the primary afferents (see Levine *et al.* 1986). (Modified from Jänig (1988).)

could be blocked or reduced relatively specifically by α_2-adrenergic antagonists (yohimbine, rauwolfcine) which suggests that the nociceptors express α_2-receptors in their receptive membrane and that their excitation is mediated (at least in part) by these receptors (Sato and Perl 1991).

Second, electrophysiological studies on cats with a long-standing 'neuroma-in-continuity' (11–20 months after the initial nerve lesion) illustrate that unmyelinated afferents can be excited by electrical stimulation of the sympathetic supply (Häbler *et al.* 1987). The proximal stump of a skin nerve was connected to the distal stump of a mixed nerve (cross-union between sural and tibial nerve), allowing most fibres to regenerate into the peripheral stump. Some afferent fibres fail to do so in this preparation and form a neuroma at the site of the nerve lesion. Some of the unmyelinated fibres excited had ongoing activity, yet it was unclear whether they ended in the 'neuroma-in-continuity' or further distally. The coupling in this experiment was α-adrenergic and, interestingly, the afferent fibres could also be excited via this chemical coupling during a reflex increase of the sympathetic activity (Fig. 13.4).

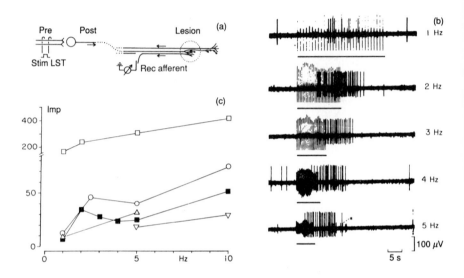

Fig. 13.4. Excitation of unmyelinated afferent units by electrical stimulation of sympathetic fibres following nerve injury. Unmyelinated primary afferents were recorded in cats 11–20 months following a nerve lesion. The central cut stump of a cutaneous nerve innervating hairy skin had been imperfectly adapted to the distal stump of a transected mixed nerve. This preparation was designed to mimic the consequences of a mixed nerve lesion. There was a 'neuroma-in-continuity' at the site of the lesion and cutaneous nerve fibres had regenerated into skin and deep somatic tissue supplied by the mixed nerve. (a) Experimental set-up. Pre, preganglionic; Post, postganglionic; LST, lumbar sympathetic trunk. (b) Record from a single unmyelinated afferent unit (conduction velocity 1.3 m/s). Supramaximal stimulation of the LST with trains of 30 pulses at 1 to 5 Hz (trains and stimulation artefacts indicated by bars). Note that the afferent unit had some low rate of ongoing activity (impulses before the trains at 1 and 4 Hz) and that a second unit was recruited at 5 Hz (marked by *). (c) Stimulus response curve for the single unit (■) and four filaments containing 2–3 (○, ▽, △) and more than 5 (□) afferent units. Ordinate scale is the total number of impulses (Imp) exceeding ongoing activity in response to variable stimulation frequency of the LST. (Taken with permission from Häbler *et al.* (1987).)

Third, it has been shown in rats that unmyelinated afferent fibres ending in a stump-end neuroma of the sciatic nerve, 8 months after cutting and ligating this nerve, can be excited by electrical stimulation of the lumbar sympathetic chain at 0.5 to 4 Hz; yet this excitation could not be mimicked by adrenaline (see Jänig and Koltzenburg 1991*a*).

Ephaptic transmission

Ephaptic coupling, i.e. direct electrical cross-talk, between postganglionic fibres and primary afferent axons has so far never been found in normal nerves, in stump neuromas, or in 'neuromas-in-continuity' after partial nerve lesions (Fig. 13.3(b)). Though ephapses between primary afferents are exceedingly rare in normal nerves and only occasionally present in partially regenerating nerves with a 'neuroma-in-continuity' (Jänig and Koltzenburg, unpublished observations), they are relatively common amongst sprouts of myelinated and unmyelinated afferent fibres in stump neuromas (see Jänig 1988).

The absence of cross-talk between sympathetic and afferent axons following nerve transection in previous experiments does not necessarily mean that this mechanism never occurs under pathophysiological conditions. It is known that the development of neuropathic disorders is not always correlated with the degree of morphological damage. A rapid and violent deformation of main nerve trunks, such as the sciatic and median nerve or the cervicobrachial plexus, without microscopically visible nerve damage might be more favourable for the generation of ephaptic contacts. Under such conditions some nerve fibres, Schwann cells, and endoneural tubes may be disrupted throughout the nerve trunk. The interrupted nerve fibres could sprout into the distal nerve between intact axons. It is conceivable that the likelihood of coupling between postganglionic axons and afferent axons might increase under such circumstances (for discussion see Jänig 1990).

Changes of neurovascular transmission and development of adaptive supersensitivity of blood vessels

Nociceptive afferents are embedded in a complex micromilieu (Fig. 13.5). The state of this micromilieu surrounding the receptive terminals depends on mediator substances that are released during inflammatory processes following trauma from non-neural cells such as mast cells, polymorphonuclear leucocytes, macrophages, fibroblasts, endothelial cells, or immune-competent cells. The microcirculation is under neural control of sympathetic vasoconstrictor neurons. Moreover, activation of nociceptive primary afferents not only causes orthodromic impulse traffic but also the release of substances from the receptive terminals (e.g. substance P and probably other vasoactive substances) that initiate the neurogenic component of inflammation (see Jänig and Koltzenburg 1991*a*).

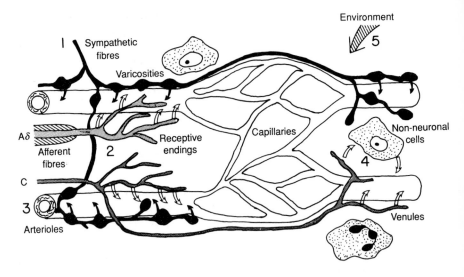

Fig. 13.5. The micromilieu of nociceptors. The microenvironment of primary afferents is thought to affect the properties of the receptive endings of myelinated (Aδ) and unmyelinated (C) afferent fibres. This has been documented in particular for inflammatory processes, but one may speculate that pathological changes in the direct surroundings of primary afferents may contribute to other pain states as well. The micromilieu depends on several interacting components. (1) Neural activity in postganglionic noradrenergic fibres supplying blood vessels causes vasoconstriction and the release of noradrenaline and possibly other substances. (2) Excitation of primary afferents causes vasodilatation in precapillary arterioles (Aδ- and C-fibres) and plasma extravasation in postcapillary venoles (C-fibres only) by the release of substance P and possibly other vasoactive compounds. (4) Some of these effects may be mediated by non-neuronal cells such as mast cells. Other factors that affect the control of the microcirculation are (3) the myogenic properties of arterioles and (5) more global environmental influences such as a change of the temperature and the metabolic state of the tissue (with permission from Jänig and Koltzenburg (1991*a*)).

The neural control of blood vessels can change dramatically after trauma with nerve lesions, but possibly also after trauma without lesions of nerves. In our laboratory we used a nerve lesion caused by suturing the central stump of the sural nerve to the distal stump of the tibial nerve. Our results showed that blood vessels in the dermis of the hairless skin of the cat hind paw, which are reinnervated after a nerve lesion (the central stump of the sural nerve was sutured to the distal stump of the tibial nerve) by the postganglionic noradrenergic fibres, exhibit normal or stronger than normal vaso-constrictions to electrical stimulation of the lumbar sympathetic chain and to reflex activation of the sympathetic neurons (Jänig and Koltzenburg 1991*b*).

1. These sympathetically reinnervated cutaneous blood vessels show stronger than normal vasoconstrictions to phenylephrine administered systemically (α_1-adrenergic agent); thus, the blood vessels appear to be supersensitive to catecholamines (see Fleming and Westfall 1988).

2. The blood vessels exhibit no or weak vasodilatation to antidromic activation of unmyelinated afferents in the lesioned nerve though these afferents have also reinnervated the plantar skin. The reinnervated blood vessels are therefore now under stronger than normal vasoconstrictor influence which cannot any longer be counteracted by a vasodilatation when nociceptors are activated.

In vitro investigations of the rat tail artery have shown that the functional recovery of neurovascular transmission may remain permanently disturbed after a nerve lesion (Jobling, McLachlan, Anderson, and Jänig, unpublished observation).

The alterations of neural control of blood vessels, which consist of supersensitivity to circulating catecholamines and possibly other circulating and local substances, of a changed noradrenergic neurovascular transmission, and of a changed influence of unmyelinated afferents on the small blood vessels, will contribute to abnormal regulation of microcirculation following trauma due to nerve lesions. For example, postcapillary constriction may increase with respect to precapillary constriction leading to an increase in filtration pressure with subsequent oedema formation. These alterations can contribute to the abnormal regulation of blood flow through skin and deep somatic tissues and possibly to the trophic changes (including the oedema) which are seen in patients with RSD. They may furthermore be a permissive factor in the generation of afferent nociceptive impulse activity and therefore in the generation of pain.

Finally, it is commonly believed that skin temperature changes during painful neuropathies (e.g. in causalgia or RSD) reflect vasoconstrictor activity. Thus, cold skin may be associated with a high level of activity in the sympathetic cutaneous vasoconstrictor neurons and warm skin with a low level of activity in them. This is probably a misconception and there is no proof at all that the relation between skin temperature and activity in sympathetic neurons holds under these pathophysiological conditions. Experimental studies by Wakisaka *et al.* (1991) support this contention. Rats with a constriction lesion at the sciatic nerve exhibit hotter skin than normal at the experimental side in the first 10 post-injury days and colder skin than normal more than 3–4 weeks postoperatively. The inter- and intraindividual variabilities of skin temperature and the overall change of the skin temperature after the nerve lesion observed in the rat are very similar to the observations on patients with neuropathic pains. The straightforward conclusion from this experimental study on rats is that the skin temperature is not necessarily correlated with the activity in sympathetic vasoconstrictor neurons. This most probably also applies to equivalent clinical situations but is generally ignored. It is therefore not correct to conclude, on the basis of the cold feet or hands of these patients, that there is a 'high sympathetic tone' or 'hypersympathetic' activity.

Indirect influence of sympathetic efferents on afferent impulse traffic by changing the micromilieu of the afferent receptors

The dependence of the micromilieu of the nociceptor in skin and deep somatic tissues on the activity of several types of non-neural cells (Fig. 13.5) and on substances produced by these cells (trophic factors, cytokines, arachidonic acid derivatives, histamine; see Table 13.2) has already been mentioned. The interaction of these cells with the primary afferent terminal is complex. It leads to a sensitization of nociceptors and therefore to an enhanced afferent impulse traffic to the CNS. It may furthermore enhance the development and maintenance of trophic changes observed in patients with RSD and with chronic inflammatory disorders (Jänig and Koltzenburg 1991a).

How is the sympathetic nervous system involved, except by its putative permissive effect via the control of the vascular bed? Answers to this question are at present at best speculative. However, this compelling possibility has recently been explored with pharmacological experiments in animal models (see Jänig and Koltzenburg 1991a). Rats were rendered hyperalgesic by repetitive chloroform treatment of the skin or by cutaneous injections of algesic chemicals. The reduction of the threshold for the flexion reflex elicited by paw pressure was used as an indicator for the presence of hyperalgesia and its modification was measured following various pharmacological treatments.

In normal control animals intradermal injection of noradrenaline and α-antagonists into the paw does not significantly change the flexion reflex threshold. This is in agreement with previous neurophysiological results showing that sympathetic efferents have little influence on nociceptive afferents under physiological conditions. In hyperalgesic rats, however, intradermal injections of noradrenaline led to a further drop of the threshold, suggesting that sympathetic activity could aggravate hyperalgesia. Conversely, an increase of the flexion reflex threshold was noted after α-receptor blockade with phentolamine. Interestingly, the reversal of the hyperalgesia was also observed after treatment with the α_2-antagonist, yohimbine, but not when the α_1-antagonists, prazosin, was applied. Moreover, the hyperalgesic effect of noradrenaline injections was absent in animals that had been chronically sympathectomized. This led to the hypothesis that catecholamines would not directly sensitize primary afferents. Rather, catecholamines might act on presynaptic α_2-receptors of postganglionic fibres thereby releasing other compounds that may subsequently affect the properties of afferent neurons (Fig. 13.3(d)). As the cyclo-oxygenase inhibitor indomethacin could also counteract the hyperalgesic effect of noradrenaline, it was suggested that prostaglandins could be the substances involved (Levine *et al.* 1986).

The exciting hypothesis developed by Levine and co-workers may indeed be relevant in chronic inflammatory conditions (e.g. rheumatoid arthritis), yet it is almost entirely based on pharmacological experiments and difficult to test directly.

Changes of the reflex pattern in sympathetic neurons

A further component that may contribute to disturbed neural control of blood vessels and sweat glands in patients with RSD is changes of the activity and reflexes in the sympathetic nervous system. Many patients with RSD cannot any longer thermoregulate with their affected extremity; furthermore, the skin of the affected extremity is usually warmer than on the contralateral side in the early stage of RSD and colder later on (Blumberg 1991). Thus, in addition to a disturbed neurovascular transmission and the development of adaptive supersensitivity of blood vessels, the activity in vasoconstrictor neurons may change after trauma caused by nerve lesions in patients with RSD. This idea is primarily based on observations of autonomic effector organ responses (reflected in changes of blood flow and sweating) in patients with RSD and would imply that the activity or activity pattern in sympathetic neurons to blood vessels and sweat glands has changed. As already mentioned above, caution is recommended in linking the skin temperature of the extremities with the activity in cutaneous vasoconstrictor neurons (see Wakisaka *et al.* 1991).

We have tested experimentally whether the reflex pattern in vasoconstrictor neurons to skin and skeletal muscle of the cat hind limb changes after nerve lesions. The lesions studied were as follows: cutting and ligating the superficial peroneal nerve (skin nerve); connecting the central stump of the superficial peroneal nerve to the distal stumps of muscle branches of the deep peroneal nerve (Blumberg and Jänig 1985); connecting the central stump of the sural nerve (skin nerve) to the distal stump of the tibial nerve (mixed nerve: Jänig and Koltzenburg 1991*b*, *c*). The neurophysiological experiments were conducted about 6 days to 18 months after the nerve lesions on anaesthetized animals. Activity was recorded from the vasoconstrictor neurons. The reflexes elicited in these neurons by stimulation of arterial chemoreceptors, arterial baroreceptors, and cutaneous nociceptors were measured. In some of the experiments the blood flow through the hairless skin of the hind paw was measured (Jänig and Koltenzburg 1991*b*, *c*).

Muscle vasoconstrictor neurons are excited during stimulation of arterial chemoreceptors and cutaneous nociceptors and inhibited by stimulation of

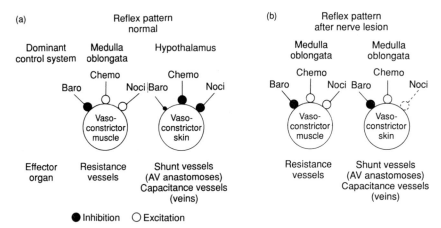

Fig. 13.6. Reflex patterns in postganglionic vasoconstrictor neurons supplying skeletal muscle and skin (a) under normal conditions and (b) after chronic nerve lesions. The patterns are simplifications and represent the pure cases. The term 'dominant control system' indicates the brain structure that controls the respective vasoconstrictor system predominantly (but not, of course, exclusively). In (b) it is proposed that the cutaneous vasoconstrictor system is under predominant control of the medulla oblongata. Note the uniformity of the reflex patterns in (b). AV, arteriovenous. Based on data from Blumberg and Jänig (1985) and Jänig and Koltzenburg (1991c). (Taken with permission from Jänig (1990).)

arterial baroreceptors in control animals under standardized experimental conditions. Most cutaneous vasoconstrictor neurons innervating blood vessels in hairy and hairless skin of the distal hind limb are inhibited during stimulation of arterial chemoreceptors and cutaneous nociceptors and are under weak or no inhibitory phasic control of the arterial baroreceptors (Fig. 13.6(a); Jänig 1985a). After the nerve lesions the reflex pattern changes in many cutaneous vasoconstrictor neurons but not in muscle vasoconstrictor neurons. Cutaneous vasoconstrictor neurons may now be excited during stimulation of arterial chemoreceptors and of cutaneous nociceptors and may exhibit a stronger than normal inhibition in their activity to stimulation of the arterial baroreceptors (Fig. 13.6(b)). Thus the differentiation between cutaneous and muscle vasoconstrictor neurons tends to disappear, though the changed reflexes are rather variable. The reflex changes were pronounced for the chemoreceptor reflex. For this reflex it has been shown that the reaction of the vascular bed of the hairless skin changes from vasodilatation in the control animals to vasoconstriction in the experimental animals. The qualitative changes of the reflex pattern in cutaneous vasoconstrictor neurons are particularly prominent in animals with a cross-union of nerves and are sustained in this preparation long after regeneration of the nerve fibres to the inappropriate target tissue has occurred (for details and discussion see Blumberg and Jänig 1985; Jänig and Koltzenburg 1991*b*, *c*).

This type of experiment illustrates that lesions of nerves can entail long-term changes of reflex activity in sympathetic neurons supplying blood vessels. It is unlikely that these changes are due to a reorganization in the sympathetic paravertebral ganglia. It appears more likely that they are due to a reorganization in the spinal cord or brainstem or both. They may reflect the plasticity of the central organization of the sympathetic nervous system. It may be speculated that activity in muscle vasoconstrictor neurons is normally under predominant control of the medulla oblongata and activity in cutaneous vasoconstrictor neurons under predominant control of the hypothalamus, resulting in the differentiated reflex patterns which are observed in these neurons (Fig. 13.6(a)). After the nerve lesion both systems may be under predominant control of the medulla oblongata (Fig. 13.6(b)). It should be kept in mind, first, that these results were obtained in anaesthetized cats under standardized experimental conditions and, second, that the expression of these central changes may look different in unanaesthetized patients.

These central changes add to the distorted regulation of the sympathetic effector organs: now a changed centrally generated signal in the sympathetic neurons contributes to the peripheral abnormalities (altered neurovascular transmission, development of adaptive supersensitivity of blood vessels, impairment of neurogenic vasodilatation mediated by unmyelinated afferents). At present it is unclear what the contribution of the central disturbance of sympathetic function to the development of RSD and related pain syndromes in patients is.

Conclusion

In healthy conditions, tissue-damaging stimuli in the periphery are encoded by nociceptive afferent neurons. The nociceptive impulse activity is transformed in the spinal cord and faithfully transmitted to the thalamocortical system and to other supraspinal brain centres leading to pain perception, control of the spinal transmission of nociceptive information, and appropriate somatomotor, autonomic, and endocrine reactions. This concerted action of the central nervous system may be disturbed under pathological conditions such as reflex sympathetic dystrophy and related states of neuropathic pain (Devor *et al.* 1991). Peripheral injury (trauma with and without obvious lesions; chronic inflammation) leads to receptor sensitization and an almost chaotic change of the afferent impulse traffic to the CNS due to peripheral nerve pathology (Jänig 1988). The peripheral changes entail changes of central neurons (globally described here as 'central sensitization') resulting in distorted sensations and distorted autonomic, somatomotor, and endocrine reactions.

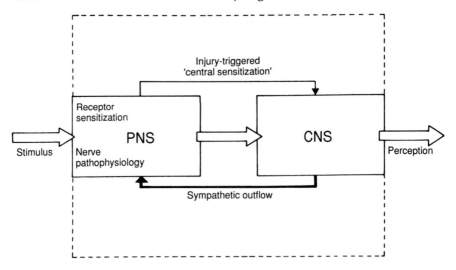

Fig. 13.7. Schematic diagram showing the components which may be important for an understanding of neuropathic pain following peripheral injury which is dependent on a positive feedback loop via the sympathetic nervous system. Peripheral injuries lead to sensitization of afferent receptors, afferent impulse activity from lesioned nerve fibres, and slow biochemical changes in the periphery (see Jänig 1988). This in turn produces central changes (generally described as central sensitization; for details see Bond *et al.* 1991; Cervero *et al.* 1989) with an abnormal activity in the neurons of the sympathetic outflow. The sympathetic loop feeds directly or indirectly back to the afferent impulse generators, this coupling being the consequence of the peripheral injury. PNS, peripheral nervous system; CNS, central nervous system. (Modified with permission from Devor *et al.* (1991).)

In consequence the sympathetic outflow to the affected peripheral part of the body may be actively involved in the generation of pain and associated processes by way of a positive feedback loop (Fig. 13.7). Stimuli which normally are non-painful may now elicit excessive painful reactions which are dependent on an intact sympathetic innervation (Price *et al.* 1989). Several pathophysiological mechanisms may be involved in this process:

(1) abnormal coupling of noradrenergic postganglionic fibres to afferent fibres and their receptors;

(2) disturbance of the micromilieu of afferent receptors by changes of the neurovascular transmission and by development of adaptive super-sensitivity of blood vessels;

(3) disturbance of the micromilieu of afferent receptors by interference of noradrenergic fibres with non-neural inflammatory and immune-competent cells;

(4) changes of the impulse pattern in neurons of the sympathetic outflow, possibly as consequence of the central changes.

The complexity of the somatosensory and autonomic abnormalities observed in patients with neuropathic pains that may be in some way or another associated with the sympathetic nervous system indicates that several pathobiological processes operate in parallel, on the sensory as well as on the efferent site, and that the actual clinical phenomenology may be dependent on the predominance of one type of pathological mechanism (Bennett 1991).

Acknowledgement

This work was supported by the Deutsche Forschungsgemeinschaft.

References

Arnér, S. (1991). Intravenous phentolamine test: diagnostic and prognostic use in reflex sympathetic dystrophy. *Pain* **46**, 17–22.

Bennett, G. J. (1991). Evidence from animal models on the pathogenesis of painful peripheral neuropathy: relevance for pharmacotherapy. In *Towards a new pharmacotherapy of pain*, Dahlem Workshop Reports (ed. A. I. Basbaum and J. M. Besson), pp. 365–79. John Wiley & Sons, Chichester.

Blumberg, H. (1991). A new clinical approach for diagnosing reflex sympathetic dystrophy. In *Pain research and clinical management: Proceedings of the VIth World Congress on Pain*, Vol. 4 (ed. M. R. Bond, J. E. Charlton, and C. J. Woolf), pp. 399–407. Elsevier, Amsterdam.

Blumberg, H. and Jänig, W. (1985). Reflex patterns in postganglionic vasoconstrictor neurones following chronic nerve lesions. *J. autonom. nerv. Syst.* **14** 157–80.

Bond, M. R., Charlton, J. E., and Woolf, C. J. (ed.) (1991). *Pain research and clinical management: Proceedings of the VIth World Congress on Pain*, Vol. 4. Elsevier, Amsterdam.

Bonica, J. J. (1990). Causalgia and other reflex sympathetic dystrophies. In *The management of pain* (2nd edn) (ed. J. J. Bonica), pp. 220–43. Lea & Febiger, Philadelphia.

Campbell, J. N., Raja, S. N., and Meyer, R. A. (1988). Painful sequelae of nerve injury. In *Pain research and clinical management: Proceedings of the Vth World Congress on Pain*, Vol. 3 (ed. R. Dubner, G. F. Gebhart, and M. R. Bond), pp. 135–43. Elsevier, Amsterdam.

Cervero, F., Bennett, G. J., and Headley, P. M. (ed.) (1989) *Processing of sensory information in the superficial dorsal horn of the spinal cord*, Nato ASI Series, Series A: Life Sciences, Vol. 176. Plenum Press, New York.

Devor, M., Basbaum, A. I., Bennett, G. J., Blumberg, H., Campbell, J. N., Dembowsky, K. P., Guilbaud, G., Jänig, W., Koltzenburg, M., Levine, J. D., Otten, U. H., and Portenoy, R. K. (1991). Mechanisms of neuropathic pain following peripheral injury. In *Towards a new pharmacotherapy of pain*, Dahlem Workshop Reports (ed. A. I. Basbaum and J. M. Besson), pp. 417–40. John Wiley & Sons, Chichester.

Fleming, W. W. and Westfall, D. P. (1988). Adaptive supersensitivity. In *Catecholamines I. Handbook of experimental pharmacology*, Vol. 90/I (ed. U. Trendelenburg and N. Weiner), pp. 509–59. Springer-Verlag, Berlin.

Frost, S. A., Raja, S. N., Campbell, J. N., Meyer, R. A., and Khan, A. A. (1988). Does hyperalgesia to cooling stimuli characterize patients with sympathetically maintained pain (reflex sympathetic dystrophy)? In *Pain research and clinical management: Proceedings of the Vth World Congress on Pain*, Vol. 3 (ed. R. Dubner, G. F Gebhart, and M. R. Bond), pp. 151–6. Elsevier, Amsterdam.

Häbler, H.-J., Jänig, W., and Koltzenburg, M. (1987). Activation of unmyelinated afferents in chronically lesioned nerves by adrenaline and excitation of sympathetic efferents in the cat. *Neurosci. Lett.* **82**, 35–40.

Hannington-Kiff, J. G. (1989). Pharmacological target blocks in painful dystrophic limbs. In *Textbook of pain* (2nd edn) (ed. P. D. Wall and R. Melzack), pp. 754–66. Churchill Livingstone, Edinburgh.

Jänig, W. (1985a). Organization of the lumbar sympathetic outflow to skeletal muscle and skin of the cat hindlimb and tail. *Rev. Physiol. Biochem. Pharmacol.* **102**, 119–213.

Jänig W. (1985b). Causalgia and reflex sympathetic dystrophy: in which way is the sympathetic nervous system involved? *Trends Neurosci.* **8**, 471–7.

Jänig, W. (1988). Pathophysiology of nerve following mechanical injury. In *Pain research and clinical management: Proceeding of the Vth World Congress on Pain*, Vol. 3 (ed. R. Dubner, G. F. Gebhart, and M. R. Bond), pp. 89–109. Elsevier, Amsterdam.

Jänig, W. (1989). Autonomic nervous system. In *Human physiology* (ed. R. F. Schmidt and G. Thews), pp. 333–70. Springer, New York.

Jänig, W. (1990). The sympathetic nervous system in pain: physiology and pathophysiology. In *Pain and the sympathetic nervous System* (ed. M. Stanton-Hicks), pp. 17–89. Kluwer Academic Publishers, Boston.

Jänig, W. and Koltzenburg, M. (1991a). What is the interaction between the sympathetic terminal and the primary afferent fiber? In *Towards a new pharmacotherapy of pain*, Dahlem Workshop Reports (ed. A. I. Basbaum and J. M. Besson), pp. 331–52. John Wiley & Sons, Chichester.

Jänig, W. and Koltzenburg, M. (1991b). Sympathetic activity and neuroeffector transmission change after chronic nerve lesions. In *Pain research and clinical management: Proceedings of the VIth World Congress on Pain*, Vol. 4 (ed. M. R. Bond, J. E. Charlton, and C. J. Woolf), pp. 365–71. Elsevier, Amsterdam.

Jänig, W. and Koltzenburg, M. (1991c). Plasticity of sympathetic reflex organization following cross-union of inappropriate nerves in the adult cat. *J. Physiol.* **436**, 309–23.

Jänig, W. and McLachlan, E. M. (1987). Organization of lumbar spinal outflow to distal colon and pelvic organs. *Physiol. Rev.* **67**, 1332–404.

Jänig, W., Blumberg, H., Boas, R. A., and Campbell, J. N. (1991). The reflex sympathetic dystrophy syndrome, Consensus statement and general recommendations for diagnosis and clinical research. In *Pain research and clinical management: Proceedings of the VIth World Congress on Pain*, Vol. 4 (ed. M. R. Bond, J. E. Charlton, and C. J. Woolf), pp. 372–5. Elsevier, Amsterdam.

Levine, J. D., Taiwo, Y. O., Collins, S. D., and Tam, J. K. (1986). Noradrenergic hyperalgesia is mediated through interaction with sympathetic postganglionic neurone terminals rather than activation of primary afferent nociceptors. *Nature, London* **323**, 158–69.

Otten, U. (1991). Nerve growth factor: a signalling protein between the nervous and the immune system. In *Towards a new pharmacotherapy of pain*, Dahlem Workshop Reports, (ed. A. I. Basbaum and J. M. Besson), pp. 353–66. John Wiley & Sons, Chichester.

Price, D. D., Bennett, G. J., and Raffii, A. (1989). Psychophysical observations on patients with neuropathic pain relieved by a sympathetic block. *Pain* **36**, 273–88.

Sato, J. and Perl, E. R. (1991). Adrenergic excitation of cutaneous pain receptors induced by peripheral nerve injury. *Science* **251**, 1608–10.

Wakisaka, S., Kajander, K. C., and Bennett, G. J. (1991). Abnormal skin temperature and abnormal sympathetic vasomotor innervation in an experimental painful peripheral neuropathy. *Pain* **46**, 299–313.

PART III

Clinical autonomic testing

14. Investigation of autonomic disorders

Christopher J. Mathias and Roger Bannister

Introduction

In a patient with a suspected autonomic disorder the major aims of investigation are:

1. to determine if autonomic function is normal or abnormal;

2. if the latter, to assess the degree of dysfunction, with an emphasis on the site of lesion and on the functional deficit;

3. to ascertain if the abnormality is of the primary variety, or secondary to recognized disorders, as the prognosis and management may depend upon the diagnostic category.

In this chapter an overview of the ways to investigate such patients is provided (Table 14.1). A range of systems is covered, with an emphasis on the cardiovascular system where there have been major advances in assessing the site of lesion and determining the functional deficit, together with recognizing the role of compensatory systems, including various neurohormones. It should be emphasized that assessment of autonomic function depends not only on reflex arcs and on efferent activity but also on end-organ responsiveness, which include the metabolic clearance and disposition of transmitters, postsynaptic receptors, postreceptor translation, and second messenger systems. Each test, and the information from it, should be considered in relation to the clinical picture, which is of particular importance in patients with generalized autonomic disorders.

In localized disorders more specific investigations may be needed. An example is Horner's syndrome where the assessment may initially concentrate on the eye; further investigation in identifying the cause is of greater importance. This may include a computerized tomography (CT) or magnetic resonance imaging (MRI) scan to exclude midbrain or medullary haemorrhage or infarction, a CT scan of the thorax and bronchoscopy to exclude Pancoast's syndrome with a lesion in the region of the apex of the lung, or carotid angiography to exclude dissection of the internal carotid artery.

Table 14.1. Outline of investigations in autonomic failure

Cardiovascular	
Physiological	Head-up tilt (45°); standing; Valsalva manoeuvre
	Pressor stimuli—isometric exercise, cold pressor, mental arithmetic
	Heart rate responses—deep breathing, hyperventilation, standing, head-up tilt, 30 : 15 ratio
	Carotid sinus massage
	Liquid meal
Biochemical	Plasma noradrenaline—supine and standing; urinary catecholamines; plasma renin activity and aldosterone
Pharmacological	Noradrenaline—α-adrenoceptors—vascular
	Isoprenaline—β-adrenoceptors—vascular and cardiac
	Tyramine—pressor and noradrenaline response
	Edrophonium—noradrenaline response
	Atropine—parasympathetic cardiac blockade
Sweating	Central regulation—increase core temperature by 1°C
	Sweat gland response—intradermal
	Acetylcholine—quantitative sudomotor
	Axon reflex test (Q-SART)—spot test
Gastrointestinal	Barium studies, video cinefluoroscopy, endoscopy, gastric emptying studies
Renal function and urinary tract	Day and night urine volumes and sodium/potassium excretion
	Urodynamic studies, intravenous urography, ultrasound examination, sphincter electromyography
Sexual function	Penile plethysmography
	Intracavernosal papaverine
Respiratory	Laryngoscopy
	Sleep studies to assess apnoea/oxygen desaturation
Eye	Schirmer's test
	Pupil function—pharmacological and physiological

Cardiovascular testing

The prime concern of the cardiovascular system is tissue perfusion, with blood pressure and blood flow therefore of critical importance. These are influenced by a number of factors, with beat-to-beat control of blood pressure dependent upon the autonomic nervous system and, in particular, the sympathetic efferent pathways. In addition, a number of secondary mechanisms, involving systemically acting hormones, such as angiotensin II and aldosterone, and locally acting substances, such as the prostaglandins, endothelium derived relaxing factor (EDRF), and endothelin, play a role.

A schematic diagram of the main neurological pathways involved in the regulation of blood pressure is provided in Fig. 14.1. There are cortical, limbic, anterior, and posterior hypothalamic and medullary centres, where the input from a range of afferents can be integrated. The major cardiovascular afferents are those from the carotid sinus, the aortic arch, and the cardiopulmonary afferents, although a range of other afferents (from skeletal muscle, skin, and viscera) also contribute. This is best seen in patients with cervical spinal cord transection, in whom control may occur at a peripheral

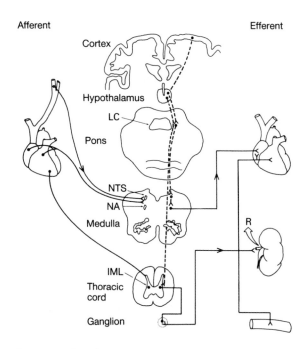

Fig. 14.1. Diagram of cardiovascular control mechanism. LC, locus ceruleus; NA, nucleus ambiguus; NTS, nucleus tractus solitarius; IML, intermediolateral column; R, renin. (Taken with permission from Bannister (1979).)

level devoid of cerebral direction (Chapter 43). Normally, from the cerebral centres the output through the vagus and the sympathetic nervous system to the heart and blood vessels is co-ordinated. A variety of investigative approaches in animals (Chapter 4) indicates that the major baroreceptor afferents pass to the nucleus tractus solitarius, that the vagal output is through the nucleus ambiguus, and that the sympathetic output is through the reticular paramedian nucleus.

Lesions resulting in autonomic dysfunction may involve the afferent pathways, the central connections, the efferent pathways, the target organs, or a combination of these, depending upon the disorder (Chapter 3). Abnormalities in cardiovascular reflex activity usually result in impairment of short-term adjustments, although long-term compensatory changes, through hormones which influence blood vessels, intravascular volume, and the kidneys, may help buffer the abnormalities. These aspects need to be borne in mind when we consider the range of tests to assess cardiovascular aspects of autonomic function, to determine the site or sites of lesions, and to ascertain hormonal factors which may be contributing to, or may be utilized for the benefit of the patient.

Physiological tests

Postural Challenge

Postural (orthostatic) hypotension is a cardinal manifestation of autonomic failure and the cardiovascular responses to head-up postural change are therefore particularly important. Postural hypotension is arbitrarily defined as a fall of more than 20 mm Hg systolic blood pressure on standing, but, as described below, a number of factors influence the fall in pressure, and a smaller fall in the presence of relevant symptoms may be of importance and will warrant further investigation. Brachial blood pressure is often measured non-invasively using a standard mercury sphygmomanometer, although there is increasing reliance on semi-automated sphygmomanometers, utilizing the auscultatory or oscillometric methods, to measure both systolic and diastolic blood pressure in addition to deriving heart rate. More recent non-invasive techniques include the measurement of finger arterial blood pressure, using a sophisticated system (Finapres; Imholz et al. 1991; Chapter 15) which provides beat-to-beat pressure. This obviates the need for invasive intra arterial (radial or brachial artery) catheterization, which was previously the only reliable means of obtaining continuous blood pressure measurements.

Basal measurements need to be performed with the subject lying supine in a quiet room and as comfortable as possible. An adequate number of readings, over a 5–10 min interval may be needed to determine the stability (or lack of stability) of supine blood pressure. Most intermittent non-invasive blood pressure measurements take around a minute and, as they involve cuff inflation, they should not be repeated too frequently. Recumbent

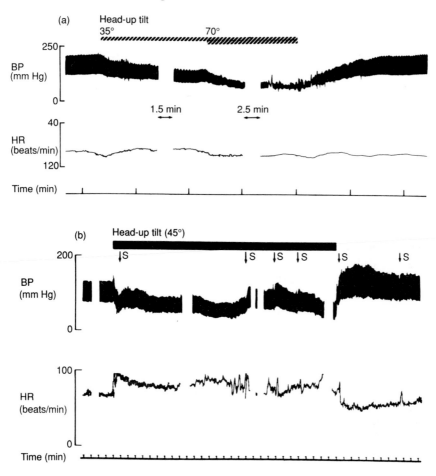

Fig. 14.2. (a) Continuous intraarterial recording of blood pressure (BP) and heart rate (HR) in a patient with postural hypotension and the Holmes–Adie syndrome. Both systolic and diastolic blood pressure fall progressively during tilt, with no recovery. There are minimal changes in heart rate. There was no change in plasma noradrenaline levels following tilt. Other investigations indicated that the lesion was likely to be on the afferent side of the baroreflex arc, (From Mathias (1987).) (b) Blood Pressure (BP) and heart rate (HR) in a tetraplegic patient before, during and after head-up tilt to 45°. Blood pressure promptly falls with partial recovery, which in this case is linked to skeletal muscle spasms (S), inducing spinal sypathetic activity. Some of the later oscillations are probably due to the rise in plasma renin, measured where there are interruptions in the intraarterial record. In the later phases, muscle spasms occur more frequently and further elevate blood pressure. On return to the horizontal, blood pressure rises rapidly above the previous basal level and slowly returns to the horizontal. Heart rate tends to move in the opposite direction. There is a transient increase in heart rate during muscle spasms. (From Mathias and Frankel (1988).)

hypertension may occur in patients with autonomic failure for reasons which include impaired baroreceptor control, supersensitivity of denervated blood vessels to even small amounts of neurotransmitters or pressor drug treatment, and fluid shifts from the periphery into the central compartment when changing posture. Postural change can be induced, using either a tilt table (45–60°), or by making the subject initially sit and then stand up, or stand directly. A tilt table is advantageous, especially in subjects who have neurological disabilities, severe postural hypotension, or both, as it enables rapid return to the horizontal. Measurements of blood pressure and heart rate should ideally be made every 2½ min, preferably for a period of 10 min, as this also enables blood collection for measurements of catecholamines and other vasoactive hormones released during postural change.

In normal subjects, head-up tilt or standing results in minimal changes in blood pressure. In autonomic disorders, however, the pressure often falls, and the degree and rapidity of fall and extent of recovery can vary considerably even within the same individual. In severe autonomic failure, the blood pressure may fall rapidly and progressively (Fig. 14.2 (a)), unlike in patients with high thoracic or cervical spinal cord transection (Fig. 14.2 (b)), especially those who have been rehabilitated, in whom there is a rapid initial fall followed by partial recovery. The latter results from activation of spinal sympathetic reflexes or humoral compensatory mechanisms which include the renin–angiotensin–aldosterone system. With an immediate and profound fall in blood pressure on postural change it may be difficult, if not impossible, to make accurate measurements using non-invasive techniques other than the Finapres, but varying the degree of tilt may help. The advantages of the Finapres are that it avoids intraarterial cannulation and provides a reliable measure of change in blood pressure.

The degree of postural hypotension is dependent upon a large number of factors. In primary autonomic failure, postural hypotension is often greater in the morning, because of nocturnal diuresis, after food ingestion because of splanchnic vasodilatation, and in hot weather because of cutaneous dilatation. Vasodilatation induced by drugs, including those normally not considered to have significant cardiovascular effects, may cause substantial changes in blood pressure when there is a baroreflex deficit. It is also necessary to consider non-neurogenic causes of postural hypotension, as outlined in Table 14.2. Twenty-four hour non-invasive ambulatory blood pressure profiles may have a role in the investigation and management of autonomic disorders (Fig. 14.3).

There is normally a small-to-moderate rise in heart rate during postural change. In the presence of a substantial fall in blood pressure, a lack of change in heart rate is indicative of a baroreflex abnormality, as in sympathetic and parasympathetic failure. In tetraplegic patients the heart rate rises in response to the fall in blood pressure, because the vagal and glossopharyngeal afferent

Table 14.2.   Non-neurogenic causes of postural hypotension

Low intravascular volume	
Blood/plasma loss	Haemorrhage, burns, haemodialysis
Fluid/electrolyte	Inadequate intake—anorexia nervosa, loss vomiting
	Diarrhoea—including losses from ileostomy
	Renal/endocrine—salt losing nephropathy, adrenal insufficiency (Addison's disease), diabetes insipidus, diuretics
Vasodilatation	Drugs—glyceryl trinitrate
	Alcohol
	Heat, pyrexia
	Hyperbradykininism
	Extensive varicose veins
Cardiac impairment	
Myocardial	Myocarditis
Impaired ventricular filling	Atrial myxoma, constrictive pericarditis
Impaired output	Aortic stenosis

and the vagal efferent pathways are intact. The heart rate, however, does not usually rise above 100 or 120 beats/min, as is seen after atropine administration and vagal blockade; further elevation is probably dependent on adrenomedullary stimulation and elevation of plasma adrenaline levels, which do not occur in such patients. This adrenal component probably accounts for the greater tachycardia observed in subjects with an intact sympathetic nervous system when they have a low blood pressure, as in haemorrhagic shock.

The responses in two special groups of patients, who do not have detectable autonomic impairment but are prone to fainting, should be mentioned. The first are those with vasovagal syncope, or emotional faints (Chapter 39). Detailed autonomic testing usually reveals no abnormalities, but patients may faint during prolonged postural change or when exposed to a variety of stimuli, including the sight or mere thought of a venepuncture needle (Fig. 14.4). In such patients the blood pressure is often maintained initially during head-up tilt, but then suddenly falls. This may be preceded by a fall in heart rate and is consistent with withdrawal of sympathetic nervous activity to blood vessels, in the presence of vagal overactivity to the heart (Wallin and Sundlöf 1982). Withdrawal of sympathetic neural activity appears to be of greater importance, as vagal blockade with atropine or maintenance of heart rate with a demand pace-maker does not protect against syncope. The second

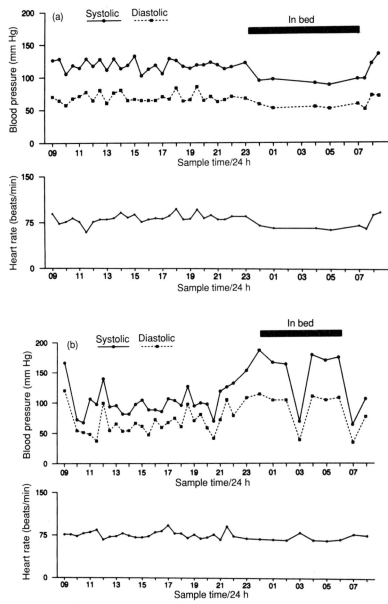

Fig. 14.3. Twenty-four hour non-invasive ambulatory blood pressure profile, showing systolic (●——●) and diastolic (■ – – – ■) blood pressure and heart rate at intervals through the day and night. (a) The changes in a normal subject with no postural fall in blood pressure; there was a fall in blood pressure at night while asleep with a rise in blood pressure on wakening. (b) The marked fluctuations in blood pressure in a patient with pure autonomic failure. The marked falls in blood pressure are usually the result of postural changes, either

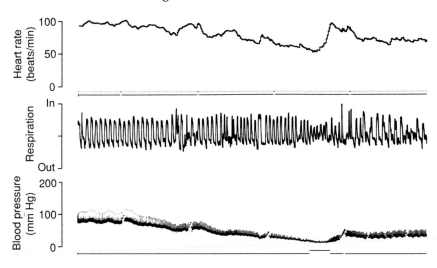

Fig. 14.4. Blood pressure changes towards the end of a period of head-up tilt in a patient with recurrent episodes of vasovagal syncope. Blood pressure which was previously maintained begins to fall. There is also a fall in heart rate. There initially are relatively minor changes in respiratory rate, which can be derived from the time signal above it, each minor dot indicating a second and the bolder mark indicating a minute. The patient was about to faint and was put back to the horizontal (indicated by elevated time signal below) and then to 5° head-down tilt. Blood pressure and heart rate recover but still remain lower than previously. This patient had no other autonomic abnormalities on detailed testing. Blood pressure was measured non-invasively by the Finapres.

special group of patients are those who have a pronounced tachycardia during postural change, following which there is a profound fall in blood pressure. Again, no autonomic deficit can be clearly defined. For reasons which are unclear, there is a marked chronotropic cardiac response which presumably results either in inadequate filling of the right side of the heart or activation of cardiac sensory receptors followed by sympathetic withdrawal (see Chapter 15), as in patients with vasovagal syncope. In some patients hyperventilation may contribute.

The '30–15 ratio' has been used as a means of quantifying the heart rate changes during standing (Chapter 16). Normally the rise in heart rate is greatest by the fifteenth beat, followed by slowing which is maximal at the

---

Fig. 14.3. (*continued*)   sitting or standing. Supine blood pressure, particularly at night, is elevated. Getting up to micturate causes a marked fall in blood pressure (at 03:00 hours). There is a reversal of the diurnal changes in blood pressure. There are relatively small changes in heart rate, considering the marked changes in blood pressure.

thirtieth beat. The ratio of the longest P-R interval of the thirtieth to the shortest interval on the fifteenth beat is thus normally over one. In the absence of change on standing it is 1.0 or < 1.0. Whether this contributes further to assessing or understanding the problem is debatable.

The Valsalva manoeuvre

The changes in blood pressure and heart rate during the Valsalva manoeuvre, when intrathoracic pressure is raised ideally to 40 mm Hg, provide a further assessment of the baroreflex pathways. To perform this the subject blows with an open glottis into a disposable syringe connected to the mercury column of a sphygmomanometer and maintains a forced expiratory pressure of up

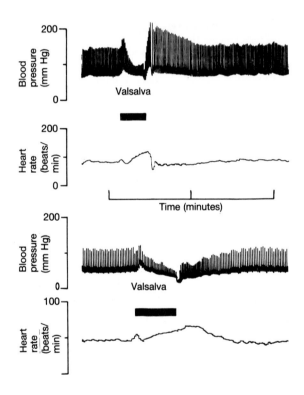

Fig. 14.5. Changes in intraarterial blood pressure and heart rate before, during, and after the Valsalva manoeuvre, when intrathoracic pressure was raised to 40 mm Hg in a normal subject (upper trace) and in a patient (lower trace). In the normal subject release of intrathoracic pressure was accompanied by an increase in blood pressure and a reduction in heart rate below basal levels. In the patient there was a gradual increase in blood pressure implying impairment of sympathetic vasoconstrictor pathways. The heart-rate scale varies in the two subjects.

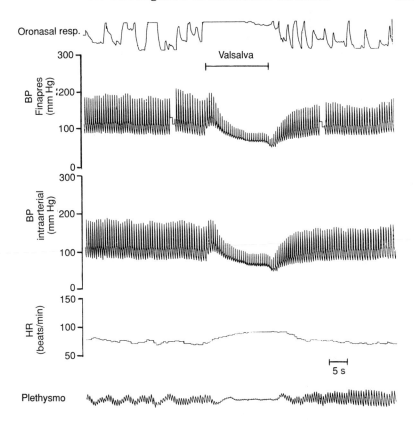

Fig. 14.6. Changes in non-invasive finger blood pressure (BP, Finapres) compared with intraarterial blood pressure (BP) in a patient with autonomic impairment, before, during, and after a Valsalva manoeuvre. Respiratory rate (oronasal resp.), heart rate (HR), and plethysmograph (Plethysmo) are also continuously recorded. The Finapres recording appears indentical to the intraarterial trace. The breaks indicate an internal calibration signal. (By courtesy of P. Cortelli and E. Zoni, University of Bologna; from Mathias (1992).)

to 40 mm Hg for 10 s. This may be difficult in some subjects, and levels of between 20–40 mm Hg often suffice to induce the necessary changes. With the rise in intrathoracic pressure the venous return falls along with blood pressure (Fig. 14.5). On releasing intrathoracic pressure there is a blood pressure overshoot because of persistence of sympathetic activity. Baroreflex activation results in a secondary fall in heart rate to below basal levels. In sympathetic vasoconstrictor failure, the Valsalva manoeuvre results in a continual fall in blood pressure with no stabilization; following release there is no blood pressure overshoot and no compensatory bradycardia. If the afferent and vagal efferent components of the baroreflex pathways are intact, as in tetraplegics and some patients with autonomic failure, heart rate rises while the blood pressure falls. There is also a sympathetic component to this response, as in normal subjects the rise in heart rate is blunted following administration of the β-adrenergic blocker propranolol.

It is often not possible to obtain beat-to-beat blood pressure during assessment of the Valsalva, and the continuous measurement of heart rate often suffices. A spuriously abnormal response may, however, occur if the cheek muscles are used to produce an apparent but false rise in intrathoracic pressure. Beat-to-beat blood pressure monitoring, as with the Finapres, is of value in these situations, as it will identify a lack of fall in blood pressure indicating that intrathoracic pressure was not elevated adequately (Fig. 14.6).

Pressor stimuli

These raise blood pressure by stimulating sympathetic efferent pathways in a variety of ways, such as isometric exercise or cutaneous cold through activation of peripheral receptors, although there is often an important cerebral component. Others, such as sudden noise or mental arithmetic, are dependent predominantly on cerebral stimulation.

Isometric exercise is performed by using either a dynamometer or a partially inflated sphygmomanometer cuff, and sustaining handgrip for 2–3 min, usually at a third of the maximum voluntary contraction pressure. The cold pressor test consists of immersing the hand for up to 2 min in ice slush, usually just below 4°C. Cortical arousal is performed by sudden noise with a starting pistol, mental arithmetic (subtraction or addition of 7 or 17), or a variety of more complex tasks. These stimuli normally elevate blood pressure and heart rate (Fig. 14.7 (a), (b)). In patients with central or efferent sympathetic lesions these stimuli do not elevate blood pressure.

In tetraplegic patients with complete cervical spinal cord lesions, mental arithmetic and stimuli above the cutaneous level of the lesion (such as with an ice pack) do not raise blood pressure, in contrast to stimuli below the lesion which activate spinal sympathetic reflexes and cause a rise in pressure, often with a fall in heart rate because of increased vagal activity. Stimuli capable

---

Fig. 14.7. Blood pressure (BP) and heart rate (HR) responses to cutaneous cold (hand up to wrist in ice slush) (a) in a normal subject and (b) in a patient with autonomic failure. The time scale is similar in (a) and (b). In the patient there is no rise in BP. Non-invasive recordings were made with the Finapres. (c) Intra-arterial BP and HR in a chronic tetraplegic before, during and after cutaneous stimulation (CS) and bladder stimulation (BS) 6 months after injury when reflex isolated spinal cord activity had returned. Cutaneous stimulation is performed by the application of ice over the chest below the level of the lesion, and urinary bladder stimulation is by suprapubic percussion of the anterior abdominal wall. There is a rise in BP with both stimuli, this being greater with bladder stimulation. (From Mathias *et al.* (1979).)

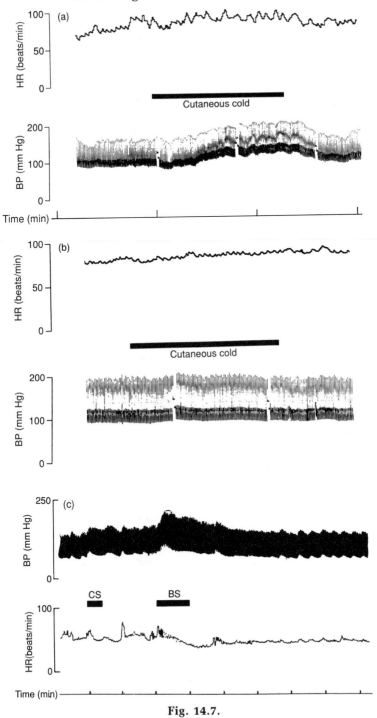

Fig. 14.7.

of such effects include cutaneous cold or other noxious cutaneous stimuli (including pin-prick), activation of abdominal or pelvic visceral reflexes by urinary bladder or large bowel contraction, and skeletal muscle spasms (Fig. 14.7 (c)). This elevation in blood pressure, along with a range of other cardiovascular changes, is an important component of the syndrome of autonomic dysreflexia and may be mistaken for a hypertensive crisis as in patients with a phaeochromocytoma, when there is excessive secretion of catecholamines from the tumour (Chapter 43).

Heart rate responses to respiratory change

Changes in respiration result in rapid responses in the cardiac vagi and variations in heart rate often provide a good guide to their activity. Normally, with inspiration there is a rise and with expiration a fall in heart rate, this being the basis of sinus arrhythmia (Fig. 14.8). A considerable number of variations to exploit and standardize this objectively are available. A single deep breath may be used, a short period of quiet breathing, or a fixed rate of 6 breaths/min; each is claimed to be a better discriminator. A heart rate variation of over 10 beats/min occurs in most normal subjects below 50 years of age; a figure below this is considered abnormal, as in diabetic autonomic neuropathy (Wheeler and Watkins 1973). Hyperventilation is

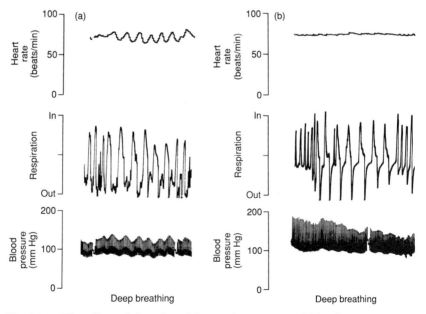

Fig. 14.8 The effect of deep breathing on heart rate and blood pressure in (a) a normal subject and (b) a patient with autonomic failure. There is no sinus arrhythmia in the patient, despite a fall in blood pressure. Respiratory changes are indicated in the middle panel.

probably a stronger stimulus to vagal withdrawal and causes a rise in heart rate. It may also lower blood pressure; the precise mechanisms of this are unclear.

In autonomic neuropathy complicating diabetes mellitus and alcoholism, cardiac vagal lesions may occur prior to sympathetic impairment, and the heart rate responses to these tests may be abnormal. Although this provides evidence of an autonomic neuropathy this should not be equated with a generalized or sympathetic deficit, or both.

Food ingestion

It is now widely recognized that food lowers supine blood pressure in a large number of patients with primary autonomic failure (Chapter 26). Postprandial hypotension in autonomic failure is linked to the release of vasodilatatory gut peptides and splanchnic vasodilatation that is not accompanied by compensatory changes in cardiac output and skeletal muscle resistance vessels, such as occur in normal subjects in whom blood pressure does not fall. In addition to the fall in supine blood pressure, food is now recognized as aggravating postural hypotension. This can be objectively measured by assessing the responses to head-up tilt before (ideally after an overnight fast) and 45 min after food ingestion. For practical reasons a liquid meal is preferable. Glucose can be used but this provides a caloric load of high osmolality which may be a problem, especially in diabetics. The alternative is a balanced liquid meal using commercially available Complan (containing various food components) and glucose, either in a milk or soya bean base made up to 300 ml. This can be easily prepared and readily ingested while lying flat, so that the effects of food ingestion independently of postural change can also be obtained (Fig. 14.9). This helps standardize postural blood pressure responses, as there are patients who in the fasting state have only modest postural hypotension which is considerably enhanced by food.

Carotid sinus massage

This should be performed if the history suggests that syncope is caused by movements of the neck or pressure over the carotid sinus by a collar or tie, especially in the presence of apparently normal autonomic function. Carotid sinus massage may provoke asystole and cardiac dysrhythmias so it is essential that adequate resuscitative measures are readily available in the event of cardiovascular collapse. Continuous monitoring of heart rate with an ECG print-out and oscilloscope, and blood pressure, ideally with a non-invasive beat-to-beat machine such as the Finapres, is needed. Only one carotid sinus should be stimulated each time, using gentle pressure which compresses the bulb against the tranverse processes of the upper cervical vertebrae. There are normally minor changes in heart rate and blood presssure. In carotid sinus hypersensitivity, severe bradycardia and hypotension may occur. The

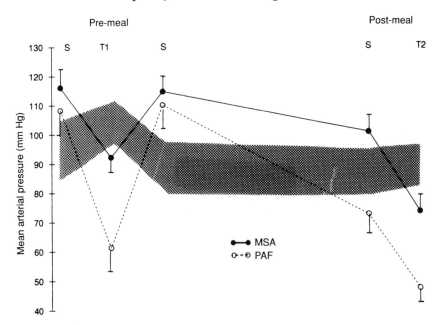

Fig. 14.9. Average levels (± SEM) of mean arterial blood pressure in 10 patients with pure autonomic failure (PAF) before and during head-up tilt to 45° pre-meal (T1) on left of panel; while supine again (S); and 45 min before and after retilting (T2) postprandially. Supine blood pressure falls to a greater degree in the PAF patients. The level of blood pressure in both groups of patients during head-up tilt and during the postprandial phase, falls to considerably lower levels and is accompanied by greater symptoms in both groups. In normal subjects (stippled area ± SEM) there is no fall in blood pressure. (Modified from Mathias *et al.* (1991*b*).)

former may precede the hypotension and, in the cardioinhibitory form, may be prevented by atropine or a demand cardiac pace-maker. There is a rare vasodepressor form, where hypotension occurs without bradycardia (Fig. 14.10 (a)); this appears to be due to withdrawal of sympathetic nerve activity, similar to that described in emotional syncope and the rare cases of syncope associated with glossopharyngeal neuralgia. Many fall into the mixed form (Fig. 14.10 (b)). In the vasodepressor and mixed forms therapeutic approaches may need to include unilateral or bilateral carotid sinus denervation. Predicting the outcome can be difficult and testing may need to be repeated after local anaesthetic infiltrated around the carotid sinus.

Specialized investigation of baroreflex and sympathetic activity

Intraneural recordings of sympathetic activity

Skin and muscle sympathetic nerve activity can be recorded using tungsten microelectrodes inserted into a cutaneous nerve in the arm or leg (Chapter 18).

Skin sympathetic activity is affected by thermal stimuli (activity increases with cold and decreases with heat), in contrast to muscle sympathetic activity which responds to manoeuvres activating baroreceptors and is time-locked to blood pressure changes within the cardiac cycle.

Microneurographic techniques have confirmed and advanced our understanding of a number of physiological and pathophysiological processes. There are, however, limitations and disadvantages to this technique. Measurements can only be made in a restricted region, and, although there is a surprisingly good correlation with plasma noradrenaline levels (Chapter 18), it may not provide specific answers when stimuli cause differential regional sympathetic responses. More important, the procedure is dependent upon considerable skill and, although safe, is an invasive one. It is likely to be unreliable or of no value when sympathoneural activity is low or absent as in autonomic failure.

Sympathetic skin response

Recordings of electric potential using recording electrodes on the foot or hand provide information on skin resistance, which is thought to be related to sympathetic activity, particularly of sudomotor function. A variety of stimuli which increase sympathetic discharge or electrical stimulation normally provoke a response. The response is usually absent in axonal neuropathies but present in demyelinating disorders (Shahani *et al.* 1984). Its value is questionable because of marked variability of responses, even in normal subjects. This partly explains the problems of using polygraph recordings as a 'lie detector', when the galvanic skin response, along with blood pressure, heart rate, and respiration rate, is obtained, usually with poor sensitivity and specificity (Brett *et al.* 1986).

Other measures of assessing baroreceptor reflex function

A variety of techniques ranging from lower-body suction to stimulation of carotid sinus afferents have been utilized. These have particular value in the research setting and can be combined with a series of investigations to assess blood flow in different regions, which is possible with accurate and sensitive non-invasive techniques (for examples see Kooner *et al.* 1989; Chaudhuri *et al.* 1991).

Negative pressure to the lower half of the body can be exerted by having the subject in a box or capsule extending up to the midthoracic region, with an air-tight seal allowing suction, usually by a vacuum cleaner which unloads and thus stimulates cardiopulmonary baroreceptor afferents. This should increase sympathetic neural activity in normal subjects, with constriction of resistance vessels and a rise in heart rate, with maintenance of blood pressure. This does not occur in sympathetic vasoconstrictor failure, when blood pressure rapidly falls (Fig. 14.11).

A specially designed cervical collar enables assessment of carotid sinus afferents which may be either inhibited or stimulated by localized elevation

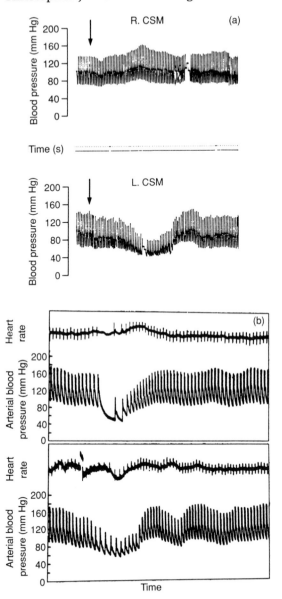

Fig. 14.10. (a) continuous non-invasive recording of finger arterial blood pressure (Finapres) before, during and after carotid sinus massage on the right (R. CSM) and left (L. CSM). The fine dots indicate the time marker in seconds. The arrow indicates when stimulation began. Stimulation on the right for 10 sec did not lower blood pressure and heart rate. On the left, carotid sinus massage caused a substantial fall in both systolic and diastolic blood pressure, during which the patient felt light-headed and had greying-out of vision. There was only a modest fall in heart rate. The syncopal attacks were abolished by left carotid

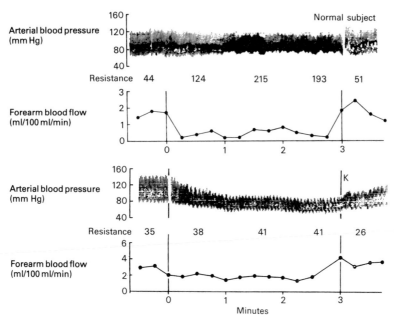

Fig. 14.11. The effect of lower body negative suction on arterial blood pressure forearm vascular resistance, and forearm blood flow in a normal subject (upper panel, and in a patient with autonomic failure (lower panel). The rise in forearm vascular resistance in the normal subject during suction is not seen in the patient, in whom there is a substantial fall in blood pressure. (From Bannister *et al.* (1967).)

or lowering of pressure. The relationship between heart rate and blood pressure helps to construct indices of baroreflex sensitivity. Pharmacological approaches using pressor agents (phenylephrine) or vasodilators (glyceryl trinitrate), given either as a bolus injection or sublingually to transiently raise or lower blood pressure, respectively, have also been used.

Biochemical and hormonal

Catecholamines and their metabolites

Noradrenaline is the major neurotransmitter at sympathetic nerve endings, while adrenaline and noradrenaline are both released from the adrenal medulla. Stimuli such as head-up tilt that result in sympathoneural activation

---

Fig. 14.10. (*continued*)   sinus denervation. (From Mathias *et al.* (1991*a*).) (b) The effect of carotid sinus massage on heart rate and blood pressure in a patient with carotid sinus hypersensitivity before (upper panel) and after (lower panel) 1 mg of atropine intravenously. The bradycardia is prevented by atropine but the blood pressure falls on repeat stimulation, indicating that vasodilatation, probably due to sympathetic withdrawal is also contributory in the mixed forms of carotid sinus hypersensitivity. (From Hutchinson and Stock (1960).)

elevate levels of noradrenaline in plasma. In sympathetic failure, there is no rise in plasma noradrenaline levels. The concentration of noradrenaline in plasma, however, is the net result of a number of processes, involving secretion, uptake mechanisms, metabolism, and clearance. As arterial measurements are not usually made, changes in a venous bed may reflect regional characteristics which may not be applicable globally (Chapter 20).

The basal supine plasma level itself may help in pointing to the possible diagnosis. In pure autonomic failure (PAF) levels are often low, because these patients are likely to have more complete distal lesions, while in multiple system atrophy (MSA) with more central lesions, levels are often within the normal range (Fig. 14.12). It should be noted that basal levels in tetraplegics with a definite preganglionic lesion are about 35 per cent of normal (Chapter 43). Levels of plasma adrenaline normally are often just at the detection limit of most assays, and basal levels do not usually provide useful information. In normal subjects stimuli such as hypoglycaemia and exercise cause a greater degree of stimulation and predominantly raise plasma adrenaline levels; this does not occur in autonomic failure.

Marked deviations from the normal basal plasma levels of catecholamines may themselves be diagnostic. An excess of plasma noradrenaline and adrenaline may suggest a phaeochromocytoma. Such patients characteristically have paroxysms of hypertension, headache, and sweating but may also suffer from postural hypotension, because of a low plasma volume and subsensitivity of α-adrenoceptors. The reverse, extremely low or virtually undetectable levels of plasma noradrenaline and adrenaline, occurs in patients with deficiency of the enzyme dopamine β-hydroxylase (Chapter 38). The characteristic difference from other groups with low levels, such as PAF, is that plasma dopamine levels are uniquely elevated (Fig. 14.12). The diagnosis can be confirmed by the absence of dopamine β-hydroxylase in both plasma and tissues.

Measurements of catecholamines and their metabolites in urine have certain advantages, as they provide a measure of secretion over a longer period, which may be of value in phaeochromocytoma where there may be intermittent secretion. They may also help in the diagnosis of rarer subgroups of autonomic failure and their treatment. In dopamine β-hydroxylase deficiency, dopamine metabolites are normal or elevated, while those of noradrenaline and adrenaline are almost undetectable; with adequate treatment with DL or L threo-DOPS, noradrenaline metabolites in urine increase (Chapter 38). A number of other urinary metabolites provide indices of central or peripheral catecholamine metabolism (Chapter 17).

Renin–angiotensin–aldosterone system

This system has a major influence on blood pressure. Renin is released from the juxtaglomerular cells of the renal afferent arteries and by a series of steps

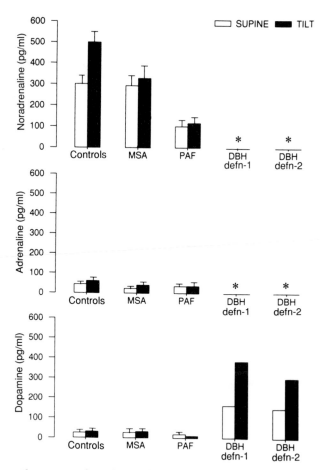

Fig. 14.12.   Plasma noradrenaline, adrenaline, and dopamine levels (measured by high-pressure liquid chromatography) in normal subjects (controls), patients with multiple system atrophy (MSA), pure autonomic failure (PAF), and two individual patients with dopamine β-hydroxylase deficiency (DBH) while supine and after head-up tilt to 45° for 10 min. The asterisk indicates levels below the detection limits for the assay, which are less than 5 pg/ml for noradrenaline and adrenaline and less than 20 pg/ml for dopamine. Bars indicate ± SEM.

results in the formation of the active pressor agent, angiotensin II, which has multiple actions: on blood vessels, sympathetic nerves, the brain and also on the adrenal cortex to cause secretion of aldosterone (Mathias *et al.* 1984). In adrenocortical deficiency (such as Addison's disease), which can also result in postural hypotension, there is a compensatory and marked elevation in renin and angiotensin II levels while plasma aldosterone levels are extremely low. In such patients plasma cortisol levels do not rise after administration of adrenocorticotrophic hormone.

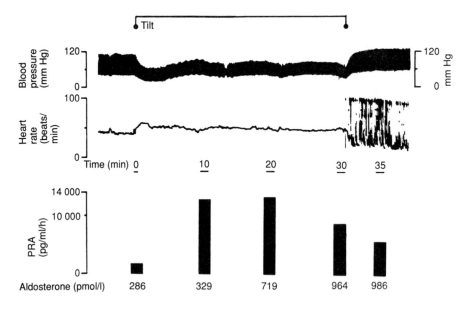

Fig. 14.13. Blood pressure (BP), heart rate, plasma renin activity (PRA), and plasma aldosterone levels in a patient with autonomic failure before, during, and after head-up tilt to 45° for 30 min. There was an immediate fall in both systolic and diastolic BP which gradually recovered. There was a small elevation in BP over previous basal levels on return to the horizontal. Heart rate rose when BP fell, but the response was modest. Following return to the horizontal, bigeminal rhythm occurred, accounting for the abnormal trace. Levels of plasma renin activity rose markedly during head-up tilt, reaching the levels often seen in severely hypertensive patients with renal artery stenosis. Plasma aldosterone levels rose later. (From Bannister *et al.* (1986).)

In autonomic disorders, the renin response to head-up tilt or standing may be of relevance to the ability to benefit from head-up tilt at night to reduce postural hypotension (Chapter 33). In some patients with primary autonomic failure the renin response is impaired, especially when related to their marked hypotension during head-up tilt (Bannister *et al.* 1979). In others, however, there may be an exaggerated rise (Mathias *et al.* 1977), as is observed also in tetraplegic patients (Chapter 43). If renin measurements are made, care should be taken to obtain an adequate basal level, keeping in mind the long half-life of renin. A 10 min period of tilt may suffice to demonstrate an exaggerated response (Fig. 14.13), although a longer period is preferable, especially if plasma aldosterone is also being measured. A variety of influences (including salt intake) and drugs (such as fludrocortisone) can modify renin release (Mathias *et al.* 1984).

Antidiuretic hormone (vasopressin)

In normal subjects there is a rise in plasma vasopressin levels with head-up tilt and with hyperosmotic stimuli (Chapter 19). Vasopressin levels have been used to assess the integrity of the afferent and central autonomic pathways. In afferent lesions, there is no rise with tilt but a preserved response following an osmotic stimulus; neither stimulus induces a response in the presence of cerebral lesions. In patients with cervical spinal cord injuries there is often an exaggerated rise in vasopressin levels with head-up tilt.

Pharmacological

Valuable information on the integrity of autonomic pathways, the number and sensitivity of receptors on target organs, and on functional components of the autonomic nervous system may be obtained by using drugs which are either agonists or antagonists. Some of these are also combined with assessment of hormonal responses, providing further information on the central and peripheral autonomic pathways and on autonomic receptors. It is important, especially in patients with suspected autonomic disorders who may have abnormal responses, that drugs to reverse their effects are available along with resuscitative facilities.

Drugs acting on the sympathetic nervous system

Noradrenaline   Noradrenaline is the major neurotransmitter at sympathetic nerve endings and predominantly stimulates α-adrenoceptors, with some effects on β-adrenoceptors. Pressor sensitivity to noradrenaline can be tested by intravenous infusion, beginning with a low dose (in case of supersensitivity) followed by increments every 5–10 min, with careful monitoring of blood pressure, heart rate, and the ECG. Construction of a dose–response curve will indicate whether there is an enhanced pressor response, when compared to normal. In more distal sympathetic lesions as in PAF, the dose–response curve is shifted considerably to the left, and there is also a greater slope, indicating that they have a greater degree of pressor supersensitivity than MSA patients (Fig. 14.14). The mechanisms responsible for pressor supersensitivity appear to be multiple. Indirect evidence from studies of α-receptors on platelets suggest that, because of the low levels of plasma noradrenaline, there is up-regulation of adrenoceptors. This may account for the difference in slope. The shift to the left that occurs in both PAF and MSA suggests that impairment of the baroreceptor reflex and the inability to compensate in different vascular beds (as also occurs in tetraplegic patients) may be major factors. Finally, clearance of noradrenaline is likely to be affected depending upon both the site and the degree of sympathetic nerve impairment.

The reverse, an impaired pressor response to noradrenaline and pressor agents, may occur in autonomic disorders such as amyloidosis because of infiltration of blood vessels by amyloid tissue.

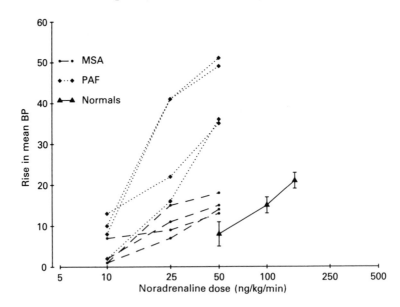

Fig. 14.14. Rise in mean blood pressure (BP) in four patients with pure autonomic failure (PAF), four patients with multiple system atrophy (MSA), and normal subjects (± SEM) during graded intravenous infusions of noradrenaline. Both groups of patients with autonomic failure had increased sensitivity to infused noradrenaline. In the PAF patients there appears to be a considerably greater response.

Assessment of sensitivity to noradrenaline is therefore of value in providing evidence of sensitivity of blood vessels and the possible response to sympathomimetic treatment. As with other pharmacological tests, they should be performed in laboratories familiar with the techniques. A large rise in pressure, especially in patients with preserved cardiac parasympathetic nerves, may result in potentially serious bradycardia. Patients with autonomic disorders may have supine hypertension, and the clinical investigator will need to decide in individual patients which level of blood pressure can be safely reached. Finally, one should be on guard for dysrhythmias. The availability of suitable drugs in an emergency is a necessity. Rapid relief of severe hypertension may be obtained by placing patients in the head-up position.

Tyramine Tyramine releases noradrenaline from both the granules and the cytosol within the sympathetic nerve terminal. A lack of rise in blood pressure and in plasma noradrenaline levels is indicative of absent noradrenaline stores and is characteristic of widespread postganglionic denervation or noradrenaline depletion, as in dopamine β-hydroxylase deficiency (Chapter 38). In incomplete lesions, however, release of even subnormal amounts of noradrenaline may cause a substantial pressor response because of super-sensitivity. The value of tyramine-induced responses is thus open to speculation.

Isoprenaline   Isoprenaline is a β-adrenoceptor agonist which acts on both the β_1 and β_2 subtypes. The β_1 subtype is predominantly concerned with raising heart rate and the β_2 with vasodilatation and bronchodilatation. Isoprenaline can be given either as a bolus or as an intravenous infusion and its effects on heart rate and blood pressure provide an indication of β-adrenoceptor responsiveness.

   In autonomic failure and tetraplegia, bolus intravenous injections cause an exaggerated but transient fall in both systolic and diastolic blood pressure (Fig. 14.15).

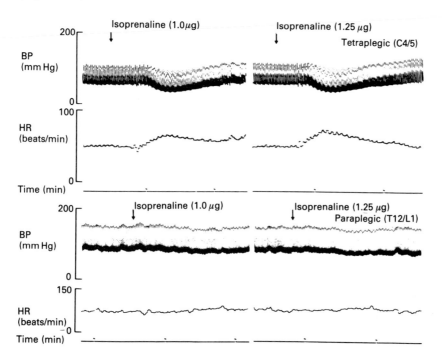

Fig. 14.15.   Blood pressure (BP) and heart rate (HR) in a tetraplegic patient (upper panel) and a paraplegic patient with an almost intact sympathetic nervous system in response to bolus injections of isoprenaline (lower panel). In the tetraplegic there is a clear fall in blood pressure after isoprenaline. This probably results from β_2-adrenoceptor mediated vasodilatation. There is a rise in heart rate before the blood pressure falls and this is likely to be a β_1-adrenoceptor mediated effect which is then enhanced by the fall in blood pressure. In the paraplegic patient there are considerably smaller changes. (From Mathias and Frankel (1986).)

Similar changes occur with intravenous infusion (Fig. 14.16). This may suggest β_2-adrenoceptor supersensitivity, that β_2-adrenoceptor-induced vasodilatation is not opposed because of the baroreceptor deficit, or that both occur. There is no chronotropic supersensitivity to isoprenaline in autonomic failure with vagal denervation (Fig. 14.17), despite indirect *in vitro* evidence from lymphocyte studies suggesting an increase in β-adrenoceptor numbers.

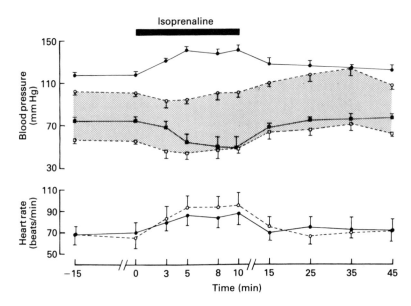

Fig. 14.16. Blood pressure and heart rate in five tetraplegic patients (open circles and squares and broken line) and five control subjects (full circles and squares and continuous line) before, during, and after intravenous infusion of isoprenaline (0.01 μg/min/kg). The shaded area indicates blood pressure in the tetraplegics; bars indicate $\pm$ SEM. In the tetraplegics there is a fall in both systolic and diastolic blood pressure. (From Mathias *et al.* (1981).)

In tetraplegics the fall in blood pressure in the presence of the preserved afferent baroreceptor and efferent vagal pathways may result in a greater rise in heart rate, not necessarily attributable to β-adrenoceptor supersensitivity.

Clonidine   Clonidine is an α_2-adrenoceptor agonist which has a number of effects, one of which includes a predominant cerebral action in reducing sympathetic neural activity and lowering blood pressure. In normal subjects after clonidine, levels of plasma noradrenaline levels fall and growth hormone levels rise. The latter appears dependent upon intact central adrenergic pathways. Clonidine can be given intravenously (2 μg/kg body weight over 10 min to avoid a transient pressor effect) with observations for a period of

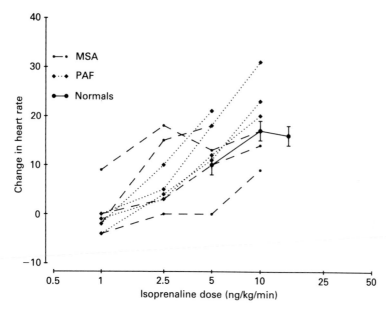

Fig. 14.17. Change in heart rate in response to incremental infusion of isoprenaline in four patients with pure autonomic failure (PAF) and in four patients with multiple system atrophy (MSA). The response in normal subjects (± SEM) is indicated. Despite a fall in blood pressure in the majority of patients with autonomic failure only a few had a greater increase in sensitivity. Chronotropic β-adrenergic supersensitivity does not therefore appear to be as marked as pressor sensitivity in autonomic failure patients.

75–90 min after administration. Its side-effects include dryness of mouth and sedation. After an hour following the intravenous infusion most subjects are awake, although drowsy.

The uses of clonidine are:

1. To determine residual sympathetic nervous activity and its contribution to the maintenance of blood pressure. In PAF there is usually a rise in blood pressure (because of supersensitivity) with no further reduction in levels of plasma noradrenaline, unlike in normal subjects in whom both blood pressure and noradrenaline levels fall. Similar changes are observed in dopamine β-hydroxylase deficiency (Chapter 38). In tetraplegia blood pressure is unchanged (Chapter 43). In patients with MSA or in incomplete lesions there is usually a fall in supine blood pressure and plasma noradrenaline levels.

2. To distinguish phaeochromocytoma patients with autonomous noradrenaline secretion from patients with essential hypertension and

labile hypertension with elevated basal noradrenaline levels. In phaeochromocytoma plasma noradrenaline levels remain elevated, unlike in normal subjects or essential hypertensive patients in whom they fall after clonidine (Fig. 14.8).

3. To assess the growth hormone response which may be a useful neuroendocrine marker of integrity of the central α-adrenergic system. In autonomic failure there appears to be no rise in plasma growth hormone levels after clonidine (Fig. 14.19). Whether there are differences between PAF and MSA, and whether this may be a valuable marker for separating patients presenting with parkinsonian features who are at an early stage of MSA from those with classical idiopathic Parkinson's disease, remains to be determined.

Drugs acting on cholinergic systems

Edrophonium This is a short-acting cholinesterase inhibitor which may help differentiate pre- from postganglionic sympathetic lesions by stimulating

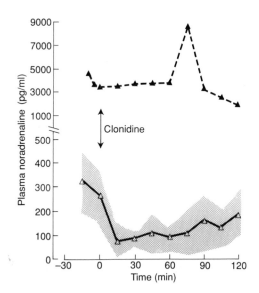

Fig. 14.18. Plasma noradrenaline levels in a patient with a phaeochromocytoma (▲--▲) and in a group of patients with essential hypertension (△—△) before and after intravenous clonidine indicated by an arrow (2 μg/kg over 10 min). Plasma noradrenaline levels fall rapidly in the essential hypertensives after clonidine and remain low over the period of observation. The stippled area indicates the ± SEM. Plasma noradrenaline levels are considerably higher in the phaeochromocytoma patient and are not affected by clonidine.

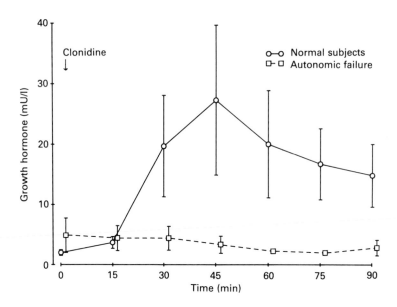

Fig. 14.19. Plasma levels of human growth hormone in normal subjects and patients with autonomic failure in response to 1.5 μg/kg of i.v. clonidine. In the normal subjects there is a significant rise within 30 min which reaches its maximum at 45 min. In the autonomic failure patients the basal levels are not different from the normal subjects but there is no change following clonidine. Vertical bars indicate ± SEM. (From da Costa *et al.* (1984).)

nicotinic receptors within autonomic ganglia (Gemmill *et al.* 1988). In PAF with distal lesions, edrophonium has no effects and there is no change in plasma noradrenaline levels. In MSA, in which it is presumed there is an intact postganglionic system, there is a rise in noradrenaline levels. The limitations and value of edrophonium testing in different autonomic disorders remain to be evaluated.

Atropine   Postsynaptic parasympathetic and sympathetic cholinergic receptors are of the muscarinic subtype and are effectively blocked by atropine sulphate. Its use has helped to determine the degree of cardiac vagal involvement. In normal subjects doses of 5 μg/kg body weight at 2 min intervals i.v. raise heart rate. Doses up to a total of 1800 μg/kg body weight are usually sufficient to assess responsiveness and construct a dose–response curve (Fig. 14.20). No further atropine should be given if the heart rate rises above about 110 beats/min, or if there is evidence of an abnormal cardiac rhythm. After atropine, side-effects are usually mild but may be troublesome. Dilatation

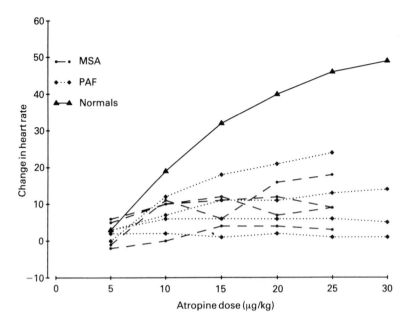

Fig. 14.20. Change in heart rate in four patients with pure autonomic failure (PAF) and four patients with multiple system atrophy (MSA) in response to atropine. In the majority of patients there is minimal change in heart rate unlike the change expected in normal subjects. Cardiac vagal impairment seems to occur equally in both groups of patients.

of the pupil and blurring of vision because of its cycloplegic effects may occur. It may impair detrusor muscle activity and those with impaired urinary bladder function should micturate before the test. Dryness of the mouth is common and usually lasts for an hour. Subjects should be cautioned not to drink fluids in excess.

In the majority of patients with primary autonomic failure (PAF and MSA) there is vagal impairment with a flat dose–response curve. This is consistent with pathological observations concerning the vagus, showing lesions in the dorsal vagal nuclei within the brainstem and/or more peripherally.

Sweat testing and thermoregulation

The regulation of body temperature is dependent upon a number of factors that influence heat generation and disposal. Heat disposal depends upon the sudomotor system and the ability of the cutaneous circulation to respond appropriately. Thermoregulatory sweating is tested by raising the core temperature by 1°C, using hot water bottles and a space blanket. Normally, sweating occurs through stimulation of eccrine sweat glands which are widely distributed over the body. This can be aided by pretreatment with a diaphoretic, paracetamol (0.5 or 1 g orally). The detection of sweat production can be enhanced by using dyes sprinkled on the skin. Quinazarine red for instance turns from pale pink to bright red on exposure to moisture. In primary autonomic failure, thermoregulatory sweating is often impaired. In dopamine β-hydroxylase deficiency, however, it is largely preserved and provides an important clue to the diagnosis (Chapter 38). Other tests of sweat gland function are described in Chapter 21.

Quinizarine powder can be used to determine local abnormalities of sudomotor function as in the patchy denervation caused by leprosy (Karat *et al.* 1969). When applied over the skin and covered by Sellotape, especially with the subject in a warm room, a colour change occurs rapidly in normal but not denervated areas. Other approaches include the acetylcholine sweatspot test (Ryder *et al.* 1988). Other local disorders of sweating may need special methods of study. In gustatory sweating (Frey's syndrome), severe and socially embarrassing sweating may occur after ingestion of spicy or acidic foods and those containing tyramine. Challenge with food, together with the use of quinazarine powder over the head, neck, and trunk, helps determine the area of distribution and the nerves which are involved.

In patients who cannot control their cutaneous circulation, hypothermia may occur in temperate or cold climates, especially in tetraplegics who are unable to shiver (Chapter 44). The reverse, hyperpyrexia, may occur in extremely hot weather especially when sweating is also impaired. It is important in the assessment of body temperature in such patients, that core temperature (for example, using a rectal thermometer) is measured. If hypothermia is suspected a low-reading thermometer should be used.

Gastrointestinal system

The gastrointestinal system is often involved in autonomic disorders. Investigations will depend on the specific problem.

The upper gastrointestinal tract may be assessed using a barium swallow, meal, and follow-through. In localized oesophageal involvement (as in Chagas' disease) a barium swallow alone may help. Specific defects of swallowing are best determined using video-cinefluoroscopy. If gastroscopy is utilized, the advantage is that biopsy of tissue is possible, which may help in the diagnosis of conditions such as systemic amyloidosis.

Assessment of gastric motility may be of importance. In some disorders, rapid gastric emptying is a problem, while in others, such as diabetes, gastroparesis may be particularly troublesome. The assessment of gut motility is described in Chapter 27.

Constipation is a common complaint in autonomic failure; occasionally other disorders need to be considered, such as neoplasia in the elderly. A barium enema or colonoscopy may be helpful. A rectal biopsy and staining with Congo red provides a definitive diagnosis in amyloidosis.

Renal function and the urinary tract

Nocturnal polyuria is common in autonomic disorders, and in autonomic failure can result in overnight weight loss of over a kilogram with a reduction in extracellular fluid volume; this appears to aggravate postural hypotension in the morning. This is best assessed by having 12-hourly evaluations (day and night) of urine volume and, if possible, of sodium and potassium secretion (Mathias *et al.* 1986). If there is urinary bladder or sphincter involvement, nocturnal polyuria may cause even greater difficulties because of the frequency of micturition and at times incontinence. The assessments are helpful in predicting the value of the antidiuretic agent, desmopressin, which may be used intranasally at night to reduce nocturnal polyuria.

Urodynamic measurements provide information on the nature of bladder dysfunction, such as detrusor areflexia or hyperreflexia. Urethral sphincter electromyography shows a distinct pattern in patients with MSA, which may help distinguish this disorder from idiopathic Parkinson's disease (Chapter 28). Urinary infections and calculi may be complications and suitable investigations, including intravenous urography and ultrasound examination, may need to be performed.

Sexual function

Impotence in the male is common in autonomic failure. Organic erectile failure can be difficult to distinguish from psychogenic impotence, though nocturnal erections do not occur in the former. Penile plethysmography may help. Intracorporeal injection of papavarine causes an erection in both groups and is not therefore a means of differentiating between the two (Chapter 24). In situations such as diabetes mellitus vascular factors may also contribute. In dopamine β-hydroxylase deficiency erection is preserved but there is a delayed ejaculation, which can be corrected by the drug l-DOPS, which replenishes noradrenaline levels (Chapter 38).

Respiratory system

Stridor, particularly at night, may occur in the later stages in MSA because of paralysis of abductors of the vocal cord (Chapter 23). This can be detected by laryngoscopy. Brainstem dysfunction causing periods of apnoea may further contribute to hypoxia and complicate the problem. Blood gas monitoring during sleep may be necessary to determine if significant oxygen desaturation warrants a tracheostomy.

The eye

Lacrimal secretion may be diminished as a result of direct involvement of the gland, as in Sjögren's syndrome. Lacrimal secretion can be tested by using a special absorbent paper, which forms the basis of Schirmer's test. Diminished secretion or alacrima may result in corneal abrasions which may need assessment using either fluorescein or Bengal red dyes and a silt lamp.

Intraocular pressure may be reduced in sympathetic lesions, as in Horner's syndrome, but has minimal clinical significance when compared with the elevation of intraocular pressure which may occur with parasympathomimetic drugs, especially in patients who are prone to glaucoma.

The pupil is involved in a number of autonomic disorders and can be assessed using either pharmacological approaches (sympathomimetics and cholinomimetics and testing for supersensitivity) or specialized physiological function tests (Chapter 22).

Miscellaneous investigations

In this section are briefly described a range of investigations which may be of value in the assessment of patients with autonomic disorders. Some of these investigations are directly concerned with diagnosis, others with elimination of disorders which may mimic autonomic failure, and there are additionally those which provide valuable information in understanding the pathophysiological basis of certain autonomic diseases.

Neurophysiological tests

Electroencephalography may be needed as the distinction between syncope (due to autonomic impairment) and epilepsy can be blurred. Occasionally epileptic seizures may be induced because of an extremely low perfusion blood pressure.

Auditory evoked responses are of value in separating patients with cerebral lesions as in MSA, from those with more distal lesions as in PAF (Chapter 28). A variety of peripheral electrophysiological studies are of value to determine the specific type of neuropathy or its absence (Chapter 35). Thermal threshold testing is a sensitive means of determining unmyelinated fibre involvement. The absence of the 'H' reflex is characteristic of patients with the Holmes–Adie syndrome, where there is a myotonic pupil and absent tendon reflexes.

Cardiac investigations

There are a number of cardiac causes of syncope, the most dramatic probably being Stokes–Adams attacks. In the elderly, in particular, cardiac dysrhythmias need to be excluded and the use of a 24-h tape with computerized analysis of cardiac rhythm may be necessary. In rare cases, postural hypotension may be the result of an atrial myxoma and two-dimensional echocardiography is probably the least invasive means of making or excluding this diagnosis.

Biopsies

Tissue can be utilized for light microscopy, electron microscopy, and a range of immunohistochemical studies. Three major sites are of value in autonomic disorders. In amyloidosis, biopsy of the kidney (if there is a renal involvement) or of a sural nerve provides the diagnosis when tissues are stained with Congo red. Sural nerve biopsies provide valuable information on the nerve fibres and on both degenerative and regenerative peripheral neural processes (Chapter 35). Skin biopsies have proven to be of value in patients with dopamine β-hydroxylase deficiency, as they have confirmed the integrity of perivascular sympathetic nerves and demonstrated normal distribution of a range of neuropeptides, some associated with sympathetic nerves (such as neuropeptide Y) and others with parasympathetic nerves (such as vasoactive intestinal polypeptide) (Chapter 38). In these patients, in skin tissue containing sympathetic nerves, there is lack of immunoreactivity to dopamine β-hydroxylase, which further confirms the diagnosis. Recently, a patient has been reported with lack of tyrosine hydroxylase, dopamine β-hydroxylase, and sensory neuropeptides (substance P and calcitonin gene-related peptide) (Anand *et al.* 1991). The abnormalities in this novel autonomic and sensory neuropeptide deficiency were confirmed by skin biopsy studies. The disorder may be due to deficiency of nerve growth factor as levels were extremely low in the patient's skin.

Skin histamine test

The use of the intradermal histamine test to assess the Lewis response (Chapter 25) may be of value in certain disorders, especially if correlation with the composition of skin tissue is possible. In the patient described above (Anand *et al.* 1991), there was a diminished histamine response consistent with low or absent sensory neuropeptide levels in skin. An abnormal skin histamine response is a characteristic feature of patients with familial dysautonomia (Riley–Day syndrome; Chapter 38).

Neuroimaging

A range of non-invasive technological advances now enable assessment of cerebral and spinal morphology. A CT scan is of value in determining cerebral atrophy in MSA but there are considerable advantages with performing an MRI scan, especially in determining abnormalities within the basal ganglia, brainstem and spinal cord (Chapter 28). In addition, positron emission tomography (PET) scans can provide details of neurotransmitters including their formation, distribution, and receptor configuration within the central nervous system. The value of PET scans in separating MSA from PAF and in the evaluation of neurochemical abnormalities is discussed in Chapter 29.

Conclusion

The autonomic nervous system innervates every organ and, in the generalized autonomic disorders, involves virtually every organ in the body. As indicated in this chapter there are a wide range of investigative approaches and, depending upon the clinical questions, specific tests need to be performed. Further details of certain tests can be found in particular chapters. It is, however, intended that this chapter, by providing an overview of the investigation of those autonomic abnormalities that cause morbidity and contribute to mortality, will help in early diagnosis and comprehensive assessment, which are important for prognosis and for appropriate management.

References

Anand, P., Rudge, P., Mathias, C. J., Springall, D. R., Ghatei, M. A., Naher-Noe, M., Sharief, M., Misra, V. P., Polak, J. M., Bloom, S. R., and Thomas, P. K. (1991). New autonomic and sensory neuropathy with loss of adrenergic sympathetic function and sensory neuropeptides. *Lancet* **337**, 1253–4.

Bannister, R. (1979). Chronic autonomic failure with postural hypotension. *Lancet* **ii**, 404–6.

Banniser, R., Ardill, L., and Fentem, P. (1967). Defective autonomic control of blood vessels in idiopathic orthostatic hypotension. *Brain* **90**,725–46.

Bannister, R., Davies, I. B., Holly, E., Rosenthal, T., and Sever, P. S. (1979). Defective cardiovascular reflexes and supersensitivity to sympathomimetic drugs in autonomic failure. *Brain* **102**, 163–76.

Bannister, R., da Costa, D. F., Hendry, W. G., Jacobs, J., and Mathias, C. J. (1986). Atrial demand pacing to protect against vagal overactivity in sympathetic autonomic neuropathy. *Brain* **109**, 345–56.

Brett, A. S., Phillips, M., and Beary, J. F. (1986). Predictive power of the polygraph: Can the "lie detector" really detect liars? *Lancet* **i**, 544–7.

Chaudhuri, K. R., Thomaides, T., Hernandez, P., Alam, M., and Mathias, C. J. (1991). Non-invasive quantification of superior mesenteric artery blood flow during sympathoneural activation in normal subjects. *Clin. autonom. Res.* **1**, 37–42.

da Costa, D. F., Bannister, R., Landon, J., and Mathias, C. J.(1984). Growth hormone response to clonidine is impaired in patients with central sympathetic degeneration. *Clin. exp. Hypertension* **6**, 1843–6.

Gemmill, J.D., Venables, G. S., and Ewing, D. J. (1988). Noradrenaline response to edrophonium in primary autonomic failure: distinction between central and peripheral damage. *Lancet* **i**, 1018–21.

Hutchinson, E. C. and Stock, J. P. P. (1960). Carotid sinus syndrome. *Lancet* **ii**, 445–9.

Imholz, B. P. M., Wieling, W., Langewouters, G. J., and van Montfrans, G. A. (1991). Continuous finger arterial pressure: utility in the cardiovascular laboratory. *Clin. autonom. Res.* **1**, 43–53.

Karat, A. B. A., Karat, S., and Pallis, C. (1969). Sweating under cellulose tape. A test of autonomic function. *Lancet* **i**, 651–2.

Kooner, J. S., Peart, W. S., and Mathias, C. J. (1989). The haemodynamic and hormonal responses after clonidine occur independently of sedation in essential hypertension. *Br. J. clin. Pharmacol.* **28**, 249–55.

Mathias, C. J. (1987) Autonomic dysfunction. *Br. J. hosp. Med.* **38**, 238–243.

Mathias, C. J. (1992). Assessment of autonomic function. In *Manual of clinical neurophysiology* (ed. J. Osselton, C. Binnie, C. Fowler, F. Maguiere, and P. Prior). Butterworth, London (in press).

Mathias, C. J. and Frankel, H. L. (1986). The neurological and hormonal control of blood vessels and heart in spinal man. *J. autonom. nerv. Syst* (suppl.), 457–464.

Mathias, C. J. and Frankel, H. L. (1988). Cardiovascular control in spinal man. *Ann. Rev. Physiol.* **50**, 577–92.

Mathias, C. J., Mathews, W. B., and Spalding, J. M. K. S. (1977). Postural changes in plasma renin activity and responses to vasoactive drugs in a case of Shy–Drager syndrome. *J. Neurol. Neurosurg. Psychiat.* **40**, 138–43.

Mathias, C. J., Christensen, N. J., Frankel, H. L., and Spalding, J. M. K. (1979). Cardiovascular control in recently injured tetraplegics in spinal shock. *Quart. J. Med.* New Series **48**, 273–87.

Mathias, C. J., Frankel, H. L., Davies, I. B., James, V. H. T., and Peart, W. S. (1981). Renin and aldosterone release during sympathetic stimulation in tetraplegia. *Clin. Sci.* **60**, 399–604.

Mathias, C. J., May, C. N., and Taylor, G. M. (1984). The renin–angiotensin system and hypertension—basic and clinical aspects. In *Molecular medicine,* Vol. 1 (ed. A. D. B. Malcolm), pp. 177–208 IRL Press, Oxford.

Mathias, C. J., Fosbraey, P. da Costa, D. F., Thornley, A., and Bannister, R. (1986). Desmopressin reduces nocturnal polyuria, reverses overnight weight loss and improves morning postural hypotension in autonomic failure. *Br. med. J.* **293**, 353–4.

Mathias, C. J., Armstrong, E., Browse, N., Chaudhuri, K. R., Enevoldson, P., and Ross-Russell, R. W. (1991*a*). Value of non-invasive continuous blood pressure monitoring in the detection of carotid sinus hypersensitivity. *Clin. autonom. Res.* **1**, 157–9.

Mathias, C. J., Holly, E. R., Armstrong, E., Shareef, M., and Bannister, R. (1991*b*). The influence of food and postural hypotension in three groups of chronic autonomic failure; clinical and therapeutic implications. *J. Neurol. Neurosurg. Psychiat.* **54**, 726–30.

Ryder, R. E. J., Johnson, K., Owens, D. R., Marshall, R., Ryder A. P. P., and Hayes, T. M. (1988). Acetylcholine sweatspot test for autonomic denervation. *Lancet* **ii**, 1303–5.

Shahani, B. T., Halpern, J. J., Boulu, P., and Cohen, J. (1984). Sympathetic skin response–a method of assessing unmyelinated axon dysfunction in peripheral neuropathies. *J. Neurol. Neurosurg. Psychiat.* **47**, 536–42.

Wallin, B. G. and Sundlof, G. (1982). Sympathetic outflow to muscles during vasovagal syncope. *J. autonom. nerv. Syst.* **6**, 287–91.

Wheeler, T. and Watkins P. J. (1973). Cardiac denervation in diabetes. *Br. med. J.* **iv**, 584–6.

15. Non-invasive continuous recording of heart rate and blood pressure in the evaluation of neurocardiovascular control

Wouter Wieling

Introduction

The basis of testing cardiovascular reflex control is to disturb the circulatory system and observe its subsequent recovery. A large number of manoeuvres is available: in the evaluation of patients suspected of suffering from autonomic disorders, forced breathing, standing, and the Valsalva manoeuvre are commonly used.

Monitoring heart rate changes induced by these manoeuvres combined with conventional blood pressure measurement in supine and standing position provides useful information on the integrity and effectiveness of neuro-cardiovascular control. For a full evaluation of disturbances in this control radial or brachial artery catheterization has been advised.

For obvious reasons the feasibility of recording of intraarterial pressure is limited. A non-invasive technique for monitoring intraarterial pressure is therefore the ideal. In this chapter such a technique is described and examples of its value in testing neurocardiovascular control are given. The advantages of continuous as opposed to intermittent recording of blood pressure by a sphygmomanometer are discussed.

The first section of this chapter is concerned with the technique of measurement of the blood pressure in the finger arteries. The second section deals with the application of a test protocol including forced breathing, standing, and the Valsalva manoeuvre. The third section focuses on the spectrum of normal and abnormal orthostatic circulatory responses.

Non-invasive finger arterial blood pressure measurement

Measurement takes place via a small inflatable cuff with a built-in infra-red emitter and sensor wrapped around the middle phalanx of the middle finger (Fig. 15.1). The cuff is connected to a small front-end box attached to the

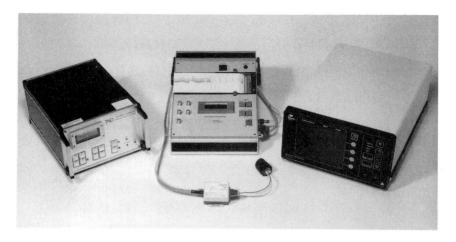

Fig. 15.1. Finapres finger blood pressure devices. On the left TNO model 4; on the right the commercially available Ohmeda 2300 NIBP monitor. Basic components of Finapres are shown in the middle, connected to the TNO model 5: a small inflatable finger cuff is connected to a small box (front-end) which is connected via a 5 m long cable to the main unit.

wrist or hand. The front-end, in turn, is connected to a main unit comprising an air pressure supply, the electronics, a recorder, and a control keyboard. Two variables are monitored: the blood volume under the cuff by the infra-red sensors and the pressure in the finger cuff by a pressure transducer.

The principle of the measurement of finger arterial blood pressure is relatively simple. The blood volume under the cuff is observed by the infra-red sensors and is clamped to a constant volume by varying cuff pressure in parallel with intraarterial pressure, using a fast servo system. For example, if intraarterial pressure were to increase by 40 mm Hg this would cause an increase in blood volume under the cuff if cuff pressure remained constant. However, the infra-red sensors detect the tendency of the blood volume to increase and the servo counteracts immediately by increasing cuff pressure to the same extent as finger intraarterial pressure. This is, in short, the volume clamp technique, invented by the Czech physiologist Peñáz; it makes it possible to monitor beat-to-beat changes in finger arterial blood pressure (Peñáz 1973). However, one additional step has to be taken: one must calibrate for the correct level of actual finger arterial pressure. This is achieved by clamping the arterial blood volume at a level corresponding to the unloaded state of the arterial wall; in this condition cuff pressure is equal to finger arterial pressure. The principle of unloading has been described in detail (Wesseling 1990) and will not be addressed here. The procedure used in Finapres™ to establish the correct volume clamp level is the Physiocal (physiological calibration) (Wesseling 1982,1990). Regularly, initially at

10-beat intervals, but, when the measurement is stabilized, at 70-beat intervals, for two or more heartbeats, cuff pressure is not varied to properly clamp blood volume, but kept constant while the then pulsatile infra-red sensor output (plethysmogram) is evaluated. The plethysmogram is judged on certain aspects such as its size and shape and, if needed, the volume clamp is adjusted to make cuff pressure nearly identical to finger arterial pressure.

Finapres recordings are similar in appearance to intraarterial blood pressure recordings (Fig. 15.2), but the measurements are not identical; it has long been known that propagation of the pressure wave towards the periphery changes the pulse wave form, and, consequently, finger blood pressure values differ from the values obtained more proximally. The physiological brachial to finger gradient causes mean and diastolic pressures to be lower in the finger compared to brachial pressure; amplification of the pulse wave, especially in young subjects, may result in higher finger systolic pressure values (Wesseling 1990).

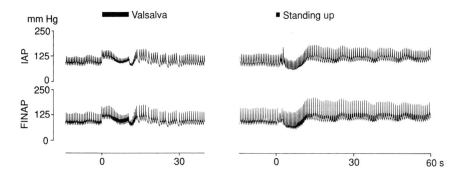

Fig. 15.2. Original recordings of intrabrachial (IAP) and finger (FINAP) arterial blood pressure responses induced by the Valsalva manoeuvre (left panel) and standing up (right panel). Duration of Valsalva strain and time needed to stand up are indicated. Note similarity between the IAP and FINAP tracings.

When results are averaged for a group of subjects, the differences between intraarterial and finger pressures are small; differences for systolic and diastolic pressure usually deviate by less than 5 mm Hg (Fig. 15.3; Imholz *et al.* 1988, 1990*a*, 1991; Parati *et al.* 1989). However, the standard deviation of the difference is not small, and therefore does not guarantee a reliable estimate of actual intrabrachial pressure in individuals any more than do conventional auscultatory methods (Imholz *et al.* 1991).

In practice, the clinician must interpret a blood pressure response in an individual patient; a reliable estimate of the changes in blood pressure within one individual is therefore of crucial importance. Finapres is an excellent device in this respect; in individuals changes in mean and diastolic pressure during steady state conditions and during manoeuvres such as Valsalva's and

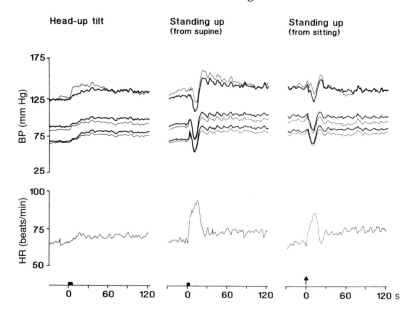

Fig. 15.3. Average intrabrachial (IAP) and finger (FINAP) arterial blood pressure (BP) and heart rate (HR) responses in 11 healthy adult subjects aged 22–40 years to three orthostatic manoeuvres. Bold trace, IAP; thin trace, FINAP. (Taken with permission from Imholz *et al.* (1990*a*).)

orthostatic stress are reliably measured. The finger to brachial differences within one subject are relatively stable; the 95 per cent individual limits of agreement of the standard deviation are between 0 and 4 mm Hg. Changes in finger systolic pressure are more variable (Imholz *et al.* 1988, 1990*a*, 1991).

Measurement of finger arterial pressure is almost always possible. Conditions that provoke severe peripheral arterial contraction and, consequently, low arterial flow to the hand are the major limitation (Wesseling 1990; Imholz *et al.* 1991). The measurement may be accompanied by a blue discoloration of the finger tip distal to the cuff due to venous congestion. However, arterial blood flow to the finger tip is not fully interrupted since the arteries under the cuff are unloaded but not completely collapsed. The measurement can usually be continued for 2–4 h without complaints. The blue discoloration of the finger tip disappears soon after the measurement has stopped.

Since intraarterial cannulation affects cardiovascular reflex function (Hainsworth 1990; Imholz *et al.* 1991), measurement of blood pressure by Finapres may be preferable to cannulation of the radial or brachial artery in physiological experiments. Moreover, Finapres can also be applied in subjects in whom, for ethical reasons, intraarterial cannulation is not allowed (Imholz *et al.* 1990*b*; Dambrink *et al.* 1991). Furthermore, the availability of the full pressure wave enables the application of new analytical methods which investigate the relation between cardiovascular function and the dynamic response of the regulatory systems; examples are the assessment of baroreflex function (Parati *et al.* 1989; Steptoe and Vogele 1990), blood pressure variability by means of spectral analysis (De Boer *et al.* 1987), or the calculation of beat-to-beat changes in stroke volume with pulse contour formulae (Sprangers *et al.* 1991*a*). Finally, the ambulatory version of Finapres, the Portapres device, may open new fields of investigation (Langewouters *et al.* 1990).

Assessment of cardiovascular reflex function

Procedures and analysis of data

In earlier studies we used the combination of continuous heart rate monitoring and conventional sphygmomanometry, to define normal and abnormal circulatory responses (Wieling 1988). Presently, in our laboratory continuous blood pressure recording by Finapres is used instead of sphygmomanometry. Both methods will be discussed here.

Experiments are performed in the morning at least 1 h after a light breakfast. Subjects are requested to abstain from coffee and cigarettes from the previous evening. The protocol is started after a test run to train the subject to perform the manoeuvres correctly. The manoeuvres are each performed after about 5 min of preceding rest.

Instantaneous heart rate is monitored with a cardiotachometer or obtained from the Finapres arterial pulse pressure interval. Blood pressure is measured supine and in the upright position with the arm relaxed at the side when sphygmomanometry is used. Using Finapres, the finger cuff is kept at heart level to avoid hydrostatic pressure influences.

Calculations are made from the original recordings. Control values for heart rate are obtained by averaging over a 10-s period prior to the manoeuvres. In case of marked fluctuations in heart rate a 10–30 s period prior to the manoeuvres should be used. Changes in heart rate from control values induced by forced breathing, standing, and the Valsalva manoeuvre are computed. Basic to the interpretation of an impaired heart rate response are the markedly different latency and time constants for the sinus node's response to changes in cardiac vagal and cardiac sympathetic nerve traffic (Fig. 15.4). Vagally mediated heart rate changes have a latency of about 0.5 s and a time constant of a few seconds, whereas these values are on the order of 1–3 and 10 s, respectively, for sympathetically mediated effects. The initial sympathetically mediated component of the heart rate response is usually completely obscured by the much larger and faster vagally mediated component. The initial sluggish

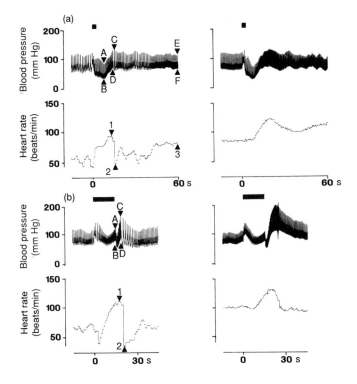

Fig. 15.4. Original tracings in a 33-year-old male subject of blood pressure (BP) and heart rate (HR) responses induced by (a) standing (■) and (b) the Valsalva manoeuvre (▬▬). Pharmacological blockade with atropine abolished the large, vagally mediated, transient heart rate changes; a sluggish sympathetically mediated heart-rate increase remains (right panels). The arrows indicate the timing of characteristic response extremes of interest. (a) For standing: A, systolic pressure and B, diastolic pressure trough; C, systolic pressure and D, diastolic pressure overshoot; E, systolic and F, diastolic pressure level after 1 min standing; 1, initial peak heart-rate increase (HR_{max}); 2, relative bradycardia (HR_{min}); 3, heart rate after 1 min standing. (b) For the Valsalva manoeuvre: A, systolic and B, diastolic pressure at the end of straining; C, systolic and D, diastolic pressure overshoot; 1, initial peak heart-rate increase (HR_{max}); 2, bradycardia (HR_{min}).

sympathetic response is unmasked, however, when parasympathetic heart rate control is blocked by atropine.

Control sphygmomanometer blood pressure values are obtained by averaging three measurements. Control values for finger arterial pressure are computed by averaging a 10–30 s period prior to the manoeuvres. Changes in blood pressure from control values induced by the three test manoeuvres are computed.

Forced breathing

In our laboratory the forced breathing test is performed supine, when vagal effects are most pronounced. The subject is instructed to perform six consecutive maximal inspiration and expiration cycles at a rate of 6 breaths/min.

Forced breathing with a frequency of 6 breaths/min induces characteristic heart rate changes in healthy subjects: a heart rate rise starting within 1 s from the start of inspiration with a peak of heart rate at about 3 s before maximal inspiration has taken place, and a minimal heart rate after about 6 s, at the beginning of expiration. Before end-expiration is reached heart rate already increases. Both cardiac vagal inhibition and activation are tested. To quantify the test score the difference between maximal and minimal heart rate for each of the six cycles is determined and averaged to obtain the inspiratory–expiratory (I–E) difference in beats/min.

An important determinant of the magnitude of the I–E difference is age as in the elderly the heart rate responses induced by forced breathing are smaller (Fig. 15.5; Table 15.1; Wieling *et al.* 1982).

The influence of the level of resting heart rate on the I–E difference is small compared to the effect of age. Thus, a correction for resting heart rate is not important in the measurement of the I–E difference (Wieling 1988). However, to observe vagally mediated changes in heart rate some vagal tone

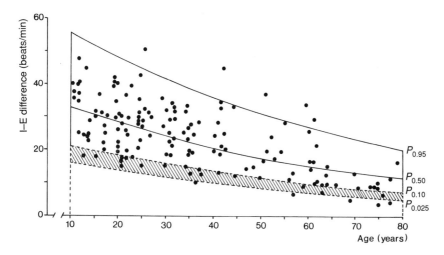

Fig. 15.5. Magnitude of the I–E difference in relation to age. The regression line ($P_{0.50}$) and confidence limits were calculated from log-transformed values. The hatched area indicates values between the lower 2.5th and 10th percentile, which we have defined as borderline. The values below this range are considered abnormally small; values above it are considered normal. (Taken with permission from Wieling *et al.* (1982) and Dambrink (1991).)

Table 15.1. Assessment of heart rate responses induced by forced breathing and the Valsalva manoeuvre

Age (years)	I–E difference* (beats/min)	Valsalva ratio[†]
10–14	< 17	< 1.53
15–19	< 16	< 1.48
20–24	< 15	< 1.43
25–29	< 14	< 1.38
30–34	< 13	< 1.33
35–39	< 12	< 1.28
40–44	< 11	< 1.24
45–49	< 11	< 1.20
50–55	< 10	< 1.16
55–60	< 9	< 1.12
60–65	< 9	< 1.08
65–70	< 8	< 1.04
70–75	< 7	< 1.00
75–80	< 7	—

*Abnormally low scores for I–E difference are defined as scores below $P_{0.025}$.
[†]Abnormally low values for heart rate changes induced by the Valsalva manoeuvre are expressed as the Valsalva ratio.

should be present. This test, therefore, cannot be interpreted when the resting heart rate is very high (> 100 beats/min). This principle applies to all tests aiming to assess cardiac vagal tone.

Circulatory response to standing

Subjects are instructed to move from supine to standing in about 3 s, if necessary with assistance. They stand for at least 2 min. The short-term circulatory adaptation to the upright position has been arbitrarily divided into an initial phase (first 30 s) with marked changes in heart rate and blood pressure and an early steady-state response (after 1–2 min standing) (Fig. 15.4(a)). Prolonged standing is defined as at least 5 min upright (Imholz *et al.* 1990*b*; Dambrink *et al.* 1991).

Initial heart rate and blood pressure responses to standing

Standing up in healthy subjects induces characteristic changes in heart rate (Fig. 15.4(a)). The heart rate increases abruptly towards a primary peak at around 3 s, increases further to a secondary peak at about 12 s, declines to a relative bradycardia at about 20 s, and then gradually rises again.

The primary heart rate peak is almost completely vagally mediated; an immediate rise (latency < 1 s) and a large primary heart rate increase exclude the presence of cardiac vagal neuropathy. However, it is not always possible to identify the primary peak separately. Therefore, in quantifying the initial heart rate response to standing, the secondary heart rate peak is generally used; the highest heart rate in the first 15 s from the onset of standing is determined and expressed as increase from control (ΔHR_{max}, peak 1 in Fig. 15.4(a)). This approach also allows quantification of the response in patients with a more gradual heart rate increase, but without a relative bradycardia and consequently without a clear secondary peak (see below). The ratio between the highest and lowest heart rate in the first 30 s from the onset of standing (1 and 2 in Fig. 15.4(a)) is generally used to quantify the relative bradycardia (HR_{max}/HR_{min} ratio).

The secondary heart rate peak is mainly, but not exclusively, vagally mediated. Enhanced sympathetic outflow to the sinus node also contributes to this response. Both are due to the concomitant initial fall in blood pressure (A and B in Fig. 15.4(a)). The relative bradycardia is the result of a vagal reflex, which depends on the presence of a recovery and overshoot of blood pressure mediated by sympathetically induced vasoconstriction (C, D in Fig. 15.4(a); Sprangers *et al.* 1991*a*).

Table 15.2. Assessment of initial heart rate response following 5–10 min resting period and assessment of early steady-state heart rate response

Age (years)	Initial heart rate response		Early steady state
	ΔHR_{max}* (beats/min)	HR_{max}/HR_{min}†	$\Delta HR_{2\ minutes}$‡ (beats/min)
10–14	< 20	< 1.20	> 35
15–19	19	1.18	> 34
20–24	19	1.17	> 33
25–29	18	1.15	> 32
30–34	17	1.13	> 31
35–39	16	1.11	> 30
40–44	16	1.09	> 29
45–49	15	1.08	> 28
50–54	14	1.06	> 27
55–59	13	1.04	> 26
60–64	13	1.02	> 25
65–69	12	1.01	> 24
70–74	12	1.00	> 23
75–80	11	—	> 22

*Abnormally low scores for ΔHR_{max} are defined as scores below $P_{0.025}$.

†Abnormally low values for relative bradycardia are numerically expressed as HR_{max}/HR_{min} ratio.

‡Heart rate increases above $P_{0.975}$ of early steady-state values (after 2 min standing) are defined as excessive increase in heart rate.

Both the ΔHR_{max} and the HR_{max}/HR_{min} ratio decrease with age (Wieling *et al.* 1982; O'Brien *et al.* 1986). Another factor that has a large influence on the initial circulatory response is the duration of the period of supine rest prior to standing (Ten Harkel *et al.* 1990). The magnitude of ΔHR_{max} after 20 min rest exceeds the maximum after 1 min rest by about 30 per cent. Our reference values (Table 15.2) are, therefore, only valid for resting periods of between 5 and 10 min. The influence of the level of resting heart rate on the magnitude of test scores is small compared to the effect of age and supine rest both in healthy subjects and in patients (Wieling 1988).

The instantaneous changes in blood pressure during the initial phase of standing (Fig. 15.4(a)) cannot be detected by sphygmomanometry. Using Finapres the magnitude of the initial blood pressure response can be quantified by determining the systolic and diastolic blood pressure trough (A and B in Fig. 15.4(a)) and the subsequent systolic and diastolic blood pressure overshoot (C and D in Fig. 15.4(a)). In patients in whom a recovery of blood pressure is not observed the value at 10 s after the onset of standing up is taken to indicate the trough and the value at 20 s to indicate the absence of an overshoot. The initial fall in blood pressure does not increase with age (Fig. 15.6).

Reference values for the magnitude of the initial blood pressure trough have not yet been established. Based on preliminary experience we consider

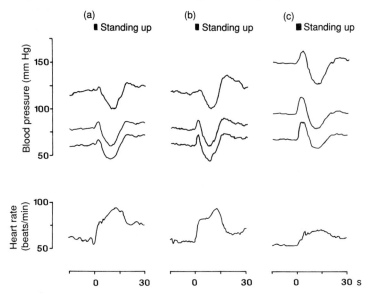

Fig. 15.6. Average systolic, mean, and diastolic blood pressure and heart rate responses upon standing in: (a) ten 10–14 year old boys; (b) ten 20–40 year old adult subjects; and (c) twenty over 70 year old male subjects. (Taken with permission from Ten Harkel *et al.* (1990), Imholz *et al.* (1990*b*), and Dambrink *et al.* (1991).)

an initial fall of more than 40 mm Hg in systolic pressure and/or more than 25 mm Hg in diastolic pressure to be abnormally large (Imholz *et al.* 1990*b*; Dambrink *et al.* 1991). An initial overshoot of systolic and or diastolic pressure is generally observed in healthy subjects.

Heart rate and blood pressure adaptation in early steady state and during prolonged standing

The early steady-state circulatory response can be expressed by single measurements of blood pressure by sphygmomanometry or by averaging 10-s periods of heart rate and finger blood pressure centred at 1 (3 and E, F in Fig. 15.4(a)) and 2 min after the change of posture. To quantify the circulatory response during prolonged standing, heart rate and blood pressure are taken at 5 and 10 min after the onset of standing up (Imholz *et al.* 1990*b*; Dambrink *et al.* 1991).

A problem with a single measurement of blood pressure by a sphygmomanometer is that the investigator is not informed about the beat-to-beat fluctuations in blood pressure that occur, especially in the upright posture (Fig. 15.2). Nevertheless, conventional sphygmomanometry is accurate enough for a routine clinical assessment of the blood pressure adjustment to standing; multiple blood pressure readings supine and standing within a single orthostatic test and/or repeated orthostatic tests provide a fair approximation of the typical blood pressure response for an individual.

The normal early steady-state blood pressure adaptation is an increase in diastolic pressure by about 10 mm Hg, with little or no change in systolic pressure. The early steady-state heart rate increase amounts to about 10 beats/min. During prolonged standing only minor further changes in heart rate and blood pressure are observed in healthy adult subjects. In healthy elderly subjects an increase in blood pressure after a relatively low value at 1 min standing has been reported (Imholz *et al.* 1990*b*).

The heart rate increase after 1–2 min standing depends predominantly on increased activity of the sympathetic nervous system; an excessive increase (postural tachycardia) indicates functionally intact neurocardiovascular control and a strong adrenergic drive to the sinus node. The early steady-state heart rate response also decreases with age (Table 15.2) (Smith and Porth 1990).

A decrease in arterial pressure in the upright position can either involve both systolic and diastolic pressure or is restricted to the systolic pressure only. A fall of systolic pressure only is most probably caused by a non-neurogenic disturbance such as central hypovolaemia. Orthostatic hypotension due to autonomic failure involves both systolic and diastolic pressure (Wieling *et al.* 1991).

Preliminary data suggest that, using Finapres, the same reference values can be applied to define normal and abnormal early steady-state blood pressure responses as with sphygmomanometry. For both methods we consider a persistent fall in systolic pressure larger than 20 mm Hg and/or a 5 mm Hg fall in diastolic pressure 1 min after a change from the supine to the upright position to be abnormal. Even in elderly subjects an orthostatic fall in systolic pressure of more than 20 mm Hg after 1 min standing appears to be rare, provided supine blood pressure is normal (Imholz *et al.* 1990*b*; Dambrink *et al.* 1991).

Head-up tilt and the assessment of autonomic circulatory control

The initial circulatory response upon passive changes of posture differs distinctly from the response on standing. A 70° head-up tilt results in a gradual rise in diastolic pressure, little change in systolic pressure, and a gradual initial heart rate rise with little or no overshoot (Figs 15.2 and 15.3). The differences in responses can be attributed to the effects of contraction of leg and abdominal muscles on the circulation during standing up; the underlying mechanisms have been addressed elsewhere (Sprangers *et al.* 1991*a,b*).

The heart rate response induced by head-up tilt does not differentiate between patients with mild vagal impairment and those whose heart rate control is normal; this is in contrast to the response induced by standing. For the assessment of short-term orthostatic neurocardiovascular control, therefore, we prefer to study the response to standing (Van Lieshout 1989). Prolonged orthostatic stress induced by tilt has been reported to be useful in identifying orthostatic disorders as in patients susceptible to vasovagal fainting.

The Valsalva manoeuvre

This is performed preferably while sitting, because the circulatory effects are larger in that position compared to the changes observed in the supine position (Fig. 15.7; Ten Harkel *et al.* 1990). In patients with autonomic failure, the manoeuvre must be performed supine if straining in sitting position induces very low blood pressures. Expiratory pressure of 40 mm Hg is maintained for 15 s. Care is taken to prevent deep breathing prior to and directly following release of the strain.

The Valsalva manoeuvre elicits typical changes in heart rate in healthy subjects (Fig. 15.4(b)). An immediate heart rate decrease during the rise in systolic and diastolic pressure at the onset of straining is usually observed. It is followed by an increase in heart rate during and directly after release of intrathoracic pressure and a subsequent bradycardia.

In quantifying the heart rate increase induced by the Valsalva manoeuvre the maximum heart rate is determined and expressed as the difference from control (ΔHR_{max}, peak 1 in Fig. 15.4(b)). The ratio between highest and

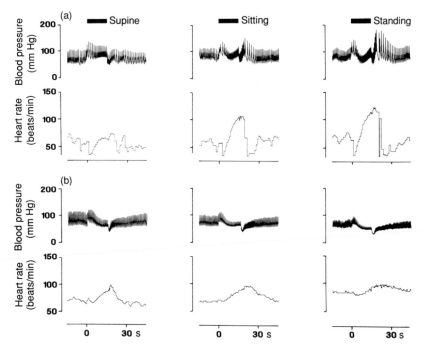

Fig. 15.7. Influence of posture on the Valsalva manoeuvre in: (a) a healthy 33-year-old subject; and (b) a 43-year-old patient with autonomic failure. Note marked influences of posture on the blood pressure responses in both subjects. The square wave response observed in the healthy adult subject in supine position is a normal finding. (Taken with permission from Ten Harkel *et al.* (1990).)

lowest heart rate directly after release of the strain (1 and 2 in Fig. 15.4(b)) is generally used to quantify the relative bradycardia (HR_{max}/HR_{min} ratio or Valsalva ratio).

The heart rate increase during and directly after release of the strain (peak 1 in Fig. 15.4(b)) is mediated by withdrawal of vagal tone and increased sympathetic outflow to the sinus node due to the fall in blood pressure. The bradycardia (2 in Fig. 15.4(b)) is the result of a vagal reflex, which depends on a blood pressure overshoot relative to control blood pressure. The magnitude of the heart rate responses induced by the Valsalva manoeuvre again decreases with age (Table 15.1) (O'Brien *et al.* 1986).

The instantaneous changes in blood pressure induced by the Valsalva manoeuvre (Fig. 15.4(b)) cannot be detected by sphygmomanometry. Using Finapres the magnitude of the blood pressure response can be quantified by determining the systolic and diastolic blood pressure at the end of straining (A and B in Fig. 15.4(b)) and the subsequent systolic and diastolic blood pressure overshoot (C and D in Fig. 15.4(b)) relative to control blood pressure.

An overshoot of systolic and or diastolic pressure is generally observed in healthy subjects. In patients without a blood pressure overshoot the highest blood pressure in the first 15 s after release of the strain is taken.

Test battery versus single test

We are in favour of using a combination of tests in the evaluation of patients suspected of suffering from autonomic disturbances. However, we feel that it is of more importance to attempt to make a physiological interpretation of test results than simply to add test scores (Van Lieshout 1989).

We use the I–E difference induced by forced breathing as a sensitive measure to assess vagal heart rate control. We have found the combination of abnormally low test scores for both the I–E difference and ΔHR_{max} to standing eminently suited to identify definite cardiac vagal neuropathy in individual patients (Wieling et al. 1982; Wieling 1988). HR_{max}/HR_{min} ratios induced by standing and the Valsalva heart rate ratios are in our experience in these conditions abnormally small as well.

In earlier studies we used the circulatory response to standing, evaluated by continuous heart rate monitoring and conventional sphygmomanometry, to define a spectrum of normal and abnormal circulatory responses. Using Finapres we have continued to use this approach (Wieling et al. 1991). Our reasons for doing so are the following. First, in patients with disturbances in autonomic circulatory control orthostatic dizziness and fainting are the main clinical problems. Second, orthostatic stress testing can be applied and interpreted both with and without sophisticated equipment. Third, orthostatic stress testing can be used not only to evaluate instantaneous, but also prolonged orthostatic circulatory responses. The Valsalva manoeuvre provides, in our experience, mainly confirmatory information (see next section).

Spectrum of normal and abnormal orthostatic responses

Five main types of responses are clinically important in the evaluation of complaints of orthostatic dizziness (Table 15.3). The first three are common and transient and are found in subjects with intact circulatory reflexes. The last two are rare and characterized by a significant and persistent fall in blood pressure in the upright position due to autonomic failure.

A careful evaluation of the patient's history and the conventional measurement of blood pressure by a sphygmomanometer and heart rate by pulse-counting supine and after 1–2 min standing are simple procedures to evaluate complaints of orthostatic dizziness in general practice. Based on the early steady-state heart rate and blood pressure responses distinctions can

Table 15.3.   Classification of patients according to their response to standing

Response	Early steady-state blood pressure		Initial heart rate response	Early steady-state heart rate response
Normal	Systolic	=	Biphasic	↑
	Diastolic	↑		
Hyperadrenergic	Systolic	↓	Large ΔHR_{max}; little or no relative bradycardia	↑↑
	Diastolic	↑↑		
Vasovagal	Systolic	↓	Normal or hyperadrenergic	↓
	Diastolic	↓		
Hypoadrenergic (vagus intact)	Systolic	↓	Large ΔHR_{max}; no relative bradycardia	↑↑
	Diastolic	↓		
Hypoadrenergic (with cardiac denervation)	Systolic	↓	Absent	=
	Diastolic	↓		

be made among: (1) normal orthostatic heart rate and blood pressure control; (2) normal orthostatic blood pressure control in combination with a postural tachycardia; and (3) orthostatic hypotension with or without postural tachycardia (Table 15.3).

It will be shown that, although continuous measurement of arterial blood pressure is no prerequisite for a classification of patients, analysis of both heart rate and blood pressure changes contributes to a more fundamental understanding of the pathophysiological mechanisms involved.

Orthostatic dizziness on standing in healthy subjects

A normal initial heart rate response, including an immediate heart rate increase, a large secondary heart rate peak, and a marked subsequent bradycardia (1 and 2 in Fig. 15.4(a)), is an important clinical finding. It indicates, for reasons explained above, that intact afferent, central, and efferent cardiac vagal and efferent sympathetic vasomotor pathways are present. Nevertheless, it should be realized that subjects with intact autonomic control can still have complaints of dizziness shortly after standing up; in fact most people experience a brief feeling of dizziness 5 to 10 s after the onset of standing up rapidly, especially after prolonged supine rest. Such common 'functional' spells of dizziness are characterized by their time of onset and short duration and appear to be more common in young subjects. An extraordinary, large initial fall in blood pressure has, for reasons unexplained, been reported in healthy young subjects with orthostatic

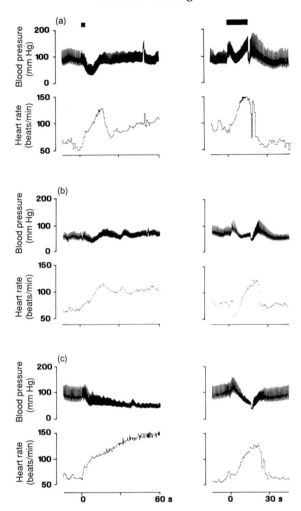

Fig. 15.8. Blood pressure and heart rate responses induced by standing (■) and the Valsalva manoeuvre (▬). (a) A 17-year-old female patient with complaints of orthostatic dizziness almost immediately upon standing and a large initial fall in blood pressure. (From Dambrink (1991).) (b) A 32-year-old female patient with a postural tachycardia. (From Wieling and Ten Harkel, unpublished.) (c) Orthostatic hypotension (hypoadrenergic) with intact heart rate control in a 23-year-old female patient. (From van Lieshout (1989).)

dizziness in the initial phase of standing (Dambrink 1991). An example is given in Fig. 15.8(a). The normal circulatory response to the Valsalva manoeuvre in this subject confirms integrity of neurocardiovascular control.

Hyperadrenergic orthostatic response

An excessive heart rate increment after 1–2 min of standing can be considered to be a compensatory response to a variety of conditions; an abnormal degree of central hypovolaemia and a strong adrenergic drive in the upright posture are common to these conditions. Classically, such a response consists of an immediate heart rate increase and a large secondary peak with little or no subsequent relative bradycardia, resulting in an excessive increase in heart rate in the upright position (Fig. 15.8(b)), together with a fall in systolic pressure and a marked increase in diastolic pressure. A marked increase in both systolic and diastolic pressure has also been described (Wieling *et al.* 1991). The normal circulatory response to the Valsalva manoeuvre in these conditions confirms functionally intact baroreflex pathways.

Vasovagal orthostatic response

Typical for a vasovagal response is a temporary phase of tachycardia in upright position, which changes into a decrease in heart rate and a fall in blood pressure due to reflex vagal facilitation and adrenergic inhibition, respectively (Fig. 15.9). The initial circulatory response is normal or hyperadrenergic, indicating integrity of neurocardiovascular control (Van Lieshout 1989). In our experience the circulatory response to the Valsalva manoeuvre in subjects with a vasovagal orthostatic response is normal.

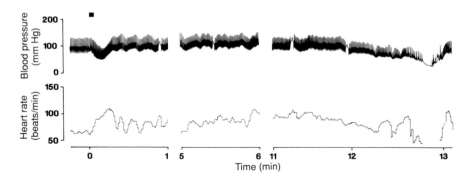

Fig. 15.9. Vasovagal fainting in a healthy 22-year-old male subject. Note normal initial heart rate and blood pressure response and marked increase in heart rate after 6 min standing. After 11–12 min standing blood pressure and heart rate start to decrease to very low values during the actual faint; the heart rate tracing in the faint is interrupted in a period of asystole of 7 s. On lying down, heart rate and blood pressure recover almost immediately. (From van Lieshout (1989).)

Hypoadrenergic orthostatic response
with intact heart rate control

In patients with sympathetic vasomotor lesions but intact vagal heart rate control, an immediate large heart rate increase without a relative bradycardia and consequently a persistent and marked heart rate rise is observed. This is accompanied by a progressive fall of both systolic and diastolic blood pressure (Fig. 15.8(c)). This response can be attributed to correct baroreceptor sensing of an absence of recovery of blood pressure due to the defective vasoconstrictor mechanisms (compare Fig. 15.4(a) with Fig. 15.8(c)). Hypoadrenergic orthostatic hypotension, combined with a marked postural tachycardia, can be found in some patients with dysautonomia, in tetraplegic patients, and after extensive sympathectomy (Van Lieshout *et al.* 1989; Wieling *et al.* 1991).

The blocked blood pressure response induced by the Valsalva manoeuvre in these patients indicates loss of sympathetic vasomotor control. If the heart rate response is considered without the simultaneous blood pressure recording, the registration may be misleading, since a reflex bradycardia and high Valsalva ratios can be observed in some of these patients (Fig. 15.8(c); Van Lieshout *et al.* 1989).

The rare combination of a hypoadrenergic orthostatic response with intact vagal heart rate control (Fig. 15.8(c)) may be interpreted as the mirror image of the common pattern of autonomic circulatory denervation, where impaired vagal heart rate control precedes overt sympathetic damage, i.e. orthostatic hypotension (Fig. 15.10(a)). However, subtle disturbances in distal sympathetic sudomotor function in the legs can be found at a much earlier stage in these patients (Low *et al.* 1986).

Hypoadrenergic orthostatic response with impairment of
vagal and sympathetic innervation of the heart

In subjects with a normal resting heart rate, a delayed and sluggish primary heart rate response upon standing indicates that vagal heart rate control is completely disrupted (Fig. 15.10(b)). The heart rate increase in these patients represents the remaining sympathetic response mentioned before. Thus, a delayed onset of cardioacceleration and a substantial heart rate increase afterwards suggest cardiac vagal denervation with intact sympathetic heart rate control. A small heart rate increase after prolonged standing in patients with orthostatic hypotension should be interpreted as a sign of impaired sympathetic heart rate control. The Valsalva manoeuvre will confirm the abnormality (compare Fig. 15.4(a,b) right and left panels and Fig. 15.10(b)).

Complete denervation of the heart can be found in patients with a cardiac transplant. The blood pressure adaptation to orthostatic stress shows that, when vasomotor innervation is intact, orthostatic blood pressure control

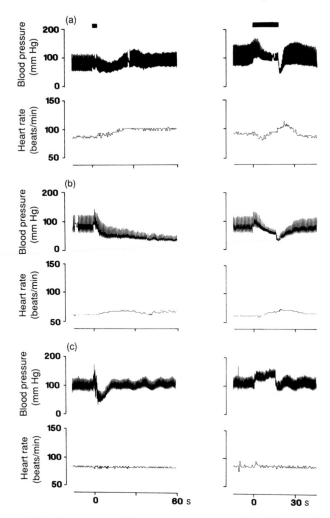

Fig. 15.10.   Blood pressure and heart rate responses induced by standing (■) and the Valsalva manoeuvre (▬). (a) A 64-year-old male patient with polyneuropathy and impairment of cardiac vagal control, but normal blood pressure responses. (b) A 69-year-old male patient with orthostatic hypotension (hypoadrenergic) with impairment of vagal and sympathetic cardiac control (the Valsalva manoeuvre is performed supine). (c) Total cardiac denervation with intact vasomotor control in a 38-year-old fit patient with a cardiac transplant. (From van Lieshout (1989).)

remains undisturbed in spite of complete denervation of the heart (Fig. 15.10(c); Wieling *et al.* 1991). A square wave response is induced by the Valsalva manoeuvre. Obviously, the marked blood pressure changes induced by standing and the Valsalva manoeuvre are missed in this patient if continuous monitoring is not available.

Conclusions

The combination of monitoring instantaneous heart rate changes to standing and the conventional recording of blood pressure by a sphygmomanometer supine and after 1–2 min standing provide sufficient information for a detailed classification of normal and abnormal circulatory responses. However, intermittent measures of blood pressure do not reflect the full impact of an acute stimulus on the circulatory system. For a more precise evaluation and documentation of the dynamics of the circulatory response it is necessary to monitor both heart rate and blood pressure continuously. In this context, the ability of Finapres to track the blood pressure signal precisely, non-invasively, and continuously makes it an important tool in clinical autonomic research.

References

Dambrink, J. H. A. (1991). Orthostatic regulation of blood pressure: a comparative study in young and old subjects. Unpublished D.Phil. thesis, University of Amsterdam.

Dambrink, J. H. A., Imholz, B. P. M., Karemaker, J. M., and Wieling, W. (1991). Circulatory adaptation to orthostatic stress in healthy 10–14 year old children. *Clin. Sci.* **81**, 51–8.

De Boer, R. W., Karemaker, J. M., and Strackee, J. (1987). Hemodynamic fluctuations and baroreflex sensitivity in humans: a beat-to-beat model. *Am. J. Physiol.* **253**, H680–9.

Hainsworth, R. (1990). Non-invasive investigations of cardiovascular reflexes in humans. *Clin. Sci.* **78**, 437–43.

Imholz, B. P. M., van Montfrans, G. A., Settels, J. J., van der Hoeven, G. M. A., Karemaker, J. M., and Wieling, W. (1988). Continuous non-invasive blood pressure monitoring: reliability of Finapres device during the Valsalva manoeuvre. *Cardiovasc. Res.* **22**, 390–7.

Imholz, B. P. M., Settels, J. J., van den Meiracker, A. H., Wesseling, K. H., and Wieling, W. (1990a). Noninvasive beat-to-beat finger blood pressure measurement during orthostatic stress compared to intra-arterial pressure. *Cardiovasc. Res.* **24**, 214–21.

Imholz, B. P. M., Dambrink, J. H. A., Karemaker, J. M., and Wieling, W. (1990b). Orthostatic circulatory control in the elderly evaluated by non-invasive continuous blood pressure measurement. *Clin. Sci.* **79**, 73–9.

Imholz, B. P. M., Wieling, W., Langewouters, G. J., and Montfrans, G. A. van (1991). Continuous finger arterial pressure; utility in the cardiovascular laboratory. *Clin. autonom. Res.* **1**, 43–53.

Langewouters, G., de Wit, B., van der Hoeven, G. *et al.* (1990). Feasibility of continuous noninvasive 24h ambulatory measurement of finger arterial blood pressure with Portapres. *J. Hypertension* **8**(S3), 87.

Low, P. A., Zimmerman, B. R., and Dyck, P. J. (1986). Comparison of distal sympathetic with vagal function in diabetic neuropathy. *Muscle Nerve* **9**, 592–6.

O'Brien, I. A. D., O'Hare, P., and Corrall, R. J. M. (1986). Heart rate variability in healthy subjects: effect of age and the derivation of normal ranges for tests of autonomic function. *Br. Heart J.* **55**, 348–54.

Parati, G., Casadei, R., Gropelli, A., Di Rienzo, M., and Mancia, G. (1989). Comparison of finger and intra-arterial blood pressure monitoring in rest and during laboratory tests. *Hypertension* **13**, 647–55.

Peñáz, J. (1973). Photoelectric measurement of blood pressure, volume and flow in the finger. In *Digest of the International Conference of Medicine and Biological Engineering*, p. 109. Conference Committee of the Xth International Conference on Medical and Biological Engineering, Dresden.

Smith, J. J. and Porth, C. J. M. (1990). Age and the response to orthostatic stress. In *Circulatory response to the upright posture* (ed. J. J. Smith), pp. 121–39. CRC Press, Boca Raton, Florida.

Sprangers, R. L. H., Wesseling, K. H., Imholz, A. L. T., Imholz, B. P. M., and Wieling, W. (1991*a*). The initial blood pressure fall upon stand up and onset to exercise explained by changes in total peripheral resistance. *J. appl. Physiol.* **70**(2), 523–30.

Sprangers, R. L. H., Veerman, D. P., Karemaker, J. M., and Wieling, W. (1991*b*). Circulatory response to changes in posture: influence of angle and speed of tilt. *Clin. Physiol.* **11**, 211–21.

Steptoe, A. and Vogele, C. (1990). Cardiac baroreflex function during postural change assessed using non-invasive spontaneous sequence analysis in young men. *Cardiovasc. Res.* **24**, 627–32.

Ten Harkel, A. D. J., van Lieshout, J. J., van Lieshout, E. J., and Wieling, W. (1990). Assessment of cardiovascular reflexes: influence of posture and period of preceding rest. *J. appl. Physiol.* **68**(1), 147–53.

Van Lieshout, J. J. (1989). Cardiovascular reflexes in orthostatic disorders. Unpublished D.Phil. thesis, University of Amsterdam.

Van Lieshout, J. J., Wieling, W., Wesseling, K. H., and Karemaker, J. M. (1989). Pitfalls in the assessment of cardiovascular reflexes in patients with sympathetic failure but intact vagal control. *Clin. Sci.* **76**, 523–8.

Wesseling, K. H. (1982). A method and a device for correcting the cuff pressure in measuring the blood pressure in a part of the body by means of a plethysmograph. European Patent EP 0-080778 AI, November 1982.

Wesseling, K. H. (1990). Finapres, continuous noninvasive finger arterial pressure based on the method of Peñáz. In *Blood pressure measurement* (ed. W. Meyer-Sabellek, M. Anlauf, R. Gotzen, and L. Steinfeld), pp. 161–72. Steinkopff Verlag, Darmstadt.

Wieling, W. (1988). Impaired vagal heart rate control in diabetes: relationship to long-term complications. *Neth. J. Med.* **33**, 260–9.

Wieling, W., van Brederode, J. F. M., de Rijk, L. G., Borst, C., and Dunning, A. J. (1982). Reflex control of heart rate in normal subjects in relation to age; a data base for cardiac vagal neuropathy. *Diabetologia* **22**, 163–6.

Wieling, W., Ten Harkel, A. D. J., and Van Lieshout, J. J. (1991). Classification of orthostatic disorders based on the short-term circulatory response to standing. *Clin. Sci.* **81**, 241–8.

16. Analysis of heart rate variability and other non-invasive tests with special reference to diabetes mellitus

David J. Ewing

Introduction

Among newer techniques for non-invasive investigation of autonomic neuropathy are those involving the detailed analysis of heart rate variation. There is, however, a bewildering variety of different approaches, and this chapter seeks to put the various 'time domain' and 'frequency domain' methods into their proper context. Basic principles are first discussed, comparison between the methods noted, and then these new analytical techniques are placed alongside the more traditional cardiovascular reflex tests for non-invasive investigation of autonomic function. The clinical relevance of these tests in diabetes mellitus is then discussed, and brief reference made to non-invasive tests that are available in other systems. For more details of the relation between abnormal cardiovascular reflexes and other diabetic complications, and to the involvement of other systems, readers are referred to a recent review article (Ewing 1991) and to other chapters in this book.

Analysis of heart variability

Time domain analysis

This approach to heart rate variability analysis involves taking a sequence of R–R intervals of whatever length, and subjecting it to relatively simple analysis to determine the variability. Several approaches have been used. The first has been recognized and applied for some time in autonomic testing, namely, to measure the reflex heart rate response to a particular stimulus. This and other cardiovascular reflex tests are considered in more detail later in this chapter.

The next approaches are based on the measurement of successive R–R

intervals, and calculation of successive R–R interval differences. This can
now be easily and accurately achieved with microcomputers. From the R–R
interval sequences a number of calculations can be made that essentially are
different ways to measure the width of the R–R interval histogram. They
include the standard deviation (SD) of a given R–R interval sequence and
the coefficient of variation (CV) about the mean R–R interval for that
sequence (CV = SD/mean × 100). A further calculation can be made from
a series of R–R interval sequences, say, of 5 min each, where the mean of
all the SDs or CVs is worked out. Similar calculations can be made for
sequences of beat-to-beat R–R interval differences. An alternative approach
has been to calculate either the mean of the square of successive R–R interval
differences (so-called MSSD method) or to take the square root of that value
(the RMSSD). A theoretical advantage of this approach is that it is
independent of the prevailing heart rate.

While these methods are easy to calculate, their exact physiological meaning
is slightly less clear. The longer the R–R interval sample, the greater the
natural variation of the signal due to all the different influences acting on
heart rate. Any 'SD' method will, therefore, include estimates of both

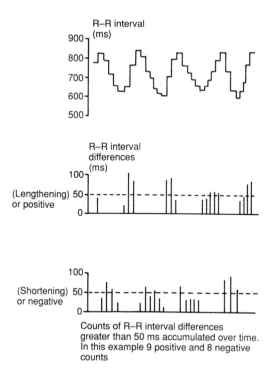

Fig. 16.1. Diagram to show how R–R interval counts are derived from the
measurement of successive R–R intervals, calculation of R–R interval differences,
and accumulation of differences greater than 50 ms.

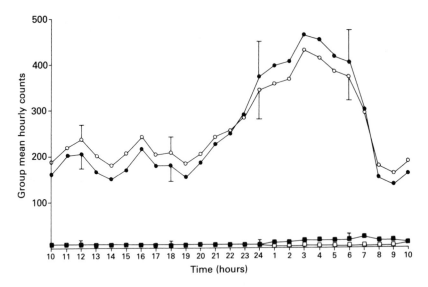

Fig. 16.2. Group mean hourly R–R interval counts in (○, positive; ●, negative) 25 normal subjects; (■) 12 diabetics with cardiac parasympathetic involvement; and (□) 6 cardiac transplant patients. Bars represent ± SEM. (From Ewing *et al.* (1984).)

parasympathetic and sympathetic inputs into heart rate control. It does not distinguish between very different patterns of heart rate; for example, a gradually increasing or decreasing rate might have the same standard deviation as a sequence where there was an abrupt change from one rate to another. The MSSD method may be more specific for parasympathetic activity.

An entirely different approach has been adopted by us, based on observation of 24-hour heart rate recordings. Examination of sequences of successive R–R intervals shows that, superimposed on cyclical variations associated with respiration (sinus arrhythmia), are a large number of bigger beat-by-beat changes in R–R interval. If a threshold of 50 ms is applied, then in normal subjects several hundred such changes over that threshold occur each hour which can then be counted (Fig. 16.1). Subjects with autonomic damage and patients with transplanted hearts have extremely low R–R interval 'counts' (Fig. 16.2). This and other evidence has suggested that this 'counts' method is a reliable and reproducible measure of cardiac parasympathetic function which can be applied as a sensitive marker for diagnostic and intervention purposes (Ewing *et al.* 1984, 1991*b*).

Frequency domain analysis

Any biological rhythm, such as heart rate, that consists of a time series of successive events can be broken down into a number of sinusoidal waves of different amplitudes and frequencies. Spectral analysis involves subjecting a series of successive R–R intervals to a mathematical transformation which separates those R–R intervals into a number of harmonics of identifiable and discrete frequencies. A non-mathematical analogy is that of a glass prism which splits white light up into a rainbow. This represents the different spectral, or frequency, components that make up the white light, and the prism is acting to separate the white light into its characteristic frequencies. Similarly, spectral analysis separates the R–R-interval time series into several characteristic frequencies.

The mathematical techniques used for this transformation are complex and beyond the scope of this chapter and readers are referred to standard mathematical texts for further details. In essence there are two alternative approaches: either using a technique known as 'fast Fourier transformation' (FFT) alone, or a two-stage approach of 'autocorrelation' followed by FFT. Autocorrelation consists of fitting the time series curve to itself with a built-in series of delays, which reveal how frequently the curve 'repeats' itself. A further technique, known as a 'Hanning window', is often applied; this is a method of smoothing out the abrupt changes at the start and finish of the R–R interval record, which might otherwise distort the spectral picture. Once the spectral analysis is complete, results are usually presented either

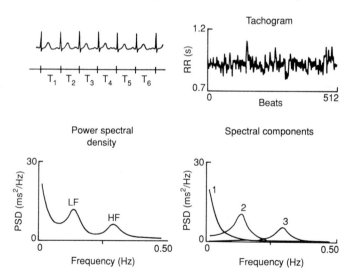

Fig. 16.3. Schematic representation of spectral analysis of heart rate variability. From the surface electrocardiogram (top left), individual R–R intervals are calculated and stored as a tachogram (top right). The power spectral density (PSD) is computed, and two major components of low and high frequencies (LF and HF) usually recognized, along with some very slow oscillations (bottom left). Different spectral components can then be selected and measured (bottom right). (From Furlan *et al.* (1990).)

as 'amplitude', which is the magnitude of the spectrum at any particular frequency, or as the 'power spectrum', which is the square of the amplitude. The latter gives a much more 'peaky' appearance to the curve.

Figure 16.3 illustrates the breakdown of a sequence of consecutive R–R intervals into its spectral components in a normal subject. Three discrete peaks are visible: at a very low frequency (below 0.05 Hz); at a low/mid frequency (LF, around 0.15 Hz); and at a high frequency (HF, around 0.3 Hz). These three peaks have generally been assumed to represent different control systems influencing heart rate. The very low frequency band has been equated with a thermoregulatory or vasomotor influence, together with some input from the renin–angiotensin system; the LF band with blood pressure and baroreflex control; and the HF band with respiration. As such, therefore, the HF band is thought to be mediated by parasympathetic pathways, while the LF band is mediated by both parasympathetic and sympathetic pathways. The very low frequency band, in addition to sympathetic control, is also thought to be influenced by neurohumoral factors.

There are several lines of evidence to support these assumptions. Parasympathetic blockade with atropine abolishes the HF heart rate fluctuations and substantially reduces the LF component. Additional propranolol further diminishes the LF band, but has no effect on its own on the HF peak (Akselrod et al. 1985; Pomeranz et al. 1985). This confirms observations made nearly 60 years ago by Rosenbleuth and Simeone (1934), who showed that the heart rate response to a change in parasympathetic efferent activity was extremely rapid, whereas the response to sympathetic activation was much slower.

Figure 16.4 shows the influence of posture on the LF and HF peaks. When a subject is supine, the HF peak is dominant, but the peak is markedly reduced when the subject stands, whereas the LF component increases in amplitude. Atropine reduces the LF peak in the supine position, while propranolol has little further effect. However, on standing, propranolol diminishes the LF peak by three-quarters, thus indicating a strong sympathetic influence on LF fluctuations in the standing position, while in the supine position this frequency is largely under parasympathetic control (Pomeranz et al. 1985).

Some measure of the HF peak, for example, using the height or the area under the curve, can therefore be used to assess parasympathetic activity. Sympathetic activity is less easy to quantify using this methodology, although some workers have claimed that the LF component acts as a sympathetic marker. Perhaps a better concept is that of 'sympathovagal balance' which recognizes both reciprocal and non-reciprocal parasympathetic and sympathetic influences on heart rate, with a further measure, the LF:HF ratio (Pagani et al. 1986; Furlan et al. 1990).

Despite enthusiastic claims about the merits of spectral analysis of heart rate as a measure of autonomic activity, some caution has to be exercised in interpreting results. The spectral signal is easily distorted by movement

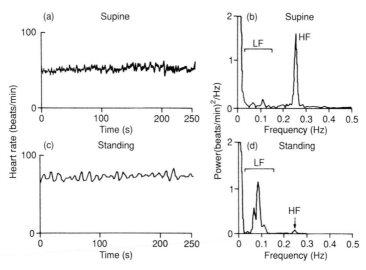

Fig. 16.4. Power spectral analysis of heart rate responses to change in posture in a normal individual. (a) Instantaneous supine heart rate; (b) Power spectrum of (a) with small low-frequency (LF) and prominent high-frequency (HF) peaks; (c) instantaneous standing heart rate; (d) power spectrum of (c) with prominent LF oscillations and a small HF peak. (From Pomeranz *et al.* (1985).)

artefacts and ectopic beats, and only short segments (for example 512 beats) can easily be computed at a time.

A further refinement of the spectral analysis technique has been to use a cross-correlation method with either blood pressure or respiration. In normal subjects there is a concordance of signals between the LF and blood pressure waves, and the HF and respiratory cycles.

Comparison of time and frequency domain methods

Relatively few studies have addressed the question of the relation between the different measures of heart rate variation. In general terms, the 'broader' methods of standard deviation and total spectral power correlate quite closely, as do the three more specific measures of cardiac parasympathetic activity, namely, the 'counts' method, MSSD, and the HF spectral component. Among diabetics, the 'counts' method and cross-correlation of heart rate and respiration appear to be more sensitive than conventional cardiovascular reflexes, while spectral analysis appears to give results that are similar to the reflex tests.

Clinical applications

The time and frequency domain methods of assessing heart rate variability require a good ECG signal, a microprocessor and the appropriate program to analyse the R–R interval signals. While these tools are readily available, the methods are not straightforward and the underlying concepts need to be grasped before valid assumptions can be made by investigators. Although some enthusiasts have claimed that spectral analysis is superior to other methods, the evidence to support this has not yet been forthcoming. However, some useful information is now emerging from the various studies using these methodologies.

In diabetes we have shown that the 'counts' method is more sensitive than conventional cardiovascular reflexes and provides a further useful way of measuring cardiac parasympathetic damage (Fig. 16.5; Ewing *et al.* 1991*b*).

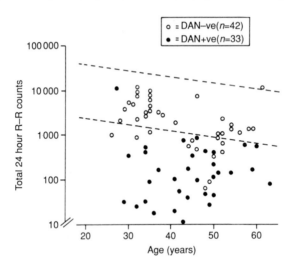

Fig. 16.5.   Total 24-h R–R counts in relation to age in: (open circles) 42 diabetics with normal cardiovascular reflexes (DAN – ve); and (filled circles) 33 diabetics with definite or severe autonomic involvement (DAN + ve). The dotted lines represent the normal 95 per cent tolerance limits for age, based on results from 57 normal subjects.

All spectral peaks are diminished in diabetic subjects with autonomic neuropathy, but debate continues about the significance of the LF peak (see Ewing 1991). In a direct comparison with the heart rate response to deep breathing, Bernardi *et al.* (1989) showed that their cross-correlation method was more sensitive (Fig. 16.6). However, none of the new methods has yet replaced conventional cardiovascular reflex tests in the objective diagnosis of autonomic neuropathy.

In cardiology a further impetus for these methods came with a study showing that long-term prognosis after myocardial infarction was linked to heart rate variability measured by SD (Kleiger *et al.* 1987). This has prompted a whole series of further studies in cardiac patients using both time and

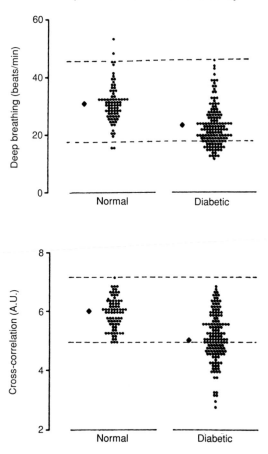

Fig. 16.6. Comparison between the heart rate response to deep breathing (maximum minus minimum heart rate) and cross-correlation (arbitrary units) in 77 normal subjects and 141 diabetics. The large diamonds represent the group mean values, and the broken lines indicate ± 2 SDs from the normal means. (From Bernardi *et al.* (1989).)

frequency domain methods. Reduced heart rate variation occurs in cardiac failure (Flapan *et al.* 1990). Drugs also affect heart rate variation; this has been demonstrated mainly using the 'counts' method (Zuanetti *et al.* 1991). However, the precise physiological significance of these changes is not altogether clear. It is likely that they indicate localized autonomic damage in the myocardium, rather than more generalized autonomic neuropathy.

In other areas, such as renal disease, alcoholism, and liver failure, these methods are also being applied, and varying degrees of abnormality are being demonstrated.

Bedside cardiovascular reflex tests—
with particular reference to diabetes

Although the newer methods of heart rate analysis provide different insights
into autonomic abnormalities, the conventional cardiovascular reflex tests
remain the cornerstone for investigation of autonomic neuropathy and its
objective diagnosis. In the report and recommendations of the San Antonio
Conference on diabetic neuropathy (1988) it was agreed that five simple non-
invasive tests were most useful. Three, the responses to the Valsalva
manoeuvre, deep breathing, and standing up, are based on the measurement
of heart rate changes, while the other two, the responses to standing up and
sustained handgrip, depend on blood pressure measurements. Other
cardiovascular tests have been proposed from time to time, but none appears
to be as reliable in distinguishing normal from abnormal or as easily
performed.

Normal ranges and repeatability

A large number of groups has reported their normal ranges for these five
tests. There are, however, some problems with lack of standardization both
of the techniques and the indices used to describe the results. For example,
tests of heart rate variation during breathing have been described with subjects
lying and sitting, breathing quietly and breathing deeply, and taking single
or repeated deep breaths. The Valsalva manoeuvre can be performed lying
down, sitting down, held for 10 s, or for 15 s.

Equally, too, the measurements used to assess these responses have
sometimes differed. The lying to standing heart rate response has been
assessed both by the 30:15 ratio and by the maximum to minimum heart rate
ratio although in practice these two ratios are almost identical. Other studies,
however, have used the rise in heart rate on standing, instead of the rebound
bradycardia. The heart rate response to breathing has revealed the most varied
measurements. Some groups have used the maximum to minimum heart rate
response, others the expiration to inspiration ratio (E:I ratio), and yet others
the coefficient of variation or standard deviation of the heart rate. There
have been no disagreements, however, about measurements of systolic blood
pressure to assess postural hypotension or diastolic blood pressure to assess
sustained handgrip or about the Valsalva ratio.

A further factor in the establishment of normal ranges has been the
relationship between the results and the ages of subjects. Heart rate variation,
however measured, declines with increasing age (Fig. 16.7). Most authors
have also found that lying to standing heart rate responses relate to age,
whereas there have been different views about the effect of age on the Valsalva
manoeuvre and the postural fall in blood pressure. The sustained handgrip

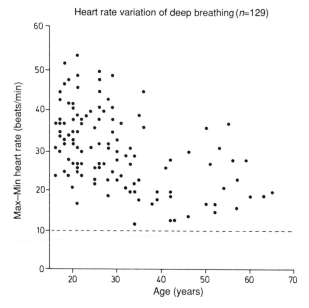

Fig. 16.7. Heart rate variation during deep breathing (maximum minus minimum heart rate) in relation to age in 129 normal subjects. The dotted line represents the lower limit of normal.

response is related more to the strength of contraction rather than to age *per se*. In view of these discrepancies it is difficult to compare different normal values. However, there is an increasing move towards standardization both in techniques used and in the actual measurements used for assessment. While there is, of course, no actual right or wrong method for performing tests or calculating the results, the following is a brief account of how the tests can be performed simply, based on our experience in Edinburgh over a number of years (Ewing *et al.* 1985).

Simple non-invasive tests

Heart rate response to the Valsalva manoeuvre

The test is performed by asking the subject to sit quietly and then blow into a mouthpiece attached to an aneroid pressure gauge at a pressure of 40 mm Hg and to hold the pressure for 15 s. The ratio of the longest R–R interval shortly after the manoeuvre (within about 20 beats) to the shortest R–R interval during the manoeuvre is then measured. The result is expressed as the Valsalva ratio which is taken as the mean ratio from three successive Valsalva manoeuvres. This test should be avoided in diabetic subjects with proliferative retinopathy.

Heart rate response to standing up

The subject is asked to lie quietly on a couch and then to stand up unaided as quickly as practicable. The characteristic heart rate response can be expressed by the 30 : 15 ratio which is the ratio of the longest R–R interval around the thirtieth beat after standing up to the shortest R–R interval around the fifteenth beat.

Heart response to deep breathing

The patient sits quietly and then breathes deeply and evenly at 6 breaths/min (5 s in and 5 s out). The maximum minus minimum heart rate during each 10-s breathing cycle is measured and the mean of the differences during three successive breathing cycles gives the 'maximum minus minimum' heart rate.

Blood pressure response to standing up

This test is performed by measuring the blood pressure (BP) while the subject is lying down, and again 1 minute after standing up. The difference in systolic blood pressure is taken as the measure of postural blood pressure change.

Blood pressure response to sustained handgrip

Handgrip is maintained at 30 per cent of the maximum voluntary contraction for up to a maximum of 5 min using a handgrip dynamometer, and the blood pressure is measured each minute. The difference between the diastolic blood pressure just before release of handgrip and before starting is taken as the measure of response.

Assessment of cardiovascular autonomic damage

Assessment of cardiovascular autonomic nerve damage can be made from the combined results of these five tests, which we have employed over several years in a large number of normal (Fig. 16.8), diabetic, and other subjects (Ewing *et al.* 1985). Table 16.1 gives the normal and abnormal values we use in Edinburgh for routine clinical and diagnostic purposes. The figures quoted do not take age into account. More stringent criteria should be applied in research studies allowing for age, particularly when one of the heart rate variation tests is used. It might be argued that, because clinical measurements such as these are not done under tightly controlled conditions, the results obtained are invalid. However, in clinical practice, provided that test conditions are standardized as much as practicable, factors such as the time of the testing, relation to meals and exercise, temperature of the laboratory, etc. appear to have little effect on the actual results obtained. Table 16.2 shows a flow plan for performing the five tests in the clinical setting. In addition, the tests have proved of considerable diagnostic use in relating autonomic abnormalities to symptoms and prognosis. Figures for repeatability

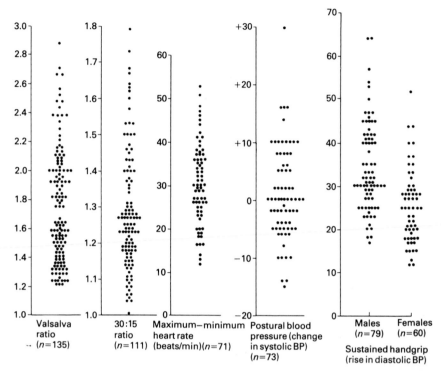

Fig. 16.8. Individual responses to five cardiovascular reflex tests in normal subjects aged 16–69 years.

Table 16.1. Normal and abnormal values for simple bedside cardiovascular reflex tests

Test	Normal	Borderline	Abnormal
Valsalva manoeuvre (Valsalva ratio)	1.21 or more	—	1.20 or less
Heart rate variation (maximum – minimum heart rate)	15 beats/min or more	11–14 beats/min	10 beats/min or less
Heart rate response to standing (30 : 15 ratio)	1.04 or more	1.01–1.03	1.00 or less
Blood pressure response to standing (postural fall in systolic BP)	10 mm Hg or less	11–29 mm Hg	30 mm Hg or more
Sustained handgrip (increase in diastolic BP)	16 mm Hg or more	11–15 mm Hg	10 mm Hg or less

Table 16.2. Flow plan for performing cardiovascular autonomic function tests

Test (in following order)	Position	Approximate time of test (min)	Apparatus required
Heart rate response to Valsalva manoeuvre	Sitting	5	Aneroid manometer, electrocardiograph
Heart rate response to deep breathing	Sitting	2	Electrocardiograph
Blood pressure response to sustained handgrip	Sitting	5	Handgrip dynamometer, sphygmomanometer
Heart rate response to standing up	Lying to standing	3	Electrocardiograph
Blood pressure response to standing up			Sphygmomanometer

are available for each of the tests. Although these are less than perfect, it must be remembered that a borderline area of uncertainty exists between normal and abnormal.

Autonomic neuropathy can be classified according to the severity of damage into one of five groups: (1) normal—all five tests normal or one borderline; (2) early involvement—one of the three heart rate tests abnormal or two borderline; (3) definite involvement—two or more of the heart rate tests abnormal; (4) severe involvement—two or more of the heart rate tests abnormal plus one or both of the blood pressure tests abnormal or both borderline; (5) atypical pattern—any other combination of abnormal tests (in the study quoted above only 6 per cent of patients tested were atypical). An alternative to this classification of severity is to give each individual test a score of 0, 1, or 2 depending on whether it is respectively normal, borderline, or abnormal. An overall 'autonomic test score' of 0–10 can then be obtained. Although increasing scores of 0–10 correlate closely with the grades of severity given above, scoring of the tests in this way allows the atypical pattern to be given an actual numerical value.

This battery of cardiovascular tests can be performed very easily in the clinic situation with only minimal equipment. All that is needed are a sphygmomanometer, an ECG machine, an aneroid pressure gauge attached to a mouthpiece by a rigid or flexible tube, and a handgrip dynamometer. With practice, a planned sequence of tests can be performed within 15–20 min. Measurement and calculation of the various ratios can be done in two ways. Before the advent of microcomputer systems, and still useful when tests are only occasionally performed, all that was required was a ruler and an ECG strip. Nowadays, however, a number of computer programs have been written which measure the R–R intervals automatically, calculate the required ratios, and group the results. Several systems have been described incorporating measurements of heart rate. In Edinburgh, a system is now in routine use based on the five tests described above and operates with a BBC or IBM PC or compatible microcomputer (AUTOCAFT, UnivEd Technologies Ltd, Edinburgh). It has the advantage of allowing blood pressure measurements to be entered and of automatically classifying the results.

The autonomic pathways involved in these cardiovascular reflexes are extremely complex and encompass both parasympathetic and sympathetic fibres to a greater or lesser extent. Most observers now agree that the heart rate response to deep breathing is mediated almost exclusively by cardiac parasympathetic pathways. Both the Valsalva manoeuvre and the lying-to-standing heart beat response rely to some extent on the integrity of sympathetic as well as parasympathetic pathways. While postural blood pressure control is predominantly dependent on intact peripheral sympathetic vasoconstriction, other factors such as blood volume may also contribute. The degree of orthostatic hypotension is also partly related to the degree of parasympathetic baroreflex dysfunction. The blood pressure response to sustained handgrip appears to be predominantly mediated by sympathetic pathways. A convincing argument has recently been put forward that abnormal cardiorespiratory reflexes may be due to a decrease in the efficacy of sensory motor nerve conduction around the reflex arc rather than simply being confined to vagal damage (Kennedy *et al.* 1989). The increased understanding of the extreme neuronal complexity of even apparently simple cardiovascular reflex pathways makes these observations particularly pertinent, as thinking moves away from the previous perhaps oversimplistic view of reflex control in the autonomic nervous system.

The classification proposed above for cardiovascular autonomic neuropathy avoids labelling reflex pathways as either precisely parasympathetic or sympathetic as it seems more logical to define autonomic involvement merely as early, definite, or severe. One trap for the unwary is to use a single cardiovascular reflex test for assessment of autonomic damage (usually the heart rate response to deep breathing) as this is misleading. It presumes that autonomic neuropathy is all or nothing and does not allow for a range of nerve damage from minimal to extremely extensive. There has also been confusion about terminology. It would seem better to use the term 'autonomic dysfunction' to refer to abnormalities of cardiovascular reflex tests, while reserving the term 'autonomic neuropathy' for the clinical syndrome of symptomatic autonomic features combined with abnormal cardiovascular reflexes.

Newer approaches to cardiovascular reflex tests

Mental arithmetic

This test has been re-evaluated recently by measuring hand skin temperature and heart rate changes after 1 min of serial subtractions. Diabetics with autonomic neuropathy showed no fall in skin temperature but this was not helpful in diagnostic terms. More reliable were the smaller heart rate changes found in the affected diabetics. As beta blockade significantly reduced the heart rate response to mental arithmetic stress in normal subjects, the authors concluded that the test might be used to evaluate sympathetic damage. When compared with sustained handgrip and postural hypotension, the mental arithmetic stress test appeared to be more sensitive than either (Locatelli *et al.* 1989).

Heart rate response to coughing

Coughing produces rapid intrathoracic pressure fluctuations with consequent haemodynamic and cardiovascular reflex effects. Normally a brief cough produces an immediate shortening of R–R interval (or increase in heart rate) reaching a peak in 2–3 s, which is followed by R–R interval lengthening back to the resting value over the next 18–20 s. The cardiac acceleration is abolished by atropine but not propranolol, showing that it is dependent on cardiac parasympathetic pathways. The heart rate response declines with age in normal subjects. One group found that diabetics with autonomic neuropathy had a response similar to normal subjects after autonomic blockade (Fig. 16.9) and suggested that this was another useful cardiovascular reflex test (Cardone *et al.* 1987, 1990). However, another group found that the heart rate responses to standing up and the Valsalva manoeuvre were superior to the heart rate response to coughing in evaluating arterial baroreflex cardiovascular function (Van Lieshout *et al.* 1989). Further studies are therefore required to see whether the cough test will, in fact, prove to be a useful non-invasive test.

Diving reflex (cold face test)

A cold compress applied to the face for 20 to 120 s produces consistent heart rate and blood flow reductions. The optimal time, before subjects found the stimulus uncomfortable, was between 40 and 60 s. This manoeuvre provides an additional test of vagal cardiac pathways, differing from the Valsalva manoeuvre and respiratory sinus arrhythmia in that its mediation is independent of pressure and stretch receptors in the thoracic cavity and

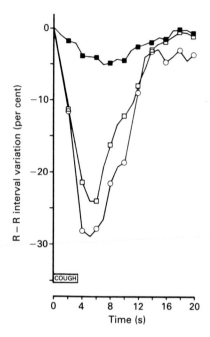

Fig. 16.9. Immediate heart rate response to coughing in: (open circles) six normal subjects; (open squares) six diabetics without; and (filled squares) six with autonomic neuropathy: group mean R–R interval variation (per cent) from baseline during the first 20 s. (From Cardone *et al.* (1987).)

afferent vagal fibres (Heath and Downey 1990). Further studies are indicated to see whether the technique is useful in autonomic damage.

Blood pressure control

Abnormal 24-h ambulatory blood pressure profiles have been found in diabetics with autonomic neuropathy, with a flattened diurnal blood pressure pattern, loss of the usual nocturnal fall, and, in some subjects, a paradoxical rise in blood pressure at night (Hornung *et al.* 1989). Another group used a beat-by-beat cuff tracking method and found less blood pressure variability in response to different stimuli in diabetics. The method appeared more sensitive than conventional heart rate and blood pressure tests. The authors claimed that the subtle blood pressure changes they found suggested signs of sympathetic dysfunction in young diabetic patients with no symptoms of neuropathy (Goldstein *et al.* 1988). They concluded that this and other beat-by-beat methods of recording blood pressure could have further research potential. This is discussed further in Chapter 15 where details of the recently developed Finapres device are reported in detail.

Cardiovascular autonomic abnormalities in diabetics

Sequence of abnormalities

The sequence of cardiovascular reflex abnormalities in diabetics is now becoming clearer. Autonomic damage is not simply present or absent but can be anywhere on the spectrum from minimal to severe. Cardiac parasympathetic function may be impaired without sympathetic damage but not the reverse, whereas detectable cardiac sympathetic lesions are usually found in longstanding diabetic subjects with extensive cardiac vagal damage.

Cardiovascular tests deteriorate with time. In a large group of diabetic patients heart rate tests were abnormal more commonly and earlier than blood pressure tests. When the tests were repeated, three-quarters were unchanged, one-quarter deteriorated, but only very few improved (Ewing *et al*. 1985). Early parasympathetic involvement may, however, be more apparent than real as heart rate tests are much more sensitive than blood pressure tests and therefore more likely to be abnormal. There is increasing evidence that deranged sympathetic function elsewhere can be found even in mild autonomic neuropathy, although within the heart it is likely that cardiac parasympathetic fibres are involved more extensively and earlier than cardiac sympathetic fibres, possibly because they are longer and therefore more liable to damage. In one recent study, heart rate variability decreased faster in diabetics than in normal subjects over time (Sampson *et al*. 1990).

Sudden death and prognosis

Mortality in diabetic autonomic neuropathy is about 50 per cent over 5 years based on our prospective Edinburgh survey. A recent survey from London, however, has concluded that the mortality of those with symptomatic autonomic neuropathy was somewhat lower at 37 per cent (Sampson *et al*. 1990). A proportion of diabetics with autonomic neuropathy die suddenly and unexpectedly but, of the possible explanations put forward, none is entirely convincing. Recently, a number of studies have shown that diabetics with autonomic neuropathy have a prolonged QT time on their ECG, and one study has shown that diabetics with autonomic neuropathy who died had longer QT times than those who survived (Ewing *et al*. 1991*a*). What the exact mechanism is for this or whether this is just an incidental finding has not yet been established.

Relation to other aspects of diabetes

Cardiac autonomic dysfunction is closely associated with other long-term diabetic complications, specifically retinal ischaemia and renal abnormalities.

Such studies add weight to previous suggestions that autonomic nerve damage is a contributory factor in the development and progression of the microvascular complications of diabetes. Obesity is an additional factor that may be associated with abnormal autonomic tests as diabetics with impaired cardiovascular reflex responses have been found to be heavier than those with normal responses. The progression of autonomic and indeed somatic neuropathy may be halted as glycaemic control is restored after pancreatic transplantation. Marked abnormalities of autonomic function are often found in painful neuropathy and, in those in whom pain later remitted, slight but significant improvement in autonomic function occurred. Hypoglycaemic unawareness, although almost always associated with autonomic neuropathy in the shorter-duration diabetics, is not necessarily associated in those of longer duration (see Ewing 1991).

Involvement of other systems

Respiratory abnormalities (see Chapter 23)

There have been further conflicting studies looking at respiratory abnormalities in diabetics with autonomic neuropathy. Bronchial reactivity has variably been found to be increased, reduced, and unchanged in response to various inhaled stimuli. Further studies examining the ventilatory responses to hypoxia and hypercapnia have also produced differing results. Although these point to abnormalities of bronchial vagal innervation, further studies are clearly needed to resolve the various discrepancies. There are therefore no reliable tests of autonomic function that can be recommended in the respiratory system in diabetes.

Pupil tests (see Chapter 22)

Two simple bedside tests to assess autonomic pupil function are available. The first measures the diameter of the dark-adapted pupil using a Polaroid photograph of the eye taken by electronic flash. When standardized against the outer diameter of the iris, the dark-adapted pupil diameter provides a quantitative estimate of sympathetic innervation. The second technique, measurement of pupil cycle time (PCT), depends on the observation that regular oscillations of the pupil can be induced with a slit lamp beam in normal subjects and timed with a stopwatch. Pharmacological testing confirms that PCT is a sensitive measure of parasympathetic dysfunction and, in diabetics with autonomic neuropathy, it is considerably prolonged. These techniques provide two additional simple methods of testing autonomic reflexes independent of cardiovascular pathways. More recently, portable systems to evaluate pupillary reflexes have been developed.

Sweat tests (see Chapter 21)

The quantification of sweating has challenged investigators for a long time. A simple sweat test, based on the local response to intradermal acetylcholine and counting the dark spots of iodine discoloration, has recently been reported. This is, in fact, a variant of the silastic mould method comprehensively described by Kennedy and Navarro (1989). Overall body sweating, using thermally induced sweating, correlates closely with another sweat test, the quantitative sudomotor axon reflex test (Q-SART).

Gastrointestinal tests (see Chapter 27)

Gastrointestinal findings in diabetics with autonomic neuropathy are included here for completeness although the tests are not strictly 'non-invasive'.

Salivary glands are richly innervated with autonomic fibres and, therefore, salivary composition might be affected by autonomic damage. One measure, the salivary glucose excretion rate, has been found to be reduced. This has been suggested as a simple screening test for diabetic autonomic neuropathy (Marchetti *et al.* 1989). Oesophageal function has been examined by the relatively new method of scintigraphy, using both liquid and solid boluses. A high proportion of diabetics have prolonged transit of a liquid bolus despite no symptoms referrable to the oesophagus. This and other studies confirm previous reports that diabetics with autonomic neuropathy frequently have diminished or disordered oesophageal peristalsis and delayed oesophageal emptying. A new observation has been that of associated abnormal pharyngeal function. Similarly, abnormal gastric emptying has frequently been found using isotope scanning and ultrasonography. Abnormalities of proximal small intestinal motility, involving both parasympathetic and sympathetic innervation, have been described in diabetics with gastric autonomic problems, including decreased intestinal transit times, and absent or grossly disordered interdigestive migrating motor complexes. Gall-bladder emptying has also been found to be significantly impaired.

Neuroendocrine disturbances (see Chapter 17)

Several different abnormalities of catecholamine metabolism have recently been reported. Plasma dihydroxyphenylglycol (DHPG), a chemical that is partly dependent on intraneural de-amination of recaptured noradrenaline in the synaptic cleft, may be useful as an alternative autonomic marker. The ratio of DHPG to noradrenaline distinguished quite well between diabetics with and without cardiovascular reflex evidence of autonomic neuropathy (Christensen *et al.* 1988). The noradrenaline response to intravenous edrophonium, which is abnormal in severe sympathetic damage, correlated with other autonomic tests and demonstrated simultaneous autonomic involvement in different systems (Matthews *et al.* 1987). The adrenaline disappearance rate is significantly longer and platelet noradrenaline efflux higher in diabetics with autonomic neuropathy.

Other studies have confirmed that diabetics with autonomic neuropathy have reduced pancreatic polypeptide secretion after a meal. Indeed, reduced pancreatic polypeptide and adrenaline responses to hypoglycaemia in early diabetics may predict later overt autonomic neuropathy. Osmotic release of vasopressin appears normal in diabetics but cardiovascular release is impaired in those with autonomic neuropathy, reflecting an afferent defect. Atrial natriuretic peptide release is probably not related to autonomic neuropathy. Renin control, however, may be. Two recent studies have found increased inactive renin in diabetics with autonomic neuropathy.

Conclusion

The place of non-invasive cardiovascular reflex tests is now firmly established for the objective bedside or out-patient assessment of diabetic autonomic neuropathy. Heart rate variability analysis, however, may have other applications, particularly in the early diagnosis of autonomic disorders and for estimation of cardiac parasympathetic activity in a number of different contexts. Over the next few years, study of heart rate variability should give rise to a number of new insights into mechanisms of disease and the way in which certain drugs work.

Some new cardiovascular tests are being developed but have not yet stood the test of time. In diabetes mellitus disordered autonomic function, although not always clinically apparent, can be detected throughout the body if techniques are sensitive enough. While tests have been described for most body systems, very few stand up to critical analysis as useful non-invasive tests with adequate repeatability, although some give valuable insights into the pathophysiology of diabetic autonomic neuropathy.

Much scope still remains for the further development and refinement of non-invasive tests to detect autonomic damage in all body systems.

References

Akselrod, S., Gordon, D., Madwed, J. B., Snidman, N. C., Shannon, D. C., and Cohen, R. J. (1985). Hemodynamic regulation: investigation by spectral analysis. *Am. J. Physiol.* **249**, H867–75.

Bernardi, L., Rossi, M., Soffiantino, F., Marti, G., Ricordi, L., Finardi, G., and Fratino, P. (1989). Cross correlation of heart rate and respiration versus deep breathing. Assessment of new test of cardiac autonomic function in diabetes. *Diabetes* **38**, 589–96.

Cardone, C., Bellavere, F., Ferri, M., and Fedele, D. (1987). Autonomic mechanisms in the heart rate response to coughing. *Clin. Sci.* **72**, 55–60.

Cardone, C., Paiusco, P., Marchetti, G., Burelli, F., Feruglio, M., and Fedele, D. (1990). Cough test to assess cardiovascular autonomic reflexes in diabetes *Diabetes Care* **13**, 719–24.

Christensen, N. J., Degjaard, A., and Hilsted, J. (1988). Plasma dihydroxy-phenylglycol (DHPG) as an index of diabetic autonomic neuropathy. *Clin. Physiol.* **8**, 577–80.

Ewing, D. J. (1991). Autonomic neuropathy. In *Diabetes annual*, Vol. 6 (ed. K. G. M. M. Alberti and L. P. Krall), pp. 326–46. Elsevier Science Publishers, Amsterdam.

Ewing, D. J., Neilson, J. M. M., and Travis, P. (1984). New method for assessing cardiac parasympathetic activity using 24 hour electrocardiograms. *Br. Heart J.* **52**, 396–402.

Ewing, D. J., Martyn, C. N., Young, R. J., and Clarke, B. F. (1985). The value of cardiovascular autonomic function tests: 10 years experience in diabetes. *Diabetes Care* **8**, 491–8.

Ewing, D. J., Boland, O., Neilson, J. M. M., Cho, C. G., and Clarke, B. F. (1991*a*). Autonomic neuropathy, QT interval lengthening, and unexpected deaths in male diabetic patients. *Diabetologia* **34**, 182–5.

Ewing, D. J., Neilson, J. M. M., Shapiro, C. M., Stewart, J. A., and Reid, W. (1991*b*). Twenty four hour heart rate variability: effects of posture, sleep, and time of day in healthy controls and comparison with bedside tests of autonomic function in diabetic patients. *Br. Heart J.* **65**, 239–44.

Flapan, A. D., Nolan, J., Neilson, J. M. M., and Ewing, D. J. (1990). Captopril therapy increases parasympathetic activity in patients with congestive cardiac failure. *Circulation* **82** (suppl. 2), 382.

Furlan, R., Guzzetti, S., Crivellaro, W., Dassi, S., Tinelli, M., Baselli, G., Cerutti, S., Lombardi, F., Pagani, M., and Malliani, A. (1990). Continuous 24-hour assessment of the neural regulation of systemic arterial pressure and RR variabilities in ambulant subjects. *Circulation* **81**, 537–47.

Goldstein, I. B., Naliboff, B. D., Shapiro, D., and Frank, H. J. L. (1988). Beat-to-beat blood pressure response in asymptomatic IDDM subjects. *Diabetes Care* **11**, 774–9.

Heath, M. E. and Downey, J. A. (1990). The cold face test (diving reflex) in clinical autonomic assessment: methodological considerations and repeatability of responses. *Clin. Sci.* **78**, 139–47.

Hornung, R. S., Mahler, R. F., and Raftery, E. B. (1989). Ambulatory blood pressure and heart rate in diabetic patients: an assessment of autonomic function. *Diabetic Med.* **6**, 579–85.

Kennedy, W. R. and Navarro, X. (1989). Sympathetic sudomotor function in diabetic neuropathy. *Arch. Neurol.* **46**, 1182–6.

Kennedy, W. R., Navarro, X., Sakuta, M., Mandell, H., Knox, C. K., and Sutherland, D. E. R. (1989). Physiological and clinical correlates of cardiorespiratory reflexes in diabetes mellitus. *Diabetes Care* **12**, 399–408.

Kleiger, R. E., Miller, J. P., Bigger, J. T., and Moss, A. J. (1987). Decreased heart rate variability and its association with increased mortality after acute myocardial infarction. *Am. J. Cardiol.* **59**, 256–62.

Locatelli, A., Franzetti, I., Lepore, G., Maglio, M. L., Gaudio, E., Caviezel, F., and Pozza, G. (1989). Mental arithmetic stress as a test for evaluation of diabetic sympathetic autonomic neuropathy. *Diabetic Med.* **6**, 490–5.

Marchetti, P., Tognarelli, M., Giannarelli, R., Crossi, C., Picardo, L., Di Carlo, A., Benzi, L., Ciccarone, A., and Navalesi, R. (1989). Decreased salivary glucose secretory rate: usefulness for detection of diabetic patients with autonomic neuropathy. *Diabetes Res. Clin. Pract.* **7**, 181–6.

Matthews, D. M., Martyn, C. N., Riemersma, R. A., Clarke, B. F., and Ewing, D. J. (1987). Noradrenaline response to edrophonium (tensilon) and its relation to other autonomic tests in diabetic subjects. *Diabetes Res.* **6**, 175–80.

Pagani, M., Lombardi, F., Guzzetti, S., Rimoldi, O., Furlan, R., Pizzinelli, P., Sandrone, G., Malfatto, G., Del'Orto, S., Piccaluga, E., Turiel, M., Baselli, G., Cerutti, S., and Malliani, A. (1986). Power spectral analysis of heart rate and arterial pressure variabilities as a marker of sympatho-vagal interaction in man and conscious dog. *Circulation Res.* **59**, 178–93.

Pomeranz, B., Macaulay, R. J. B., Caudill, M. A., Kutz, I., Adam, D., Gordon, D., Kilborn, K. M., Barger, A. C., Shannon, D. C., Cohen, R. J., and Benson, H. (1985). Assessment of autonomic function in humans by heart rate spectral analysis. *Am. J. Physiol.* **248**, H151–3.

Rosenbleuth, A. and Simeone, F. A. (1934). The interrelations of vagal and accelerator effects on the cardiac rate. *Am. J. Physiol.* **110**, 42–55.

Sampson, M. J., Wilson, S., Karagiannis, P., Edmonds, M., and Watkins, P. J. (1990). Progression of diabetic autonomic neuropathy over a decade in insulin-dependent diabetics. *Quart. J. Med.* **75**, 635–46.

San Antonio Conference on Diabetic Neuropathy (1988). Report and recommendations of the San Antonio conference on diabetic neuropathy. *Diabetes* **37**, 1000–4.

Van Lieshout, E. J., Van Lieshout, J. J., Ten Harkel, A. J. D., and Wieling, W. (1989). Cardiovascular response to coughing: its value in the assessment of autonomic nervous control. *Clin. Sci.* **77**, 305–10.

Zuanetti, G., Latini, R., Neilson, J. M. M., Schwartz, P. J., and Ewing, D. J. (1991). Heart rate variability in patients with ventricular arrhythmias: effect of antiarrhythmic drugs. *J. Am. Coll. Cardiol.* **17**, 604–12.

17. Neuropharmacological investigation of autonomic failure

Ronald J. Polinsky

Introduction

Autonomic nervous system testing has evolved over the last 20 years in conjunction with advances in analytical capability in the laboratory. Development of sensitive specific assays for measuring neurotransmitters and neuropeptides in various biological fluids has fostered a new era in clinical neuroscience. It is now feasible to carry out investigations in man that parallel studies in experimental animals. Neuropharmacological assessment of

Table 17.1. Neuropharmacological approaches for investigating autonomic failure

Target	Strategy
Postganglionic sympathetic neuron	Plasma NA at rest and in response to stimuli NA metabolites in plasma, urine Clearance of NA Pressor responsivity
Peripheral parasympathetic function	Pancreatic polypeptide response to hypoglycaemia Basal gastrin levels
Adrenal medullary activity	Plasma A responses to hypoglycaemia, cholinergic stimulation
Sympathetic ganglia	Plasma NA responses to acetylcholine
CNS pathways	Cardiovascular responses to various drugs PET scanning Neurotransmitters, metabolites, enzymes, peptides in CSF Plasma and/or urinary levels of hormones, peptides, metabolites following activation

NA, noradrenaline; A, adrenaline.

autonomic function has a distinct advantage over the physiological approach. Although both strategies yield useful information that help to localize lesion(s), the pharmacological characteristics of the disorder often provide a rational foundation for treatment.

The contrast between two distinct disorders, pure autonomic failure (PAF) and multiple system atrophy (MSA), illustrates the value of a neuropharmacological approach. Despite similar clinical manifestations of autonomic failure the underlying lesion(s) have different characteristics in these two syndromes. Application of the various tests listed in Table 17.1 has substantially increased our understanding of PAF and MSA. Abnormal functioning of the nervous system and related control mechanisms contributes to the pathophysiology in these disorders.

Much work in this area has been directed towards postural hypotension, the most disabling aspect of autonomic failure. Consequently, post-ganglionic noradrenergic neuronal function is a major focus of research efforts since this unit is the primary link between the nervous system and blood pressure control. Several neurological and neuroendocrine mechanisms participate in the regulation of other vital functions under automatic control. This chapter summarizes the neuropharmacological approach to evaluating the autonomic nervous system. A discussion of neurotransmitter and neuropeptide function in patients with autonomic failure emphasizes the distinction between peripheral and central disorders.

Peripheral mechanisms

Relatively simple, non-invasive access to the appropriate biological compartments facilitates evaluation of the peripheral components of autonomic control. In addition, the peripheral origins of neurotransmitters and their metabolites in plasma and urine have been more clearly defined in comparison with central nervous system contributions.

Sympathetic noradrenergic neuronal function

Noradrenaline is the primary neurotransmitter released from most postganglionic sympathetic neurons. Several aspects of sympathetic neuronal function provide the basis for characterizing abnormalities in autonomic failure: synthesis, storage, release, uptake, and metabolism. The general approach for evaluating these functional characteristics involves measurement of noradrenaline and metabolite levels in plasma and urine under baseline conditions and after application of various physiological and pharmacological stimuli.

Plasma noradrenaline

Following release of noradrenaline into the synaptic cleft in response to nerve impulses, a small amount (approximately 10 per cent) reaches the plasma. This 'spillover' of noradrenaline provides a biochemical window to view sympathetic nerve activity. Great care must be observed in obtaining and handling blood samples for plasma noradrenaline measurement. The levels in blood change very rapidly and are extremely responsive to external and internal stimuli. The age of the subject and site of sampling also affect plasma noradrenaline. Despite these limitations the neurotransmitter levels in plasma can be used as an index of sympathetic function as long as the experimental protocol and methods for analysis are rigorously controlled and standardized. Plasma noradrenaline levels correlate with electrophysiological measurements of muscle sympathetic nerve activity in man (Wallin *et al.* 1981).

Plasma noradrenaline levels in PAF and MSA reflect distinct pathophysiological consequences of autonomic failure in the two disorders. MSA patients generally have normal (150–300 pg/ml) or slightly elevated supine plasma noradrenaline levels. Occasional patients manifest low levels (less than 100 pg/ml), suggestive of peripheral involvement. Although direct recording of sympathetic nerve activity in a single patient with MSA reveals evidence of preganglionic dysfunction (Dotson *et al.* 1990), electromyographic studies have demonstrated denervation changes in selected muscle groups. Cohen *et al.* (1987) identified somatic neuropathy in approximately 20 per cent of their MSA patients. In contrast to MSA, the basal supine plasma noradrenaline levels in PAF are lower than normal. The only group of PAF patients reported to have nearly normal noradrenaline levels also manifested significantly decreased clearance which could elevate the plasma level (Esler *et al.* 1980). This aspect of sympathetic neuronal function will be discussed later in the chapter.

Most studies confirm the above difference in supine plasma noradrenaline levels; however, the diagnostic value of this neurochemical measure is limited by substantial overlap among normal, MSA, and PAF groups. In the author's experience, only 4 per cent of patients with MSA have a plasma level less than 100 pg/ml. In contrast, approximately 20 per cent of PAF patients manifest levels greater than 100 pg/ml. Thus, a normal plasma noradrenaline level supports the clinical diagnosis of MSA. However, a low value has much greater significance in establishing the diagnosis of PAF, especially if observed early in the course of the disease.

It must be emphasized that this index of sympathetic activity should be used in conjunction with the results of other investigative procedures. A single value for plasma noradrenaline is analogous to an individual frame of a moving picture. Although it bears a relationship to the preceding and subsequent frames, an isolated shot contributes little to understanding the entire sequence. Consider the example of measuring plasma noradrenaline after a venipuncture: the level rises dramatically following needle insertion and then gradually declines to basal levels in approximately 15–20 min. Without knowledge of the basal level and time from the stimulus, measurement of noradrenaline levels could lead to drastically different conclusions about clinical status. Postural change is a standardized stimulus which elicits an increase in sympathetic nerve activity; at least 5 min should elapse before samples are taken to assess the plasma noradrenaline response. This protocol is based on the relatively short half-life of noradrenaline in plasma; interpretation is facilitated by sampling after a steady state has been achieved. Plasma noradrenaline levels double when normal subjects stand. This increment reflects the increased sympathetic nerve activity required to maintain blood pressure despite gravity-induced pooling of blood in the lower extremities. Neither patients with MSA nor PAF manifest an adequate increase in plasma noradrenaline on standing. The implication of these observations is that both groups have lesion(s) that prevent normal operation of the baroreflex arc. Low basal supine noradrenaline levels in PAF suggest primary involvement of postganglionic sympathetic neurons, whereas the normal or slightly elevated levels in MSA are consistent with a more central lesion that causes failure to activate relatively intact peripheral noradrenergic neurons.

Neuronal uptake of noradrenaline

As mentioned above, plasma noradrenaline levels are affected by a variety of factors, including the processes involved with its disposition following release at the nerve ending. The neuronal uptake mechanism can be qualitatively evaluated by measuring the physiological and biochemical effects of an indirectly acting sympathomimetic drug. Such agents require: (1) an intact uptake mechanism to enter the nerve ending; and (2) adequate neuronal stores of noradrenaline. Their pharmacological effects are exerted through release of endogenous neurotransmitter. This approach is more relevant to the distinction between denervation and decentralization which will be discussed in a subsequent section. An alternative strategy, though not practical at most institutions, consists of measuring the kinetic disposition of radiolabelled catecholamines. In theory it is necessary to achieve steady-state conditions so that the various processes which determine the plasma noradrenaline concentration are at equilibrium. From a practical standpoint, tracer infusion should be maintained for at least 3 half-lives of the substance under investigation. The advantage of this method lies in the quantitative values that can be derived from equations for calculating the clearance of noradrenaline and its endogenous secretion rate into plasma. Since neuronal uptake is the primary mechanism for terminating the effects of released noradrenaline, assessment of clearance provides a useful index of sympathetic function.

Despite the importance of evaluating neuronal uptake, there have been only two studies of noradrenaline kinetics in autonomic failure (Esler *et al.* 1980; Polinsky *et al.* 1985). Although both groups found reduced noradrenaline clearance in PAF, the patients studied by Esler *et al.* (1980) had normal basal levels of the catecholamine. Uptake may have been affected out of proportion to synthesis and release so that the slower removal of noradrenaline resulted in an increase of the plasma level into the normal range. These findings highlight the need to investigate clearance. Delayed clearance could also explain the prolonged pressor effect observed following injection of sympathomimetic amines in some patients with autonomic failure. Polinsky *et al.* (1985) demonstrated a striking deficit of neuronal uptake in PAF by comparing the disappearance rates of radiolabelled noradrenaline and isoproterenol. The latter compound is only cleared through extraneuronal mechanisms; hence, its disappearance from plasma is normally much slower than noradrenaline. In patients with PAF, noradrenaline and isoproterenol are removed from plasma at similar rates. The very low plasma levels and clearance in these patients reflect severe involvement of postganglionic sympathetic neurons. Normal noradrenaline clearance in MSA indicates that these neurons remain functionally intact.

Noradrenaline metabolism

Another approach to evaluating sympathetic function is based on the dissociation in metabolic fate between noradrenaline taken up into sympathetic neurons and that which escapes into plasma. Intraneuronal metabolism results in the formation of de-aminated metabolites following the action of monoamine oxidase on cytoplasmic noradrenaline. Neuronal uptake and leakage of vesicular noradrenaline contribute to the cytoplasmic pool of neurotransmitter. Dihydroxyphenylglycol (DHPG) results from intraneuronal noradrenaline metabolism; subsequent enzymatic reactions yield vanillylmandelic acid (VMA) and 3-methoxy,4-hydroxyphenylglycol (MHPG). Through the action of extraneuronal catechol-O-methyltransferase,

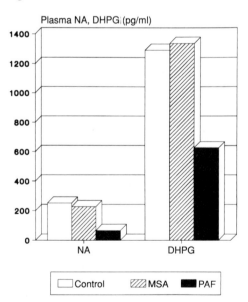

Fig. 17.1. Plasma noradrenaline (NA) and dihydroxyphenylglycol (DHPG) levels in control subjects and patients with autonomic failure.

normetanephrine is formed from released noradrenaline that is not taken up into sympathetic nerve endings. Conjugation protects a small portion of normetanephrine from de-amination; this conjugated normetanephrine is excreted by the kidney.

In MSA there is a disproportionate reduction in the urinary excretion of normetanephrine; total metabolites are normal or slightly decreased (Kopin et al. 1983b). This metabolite pattern is consistent with failure to activate functionally intact noradrenergic neurons since the selective decrease in normetanephrine reflects a reduction in noradrenaline release. All noradrenaline metabolites are decreased in PAF consistent with an overall reduction in noradrenergic neurons. These results have been confirmed and extended through measurement of plasma catechol patterns (Fig. 17.1). The rate-limiting step in catecholamine synthesis involves tyrosine hydroxylase; thus, plasma levels of dihydroxyphenylalanine (dopa) may serve as an index of noradrenaline synthesis. Although plasma dopa levels are normal, noradrenaline and DHPG are low in PAF as anticipated (Goldstein et al. 1989). A preganglionic dysfunction in MSA is supported by the observation of normal catechol levels in plasma; basal levels of dopa, noradrenaline, and DHPG confirm normal operation of synthetic and degradative pathways in sympathetic neurons. Although the number of patients is small, Goldstein et al. (1989) suggest that peripheral involvement may occur in MSA. The relationship between DHPG and noradrenaline in MSA patients differs from that in normal subjects; less noradrenaline may be released through exocytosis relative to the amount of noradrenaline synthesized. In one subgroup, low noradrenaline attended by normal dopa and DHPG levels reflects a greater discrepancy between synthesis and release. Another pattern in MSA consists of normal noradrenaline and low dopa and DHPG; this is consistent with a reduction in synthesis accompanied by a compensatory increase in exocytotic release of noradrenaline.

In PAF the DHPG/noradrenaline ratio was much higher than in control subjects. Since newly synthesized noradrenaline preferentially leaks into the cytoplasm, DHPG formation continues in the absence of noradrenaline release. Two subgroups of PAF patients were identified: (1) low noradrenaline and normal dopa and DHPG; and (2) low noradrenaline and DHPG and substantially reduced dopa. The former group may have increased noradrenaline synthesis in remaining neurons as a compensatory mechanism but the high DHPG/noradrenaline ratio suggests either decreased postganglionic sympathetic activity or defective exocytotic release. In the latter group vesicular uptake might be affected. Of special importance are the findings in patients with dopamine β-hydroxylase deficiency which causes a selective disturbance in noradrenaline production. As predicted, noradrenaline and DHPG are virtually absent from plasma. However, high dopa levels suggest an attempt to increase synthesis, consistent with the increase in sympathetic nerve activity identified by microneurography. These results demonstrate the value of examining noradrenaline metabolism, which may not only facilitate the distinction between central and peripheral lesions but may elucidate intraneuronal abnormalities as well.

Noradrenergic cardiovascular responses

Pharmacological assessment of sympathetic nervous system function is based on the descriptions of supersensitivity that appeared in the literature more than a century ago. This important facet depends indirectly on the function of noradrenergic neurons since postsynaptic end-organ changes may be secondary to noradrenaline output. The ability of the baroreflex to modulate changes in cardiovascular parameters is also critical. Drugs with selective mechanisms of action test various components of the system. A non-adrenergic pressor drug, e.g. angiotensin, may be used to assess the end-organ response (vaso-constriction). Noradrenaline and isoproterenol effect cardiovascular changes through stimulation of α- and β-adrenoceptors, respectively. Tyramine causes a pressor effect through release of endogenous noradrenaline stores.

The neuropharmacological consequences of lesioning experiments in animals provide a basis for interpreting the results of pressor infusion studies in patients with autonomic failure. A postganglionic lesion (denervation) enhances the response to noradrenaline; there is also a loss of sympathetic neuronal noradrenaline stores. A more modest increase in pressor responsivity follows a preganglionic lesion; however, this change is non-specific and is not attended by a reduction in the response to indirectly acting sympatho-mimetics. Both types of lesions interrupt the sympathetic nervous system component of the baroreflex arc. Several principles regarding interpretation of pharmacological dose–response curves are relevant to understanding clinical investigations. Although these relationships have a sigmoidal shape when appropriately plotted on a semi-logarithmic scale, it is the linear portion that has clinical importance. Two characteristics, threshold and gain, are crucial to the distinction between denervation and decentralization. Gain is the slope of the dose–response curve and threshold is the dose at which the response begins. With respect to blood pressure–log dose relationships, gain and threshold, respectively, reflect baroreflex modulation and adrenoceptor sensitivity. Discussion of the results obtained using the pharmacological approach in patients with autonomic failure will illustrate this type of analysis.

Exaggerated cardiovascular responses to a variety of drugs have been reported in MSA and PAF. These include noradrenaline, angiotensin, isoproterenol, dopamine, tyramine, methoxamine, vasopressin, and somato-statin (and its analogues). The wide array of pharmacological agents reflects the non-specific nature of this hyperresponsivity. An increase in gain of the blood pressure–dose response curves to noradrenaline and angiotensin is manifested in patients with PAF and MSA (Fig. 17.2). The increased slope of the pressor response is consistent with a lesion in the baroreflex arc preventing normal modulation of blood pressure (Polinsky *et al.* 1981*a*). Bannister *et al.* (1979) found that the magnitude of the pressor response to

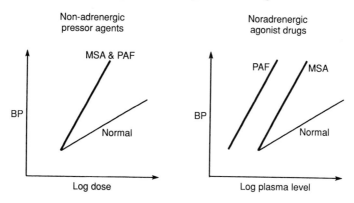

Fig. 17.2. Schematic representation of pressor responses to different drug classes in autonomic failure.

noradrenaline appeared to correlate with the degree of baroreflex impairment. They also observed the greatest sensitivity to noradrenaline in a PAF patient who had a prolonged pressor effect following a bolus injection, suggesting that the mechanism of hyperresponsivity in PAF might differ from MSA. In contrast to MSA, the blood pressure response to intravenous noradrenaline in PAF is characterized by a shift to the left (Fig. 17.2). This leftward shift is a manifestation of true adrenoceptor supersensitivity, presumably the result of a postganglionic lesion (Polinsky *et al.* 1981*a*). Chronotropic and vasodepressor responses to isoproterenol in PAF are characterized by similar evidence of β-adrenergic supersensitivity (Baser *et al.* 1991). These results further confirm the pharmacological distinction between PAF and MSA observed by Kontos *et al.* (1976). In their study, both groups decreased forearm blood flow in response to intraarterial administration of noradrenaline, but only those with MSA responded to tyramine. Polinsky *et al.* (1981*a*) found that patients with PAF manifested a significantly smaller increment in plasma noradrenaline following intravenous bolus injections of tyramine compared to normal subjects or patients with MSA. The reduced response to an indirectly acting sympathomimetic in PAF gives additional support for the presence of a postganglionic lesion in this disorder.

In summary, pressor responsivity is increased in both PAF and MSA, but the mechanism underlying this change differs in the two disorders. Low resting plasma noradrenaline and metabolites, decreased neuronal uptake, leftward shift of the cardiovascular dose–response curves to adrenergic agonist drugs, and diminished responses to tyramine provide clear evidence for postganglionic noradrenergic dysfunction in PAF. Normal indices of peripheral noradrenergic function together with a non-specific increase in pressor responsivity point to a primary involvement of the central nervous system in MSA. Thus, pharmacological investigations can be used to localize lesions within the nervous system pathways that control cardiovascular function.

In addition, assessment of plasma catechol patterns shows promise for further defining abnormalities of the sympathetic nervous system.

Peripheral parasympathetic function

Neurochemical research on autonomic failure has focused on the nor-adrenergic nervous system because biochemical indices are available for evaluating sympathetic neuronal function. Acetylcholine, the neurotransmitter of parasympathetic neurons in the periphery, is extremely labile in plasma and attempts to measure and use it as a meaningful index, analogous to noradrenaline, have been unsuccessful. Another approach which overcomes these limitations is the assessment of hormonal mechanisms controlled by the parasympathetic nervous system; pancreatic polypeptide and gastrin are two examples which illustrate this strategy. Unlike true circulating hormones, these peptides are released locally through nerve stimulation and produce functional changes in nearby structures. Their levels in plasma may have little to do with physiological parameters (e.g. blood pressure, heart rate) but may serve as an index of parasympathetic activity.

Although the physiological importance of pancreatic polypeptide is unclear, it is one of several gut peptides released during insulin hypoglycaemia. Release of pancreatic polypeptide appears to be mediated through a vagal, cholinergic mechanism (see Polinsky *et al.* 1982 for references). The increase in plasma levels of pancreatic polypeptide induced by insulin is blocked by muscarinic

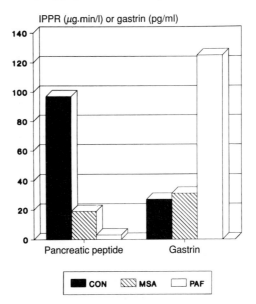

Fig. 17.3. Integrated pancreatic polypeptide response (IPPR) to hypoglycaemia and basal gastrin levels in normal controls (CON) and patients with MSA or PAF.

anticholinergic drugs and truncal vagotomy. Since hypoglycaemia also elicits elevation of plasma catecholamines, insulin administration can be used to simultaneously assess sympathetic and parasympathetic function. In normal subjects hypoglycaemia is attended by a precipitous rise in plasma levels of pancreatic polypeptide. This response is virtually absent in PAF and in most patients with MSA (Fig. 17.3). Polinsky *et al.* (1982) found no correlation between catecholamine and peptide responses, consistent with their independent neural control. In the few MSA patients who manifested an increment in pancreatic polypeptide, subsequent testing revealed a loss of this response as the illness progressed. Deficient or absent pancreatic polypeptide responses provide biochemical evidence for parasympathetic involvement in PAF and MSA. Unfortunately, this test has no localizing value since the response to hypoglycaemia depends on the functional integrity of central and peripheral pathways.

Control of gastrin release is more complicated. Although vagal stimulation increases gastrin release, basal levels are increased following vagotomy. The physiological consequences of vagotomy, i.e. gastric distension and increased stomach pH, predominate in this situation. Hypoglycaemia continues to elicit a gastrin response even after highly selective vagotomy. An adrenergic mechanism appears to be involved in mediating the response during hypoglycaemia. Infusion of adrenaline releases gastrin through β-adrenergic stimulation; there is also a correlation between the gastrin increment and the plasma adrenaline response during hypoglycaemia. The pattern of basal and stimulated gastrin levels differs in PAF and MSA (Polinsky *et al.* 1988*b*). High basal levels in PAF reflect peripheral parasympathetic involvement (Fig. 17.3); in fact, gastrin levels in some patients are similar to those observed in achlorhydric subjects. Gastrin responses during hypoglycaemia are respectively lower and higher than normal in MSA and PAF. As discussed earlier in this chapter, only patients with PAF have adrenoceptor supersensitivity. Thus, although both groups have deficient catecholamine responses, the effects on gastrin release differ since β-adrenergic sensitivity is normal in MSA. Infusion studies with isoproterenol confirm this pathophysiological distinction. Only patients with PAF manifest a greater than normal increase in plasma gastrin levels during isoproterenol administration. Hence, measurement of basal and isoproterenol-induced gastrin levels permits assessment of peripheral vagal and β-adrenoceptor function. The response to hypoglycaemia may give an indirect indication of the latter.

Adrenal medullary activity

In accord with its teleological function, the adrenal gland secretes adrenaline and a small amount of noradrenaline into the bloodstream in response to stressful stimuli. Although adrenaline plays a critical role during catastrophic circulatory compromise, adrenal medullary activity is more directly related to metabolic control. Catecholamines can effect an increase in various metabolic mechanisms to counter the consequences of hypoglycaemia. In this manner, adrenaline functions more like a hormone than a neurotransmitter. The primacy of this protective response is highlighted by the order in which glucose counterregulatory hormones are secreted: adrenaline, noradrenaline, glucagon, growth hormone, and cortisol. Studies of insulin-induced hypoglycaemia as a stimulus for evaluating adrenal medullary activity began in the early part of this century. Despite the importance of this specialized ganglion, few additional studies have been conducted since Luft and von Euler (1953) reported a lack of catecholamine excretion in response to insulin-induced hypoglycaemia in two patients with postural hypotension.

Investigation of catecholamines during insulin-induced hypoglycaemia has yielded valuable insight into the normal physiological response (Polinsky *et al.* 1980). The glucose recovery curve following the nadir of hypoglycaemia is characterized by two phases in normal subjects: an initial rapid rise precedes a slower return towards euglycaemia. The fall in blood glucose is attended by a dramatic rise in plasma adrenaline which peaks within minutes of the lowest blood sugar. This striking adrenaline response is analogous to an intravenous injection of the neurotransmitter. Its importance is exemplified by the absence of the initial rapid phase of glucose recovery in patients who lack catecholamine responses during hypoglycaemia. Fortunately, other counterregulatory mechanisms, including glucagon, growth hormone, and cortisol, function normally in these patients (Polinsky *et al.* 1981*b*). Most patients with MSA or PAF manifest deficient catecholamine responses to hypoglycaemia because a lesion at any point in the pathway from central glucose receptors to the adrenal medulla would block the reflex. Thus, assessment of the adrenal medullary response has important clinical and therapeutic implications but cannot be used to identify the site of lesions in autonomic failure. It is possible, however, to employ a pharmacological strategy to further characterize an abnormal adrenaline response. Arecoline, a cholinergic agonist, stimulates muscarinic and nicotinic receptors. Following pre-treatment with a muscarinic blocking drug, only patients with MSA increase their plasma adrenaline levels, consistent with a central lesion preventing the response to hypoglycaemia (Polinsky *et al.* 1991*a*). Primary involvement of adrenal medullary innervation probably occurs in PAF since these patients do not respond to arecoline or hypoglycaemia (Fig. 17.4).

Counterregulatory mechanisms can be examined in the absence of cate-cholamine responses in patients with adrenergic insufficiency. As indicated above, their glucose recovery curves demonstrate that adrenaline is responsible for the initial rapid phase of glucose elevation in man. This is consistent with the view that adrenaline release protects against severely stressful insults until other more slowly responsive mechanisms come into play. Furthermore, these patients are able to recover from severe hypoglycaemia, indicating that adrenaline is not essential for restoring euglycaemia or eliciting other glucose

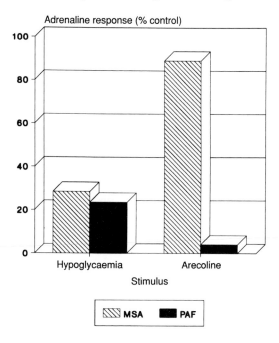

Fig. 17.4.   Adrenal medullary responses to hypoglycaemia and intravenous arecoline in patients with autonomic failure.

counterregulatory hormones. The noradrenaline response during hypoglycaemia may be a compensatory mechanism to counter the hypotensive effect of insulin.

Central mechanisms

Although sympathetic ganglia are anatomically located in the periphery, their synaptic function is primarily governed by cholinergic neurons whose cell bodies are in the intermediolateral cell column of the spinal cord. Thus, evaluation of ganglion function provides a natural transition from peripheral to central mechanisms.

Sympathetic ganglia

As discussed earlier in this chapter, tests of peripheral noradrenergic function in MSA reveal findings characteristic of decentralization. Furthermore, the number of intermediolateral column neurons is reduced in MSA. In order to investigate ganglionic function, Polinsky *et al.* (1991*c*) measured plasma noradrenaline responses to intravenously administered acetylcholine in patients with autonomic failure. Peripheral muscarinic effects were blocked to study ganglionic (nicotinic) effects of the drug. Normal subjects increase their plasma noradrenaline levels in proportion to the acetylcholine infusion rate. Lack of a noradrenaline increase in PAF is consistent with postganglionic sympathetic involvement, previously demonstrated by a variety of neuro-chemical and pharmacological methods. However, two distinct response patterns were evident in the MSA patients. One group did not increase their plasma noradrenaline levels while the other MSA patients manifested an exaggerated response at low doses followed by a decrease to normal levels as the infusion rate was increased. The biphasic response in the latter group suggests cholinergic supersensitivity with depolarization blockade at higher doses. Although the lack of response in the former group might indicate peripheral involvement as in PAF, extreme supersensitivity could produce blockade at even the lowest acetylcholine doses. Pharmacological demonstra-tion of ganglionic supersensitivity further distinguishes peripheral and central lesions of the sympathetic nervous system. Although somewhat speculative, lesions more central than the intermediolateral column might not result in cholinergic ganglionic supersensitivity.

Central nervous system neurotransmitter pathways

Three general approaches have been utilized to overcome the inherent difficulties in studying central nervous system (CNS) neurotransmitter function in man: (1) neuroimaging; (2) neurochemical; and (3) neuro-endocrine. Each strategy has limitations which differ according to practical and theoretical issues. Functional neuroimaging studies are very expensive and depend critically upon access to a cyclotron, required to produce neurotransmitter precursors and ligands labelled with positron-emitting isotopes. From a theoretical standpoint it is important to verify the behaviour of these compounds. The primary advantage of this positron emission tomography (PET) application is that technological advances permit direct visualization and quantitation of regional brain function. Although less direct than the previous approach, measurement of neurotransmitter-related substances in the cerebrospinal fluid (CSF) provides an opportunity to simultaneously study multiple systems with little risk or inconvenience to the patient. However, standardized methods for collection and storage are imperative. In addition, the use of particular substances as indices of specific neuronal systems requires a thorough knowledge of their origin in CSF and the various factors that affect interpretation of the findings. The most indirect method involves the application of neuroendocrine paradigms. In some instances, it is possible to measure the levels of substances in plasma or urine. Otherwise, drugs with specific mechanisms of action must be employed to elicit hormonal/peptide responses. In this approach peripheral effects should be blocked to facilitate interpretation.

Neuroimaging studies

This strategy will only be briefly discussed since PET studies are included in Chapter 29. Cerebral glucose metabolism is decreased in those areas primarily involved with the degenerative process in MSA; patients with PAF do not exhibit abnormal metabolism (Fulham *et al.* 1991). Unfortunately, only indirect inferences about neurotransmitter systems can be made from these results. Although cerebral glucose metabolism has been investigated extensively over the last decade in various neurological disorders, PET studies of neurotransmitter systems have only been possible within the last few years. Bhatt *et al.* (1990) observed a reduction of ^{18}F-fluorodopa uptake in two patients with MSA; another patient with normal uptake manifested mild parkinsonism which had been present for only a short time. Brooks *et al.* (1990) applied this approach to patients with PAF and MSA. In addition to ^{18}F-fluorodopa, they used S-^{11}C-nomifensine, which binds to thalamic dopamine uptake sites. A reduction in putaminal ^{18}F-fluorodopa uptake correlated with locomotor disability in MSA; caudate uptake was also impaired. Normal caudate function in Parkinson's disease differentiated the two disorders. It appears that the striatal abnormality was attended by a loss of nigrostriatal nerve terminals as indicated by the reduction in nomifensine binding. Patients with PAF generally have normal striatonigral function. Thus, this approach not only distinguishes among patients with MSA, PAF, and Parkinson's disease but points to regional localization of lesions involving specific CNS neurotransmitters.

Neurochemical measurements in CSF

Despite limitations which hamper application of this approach, the levels of neurotransmitters, metabolites, and neuronal enzymes have been used to examine the functional integrity of CNS pathways. Since access is generally limited to lumbar CSF, it is important not to overinterpret the significance of abnormalities. This strategy has been most extensively employed in the investigation of monoamine systems; however, the development of sensitive, specific radioimmunoassay methods permits measurement of peptides in CSF as well.

Noradrenaline plays an important role as a central neurotransmitter in addition to its role in the periphery. Noradrenergic neurons in the locus ceruleus, one of the nuclei consistently affected by the degenerative process in MSA, innervate the hypothalamus; other fibres project to the cerebellum, hippocampus, cerebral cortex, and hypothalamus. Another pathway originates from diffuse brainstem areas to innervate the hypothalamus, limbic system, and other brainstem centres. Descending bulbospinal fibres project to preganglionic sympathetic neurons and anterior horn cells.

In man, MHPG is the predominant metabolite of noradrenaline in the central nervous system. Approximately one-third of the total MHPG in plasma is unconjugated; most of the metabolite in CSF is in the free form. Although there is a significant correlation between CSF and plasma MHPG, the levels in CSF are consistently higher than in plasma (Kopin *et al.* 1983*a*). This is true even in patients with phaeochromocytoma, a rare tumour of the adrenal medulla that secretes large amounts of catecholamines and is not under nervous system control. Since free MHPG readily crosses the blood-brain barrier, it appears that a component of CSF MHPG is derived from peripheral sources. In order to use CSF levels of MHPG as an index of central noradrenaline metabolism, a correction for the contribution from free plasma MHPG must be made. A method for estimating the central component of CSF MHPG has been derived from a kinetic model in which the plasma and CSF are considered as a two-compartment system with similar rate constants for entry into and exit from the CSF. The slope of the line relating CSF to plasma MHPG in normal subjects and patients with phaeochromocytoma gives the proportion of plasma MHPG which must be subtracted from the total CSF level since the elevation of CSF MHPG in the latter group results solely from diffusion of free MHPG from plasma into CSF. The empirically determined value for the slope, 0.9, fits well with theoretical predictions since it represents the ratio of entry and exit constants for MHPG. The constant for exit of MHPG from CSF should be slightly greater than the entry constant due to bulk flow of CSF.

Application of this strategy to patients with autonomic failure illustrates the importance of understanding the various factors required to interpret CSF neurotransmitter metabolite levels. Patients with MSA and PAF have low total CSF MHPG levels (Polinsky *et al.* 1984). As expected on the basis of their low plasma noradrenaline, patients with PAF have low levels of plasma MHPG. In contrast, plasma MHPG is normal in MSA. Thus, when the low total CSF MHPG levels are corrected for the respective plasma contributions in these two disorders, only those with MSA manifest a decrease in the component due to central nervous system noradrenaline metabolism (Fig. 17.5). Low total CSF MHPG in PAF results from the small contribution of peripheral noradrenaline metabolism. The findings in MSA are in accord with the neuropathology; several brain areas innervated by noradrenergic pathways are involved. Furthermore, Spokes *et al.* (1979) found reduced noradrenaline content in the locus ceruleus, hypothalamus, and septal nuclei in MSA. Although corrected CSF levels of MHPG provide clinical evidence of central noradrenergic lesions in MSA, this approach cannot be used at present to further localize the lesion(s). Normal central nervous system metabolism in PAF is consistent with primary postganglionic involvement demonstrated through investigations of peripheral mechanisms.

Two other brain monoamine systems have also been investigated in patients with MSA and PAF. Dopaminergic involvement is the likely cause of parkinsonism in MSA. The importance of the serotonergic system is highlighted by its regional distribution in the CNS; high concentrations

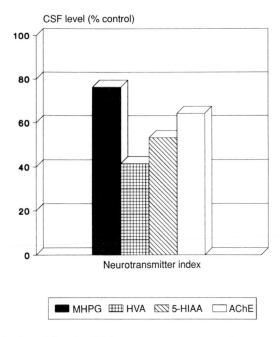

Fig. 17.5. Reduced levels of CSF neurotransmitter indices in multiple system atrophy.

parallel the pathways responsible for wakefulness and vegetative control. Brainstem serotonergic neurons with spinal cord projections make this system a likely neurochemical target for the degenerative process. The primary brain metabolites in man of dopamine and serotonin are, respectively, homovanillic acid (HVA) and 5-hydroxyindoleacetic acid (5-HIAA); both acid metabolites are removed from CSF through the same mechanism. Interpretation of their measurements in CSF is less complicated than for MHPG since there does not appear to be a contribution from the periphery. However, the collection method must be standardized because of the rostral–caudal concentration gradient. Both metabolites are reduced to approximately 50 per cent of control values in patients with MSA (Fig. 17.5; Polinsky *et al.* 1988*a*). A deficit in turnover rather than transport is supported by the observation that probenecid elevates both metabolites in MSA. Bromocryptine lowers CSF HVA in patients with MSA (Williams *et al.* 1979), consistent with the functional integrity of dopaminergic receptors. The increase in CSF HVA following treatment with Sinemet® suggests that some synthesis, release, and metabolism of dopamine may continue despite degeneration in the areas of dopaminergic projections (Polinsky *et al.* 1988*a*). This latter observation may explain the modest therapeutic benefit from antiparkinsonian drugs during the early and middle stages of the illness.

Polinsky *et al.* (1988*a*) noted some interesting clinical correlations among the patients with MSA in their study. Patients were subdivided according to the presence and severity of parkinsonian features. All subgroups, including those without clinical signs of parkinsonism, manifested low CSF levels of HVA. The MSA subgroup with olivopontocerebellar atrophy may not have exhibited clinical evidence of dopaminergic deficiency because the degree of involvement may not have reached the 80 per cent threshold estimated for appearance of symptoms in idiopathic Parkinson's disease. In addition, other brain dopamine systems unrelated to motor control might be affected since there are widespread neuropathological lesions in olivopontocerebellar atrophy. As anticipated, MSA patients with the most severe parkinsonism had the lowest CSF HVA levels. The reductions in CSF HVA in MSA are consistent with neuronal loss and decreased dopamine content in the striatum and substantia nigra. Although low CSF 5-HIAA in MSA probably reflects decreased serotonin turnover, the significance of this finding is unclear. Neurochemical studies of post-mortem brain tissue have not revealed consistent changes in serotonin content in MSA. Reductions in various brain regions have been observed, however, in Parkinson's disease. Since the rostral–caudal gradient is less than for HVA, the spinal cord may make a larger contribution to the CSF level (perhaps as much as one-third of the total). Thus, low CSF 5-HIAA in MSA may result from the well-documented neuropathological involvement in spinal cord pathways. Similar levels of the serotonin metabolite in the various MSA subgroups adds further support to the notion that this deficit is not related to the abnormality in motor control. Normal levels of HVA and 5-HIAA in patients with PAF provide further evidence that this disorder is limited to peripheral autonomic involvement. In addition, these neurochemical results do not support an association between PAF and Parkinson's disease. The changes in MSA confirm central nervous system dysfunction in dopaminergic and serotonergic systems but this strategy does not allow a more precise definition or characterization of the areas responsible for these functional deficits.

Cholinergic function is important for the normal operation of several brain regions including the cerebral cortex, basal ganglia, hypothalamus, and brainstem nuclei. Involvement of this neurotransmitter system in MSA has been demonstrated by measuring decreases in the regional concentration of choline acetyltransferase, a marker of cholinergic neuronal integrity. Assessment of the cholinergic system in man presents a greater challenge in comparison with the monoamine systems discussed above. There is not a comparable index of central acetylcholine turnover. This neurotransmitter is extremely labile in biological fluids due to the ubiquitous presence of degradative enzymes. Efforts to measure CSF levels of choline acetyltransferase have been unsuccessful. However, acetylcholinesterase (AChE) is present in CSF and appears to be derived from a neuronal source. The enzyme may be a marker of cholinergic innervation since its activity in frontal cortex parallels that of choline acetyltransferase. Various drugs and electrical stimulation cause secretion of AChE into the spinal fluid. The rates of recovery for various molecular forms of the enzyme following irreversible inhibition support a brain tissue source for AChE. It is important to separate AChE activity from butyrylcholinesterase although there is little activity of the latter enzyme in CSF. Polinsky *et al.* (1989*a*) found low levels of CSF AChE in patients with MSA (Fig. 17.5) but not PAF. This observation is consistent with central cholinergic involvement in MSA; since the low enzyme levels did not correlate with reduced monoamine metabolites it appears that these neurotransmitter systems are independently affected by the degenerative disorder. Dopaminergic dysfunction could contribute to the low CSF AChE in MSA since nigral neurons appear to release the enzyme. Specific localization of the lesion(s) responsible for the decrease in CSF AChE activity would be speculative. Patients with Parkinson's disease do not have low levels of the enzyme. Thus, it would appear that extrapyramidal lesions do not contribute to the abnormality; furthermore, reduced cholinergic turnover in the basal ganglia would yield the opposite clinical effects in MSA since anticholinergic drugs improve the parkinsonian features. Cholinergic dysfunction may involve cortical, hypothalamic, brainstem, or spinal cord pathways.

Peptides may function as neurotransmitters or neuromodulators throughout the nervous system. Many gut peptides are present in the brain. In addition, pituitary peptides appear to act in other non-hormonal capacities. Autonomic pathways in the spinal cord also contain a variety of neuropeptides. Substance P was perhaps the first peptide proposed as a neurotransmitter. Its importance in the control of blood pressure is underscored by its potential role as a neurotransmitter in the baroreflex arc. It also appears to be released by unmyelinated sensory fibres in the skin. Despite their role in mediating a variety of actions, relatively few studies of CSF peptides have been conducted in patients with autonomic failure. The levels in CSF of substance P (Nutt *et al.* 1980), somatostatin (Polinsky *et al.* 1989*b*), and corticotrophin releasing factor (CRF) (Polinsky *et al.* 1991*b*) are low only in patients with MSA. Low levels of substance P and somatostatin are consistent with the reductions in their spinal cord concentration. However, Kwak (1985) also demonstrated markedly decreased levels of substance P in the basal ganglia. In view of the postulated role for substance P in producing the skin flare, it is interesting that histamine-induced flares are normal in patients with MSA (Anand *et al.* 1988). The CSF levels of somatostatin and CRF in MSA do not correlate with dysfunction in the other neurotransmitter systems described earlier in this section. Although Polinsky *et al.* (1989*b*) found a significant negative correlation between CSF somatostatin and a clinical rating of parkinsonism, low levels in those patients without parkinsonian features suggest that the relationship may be a reflection of disease progression. The levels of CRF are not related to clinical ratings of parkinsonism, depression, or dementia.

Normal CSF peptide levels in PAF are consistent with the known patho-physiology in this disorder and indicate that autonomic dysfunction does not affect the levels of these peptides in CSF.

Neuroendocrine strategies

The release of endocrine substances into the plasma from specific brain regions justifies their measurement to investigate pathways that mediate these responses. Various physiological and pharmacological stimuli comprise strategies to probe these central nervous system mechanisms. Several hormonal/peptide substances have been studied in patients with autonomic failure.

Although the function of melatonin in man is not known, its diurnal pattern of secretion by the pineal gland permits an indirect assessment of the central mechanisms and peripheral pathways that mediate its release. The rhythmic pattern is controlled by an endogenous circadian oscillator (perhaps the 'biological clock') located in the suprachiasmatic nucleus. Light plays a major role in modulating the diurnal cycle; the effects of environmental illumination are transmitted via retinohypothalamic pathways. A projection from the suprachiasmatic nucleus terminates in the hypothalamus. The central pathways that provide pineal innervation arise from the medial forebrain bundle and midbrain reticular formation, terminating on the cells of the intermediolateral column in the thoracic spinal cord. Preganglionic fibres innervate the superior cervical ganglion which sends ascending sympathetic nerve fibres to the pineal gland. These postganglionic neurons release increased amounts of noradrenaline at night; pineal noradrenergic receptors respond to β-adrenergic stimulation by increasing melatonin synthesis and release. Plasma melatonin is rapidly metabolized to 6-hydroxymelatonin and subsequently excreted as a conjugate through the kidney. Urinary levels of the metabolite can be used to assess pineal activity.

Normal subjects excrete most of their melatonin during the night with relatively little during the day. Distinct differences between MSA and PAF reflect the underlying pathophysiology in these disorders (Tetsuo *et al.* 1981). Although the total daily amount of 6-hydroxymelatonin is low in PAF, the diurnal pattern appears to be preserved; this finding suggests that pineal innervation may be affected. Presumably, reduced synthesis and release results from a decrease in nocturnal stimulation since postganglionic activity would be diminished in PAF. In contrast, the daytime excretion in many MSA patients was equal to or in excess of the nocturnal amount. This alteration in the pattern is consistent with disruption in central pathways which control the timing of synthesis and release. Decentralization of the pineal is further supported by the findings in patients with cord transection: complete cervical but not a lumbar lesion alters the normal day–night pattern of melatonin excretion. Thus, investigation of this β-adrenergic sympathetically controlled substance biochemically distinguishes central and peripheral autonomic nervous system disorders.

The pituitary peptides, β-endorphin and adrenocorticotrophic hormone (ACTH), are among the many central and peripheral hormonal responses activated during hypoglycaemia. Insulin only releases these peptides if hypoglycaemia occurs. Although hypothalamic releasing factors primarily control anterior pituitary hormones, neurotransmitters also modulate their release. Arecoline, a cholinergic agonist, increases β-endorphin even after peripheral effects of the drug are blocked; atropine prevents the rise in β-endorphin during insulin hypoglycaemia. Thus, it appears that a central cholinergic pathway mediates the β-endorphin and ACTH responses to hypoglycaemia. Polinsky *et al.* (1987) found that patients with MSA but not PAF had essentially absent β-endorphin and ACTH responses to insulin-induced hypoglycaemia. This observation suggests CNS involvement, probably at the level of the hypothalamus. Normal responses in PAF would be expected on the basis of a peripheral disorder.

The abnormality in β-endorphin and ACTH indicates that at least one central cholinergic pathway is affected in MSA. In order to further examine

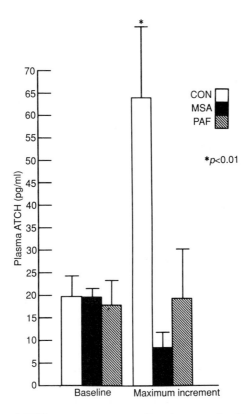

Fig. 17.6. Plasma ACTH responses to arecoline in normal subjects (CON) and patients with autonomic failure.

this possibility, Polinsky *et al.* (1991*a*) administered arecoline to patients with autonomic failure. Patients with MSA and PAF failed to increase plasma ACTH in response to the drug (Fig. 17.6). This paradoxical result emphasizes the importance of considering interactions among various neurotransmitter and peptide control systems. As mentioned in the discussion of adrenal medullary function, patients with MSA but not PAF manifested an increase in plasma adrenaline following administration of arecoline. Peripheral administration of isoproterenol releases ACTH in intact rats and in those who have either pituitary stalk sectioning or lesioning of the median eminence. The effects of insulin hypoglycaemia or isoproterenol on ACTH release can be blocked by propranolol. Since adrenaline crosses the blood–brain barrier in the region of the hypothalamus, it appears that peripheral adrenergic activity may be required for cholinergic-mediated release of ACTH. Thus, PAF patients do not increase their plasma ACTH levels following arecoline because they lack the adrenaline increment. In MSA, the response is absent due to the degenerative process that is known to affect several areas with dense, cholinergic innervation including the hypothalamus. Choline acetyltransferase activity is reduced in the brains of MSA patients. Surprisingly, no evidence of central cholinergic supersensitivity was observed in relation to the ACTH responses to arecoline. Degeneration may have also affected postsynaptic elements.

Growth hormone is produced by acidophil cells of the anterior pituitary and is released by stimulation of the hypothalamopituitary axis. Variable plasma growth hormone responses to insulin-induced hypoglycaemia in MSA have been reported. This inconsistency limits the localizing value of this approach. Normal growth hormone responses in PAF patients with adrenergic insufficiency suggest that peripheral catecholamines are not required to mediate the response to hypoglycaemia (Polinsky *et al.* 1981*b*). A pharmacological challenge with intravenous clonidine was carried out by da Costa *et al.* (1984) in six patients with autonomic failure. Although only two patients had PAF, all patients were reported to have low plasma noradrenaline levels. Patients with autonomic failure did not increase their plasma growth hormone levels as observed in normals. The rather large standard errors in the control group suggest sufficient variability which decreases the utility of this approach in individual patients. Presumably, the lack of response in the MSA patients could result from a central lesion though these patients are atypical because their basal noradrenaline levels were low. However, the results in PAF are analogous to the findings with arecoline discussed above. Although it is tempting to speculate about the possibility of a central lesion in PAF, it may be necessary to assess other possible interactions that could explain this abnormality. Clonidine-induced growth hormone release may be useful as an index of central α-adrenergic function but further development is required before this strategy can be used to unequivocally localize lesion(s).

Vasopressin, named for its potent vasoconstrictor actions, is released by the posterior pituitary in response to water deprivation or extracellular fluid volume depletion. Although the peptide also serves as a central neuro-transmitter, plasma levels reflect its hormonal function. Localizing value is diminished by the spectrum of general and local stimuli that effect its release: primary stimuli include serum osmolality and activation of thoracic stretch receptors. A brisk rise in plasma vasopressin occurs when normal subjects stand. The postural increment is blunted in patients with autonomic failure

Table 17.2. Neurochemical and pharmacological differences between PAF and MSA

	PAF	MSA
Peripheral		
Supine plasma NA	Low	Normal
Neuronal uptake	Decreased	Normal
Neuronal NA stores	Low	Normal
Urinary NA metabolites		
Total	Decreased	Normal
NM/Total	Normal	Decreased
Plasma NA metabolites	Low	Normal
NA receptor sensitivity	Increased	Normal
Gastrin		
Basal level	Increased	Normal
Response to hypoglycaemia	Increased	Decreased
Response to isoproterenol	Increased	Normal
Adrenaline response to arecoline	Absent	Normal
Central		
Plasma NA response to acetylcholine	Absent	Increased
Neuroimaging		
Glucose metabolism	Normal	Decreased
Dopamine uptake	Normal	Decreased
CSF studies		
MHPG	Normal	Low
HVA	Normal	Low
5-HIAA	Normal	Low
AChE	Normal	Low
Substance P	?	Low
Somatostatin	Normal	Low
CRF	Normal	Low
Neuroendocrine mechanisms		
Melatonin		
Total	Low	Normal
Diurnal pattern	Normal	Reversed
β-endorphin/ACTH	Normal	Decreased

NA, noradrenaline; NM, normetanephrine; all other abbreviations defined in text.

(Zerbe *et al.* 1983; Williams *et al.* 1985). Williams *et al.* (1985) suggested an afferent lesion since the response to infusion of normal saline was preserved. Central lesions in MSA presumably prevent the suppression of vasopressin by levodopa or naloxone. Normal vasopressin responses to osmotic and cardiovascular stimuli in tetraplegic patients provide additional support for localizing the deficit. Unfortunately, this information only points out the areas that are not functionally involved.

Summary

Neurochemical and pharmacological strategies clearly distinguish patho-physiological differences between central and peripheral disorders of the autonomic nervous system. In addition, underlying deficits in circulatory and metabolic homeostasis have been elucidated. Investigation of patients with autonomic failure provides an opportunity to study lesions involving various neurotransmitter and neuropeptide pathways in man. Their results have often enlightened our understanding of normal function and metabolism and allowed us to validate hypotheses otherwise tested only in experimental animal preparations. Table 17.2 summarizes the results of applying these methods to patients with MSA and PAF. Some of the results clarify functional abnormalities while others contribute to the development of rational therapeutic approaches. Unfortunately, progress in our understanding and management of these patients has not been attended by comparable advances in improving the prognosis, particularly in MSA. Sustained efforts to further define the cause and consequences of these disorders will undoubtedly focus our attempts to succeed in that regard.

References

Anand, P., Bannister, R., McGregor, G. P., Ghatei, M. A., Mulderry, P. K., and Bloom, S. R. (1988). Marked depletion of dorsal spinal cord substance P and calcitonin gene-related peptide with intact skin flare responses in multiple system atrophy. *J. Neurol. Neurosurg. Psychiat.* **51**, 192–6.

Bannister, R., Crowe, R., Eames, R., Rosenthal, T., and Sever, P. (1979). Defective cardiovascular reflexes and supersensitivity to sympathomimetic drugs in autonomic failure. *Brain* **102**, 163–76.

Baser, S. M., Brown, R. T., Curras, M. T., Baucom, C. E., Hooper, D. H., and Polinsky, R. J. (1991). Beta-receptor sensitivity in autonomic failure. *Neurology* **41**, 1107–12.

Bhatt, M. H., Snow, B. J., Martin, W. R. W., Cooper, S., and Calne, D. B. (1990). Positron emission tomography in Shy–Drager syndrome. *Ann. Neurol.* **28**, 101–3.

Brooks, D. J., Salmon, E. P., Mathias, C. J., Quinn, N., Leenders, K. L., Bannister, R., *et al.* (1990). The relationship between locomotor disability, autonomic dysfunction, and the integrity of the striatal dopaminergic system in patients with multiple system atrophy, pure autonomic failure, and Parkinson's disease, studied with PET. *Brain* **113**, 1539–52.

Cohen, J., Low, P., Fealey, R., Sheps, S., and Jiang, N.-S. (1987). Somatic and autonomic function in progressive autonomic failure and multiple system atrophy. *Ann. Neurol.* **22**, 692–9.

da Costa, D. F., Bannister, R., Landon, J., and Mathias, C. J. (1984). Growth hormone response to clonidine is impaired in patients with central sympathetic degeneration. *Clin. exp. Hypertension* **6**, 1843–6.

Dotson, R., Ochoa, J., Marchettini, P., and Cline, M. (1990). Sympathetic neural outflow directly recorded in patients with primary autonomic failure: clinical observations, microneurography, and histopathology. *Neurology* **40**, 1079–85.

Esler, M., Jackman, G., Kelleher, D., Skews, H., Jennings, G., Bobik, A., *et al.* (1980). Norepinephrine kinetics in patients with idiopathic autonomic insufficiency. *Circulation Res.* **46** (suppl. 1), 47–8.

Fulham, M. J., Dubinsky, R. M., Polinsky, R. J., Brooks, R. A., Brown, R. T., Curras, M. T., *et al.* (1991). Computerized tomography, magnetic resonance imaging and positron emission tomography with [^{18}F]flurodeoxyglucose in the assessment of multiple system atrophy and pure autonomic failure. *Clin. autonom. Res.* **1**, 27–36.

Goldstein, D. S., Polinsky, R. J., Garty, M., Robertson, D., Brown, R. T., Biaggioni, I., *et al.* (1989). Patterns of plasma levels of catechols in neurogenic orthostatic hypotension. *Ann. Neurol.* **26**, 558–63.

Kontos, H. A., Richardson, D. W., and Norvell, J. E. (1976) Mechanisms of circulatory dysfunction in orthostatic hypotension. *Trans. Am. Clin. Climatol. Ass.* **87**, 26–33.

Kopin, I. J., Gordon, E. K., Jimerson, D. C., and Polinsky, R. J. (1983*a*). Relationship between plasma and cerebrospinal fluid levels of 3-methoxy-4-hydroxyphenylglycol. *Science* **219**, 73–5.

Kopin, I. J., Polinsky, R. J., Oliver, J. A., Oddershede, I. R., and Ebert, M. H. (1983*b*). Urinary catecholamine metabolites distinguish different types of sympathetic neuronal dysfunction in patients with orthostatic hypotension. *J. clin. Endocrinol. Metab.* **57**, 632–637.

Kwak, S. (1985). Biochemical analysis of transmitters in the brains of multiple system atrophy. *No Shinkei* **37**, 691–4.

Luft, F. and von Euler, U. (1953). Two cases of postural hypotension showing a deficiency in release of norepinephrine and epinephrine. *J. clin. Invest.* **32**, 1065–9.

Nutt, J. G., Mroz, E. A., Leeman, S. E., Williams, A. C., Engel, W. K., and Chase, T. N. (1980). Substance P in human cerebrospinal fluid: reductions in peripheral neuropathy and autonomic dysfunction. *Neurology* **30**, 1280–5.

Polinsky, R. J., Kopin, I. J., Ebert, M. H., and Weise, V. (1980). The adrenal medullary response to hypoglycaemia in patients with orthostatic hypotension. *J. clin. Endocrinol. Metab.* **51**, 1401–6.

Polinsky, R. J., Kopin, I. J., Ebert, M. H., and Weise, V. (1981*a*). Pharmacologic distinction of different orthostatic hypotension syndromes. *Neurology* **31**, 1–7.

Polinsky, R. J., Kopin, I. J., Ebert, M. H., Weise, V., and Recant, L. (1981*b*). Hormonal responses to hypoglycaemia in orthostatic hypotension patients with adrenergic insufficiency. *Life Sci.* **29**, 417–25.

Polinsky, R. J., Taylor, I. L., Chew, P., Weise, V., and Kopin, I. J. (1982). Pancreatic polypeptide responses to hypoglycaemia in chronic autonomic failure. *J. clin. Endocrinol. Metab.* **54**, 48–52.

Polinsky, R. J., Jimerson, D. C., and Kopin, I. J. (1984). Chronic autonomic failure: CSF and plasma 3-methoxy-4-hydroxyphenylglycol. *Neurology* **34**, 979–83.

Polinsky, R. J., Goldstein, D. S., Brown, R. T., Keiser, H. R., and Kopin, I. J. (1985). Decreased sympathetic neuronal uptake in idiopathic orthostatic hypotension. *Ann. Neurol.* **18**, 48–53.

Polinsky, R. J., Brown, R. T., Lee, G. K., Timmers, K., Culman, J., Foldes, O., *et al.* (1987). Beta-endorphin, ACTH, and catecholamine responses in chronic autonomic failure. *Ann. Neurol.* **21**, 573–7.

Polinsky, R. J., Brown, R. T., Burns, R. S., Harvey-White, J., and Kopin, I. J. (1988*a*). Low lumbar CSF levels of homovanillic acid and 5-hydroxyindoleacetic acid in multiple system atrophy with autonomic failure. *J. Neurol. Neurosurg. Psychiat.* **51**, 914–19.

Polinsky, R. J., Taylor, I. L., Weise, V., and Kopin, I. J. (1988*b*). Gastrin responses in patients with adrenergic insufficiency *J. Neurol. Neurosurg. Psychiat.* **51**, 67–71.

Polinsky, R. J., Holmes, K. V., Brown, R. T., and Weise, V. (1989*a*). CSF acetylcholinesterase levels are reduced in multiple system atrophy with autonomic failure. *Neurology* **39**, 40–4.

Polinsky, R. J., Hooper, D., and Baser, S. M. (1989*b*). Reduced CSF somatostatin in multiple system atrophy with autonomic failure. *Neurology* **39** (suppl. 1), 142.

Polinsky, R. J., Brown, R. T., Curras, M. T., Baser, S. M., Baucom, C. E., Hooper, D. R., *et al.* (1991*a*). Central and peripheral effects of arecoline in patients with autonomic failure. *J. Neurol. Neurosurg. Psychiat.* **54**, 807–12.

Polinsky, R. J., Hooper, D., Nee, L., Marini, A., and Scott, J. (1991*b*). CSF corticotropin releasing factor in patients with autonomic failure. *Neurology* **41** (Suppl. 1), 283.

Polinsky, R. J., Baser, S. M., Brown, R. T., Marini, A. M., and Baucom, C. E. (1991*c*). Ganglionic responsivity in patients with autonomic failure. *Clin. autonom. Res.* **1**, 83.

Spokes, E. G. S., Bannister, R., and Oppenheimer, D. R. (1979). Multiple system atrophy with autonomic failure: clinical, histological and neurochemical observations on four cases. *J. Neurol. Sci.* **43**, 59–82.

Tetsuo, M., Polinsky, R. J., Markey, S. P., and Kopin, I. J. (1981). Urinary 6-hydroxymelatonin excretion in patients with orthostatic hypotension. *J. clin. Endocrinol. Metab.* **53**, 607–10.

Wallin, B. G., Sundlöf, G., Eriksson, B.-M., Dominiak, P., Grobecker, H., and Lindblad, L.-E. (1981). Plasma noradrenaline correlates to sympathetic muscle nerve activity in normotensive man. *Acta physiol. scand.* **111**, 69–73.

Williams, A. C., Nutt, J., Lake, C. R., Pfeiffer, R., Teychenne, P. E., Ebert, M., *et al.* (1979). Actions of bromocriptine in the Shy–Drager and Steele–Richardson–Olszewski syndromes. In *Dopaminergic ergots and motor control* (ed. K. Fuxe and D. B. Calne), pp. 271–83. Pergamon Press, New York.

Williams, T. D. M., Lightman, S. L., and Bannister, R. (1985). Vasopressin secretion in progressive autonomic failure: evidence for defective afferent cardiovascular pathways. *J. Neurol. Neurosurg. Psychiat.* **48**, 225–8.

Zerbe, R. L., Henry, D. P., and Robertson, G. L. (1983). Vasopressin response to orthostatic hypotension: etiologic and clinical implications. *Am. J. Med.* **74**, 265–71.

18. Intraneural recordings of normal and abnormal sympathetic activity in man

B. Gunnar Wallin

Introduction

Sympathetic neural activity is difficult to evaluate in humans. The most common method has been to record sympathetic effector activities, such as heart rate, blood flow, blood pressure, and sweat production, and use the data to draw conclusions about the neural drive. With such recordings a battery of clinical tests has been developed for detecting autonomic dysfunction (see Chapters 4 and 15). The main drawback with this approach is that data are difficult to interpret because effector organs react slowly to variations in sympathetic neural drive and because they also react to hormonal, local chemical, and mechanical stimuli. For the same reason our understanding of the neurophysiological mechanisms underlying different autonomic reflexes is still incomplete. However, with the development of a microelectrode technique for recording sympathetic action potentials in human peripheral nerves, many of these difficulties have been eliminated. With this new method direct information can be obtained about sympathetic impulse traffic to skin and muscle both at rest and during various manoeuvres (visceral sympathetic activity and parasympathetic activity are still inaccessible). The technique is too complex for routine diagnostic work but well suited to study sympathetic pathology and pathophysiology. This chapter will review first the characteristics of normal sympathetic outflow to skin and muscle and then the abnormalities found in certain diseases investigated with the microneurographic technique. Specific references will be given only to recent work and pathophysiological findings. Other references can be found in Vallbo *et al.* (1979), Wallin and Fagius (1988), and Mano (1990).

Methods

Nerve recordings are made with tungsten microelectrodes with tip diameters of a few micrometres. The recording electrode is inserted manually through intact skin into an underlying nerve with a reference electrode placed subcutaneously 1–2 cm away. Usually multiunit activity is obtained, but occasionally single units may be recorded. Most recordings are made in large nerves such as the peroneal (at the fibular head), median (at wrist or elbow), or tibial (in the popliteal fossa) nerves, but sometimes small cutaneous arm and leg nerves have been used. Recently, sympathetic recordings have also been made from the supraorbital branch of the trigeminal nerve in the face (Nordin 1990). In man, peripheral nerves are composed of a varying number of fascicles, each of which is surrounded by a barrier of connective tissue. With the electrodes used, action potentials can be recorded only when the tip has penetrated a fascicle and there is no cross-talk from neighbouring fascicles. Fascicles are most numerous distally where each contains fibres connected only to skin or only to a muscle, but in the proximal part of an extremity all fascicles are composed of a mixture of skin and muscle nerve fibres. For this reason mixed nerves are impaled as far distally as possible in order to obtain recordings from relatively 'pure' muscle or skin nerve fascicles. Usually nerve recordings cause minimal discomfort and no or negligible, transient after-effects (such as skin paraesthesia or mild muscle tenderness). Detailed descriptions of the techniques as well as evidence for the sympathetic nature of the recorded impulses were given previously (Vallbo *et al.* 1979).

Intraneural stimulation

In addition to its use for *recording* nerve impulses, the microelectrode can also be used for *evoking* action potentials by means of intraneural electrical stimulation. All types of nerve fibres (i.e. afferent and efferent, myelinated and unmyelinated) can be stimulated; weak pulses activate preferentially myelinated axons but, with higher stimulus strength, action potentials are induced also in unmyelinated (afferent and sympathetic) fibres. Stimulation-induced cutaneous sympathetic effector responses can be detected by monitoring blood flow, skin resistance, and/or water evaporation. Local anaesthetic blocks of the nerve proximal or distal to the stimulation site can be used to differentiate between effector responses caused by reflexes and those caused by centrifugally conducted impulses (see Blumberg and Wallin 1987).

Normal sympathetic outflow

Sympathetic skin nerve activity

Skin blood vessels and sweat glands are innervated by separate sympathetic fibres, which are intermingled and can be recorded from in the same intrafascilular site. At rest at normal room temperature, spontaneously occurring skin nerve sympathetic activity (SNSA) in nerves to hand and foot consists of irregular bursts of impulses, varying in strength and duration and without clear relationship to the heart rhythm. The bursts may be followed by changes of skin resistance (i.e. sweating) and/or plethysmographic signs of vasoconstriction, indicating that they contain sudomotor and/or vasoconstrictor impulses. Impulses causing active vasodilatation may also be present (see below). Arterial baroreceptor modulation of the outflow of skin vasoconstrictor impulses to hand and foot is weak or absent: impulse bursts are not pulse synchronous, they show no systematic correlation to spontaneous blood pressure fluctuations, and they are not affected in a reproducible way by electrical stimulation of the carotid sinus nerves or temporary baroreceptor deafferentation. Surprisingly, however, sudomotor activity displays cardiac rhythmicity but the functional significance of this finding is unknown. There is also a coupling between the occurrence of sympathetic bursts and the respiratory rhythm, and a deep breath will regularly evoke a strong burst of impulses.

Early recordings of cutaneous effector responses showed that spontaneous electrodermal and plethysmographic activity occurs in parallel in hands and feet, and there is also a similar parallelism and synchrony of the underlying sympathetic discharges. The parallelism does not apply to all skin areas, however, and differences in sympathetic drives have been found between nerves to glabrous and hairy skin.

Effects of manoeuvres

The skin is important for *thermoregulation* and SNSA is sensitive to thermal stimuli. Body cooling increases outflow of vasoconstrictor impulses (Fig. 18.1) and during moderate warming the strength of this activity is reduced to a minimum. When body heating is associated with sweating, there is again an increase of SNSA, but this time due to activation of sudomotor impulses. Thus, changes of environmental temperature lead to selective activation of either the vasoconstrictor or the sudomotor neural system with suppression of activity in the other system.

Stimuli with *emotional* effects may change skin colour and moisture and such stimuli cause an increase of SNSA. Any arousal stimulus regularly evokes a single burst of impulses, and mental stress (e.g. mental arithmetic) leads to a more long-lasting increase of activity. Reflex discharges induced by arousal occur after a latency of 0.5 to 1.0 s, depending on the recording site and the subject's height. The latency differences are due mainly to differences in conduction time in postganglionic C fibres, and the reflex latency can be used as an indirect measure of sympathetic conduction velocity. Sudomotor fibres have higher conduction velocity (around 1.3 m/s) than vasoconstrictor fibres (around 0.8 m/s). Changes of electrodermal activity (skin resistance or potential) in response to arousal stimuli have been used as an indirect measure of the strength of SNSA. Such data have to be interpreted with

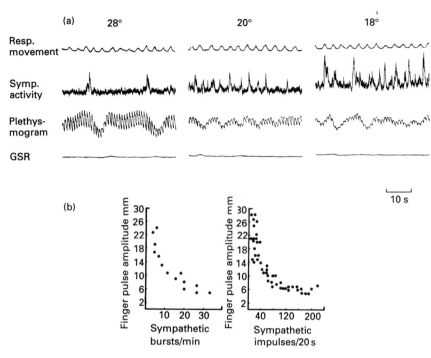

Fig. 18.1. Relationship between skin vasoconstrictor bursts and accompanying finger plethysmographic events. (a) Sympathetic activity recorded from median nerve at external temperatures of 28, 20, and 18 °C. Traces are from above: respiration, integrated neural signal, plethysmogram, and skin resistance (b) Left, diagram showing quantitative relationship between burst incidence/min (abscissa) and finger-pulse amplitude (ordinate). Right, diagram showing quantitative relationship between sympathetic impulses per 20 s (abscissa) and finger-pulse amplitude (ordinate). (Taken with permission from Bini *et al.* (1980).)

caution, however, since the relationship between the number of sudomotor impulses and the skin resistance response is highly non-linear (Kirnö *et al.* 1991).

There are powerful interactions between thermoregulatory and other cutaneous reflex effects. In the extremities of thermoneutral or warm subjects arousal, a deep breath or mental stress will cause simultaneous activation of vasoconstrictor and sudomotor fibres and this constitutes the basis for 'cold sweat'. In cold subjects, on the other hand, the same stimuli induce vasodilatation. Consequently, skin nerves may also contain sympathetic fibres causing vasodilatation. In agreement with this, painful intraneural electrical stimulation causes reflex vasodilatation (Blumberg and Wallin 1987), and in the supraorbital nerve in the face arousal stimuli may induce bursts of impulses followed by plethysmographic signs of vasodilatation (Nordin 1990). Direct confirmation of the presence of vasodilator fibres has also been obtained. Electrical stimulation of the lumbar sympathetic chain in humans may induce increases of skin blood flow in the sole of the foot and at the ankle (Lundberg *et al.* 1989). This finding provides evidence that vasodilatation may be induced actively not only in hairy skin (which has been known previously) but also in glabrous skin. On the other hand, it is still unclear whether there are specific vasodilator fibres in humans (known to exist in cats) or if active vasodilatation is secondary to sweating.

Isometric handgrip

This has been found to increase SNSA in forearm nerves and recently also in the tibial nerve to the sole of foot. The increase of activity seems to be dominated by sudomotor impulses and occurs with short latency. It is probably influenced more by central command and the thermal state of the subject than by intramuscular chemoreceptors.

Metabolic-hormonal effects

A series of studies on the coupling between the glucose metabolism and sympathetic outflow has been performed by Fagius and co-workers (see also below). Intravenous infusion of insulin or 2-deoxy-D-glucose was found to increase sudomotor and inhibit vasoconstrictor outflow to the skin, probably due to CNS glucopenia. Oral intake of D-glucose did not change SNSA.

Sympathetic muscle nerve activity

In muscle nerve fascicles sympathetic impulses are also grouped in bursts, but the temporal pattern of activity differs from that found in skin nerve fascicles. Most bursts have similar duration, display cardiac rhythmicity, and occur intermittently, sometimes as single discharges, sometimes in short sequences with interposed silent periods, and sometimes more continuously. There is also a relationship to respiration, and bursts occur most frequently during expiration. The activity is dominated by vasoconstrictor impulses. The level of activity is reduced during non-REM sleep and increases during REM sleep (Hornyak *et al.* 1991). In a given awake individual the strength of the activity at rest (expressed as bursts/100 heart beats or bursts/min) is remarkably constant over many months but there are wide interindividual differences.

Relationship to blood pressure

The occurrence of sympathetic bursts in muscle nerves shows an intimate relationship to spontaneous blood pressure variations. Bursts occur more frequently during reductions of blood pressure and disappear when blood pressure rises (Fig. 18.2). These findings and the facts that electrical stimulation of the carotid sinus nerves inhibits muscle nerve sympathetic activity (MNSA) and that cardiac rhythmicity is eliminated by temporary baroreceptor deafferentation show that the activity is influenced by arterial

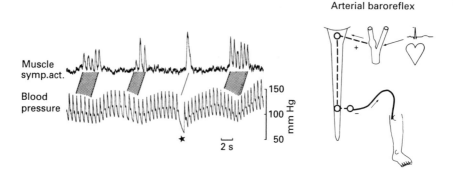

Fig. 18.2. Relationship between spontaneous fluctuations of blood pressure and muscle nerve sympathetic activity (left) recorded in right peroneal nerve. Baroreflex accounts for the pulse synchrony of nerve activity and the inverse relationship to blood-pressure fluctuations. ★ indicates diastolic blood-pressure fall due to sudden atrioventricular block. Stippling indicates corresponding sequences of bursts and heart beats. (Taken with permission from Wallin *et al.* (1980).)

baroreflexes. This implies that bursts correspond to diastolic pressure reductions, whereas pauses between successive bursts correspond to systolic inhibitions. In agreement with this an atrioventricular block with a sudden fall of diastolic blood pressure in a single heart beat is regularly followed by an unusually strong sympathetic burst. In the peroneal nerve the latency between pressure fall and burst is approximately 1.3 s, which corresponds to the delay in the baroreflex arc. Although the delay may vary with some manoeuvres, mean latency at rest is related to the subject's height and can be used as an indirect measure of sympathetic conduction velocity. Variations of MNSA are determined primarily by fluctuations of diastolic blood pressure, whereas other blood pressure parameters seem to be of little importance. The mean level of MNSA at rest is not influenced by physical conditioning but increases with age. Studies of the relationship between mean levels of MNSA and blood pressure at rest have given varying results. In an early report on normotensive subjects no significant relationship was found but in a recent study of a much larger group of subjects there was a positive correlation between mean levels of blood pressure and MNSA (Yamada *et al.* 1989). For data concerning hypertension, see below.

Reflex effects on MNSA

1. *Arterial baroreceptors* have complex effects on MNSA. Dynamic stimulation of carotid baroreceptors is effective in influencing the activity whereas static stimuli only have minor effects. In contrast, static stimulation of aortic baroreceptors seems to cause long-lasting changes of MNSA. This suggests that changes of MNSA evoked by changes of posture (which can be

assumed to alter carotid but not aortic arterial baroreceptor firing) are evoked only to a minor degree from arterial baroreceptors.

2. *Cardiopulmonary baroreceptors*, which are volume receptors in the heart and the vessels entering the heart, are stimulated by changes of central blood volume. Reduction of central blood volume increases the level of MNSA and the increase is similar in arm and leg nerves. Conversely, head-out water immersion, which increases central blood volume, leads to a sustained decrease of MNSA. These findings agree with the notion that postural changes of MNSA are evoked mainly from cardiopulmonary baroreceptors.

3. *Systemic chemoreceptors*. Both hypoxia and hypercapnia increase MNSA. The sympathoexcitatory effects of chemoreceptor stimulation are blunted, presumably from pulmonary stretch receptors if there are simultaneous increases of ventilation.

4. *Intramuscular chemoreceptors*. During isometric hand contractions at 30 per cent of maximum power, MNSA recorded in a peroneal nerve (i.e. supplying non-contracting muscles) is unchanged during the first minute but increases successively thereafter. The increase of MNSA can be maintained for minutes after the end of contraction if circulation to the contracting muscles is arrested. Presumably, therefore, the response is evoked from chemoreceptors in the contracting muscles and there is a coupling between changes of intramuscular pH and increases of MNSA. In agreement with this, patients with muscle phosphorylase deficiency (McArdle's disease), whose intramuscular pH does not change with ischaemic contractions, did not increase their MNSA (Pryor *et al.* 1990). Central command does not contribute significantly to the increase of MNSA until near maximal efforts.

5. *Miscellaneous receptors*. Immersion of a hand in cold water ('cold pressor test') leads to increases of MNSA, heart rate, and blood pressure, presumably evoked from cutaneous cold and/or pain receptors. Face immersion in cold water also increases MNSA. Although evoked in part from cutaneous receptors in the face this 'diving reflex' is more complex and differs functionally from the reflex response evoked by the cold pressor test. Mechanical stimulation of receptors in the pharynx and larynx in paralysed patients under general anaesthesia causes pronounced and long-lasting sympathetic excitation both in muscle (Sellgren *et al.* 1990) and skin nerves. Accumulation of urine in the bladder increases MNSA, an effect which may be induced from stretch receptors in the bladder wall.

Mental stress

Stimuli which cause mental stress evoke complex sympathetic reactions. MNSA does not change significantly during mental arithmetic lasting 1 min or less but with stress of longer duration MNSA increases in the peroneal nerve in the leg but remains unchanged in the radial nerve in the arm. Presumably, the difference between arm and leg nerves is of central origin. If plasma adrenaline concentrations increase during the stress this may also contribute to an increase of peroneal MNSA (see next section).

Hormonal influence

Several hormones influence MNSA. Insulin-induced hypoglycaemia increases the activity as does infusion of 2-deoxy-D-glucose. The underlying mechanisms are complex but central nervous system glucopenia may be an important factor. MNSA increases moderately during and markedly after infusion of high concentrations of adrenaline; the underlying mechanism is unclear. A central nervous mechanism has been implied for the transient (less than 10 min) increase of MNSA following subcutaneous injections of thyrotrophin-releasing hormone. A central (or ganglionic) mechanism may also explain the reduction of MNSA by atrial natriuretic factor. In contrast, the decrease of MNSA induced by infusion of arginine–vasopressin may be due to reflex inhibition from arterial and cardiopulmonary baroreceptors.

Drug effects

The effects of a few antihypertensive drugs on MSNA have been studied. Clonidine reduced the activity in some hypertensive patients but at low plasma concentrations an increase was seen. Acute administration of the β-selective adrenoceptor antagonist metoprolol increased MNSA in patients with essential hypertension but with long-term treatment the activity was reduced, possibly via a central mechanism. MNSA increased when nifedipine (a calcium channel blocker) was given acutely to normal subjects, possibly because of potentiation of cardiopulmonary baroreceptors (Ferguson and Hayes 1989). In addition, digitalis glycosides have been studied in patients with heart failure and were found to inhibit MNSA, presumably partly via low- and/or high-pressure baroreflex mechanisms (Ferguson *et al.* 1989). Anaesthetics have varying effects. General anaesthesia with isoflurane was found to cause a dose-dependent reduction and nitrous oxide an increase of MNSA both in subanaesthetic and anaesthetic concentrations (see Sellgren *et al.* 1990).

'Sympathetic tone'

Functional organization of sympathetic outflow

Traditionally, sympathetic reactions were thought to be slow and protracted and occur in parallel in different parts of the body. This view of a diffusely acting system led to the term 'sympathetic tone' to describe the strength of a presumed global level of activity in sympathetic nerves. Unfortunately, the concept is not tenable. Direct nerve recordings both in animal and man reveal clear differences in nerve traffic between different sympathetic subdivisions indicating that sympathetic outflows to different regions are controlled differentially. On the other hand, there is a remarkable parallelism between two neurograms when resting sympathetic activity is recorded simultaneously in different muscle nerves (or in different skin nerves innervating hands and feet). These findings suggest that there are different populations of sympathetic neurons, each of which is subjected to its own homogeneous supraspinal drive which is different from that of other populations. Consequently there is no common 'sympathetic tone'; if the term is to be retained, it should be used only when considering the sympathetic drive in specified nerves supplying well-defined effector organs.

With some reflex stimuli there is still a high degree of parallelism between neurograms of MNSA recorded simultaneously in arm and leg nerves. Other manoeuvres induce quantitative differences between outflows of MNSA to arm and leg muscles. Differences have also been found between SNSA in hand and forearm nerves. Thus the degree of sympathetic differentiation is even greater than previously known; it occurs not only between different tissues but may also occur between different regions of the same tissue. Probably such differences may originate both at spinal and supraspinal levels.

Relationship between MNSA and plasma noradrenaline

Noradrenaline is the principal transmitter released from postganglionic sympathetic neurons and the plasma level of noradrenaline is often used as an index of sympathetic activity. There is a linear correlation between the sympathetic burst incidence of MNSA at rest and the plasma concentration of noradrenaline in forearm venous plasma in normotensive and hypertensive subjects and in cardiac failure. MNSA also correlates to spillover of tritiated noradrenaline to venous plasma (Hjemdahl *et al.* 1989) and, during several manoeuvres, increases of MNSA are followed by increases of forearm venous plasma noradrenaline concentration. The probable reasons that plasma noradrenaline levels seem to reflect in particular the strength of MNSA are: (1) skeletal muscle is a large tissue responsible for about 20 per cent of the total spillover to blood; and (2) the contribution of noradrenaline from muscle is disproportionately high in forearm venous blood. There is, however, an exception in that the increase of MNSA that occurs with systemic hypoxia is not associated with increased plasma noradrenaline levels (Rowell *et al.* 1989). The reason is unclear but since plasma concentrations are influenced also by other factors than noradrenaline spillover (e.g. plasma clearance) the finding is not surprising.

Abnormal sympathetic outflow

Many nervous lesions may result in pathological sympathetic activity which should be possible to detect in microneurographic recordings. The technique is inappropriate, however, for abnormalities which arise distal to the recording site, i.e. in the most distal parts of the postganglionic sympathetic neurons or in the neuroeffector junction. In such cases intraneural stimulation of sympathetic fibres combined with effector recordings (Blumberg and Wallin 1987) may provide a methodological alternative. In principle, sympathetic abnormalities may be quantitative or qualitative. Quantitative abnormalities arise if the number of sympathetic action potentials reaching the effector is reduced (or increased) resulting in weakened (or exaggerated) but qualitatively normal reflex responses. Such effects may be induced either from the afferent limb of a reflex arc or in the central nervous system. A qualitative abnormality implies that reflex effects are evoked from a stimulus which normally is ineffective, or that the 'sign' of a reflex effect is reversed, e.g. if a normally excitatory response is turned into an inhibitory one.

Examples of how qualitative abnormalities may arise have been demonstrated. Fagius *et al.* (1985) found that temporary baroreceptor deafferentation eliminated cardiac rhythmicity of MNSA. During this period arousal stimuli gave rise to clear sympathetic reflex responses both in skin and muscle nerve fascicles (Fig. 18.3). Normally, such responses occur only in skin nerves and the muscle nerve responses also disappeared as the anaesthesia wore off. Consequently, it appears that afferent baroreceptor activity, in addition to being involved in blood pressure homeostasis, also serves as a

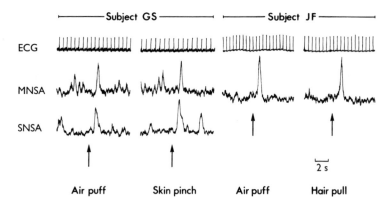

Fig. 18.3. Examples of arousal stimuli evoking distinct single bursts of MNSA (and SNSA) following bilateral block of glossopharyngeal and vagus nerves. Arrows indicate stimulus. Same time-scale in all panels. (Taken with permission from Fagius *et al.* (1985).)

powerful brake on reflex effects in MNSA from other afferent inputs; therefore, when baroreceptor inhibition was eliminated by the anaesthesia, such reflexes were unmasked. Another example was reported by Blumberg and Jänig (1983) who found that, some time after a peripheral nerve had been cut in the cat, the normal differences between muscle and skin vasoconstrictor activity were reduced and reflex effects became more similar in the two types of nerves (proximal to the lesion). These findings show that interruption of afferent pathways may result in abnormal sympathetic reflex patterns. If such effects would occur during a disease, clinical symptoms may arise. This hypothesis is in accordance with other examples of lesions in the nervous system revealing patterns which normally are concealed due to inhibitory regulation, e.g. the Babinski sign and reflex grasping.

Our knowledge of the precise mechanisms underlying pathological sympathetic reactions is limited but the character of an abnormality should depend on which reflex(es) and where in the reflex arc(s) the pathological influence occurs. In some of the conditions presented in the rest of this chapter this is known; in others not.

Peripheral efferent lesions: polyneuropathy

In most cases of polyneuropathy sensory disturbances dominate but some patients have symptoms suggesting autonomic involvement. In somatic

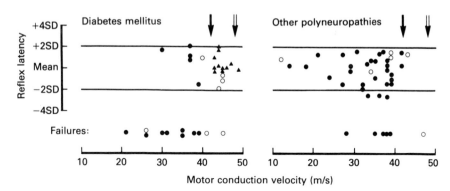

Fig. 18.4. Sympathetic reflex latencies (proportional to conduction velocity in postganglionic sympathetic fibres) expressed as standard deviations from normal and related to motor conduction velocity of the nerve recorded from in patients with polyneuropathy. The reflexes used were the arterial baroreflex (for muscle sympathetic activity) and an arousal reflex (for skin sympathetic activity). (○ and ●) patients with polyneuropathy, peroneal and median nerve, respectively, and (▲) diabetic patients without polyneuropathy, peroneal nerve. Failures, motor conduction velocity of the nerves in which no sympathetic activity could be found. Lower normal limit for motor conduction velocity in the peroneal and median nerve indicated by filled and open arrows, respectively.

SD, standard deviation (Taken with permission from Fagius (1982).)

myelinated fibres, conducting velocity is usually lowered but slowing does not seem to occur in sympathetic fibres. In patients with polyneuropathy of different aetiology, the general character of SNSA and MNSA was normal and sympathetic conduction velocities were also normal, even if patients had autonomic symptoms and marked slowing of skeletomotor conduction velocity (Fig. 18.4). However, failure to find sympathetic activity was significantly increased especially in diabetic polyneuropathy (Fagius 1982). The findings suggest that, in polyneuropathy, sympathetic conduction velocity is normal as long as the fibres conduct. With sympathetic involvement in the disease successive loss of functioning fibres leads to disappearance of detectable activity. It cannot be excluded, however, that fibres on the afferent side of various reflex arcs also may become engaged in the disease. If so, symptoms due to failure of conduction in postganglionic sympathetic fibres may be mixed with symptoms due to the afferent lesion.

Peripheral afferent lesions

If nerve fibres on the afferent side of a sympathetic reflex arc are damaged, different effects will arise if the reflex is excitatory or inhibitory. The following diseases involve defects in arterial and/or cardiopulmonary baroreflexes which have inhibitory effects on MNSA.

Decreased afferent activity

If afferent nerve traffic from arterial and cardiopulmonary baroreceptors should decrease, one would expect increases of sympathetic activity, heart rate, and blood pressure. This may occur in the *Guillain–Barré syndrome* (Fagius and Wallin 1983). In three such patients the character of MNSA was qualitatively normal, i.e. pulse synchrony was preserved, but quantitatively all patients had higher activity during the acute phase than after recovery. However, when recordings were repeated after clinical recovery the incidence of sympathetic bursts was reproducible: in other words, when symptoms disappeared results of repeated sympathetic recordings became normal (Fig. 18.5). The abnormality can be explained by reduced inhibition of brainstem vasomotor centres caused by involvement of afferent baroreceptor fibres in the disease. Since cardiac rhythmicity was maintained it is likely that mainly fibres from cardiopulmonary receptors were affected.

Paroxysmal attacks of hypertension have also been described in a patient with a history of neck and mediastinal radiation who had loss of cardiac rhythmicity in MNSA but preserved MNSA responses to lower body negative pressure (Aksamit *et al.* 1987). In this case selective loss of arterial baroreceptor function may explain the findings.

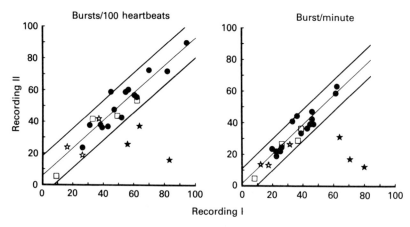

Fig. 18.5. Quantity of sympathetic bursts at two consecutive recordings of MSNA plotted against each other. ★, Guillain–Barré syndrome with tachycardia and hypertension; acute and first follow-up recording. ☆, Guillain–Barré syndrome with tachycardia and hypertension; both recordings after recovery. □, Guillain–Barré syndrome without autonomic involvement. ●, Healthy subjects. Thick lines indicate 2 standard deviations (SD) from the regression line. $r = 0.94$ for both graphs. Note clear aberration of the three Guillain–Barré syndrome patients with hypertension and tachycardia at the recording during their acute illness. (Taken with permission from Fagius and Wallin (1983).)

In *heart failure* baroreflexes are thought to be impaired at least partly because of decreased afferent activity. This may contribute to the increase of MNSA in this condition (Leimbach *et al.* 1986).

Increased afferent activity: syncope

Increased afferent nerve traffic from baroreceptors should be expected to inhibit sympathetic activity, decrease heart rate, and lower blood pressure. Physiologically, this occurs as part of normal homeostatic blood pressure regulation whenever a transient blood pressure increase is buffered by baroreceptor mechanisms. If buffering reactions become exaggerated, they will cause more pronounced blood pressure falls and ultimately syncope. A syncopal reaction can probably be induced by increased activity both from arterial and cardiopulmonary receptors and it has been suggested that activation of sympathetic vasodilator fibres also forms part of the syncopal reaction. MNSA has been recorded both during typical *vasovagal syncope* (Wallin and Sundlöf 1982) and in atypical long-lasting vasodepressive attacks (Yatomi *et al.* 1989). In all patients sympathetic activity suddenly disappeard when syncope occurred. This does not exclude activation of vasodilator fibres but it shows that withdrawal of vasoconstrictor activity contributes importantly to muscle vasodilatation during syncope. The sympathetic withdrawal may be a reflex effect evoked by increased activity from cardiac ventricular receptors. However, since syncope with cessation of MNSA may occur also in patients without innervated ventricular receptors (after heart transplantation; Scherrer *et al.* 1990*a*), vasovagal syncope is not always dependent on ventricular baroreceptor activation.

Increased afferent activity from arterial baroreceptors may be the cause of sympathetic inhibition and syncope in patients with so-called hypersensitive carotid-sinus baroreceptors but no direct evidence from human nerve recordings is available. However, in a case of *glossopharyngeal neuralgia with syncope* (Wallin *et al.* 1984) each syncope was associated with cessation of MNSA (Fig. 18.6). In glossopharyngeal neuralgia the patient gets short-lasting severe pain attacks in the throat evoked by chewing, swallowing, coughing, etc. In rare cases fainting is precipitated simultaneously with the pain. Since afferent sensory fibres from the throat and from carotid baroreceptors both run in the glossopharyngeal nerve it has been suggested that there is a pathological 'synapse', a so-called ephapse, in the glossopharyngeal nerve at which pain impulses are misdirected and jump over to baroreceptor fibres. Presumably when this barrage of afferent impulses reaches brainstem vasomotor centres there is profound inhibition and fainting occurs.

Hypertension

To compare the strength of MNSA at rest between groups is complicated by the large interindividual variability and the increase of MNSA that normally occurs with age. In early comparisons between fairly small samples

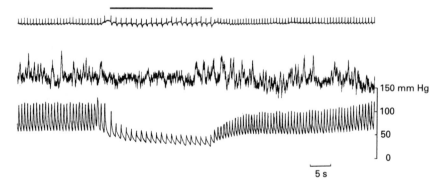

Fig. 18.6. Recordings of ECG (upper trace), MSNA (middle trace), and intra-arterial blood pressure (bottom trace) during attack of glossopharyngeal neuralgia associated with syncope. Sympathetic activity displayed in mean voltage neurogram (time constant 0.1 s). Horizontal bar indicates period when cardiac pacemaker was activated. (Taken with permission from Wallin *et al.* (1984).)

of established hypertension and controls a slightly higher level in the patients could have been an effect of differences in age between the groups. Recently, however, a significant increase of MNSA at rest was found at all ages in a much larger sample of patients with essential hypertension (Yamada *et al.* 1989). In borderline hypertension one study has shown an increased MNSA at rest and another study no increase. Subjects with borderline hypertension who developed postexercise hypotension were found to have a reduced MNSA when examined 60 min after exercise. Some reflex abnormalities have also been demonstrated in borderline and essential hypertension. Increased MNSA responsiveness was found with apnoea during hypoxia, the cold pressor test, and lower body negative pressure, but not with isometric handgrip. For a detailed discussion of hypertensive mechanisms and references to recent microneurographic findings see Chapter 41.

It is known that the immunosuppressive agent cyclospirin may cause hypertension. In a recent microneurographic study on cylcosporin-induced hypertension both heart transplant patients and patients with myasthenia gravis had increased MNSA at rest (Scherrer *et al.* 1990*b*). Since the abnormalities were present after heart transplantation they do not depend on activity in ventricular baroreceptors; in fact, these receptors may have a protective effect since the increases of blood pressure and MNSA were higher after heart transplantation than in myasthenia gravis.

Central nervous system

Several abnormalities of sympathetic outflow have been found in patients with traumatic *spinal cord injury* (Wallin and Stjernberg 1984; Stjernberg *et al.* 1986).

1. Both in skin and muscle nerves spontaneous sympathetic activity was virtually absent and, when it occurred in muscle nerve fascicles, there was no cardiac rhythmicity.

2. Sympathetic reflex discharges were more difficult to evoke and not stronger than normal; nevertheless, long-lasting pronounced blood pressure increases occurred. Thus, attacks of high blood pressure in these patients are probably not due to sympathetic hyperactivity.

3. Sudden pressure over the bladder and arousal-like skin stimuli (skin pinching, electrical skin stimulation) below the lesion gave rise to excitatory responses both in skin and muscle nerve fascicles (Fig. 18.7). The responses in muscle nerves represent a qualitative abnormality similar to that reported after temporary baroreceptor denervation (Fagius *et al.* 1985).

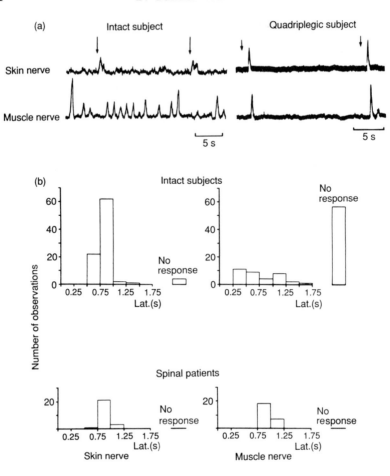

Fig. 18.7. (a) Mean voltage neurograms from simultaneous recordings in peroneal nerve fascicle to skin in the right leg and to muscle in the left leg in an intact subject (left) and a patient with complete cervical spinal cord lesion (right). Arrows indicate electrical stimulations to the left upper thigh, inducing synchronous neural responses in skin and muscle nerve fascicles in the quadriplegic patient but responses only in the skin fascicle in the intact subject. (b) Relationship between electrical skin stimuli applied to the upper part of the thigh and sympathetic discharges in nerves to skin and muscle in five intact subjects (upper) and two patients with spinal cord lesion (lower). Sympathetic discharges recorded simultaneously from the two peroneal nerves. In skin nerves of intact subjects, bursts were usually (85 cases, 93 per cent) recorded 0.5–1.0 s after stimuli and only in four cases (4 per cent) were there no bursts within 0.25–1.75 s after stimuli. In muscle nerves bursts were often lacking (56 cases, 61 per cent) and the bursts recorded showed no systematic relationship to the stimuli. In patients with spinal cord lesions all stimuli evoked bursts in both skin and muscle nerves (Data from Stjernberg *et al.* (1986).)

MNSA has been recorded before and after oral administration of 200 mg L-threo-3,4-dihydroxyphenylserine in a case of the *Shy–Drager syndrome* (Kachi *et al.* 1988). In the control situation MNSA was weak (but surprisingly displayed cardiac rhythmicity) and there was only a weak response to head-up tilting; 30 min after the drug was given both resting activity and tilting response were markedly enhanced. The result suggests that at least in some Shy–Drager patients loss of sympathetic function may be due to a biochemical defect rather than an anatomical loss of central or peripheral sympathetic neurons. Dotson *et al.* (1990) attempted to record SNSA in one patient with primary autonomic failure and one with the Shy–Drager syndrome. In 1 of 7 fascicles and 3 of 12 fascicles, respectively, spontaneous multiunit activity was found which may have been of sympathetic origin but which could not be influenced by manoeuvres. No conclusion can be drawn from the data but if the activity was of sympathetic origin, the results are compatible with the idea that spinal sympathetic neurons are decentralized in both conditions.

Miscellaneous conditions

Sympathetic activity has been recorded in patients with migraine (MNSA) and in patients with the Raynaud phenomenon (SNSA) but no abnormality was detected. In cirrhosis of the liver MNSA was reported to be increased only if the patients had ascites (Floras *et al.* 1991). MNSA was also increased in hypothyroidism but was normal in hyperthyroidism (Fagius *et al.* 1990). The mechanisms are unknown.

Acknowledgement

This work was supported by the Swedish Medical Research Council, Grant No B91-04X-03546-20A.

References

Aksamit, T. R., Floras, J. S., Victor, R. G., and Aylward, P. E. (1987). Paroxysmal hypertension due to sinoaortic baroreceptor denervation in humans. *Hypertension* **9**, 309–14.

Bini, G., Hagbarth, K.-E., Hynninen, P., and Wallin, B. G. (1980). Thermoregulatory and rhythm-generating mechanisms governing the sudomotor and vasoconstrictor outflow in human cutaneous nerves. *J. Physiol., Lond.* **306**, 537.

Blumberg, H. and Jänig, W. (1983). Changes of reflexes in vasoconstrictor neurons supplying the cat hindlimb following chronic nerve lesions: a model for studying mechanisms of reflex sympathetic dystrophy? *J. autonom. nerv. Syst.* **7**, 399–411.

Blumberg, H. and Wallin, B. G. (1987). Direct evidence of neurally mediated vasodilatation in hairy skin of the human foot. *J. Physiol. London* **382**, 105–21.

Dotson, R., Ochoa, J., Marchettini, P., and Clive, M. (1990). Sympathetic neural outflow directly recorded in patients with primary autonomic failure: clinical observations, microneurography and histopathology. *Neurology* **40**, 1079-85.

Fagius, J. (1982). Microneurographic findings in diabetic polyneuropathy with special reference to sympathetic nerve activity. *Diabetologia* **23**, 415-20.

Fagius, J. and Wallin, B. G. (1983). Microneurographic evidence of excessive sympathetic outflow in the Guillain-Barré syndrome. *Brain* **106**, 589-600.

Fagius, J., Wallin, B. G., Sundlöf, G., Nerhed, C., and Englesson, S. (1985). Sympathetic outflow in man after anaesthesia of glossopharyngeal and vagus nerves. *Brain* **108**, 423-38.

Fagius, J., Westermark, K., and Karlsson, A. (1990). Baroreflex-governed sympathetic outflow to muscle vasculature is increased in hypothyroidism. *Clin. Endocrinol.* **33**, 177-85.

Ferguson, D. W. and Hayes, D. W. (1989). Nifedipine potentiates cardiopulmonary baroreflex control of sympathetic nerve activity in healthy humans. *Circulation* **80**, 285-98.

Ferguson, D. W., Berg, W. J., Sanders, J. S., Road, P. J., Kempf, J. S., and Kienzle, M. G. (1989). Sympathoinhibitory responses to digitalis glycosides in heart failure patients. *Circulation* **80**, 65-77.

Floras, J. S., Legault, L., Morali, G. A., Hara, K., and Blendis, L. M. (1991). Direct evidence from intraneural recordings for increased sympathetic outflow in patients with cirrhosis and ascites. *Ann. intern. Med.* **114**, 373-80.

Hjemdahl, P., Fagius, J., Freyschuss, U., Wallin, B. G., Daleskog, M., Bohlin, G., and Perski, A. (1989). Muscle sympathetic activity and norepinephrine release during mental challenge in humans. *Am. J. Physiol.* **257**, E654-64.

Hornyak, M., Cejnar, M., Elam, M., Matousek, M., and Wallin, B. G. (1991). Sympathetic muscle nerve activity during sleep in humans. *Brain* **114**, 1281-95.

Kachi, T., Iwase, S., Mano, T., Saito, M., Kunimoto, M., and Sobue, I. (1988). Effect of L-threo-3, 4-dihydroxyphenylserine on muscle sympathetic nerve activities in Shy-Drager sydrome. *Neurology* **38**, 1091-4.

Kirnö, K., Kunimoto, M., Lundin, S., Elam, M., and Wallin, B. G. (1991). Can galvanic skin response (GSR) be used as a quantitative estimate of sympathetic nerve activity in regional anaesthesia? *Anaesthesia Analgesia.* **73**, 138-42.

Leimbach, W. N., Wallin, B. G., Victor, R. G., Aylward, P. E., Sundlöf, G., and Mark, A. L. (1986). Direct evidence from intraneural recordings for increased central sympathetic outflow in patients with heart failure. *Circulation* **73**, 913-19.

Lundberg, J., Norgren, L., Ribbe, E., Rosén, I., Steen, S., Thörne, J., and Wallin, B. G. (1989). Direct evidence of active sympathetic vasodilatation in the skin of the human foot. *J. Physiol. London* **417**, 437-46.

Mano, T. (1990). Sympathetic nerve mechanisms of human adaptation to environment—findings obtained by recent microneurographic studies. *Environ. Med.* **34**, 1-35.

Nordin, M. (1990). Sympathetic discharges in the human supraorbital nerve and their relation to sudo- and vasomotor responses. *J. Physiol., London* **423**, 241-55.

Pryor, S. L., Lewis, S. F., Haller, R. G., Bertocci, L. A., and Victor, R. G. (1990). Impairment of sympathetic activation during static exercise in patients with muscle phosphorylase deficiency (McArdle's disease). *J. clin. Invest.* **85**, 1444-9.

Rowell, L. B., Johnson, D. G., Chase, P. B., Comess, K. A., and Seals, D. R. (1989). Hypoxemia raises muscle sympathetic activity but not norepinephrine in resting humans. *J. appl. Physiol.* **66**, 1736-43.

Scherrer, U., Vissing, S., Morgan, B. J., Hanson, P., and Victor, R. G. (1990*a*). Vasovagal syncope after infusion of a vasodilator in a heart-transplant recipient. *New Eng. J. Med.* **322**, 602–4.

Scherrer, U., Vissing, S. F., Morgan, B. J., Rollins, J. A., Tindall, R. S. A., Ring, S., Hanson, P., Mohanty, P. K., and Victor, R. G. (1990*b*). Cyklosporineinduced sympathetic activation and hypertension after heart transplantation. *New Eng. J. Med.* **323**, 693–9.

Sellgren, J., Pontén, J., and Wallin, B. G. (1990). Percutaneous recording of muscle nerve sympathetic activity during nitrous oxide and isoflurane anaesthesia in man. *Anaesthesiology* **73**, 20–7.

Stjernberg, L., Blumberg, H., and Wallin, B. G. (1986). Sympathetic activity in man after spinal cord injury. Outflow to muscle below the lesion. *Brain* **109**, 695–715.

Vallbo, Å. B., Hagbarth, K.-E., Torebjörk, H. E., and Wallin, B. G. (1979). Somatosensory, proprioceptive and sympathetic activity in human peripheral nerves. *Physiol. Rev.* **59**, 919–57.

Wallin, B. G. and Fagius, J. (1988). Peripheral sympathetic neural activity in conscious humans. *Ann. Rev. Physiol.* **50**, 565–76.

Wallin, B. G. and Stjernberg, L. (1984). Sympathetic activity in man after spinal cord injury. Outflow to skin below the lesion. *Brain* **107**, 183–98.

Wallin, B. G. and Sundlöf, G. (1982). Sympathetic outflow to muscles during vasovagal syncope. *J. autonom. nerv. Syst.* **6**, 287–91.

Wallin, B. G., Sundlöf, G., and Linblad, L.-E. (1980). Baroreflex mechanisms controlling sympathetic outflow to the muscles in man. In *Arterial baroreceptors and hypertension* (ed. P. Sleight) p. 101. Oxford University Press.

Wallin, B. G., Westerberg, C.-E., and Sundlöf, G. (1984). Sympathetic outflow to muscles during syncope induced by glossopharyngeal neuralgia. *Neurology* **34**, 522–4.

Yamada, Y., Miyajima, E., Tochikubo, O., Matsukawa, T., and Ishii, M. (1989). Age-related changes in muscle sympathetic nerve activity in essential hypertension. *Hypertension* **13**, 870.

Yatomi, A., Iguchi, A., Uemura, K., Sakamoto, N., Iwase, S., and Mano, T. (1989). A rare case of recurrent vasodepressive attacks of two hours duration: analysis of the mechanisms by muscle sympathetic nerve activity recording. *Clin. Cardiol.* **12**, 164–8.

19. Hypothalamic and pituitary function in autonomic failure

Stafford L. Lightman and T. D. M. Williams

Introduction

Post-mortem studies of brain tissue from patients with autonomic failure (AF) with multiple system atrophy (MSA) reveal marked reductions in hypothalamic noradrenaline, dopamine, and tyrosine hydroxylase (Spokes *et al.* 1979). Although the cell bodies of the tuberoinfundibular dopamine system are located within the mediobasal hypothalamus, there are no noradrenaline or adrenaline cell bodies in spite of the high concentration of these amines. The rich network of noradrenaline and adrenaline terminals in the hypothalamus is derived from cell bodies in the pons and medulla, and it is therefore not surprising that the decreased hypothalamic noradrenaline and adrenaline in AF is also associated with a decrease in brainstem catecholamines, notably in the locus ceruleus (Spokes *et al.* 1979). The catecholamine brainstem nuclei play an important role in the

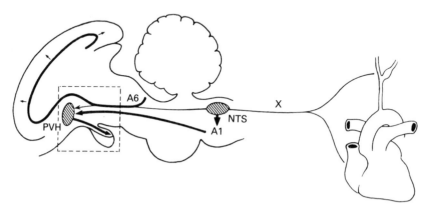

Fig. 19.1. Schematic representation of the catecholamine projections from the brainstem to the paraventricular nucleus of the hypothalamus (PVH) and of neurosecretory fibres from the hypothalamus to the pituitary neural lobe. The dorsal noradrenergic bundle runs between A6 (the locus ceruleus) and the hypothalamus, the ventral noradrenergic bundle between A1 and the hypothalamus. NTS, nucleus of the tractus solitarius.

communication of visceral information from the ninth and tenth nerves to the hypothalamus. These nerves synapse in the nucleus of the tractus solitarius (NTS) in the dorsomedial medulla (Fig. 19.1), whence catecholamine pathways radiate to the hypothalamus and forebrain structures. It would therefore be expected that derangements of these ascending catecholamine pathways and of the local dopaminergic tuberoinfundibular system would result in changes in neuroendocrine control. Before we consider our clinical studies in patients with autonomic failure, it is important to summarize our current understanding of the role of catecholamines in hypothalamic function (Fig. 19.2 (a), (b)).

Dopamine

The dopaminergic neurons in the hypothalamic arcuate nucleus have long been of major interest to neuroendocrinologists. They are the source of dopamine in the external layer of the median eminence (Everitt and Hökfelt 1986) and thus of dopamine in the hypothalamo–hypophyseal portal blood. This dopamine is recogized to be the major prolactin inhibitory factor, and dopamine antagonists cause hyperprolactinaemia in man and experimental animals while dopaminergic agonists suppress prolactin release. These are direct actions on the pituitary lactotroph cells.

In the hypothalamus there is immunocytochemical evidence for an association between dopamine and luteinizing hormone releasing hormone (LHRH) neurons, and the demonstration that many of the arcuate nucleus dopaminergic neurons accumulate the sex steroid oestradiol (Heritage et al. 1975) suggests that these cells may have an important role in the feedback regulation of LHRH secretion. It has been demonstrated that noradrenaline turnover in the preoptic area and median eminence bears a consistent relationship with LHRH secretion (Barraclough et al. 1984) and hypothalamic adrenaline concentrations also co-vary with plasma luteinizing hormone (LH) concentrations (Kalra and Kalra 1985). In vivo studies indeed suggest that dopamine inhibits LHRH secretion but, unfortunately, in vitro studies contradict this. In man dopamine usually reduces LH secretion and in females this effect depends upon the oestrogen status or time of the menstrual cycle.

Dopamine inhibits thyroid stimulating hormone (TSH) secretion in vitro with the same specificity and sensitivity as it does prolactin (Foord et al. 1986) and dopamine antagonists increase TSH secretion by an action on pituitary thyrotrophs. In man inhibitory effects of dopamine on TSH secretion can be demonstrated, but the effect is small and the physiological significance uncertain.

Dopamine has both stimulatory and inhibitory effects on growth hormone secretion, with stimulation of growth hormone release in vivo and an inhibitory effect both at the hypothalamus and directly at the level of the

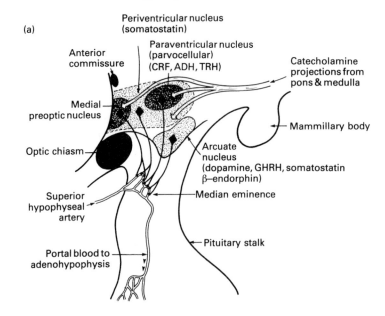

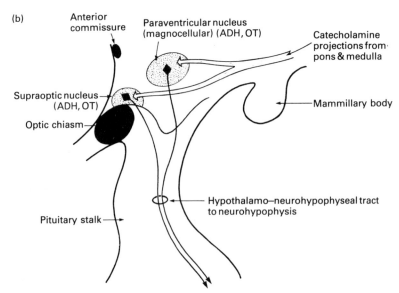

Fig. 19.2. Schematic representation of the hypothalamic nuclei which project to the external layer of the median eminence where hypophyseotrophic factors are secreted into the portal circulation. CRF, corticotrophin releasing factor; ADH, arginine vasopressin; TRH, thryotophin release hormone; GHRH, growth hormone releasing hormone. (b) Schematic representation of the hypothalamic nuclei which send axons to the neurohypophysis where vasopressin and oxytocin are neurosecreted directly into the circulation. ADH arginine vasopressin: OT, oxytocin.

pituitary (Quabbe 1986). Dopamine has recently been demonstrated to coexist with growth hormone releasing hormone (GHRH) in arcuate neurons and this suggests that a significant interaction may occur between these agents. In man administration of dopamine results in increased basal growth hormone but a reduced growth hormone response to hypoglycaemia, while in acromegaly dopamine usually reduces growth hormone secretion.

Dopamine does not seem to be an important component of the control of basal or stress-induced adrenocorticotrophic hormone (ACTH) secretion in the rat. In man dopamine can result in ACTH and cortisol (Lightman 1981) release, but it is unclear whether this is a direct effect of the amine or an indirect effect via other neurotransmitters in the hypothalamus.

Dopamine also plays a role in the control of neurohypophyseal secretion. Dopamine inhibits electrical activity in vasopressinergic neurons and has direct effects on the neural lobe, inhibiting the release of vasopressin (see Carter and Lightman 1985). In man there is also evidence that L-dopa diminishes arginine vasopressin (ADH) secretion by a direct effect at the level of the neural lobe.

Noradrenaline and adrenaline

There is little evidence that adrenaline or noradrenaline are involved in the physiological control of prolactin secretion either in man or experimental animals. There is, however, a close relationship between noradrenaline turnover and LHRH secretion in the rat suggesting that medullary catecholamine nuclei modulate hypothalamic LHRH secretion. Since these medullary nuclei accumulate oestradiol, the phenomenon of oestrogen positive feedback may even occur at this level. Hypothalamic adrenaline also correlates with plasma LH and this amine may also influence pre-ovulatory and oestrogen-induced LH release. Studies are difficult in man since catecholamines do not cross the blood–brain barrier, but neither α-adrenoceptor agonists or antagonists affect pulsatile LH secretion.

The role of noradrenaline and adrenaline in TSH secretion is unclear (Foord *et al.* 1986). Noradrenaline has been reported to release thyrotrophin releasing hormone (TRH) from hypothalamic slices and depletion of hypothalamic amines by 6-hydroxydopamine abolishes the TSH response to cold exposure. Rat pituitary cells release TSH in response to α_1-adrenoceptor stimulation, and adrenaline and TRH act additively to release TSH. Since hypophyseal blood adrenaline levels are higher than those in peripheral blood, this may represent an additional mechanism for the control of TSH. In man α_1-antagonists have been shown to decrease basal TSH and prevent the nocturnal rise found in mildly hypothyroid subjects.

There is considerable evidence for a major role of noradrenaline in the control of growth hormone secretion (Quabbe 1986). Noradrenaline stimulates the release of growth hormone through an α-adrenergic mechanism and inhibits growth hormone via β-receptors. These effects are probably indirect via actions on somatostatin neurons in the periventricular hypothalamus—an area innervated by the locus ceruleus. In man the α_2-agonist clonidine and the β-blocker propranolol stimulate growth hormone secretion while the α_1-antagonist phentolamine reduces and clonidine increases the growth hormone responses to hypoglycaemia.

Activation of catecholaminergic pathways facilitates the release of CRF-41 into portal blood (Plotsky 1987) and lesions of these pathways reduce portal CRF-41 but not portal vasopressin concentrations (Eckland *et al.* 1988). Furthermore, stress increases brain catecholamine turnover and direct lesions of hypothalamic catecholamine terminals prevent the CRFmRNA response to stressful stimuli (Harbuz *et al.* 1991). In man α_1-agonists have been shown to increase ACTH secretion (Al-Damluji 1987), α_2-agonists decrease ACTH release and β-blockers enhance the cortisol response to hypoglycaemia or to amphetamines. This suggests that α_1-receptors may be stimulatory and α_2 and β-receptors inhibitory to ACTH secretion at the hypothalamic level.

The role of brainstem catecholamine pathways has been much more clearly defined in the control of neurohypophyseal activity. The cell bodies which secrete vasopressin and oxytocin are easy to locate and can be recorded electrophysiologically. Although there has been some dispute about the effects of amines on these cells, it is now generally agreed that noradrenaline facilitates the firing of vasopressinergic cells and the release of vasopressin (Day *et al.* 1984). The adrenergic and noradrenergic pathways which relay the hypothalamic response to changes in NTS activity have now been mapped and it is clear that two major tracts are involved: the ventral noradrenergic bundle in the ventral brainstem and the dorsal noradrenergic bundle in the dorsal midbrain. Selective lesions with the neurotoxin 6-hydroxydopamine have demonstrated that the dorsal noradrenergic bundle (which includes fibres from the locus ceruleus) plays an important role in the vasopressin response to cardiovascular stimuli (Lightman *et al.* 1984*a*). These results confirm the facilitatory nature of noradrenaline on vasopressin release. It is difficult to obtain any data in man since not only do adrenaline and noradrenaline fail to cross the blood–brain barrier, but they also have major cardiovascular effects which result in secondary changes in vasopressin secretion. Thus, although infusions of noradrenaline and adrenaline have been shown to increase free water clearance with negligible effects on renal plasma flow and glomerular filtration rate, these results are difficult to interpret.

Studies in autonomic failure

It is with a background of the great difficulties encountered in the study of the role of amines in the control of hypothalamic function in normal man that we must consider our patients with autonomic failure and multiple system atrophy. Patients with AF and MSA have a major loss of ascending catecholamine pathways with an associated decrease in hypothalamic amines. There is also a marked decrease in intrinsic hypothalamic dopamine. Although these subjects present us with a complex pathology, they also provide us with the unique situation of human subjects with abnormal hypothalamic catecholamines, and it is clearly very interesting to assess whether this is associated with any changes in the control of their hypothalamopituitary function. Since the experimental animal data is clearest for neurohypophyseal function, we shall consider this first.

Posterior pituitary function

Vasopressin is secreted in response to both osmotic and cardiovascular stimuli, as well as to oropharyngeal and non-specific stimuli such as nausea and hypoglycaemia (Lightman and Everitt 1986). Since the osmoreceptors are located within the hypothalamus, probably in the area anterior and ventral to the third ventricle, they have relatively direct neuronal access to the vasopressin-containing cells of the magnocellular supraoptic and paraventricular nuclei. Cardiovascular information, however, travels from the thorax in the ninth and tenth nerves to synapse in the NTS in the dorsomedial medulla. Two major pathways—the dorsal and ventral noradrenergic bundles—have been described in the rat (Sawchenko and Swanson 1982), and we have demonstrated (Lightman et al. 1984a) that lesions of the dorsal bundle very markedly reduce the vasopressin response to haemorrhage. Interestingly, the lesion is specific for the cardiovascular stimulus to vasopressin release since the responses to osmotic and nicotine stimuli are unaffected (Lightman et al. 1984a, b). Thus, we have evidence in rats that the integrity of the brainstem noradrenergic pathways is important for the relay of cardiovascular information from the dorsomedial medulla to the vasopressin cells of the hypothalamus.

The loss of brainstem catecholamine pathways in AF is probably the closest we shall be able to get in man to our model of 6-hydroxydopamine lesioned brainstem pathways in the rat. Any studies on these subjects, however, are complicated by the associated degeneration of their sympathetic nervous system which present major problems for the assessment of any cardiovascular stimulus to vasopressin secretion. In order to get over this problem we have now studied three groups of subjects with AF and patients with midcervical spinal cord transections. This last group of subjects has no sympathetic output and can act as a control for the sympathetic nervous system loss in the patients with AF.

The integrity of the vasopressin response to hypertonic saline is good evidence for normal function of the hypothalamo-neurohypophyseal system itself. We tested the vasopressin response to an osmotic stimulus in all three groups of subjects (Williams et al. 1985; Poole et al. 1987). Hypertonic

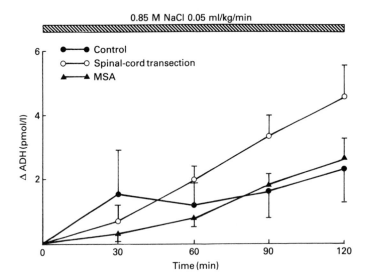

Fig. 19.3. Changes in plasma vasopressin Δ (ADH) during intravenous infusion of 0.85 mol saline, 0.05 ml/kg/min over 2 h in control subjects, patients with AF, and patients with spinal cord transection.

(0.85 M) saline was infused i.v. at a rate of 0.05 ml/kg/min over a period of 2 h, and blood samples were taken every 30 min for assessment of plasma osmolality and vasopressin concentrations. There was a similar change in plasma osmolality in all three groups, and the changes in plasma vasopressin can be seen in Fig. 19.3. Although the increase in the subjects with spinal cord transection is greater than for the other two groups, the difference was not significant.

In the knowledge that all three groups of subjects have a normal vasopressin response to an osmotic stimulus, any differences in their vasopressin response to a cardiovascular stimulus must result from abnormalities proximal to the hypothalamo-neurohypophyseal unit itself. In order to assess the functioning of the vasopressin response to changes in blood pressure and plasma volume we tested the response of all three groups to head-up tilt (Fig. 19.4) (Puritz et al. 1983; Poole et al. 1987). Normal subjects show a significant rise in plasma vasopressin following tilt, while the additional stimulus of postural hypotension in the subjects with spinal cord transection resulted in a markedly increased release of vasopressin. In marked contrast to this—and in spite of a very similar hypotensive response to tilt—the patients with AF have a minimal vasopressin response amounting to only 10 per cent of the rise found in their control group.

It is clear from these studies that patients with AF have abnormalities of vasopressin secretion very similar to those found in our rats with lesions of the dorsal noradrenergic bundle. The response to an osmotic stimulus is intact

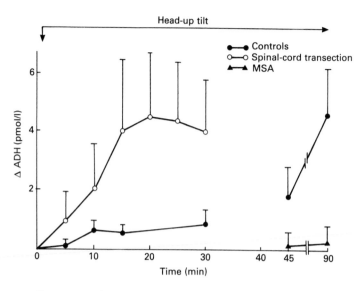

Fig. 19.4. Changes in plasma vasopressin (Δ ADH) during head-up tilt in control subjects, patients with AF, and patients with spinal cord transection.

but there is a severely blunted response to a cardiovascular stimulus. This suggests that in man, as in the rat, ascending catecholamine pathways are important in mediating the vasopressin response to cardiovascular stimuli.

Anterior pituitary function

Hypothalamo-anterior pituitary function has been assessed in five male subjects with AF and compared with five age- and sex-matched controls (Williams *et al.* 1989). Four investigations were carried out on separate occasions: (1) TRH (200 μg) plus LHRH (100 μg) were given i.v. and serum LH, follicle-stimulating hormone (FSH), TSH, and prolactin were measured every 30 min for 2 h; (2) metoclopramide (10 mg) was given i.v. and prolactin and TSH measured every 30 min for 2 h; (3) blood samples were taken at 09.00 and 24.00 h for assessment of cortisol rhythm; (4) a control infusion of saline was administered between 09.00 and 13.00 h followed by an infusion of the opiate antagonist naloxone (10 mg) in 25 ml of 0.17 mol/l saline between 13.00 and 17.00 h; LH, FSH, prolactin, cortisol, and growth hormone (GH) were measured at 30 min intervals.

TRH/LHRH test (Fig. 19.5)

Both controls and AF subjects showed a normal response of TSH and prolactin to TRH, with maximal responses at 30 min in nearly all cases. There was a decrease or reversal in the normal basal LH:FSH ratio in both groups

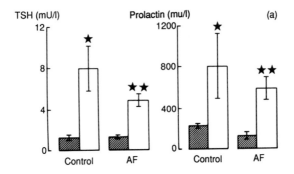

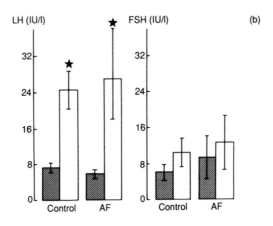

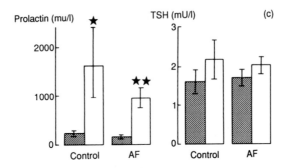

Fig. 19.5. Basal hormone concentrations and maximal responses (mean ± SEM) following intravenous administration of: (a) TRH (200 μg); (b) LHRH (100 μg); and (c) metoclopramide (10 mg) in five subjects with AF and five controls.

due to an increase in basal FSH in these elderly subjects. There was a brisk LH response to LHRH (maximal at 30 min in nearly all cases) with relatively poor stimulation of FSH in both groups.

Metoclopramide test (Fig. 19.5)

There was a good prolactin response to metoclopramide, maximal at 30 min in nearly all cases, and no significant change in TSH in both groups.

Cortisol rhythm

Diurnal cortisol estimation in AF patients confirmed that the cortisol rhythm was intact in spite of the central defects in these patients (09.00 h, cortisol 415 ± 42 nmol/l; 24.00 h, cortisol 199 ± 83 nmol/l).

Naloxone infusion

Mean plasma cortisol concentrations in both groups were not significantly different during the saline and naloxone infusion periods (data not shown), indicating a loss of diurnal fall in plasma cortisol during naloxone infusion in both groups. Naloxone had no effect on mean FSH or prolactin levels in either group of subjects (data not shown).

The pattern of growth hormone (GH) secretion during naloxone and saline infusion was similar in both groups, with overall mean levels increasing during naloxone infusion from 1.7 ± 0.7 to 3.9 ± 1.0 mU/l in AF subjects ($p < 0.01$) and from 1.8 ± 0.8 to 3.8 ± 1.2 mU/l in the controls (not significant). The overall number of neurosecretory pulses also increased in both groups during naloxone infusion.

In control subjects, naloxone caused a significant rise in overall LH concentrations (saline, 4.7 ± 0.4 U/l; naloxone 7.2 ± 0.8U/l; $p < 0.01$) as well as increased frequency and amplitude of LH pulses (Fig. 19.6). In marked contrast, in AF subjects naloxone did not increase overall LH concentrations (saline, 5.1 ± 1.0 U/l; naloxone, 5.9 ± 1.4 U/l; not significant), nor did it alter the frequency of LH pulses. LH pulse frequency was markedly depressed in these subjects. Indeed, three of the subjects showed no LH pulses during the 8 h of testing and the other two subjects showed no LH pulses during the 8 h of testing and the other two had a total of only five pulses between them.

Conclusions

Although there is a reported decrease in hypothalamic dopamine content in AF, we do not find evidence for a lack of hypothalamo-hypophyseal portal dopamine, as evidenced by a normal prolactin response to the dopamine antagonist metoclopramide. TSH and prolactin responses to TRH are also normal as was the loss of cortisol rhythm during naloxone infusion.

There is very little data on the effects of age on GH secretion (Ho *et al.* 1987). We clearly demonstrated that basal GH levels were low, and responded

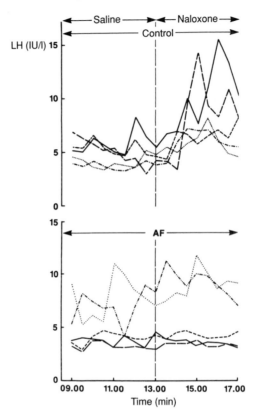

Fig. 19.6. Individual serum LH values during infusion of 25 ml of 0.17 mol/l saline between 09.00 and 13.00 h followed by naloxone (10 mg) between 13.00 and 17.00 h in (above) five controls and (below) five subjects with AF.

to naloxone in the same way in both controls and patients with AF. Furthermore, other studies have confirmed normal GH responses to hypoglycaemia in patients with AF (Polinsky and Recant 1981). On the other hand there is much experimental data for an important role of catecholamines in the regulation of GH secretion and it is interesting that a complete absence of GH response to clonidine has been reported in AF (da Costa *et al.* 1984) suggesting a selective loss of the α_2-adrenoceptor mediated response.

The relatively high FSH and the brisk LH response to LHRH in both AF and control groups is related to the poor functioning of the ageing testis presumably related to diminished feedback from testicular inhibin and testosterone (Desylpere *et al.* 1987). In light of the evidence for a major role of catecholamines in the regulation of gonadotrophins in experimental animals, it was of particular interest that AF patients who have pathological changes to their ascending catecholamine pathways had abnormal hypothalamic control of gonadotrophin secretion during the naloxone infusion.

Summary

Patients with AF provide a unique opportunity to study the neuroendocrine effects of a condition associated with abnormal hypothalamic amines. The clearest abnormalities are found in the control of posterior pituitary secretion of vasopressin where there are very similar abnormalities to those found in rats with lesions of their dorsal noradrenergic bundles. Abnormalities of anterior pituitary function are less clear, but there is evidence for altered regulation of two hormones known to be responsive to catecholamines— luteinizing hormone and growth hormone. It seems likely that these abnormalities are related to the degeneration of ascending noradrenergic and adrenergic pathways. Although hypothalamic dopamine concentrations are decreased, dopaminergic neuroendocrine control appears intact as evidenced by the normality of prolactin responses.

References

Al-Damluji, S., Perry, L., Tomlin, S., Bouloux, P., Grossman, A., Rees, L. H., and Besser, G. M. (1987). Alpha-adrenergic stimulation of corticotrophin secretion by a specific central mechanism in man. *Neuroendocrinology* 45, 68–76.

Barraclough, C. A., Wise, P. M., and Selmanoff, M. K. (1984). A role of hypothalamic catecholamines in the regulation of gonadotrophin secretion. *Recent Prog. Hormone Res.* 40, 487–520.

Carter, D. A. and Lightman, S. L. (1985). Neuroendocrine control of vasopressin secretion. In *The posterior pituitary* (ed. P. H. Bayliss and P. L. Padfield), pp. 53–118. Marcel Dekker, New York.

da Costa, D. F., Bannister, R., Landon, J., and Mathias, C. J. (1984). Growth hormone response to clonidine is impaired in patients with central sympathetic degeneration. *J. clin. exp. Hypertension* 6, 1943–6.

Day, T. A., Ferguson, A. V., and Renaud, L. P. (1984). Facilitatory influence of noradrenergic afferents on the excitability of rat paraventricular nucleus neurosecretory cells. *J. Physiol.* 355, 237–49.

Desylpere, J. P., Kaufman, J. M., Vermeulen, T., Vogelaers, D., Vandalem, J. L., and Vermeulen, A. (1987). Influence of age of pulsatile luteinizing hormone release and responsiveness of the gonadotrophs to sex hormone feedback in men. *J. clin. Endocrinol. Metab.* 64, 68–73.

Eckland, D. J. A., Todd, K., Jessop, D. S., Biswas, S., and Lightman, S. L. (1988). Differential effects of hypothalamic catecholamine depletion on the release of arginine vasopressin and CRF-41 into hypothalamo-hypophyseal portal blood. *Neurosci. Letts.* 90, 292–6.

Everitt, B. J. and Hökfelt, T. (1986). Neuroendocrine anatomy of the hypothalamus. In *Neuroendocrinology* (ed. S. L. Lightman and B. J. Everitt), pp. 5–31. Blackwell Scientific, Oxford.

Foord, S. M., Peters, J. R., Dieguez, C., Lewis, M. D., Lewis, B. M., Hall, R., and Scanlon, M. F. (1986). Thyroid stimulating hormone. In *Neuroendocrinology* (ed. S. L. Lightman and B. J. Everitt), pp. 450–71. Blackwell Scientific, Oxford.

Harbuz, M. S., Chowdrey, H. S., Jessop, D. S., Biswas, S., and Lightman, S. L. (1991). Role of catecholamines in mediating messenger RNA and hormonal responses to stress. *Brain Res.* **551**, 52–7.

Heritage, A. S., Grant, L. D., and Stumpf, W. E. (1975). Oestradiol in catecholamine neurons of the rat brainstem: combined localisations by autoradiography and formaldehyde-induced fluorescence. *J. comp. Neurol.* **176**, 607–30.

Ho, K. Y., Evans, W. S., Blizzard, R. M., Veldhuis, J. D., Merriam, G. R., Samojlik, E., Fulanetto, R., Rogol, A. D., Kaiser, D. L., and Thorner, M. O. (1987). Effects of sex and age on the 24-hour profile and growth hormone secretion in man: importance of endogenous oestradiol concentrations. *J. clin. Endocrinol. Metab.* **64**, 51–8.

Kalra, P. S. and Kalra, S. P. (1985). Control of gonadotrophin secretion. In *The pituitary gland* (ed. H. Imura), pp. 189–220. Raven Press, New York.

Lightman, S. L. (1981). Studies on the responses of plasma renin activity and aldosterone and cortisol levels to dopaminergic and opiate stimuli in man. *Clin. Endocrinol.* **15**, 45–52.

Lightman, S. L., Jacobs, H. S., Maguire, A. K., McGarrick, G., and Jeffcoate, S. L. (1981). Constancy of opioid control of luteinising hormone in different pathophysiological states. *J. clin. Endocrinol. Metabl.* **52**, 1260–3.

Lightman, S. L. and Everitt, B. J., and Todd, K. (1984a). Ascending noradrenergic projections from the brainstem; evidence for a major role in the regulation of blood pressure and vasopressin secretion. *Exp. Brain Res.* **55**, 145–51.

Lightman, S. L., Todd, K., and Everitt, B. J. (1984b). Role for lateral tegmental noradrenergic neurons in the vasopressin response to hypertonic saline. *Neurosci. Lett.* **42**, 55–9.

Plotsky, P. M. (1987). Facilitation of immunoreactive corticotropin releasing factor secretion into the hypophysial portal circulation after activation of catecholaminergic pathways or central norepinephrine injection. *Endocrinology* **121**, 924–30.

Polinsky, R. and Recant, L. (1981). Hormonal responses to hypoglycaemia in orthostatic hypotension patients. *Life Sci.* **28**, 417–25.

Poole, C. J. M., Williams, T. D. M., Lightman, S. L., and Frankel, H. L. (1987). Neuroendocrine control of vasopressin secretion and its effect on blood pressure in subjects with spinal cord transection. *Brain* **110**, 727–35.

Puritz, R., Lightman, S. L., Wilcox, C. S., Forsling, M., and Bannister, R. (1983). Blood pressure and vasopressin in progressive autonomic failure. *Brain* **106**, 502–11.

Quabbe, H. J. (1986) Growth hormone. In *Neuroendocrinology* (ed. S. L. Lightman and B. J. Everitt), pp. 409–49. Blackwell Scientific, Oxford.

Sawchenko, P. E. and Swanson, L. W. (1982). The organisation of noradrenergic pathways from the brainstem to the paraventricular and supraoptic nuclei in the rat. *Brain Res. Rev.* **4**, 275–325.

Spokes, E. G., Bannister, R., and Oppenheimer, D. R. (1979). Multiple system atrophy with autonomic failure: clinical histological and neurochemical observations on four cases. *J. neurol. Sci.* **43**, 59–82.

Williams, T. D. M., Lightman, S. L., and Bannister, R. (1985). Vasopressin secretion in progressive autonomic failure; evidence for defective afferent cardiovascular pathways. *J. Neurol. Neurosurg. Psychiat.* **48**, 225–9.

Williams, T. D. M., Lightman, S. L., Johnson, M. R., Carmichael, D. J. S., and Bannister, R. (1989). Selective defect in gonadotrophin secretion in patients with autonomic failure. *Clin. Endocrinol* **30**, 285–92.

20. A commentary on clinical tests of autonomic function with particular reference to recent developments

Terence Bennett and Sheila M. Gardiner

Introduction

The present commentary is confined largely to disorders of cardiovascular regulation, predominantly in patients with diabetes mellitus, but the points made have a more general relevance to the interpretation of responses to clinical tests of autonomic neuronal function in normal and disordered states.

What is normal?

One of the main questions that must tax any investigator can be considered under the subheading 'conditions under which the measurement is made'. Intuitively, most of us feel that these conditions should be controlled. Indeed, in animal studies, care is taken to ensure that individuals are of the same sex, genotypically homogeneous, eating the same food, exposed to the same housing conditions, and studied at the same time of day using the same experimental protocol. In studies of normal man, experiments are often confined to the same time of day on fasted subjects, of the same sex, and under the same environmental conditions. Evidence that such caution is justified comes from investigations of the influence of factors such as starvation or exercise on cardiovascular reflexes. Following a 48-h fast in normal male subjects, a reduction in supine diastolic blood pressure and forearm vascular resistance occur with abnormal baroreflex responses to lower body negative pressure or to standing. While 48 h starvation may seem an unlikely stress in normal subjects, it may be highly relevant to the acute metabolic disturbances experienced in diabetes mellitus.

A more frequently encountered and difficult to control variable is exercise. In both normotensive and hypertensive subjects, moderate levels of exercise produce effects on cardiovascular reflexes for 8 h or more. Exercise lowers systemic arterial blood pressure, partly due to resetting and sensitization of cardiac and vascular reflexes. However, our understanding of this phenomenon is incomplete, since muscle sympathetic efferent activity is suppressed 60 min after exercise, whereas observed forearm vascular resistance is elevated at this time. The greater effect of exercise on cardiovascular reflexes in hypertensive patients is noteworthy in the context of the frequent occurrence in diabetic patients of elevated systemic arterial blood pressures. There have been no studies of the influence of exercise on cardiovascular reflexes in diabetes mellitus, although exercise may be an important factor in the treatment of this disease.

Recently, it has been demonstrated that the blood pressure and heart rate responses to standing up in normal subjects are influenced, quantitatively, by the period of preceding rest, possibly due to differences in the volume of blood shifting on account of an increase in venous capacitance. In subjects with abnormal cardiovascular regulation it is feasible that the period of preceding rest might have greater effects than usual on the orthostatic responses.

Environmental temperature is an important variable not usually considered in studies of cardiovascular reflexes. Patients with diabetes mellitus may show substantial abnormalities of thermoregulatory reflexes, e.g. impaired vasoconstriction and disordered sweating, emphasizing the need for thermally controlled conditions. Furthermore, it would be of great value if all laboratories reported data obtained at agreed thermoneutral temperatures.

Examination of the literature gives the impression that there are currently available large data bases for normal responses to a variety of manoeuvres that take into account age and sex. However, most of these data have been collected under uncontrolled conditions. None of us have yet taken the trouble to establish normal ranges for a spectrum of cardiovascular reflexes in the same normal subjects, assessing the responses under controlled conditions through time. The latter point raises the spectre of reproducibility and the appropriateness of control values established in others' studies. Given the variability encountered in patients and the ways in which they can differ from normal subjects, it would be most correct scientifically if each investigator generated the control data apposite for the study in hand. An inevitable consequence of this approach is the acceptance that data obtained from normal volunteers (often the investigators and their colleagues) may not be suitable as control values for clinical patients who, apart from other problems, might be very apprehensive about their circumstances.

It is accepted generally that it would be inappropriate to decide whether or not a particular patient had hypertension on the basis of blood pressure measurements made on a single occasion. We suggest similar caution should be applied in circumstances where more sophisticated clinical investigations are being carried out in order to diminish the possible contributions that the emotional state of the patient might make to the results obtained. For example, variables such as heart rate and forearm blood flow and their responses to clinical tests may be influenced substantially by elevated circulating catecholamine levels.

Another aspect of this general problem is the obsession with the statistical significance of differences between data sets, regardless of whether or not any clinical or functional meaning can be attached to such differences. (An example of this problem is seen in a recent study in which active drug treatment produced a statistically significant increase of 0.7 ± 0.24 m/s in peroneal motor nerve conduction velocity in a group of diabetic patients, against a background of the two 'normal' groups in the study having values of 46.5 ± 3.9 and 49.1 ± 2.4 m/s for this variable.)

What is abnormal?

In the light of the above comments it is worthwhile considering the particular problems in assessing what is abnormal when studying cardiovascular reflexes in diabetes mellitus. It is clear that those variables one tries to control for in normal subjects may be more important in patients. For example, it is not necessarily true that an overnight-fasted (or fed) diabetic patient has normal fluid and electrolyte balance or, if studied under something other than thermoneutral conditions, would be in a comparable thermal state to a normal subject. However, the biggest problem arises with those variables, such as glucose and insulin 'status', which are likely to be abnormal. Many past and recent studies in diabetic patients have been under conditions in which metabolic variables must have been changing throughout the experimental period. This problem could have been avoided by admitting the patient to hospital the night before the study and controlling blood glucose by continuously adjusting the rate of intravenous glucose and insulin until the study was finished (Scott *et al.* 1987, 1988*a,b*). However, this does not avoid the important question: how long before the study should one attempt such control to distinguish between disorders attributable to acute or chronic metabolic abnormalities? None the less, attempting to control glycaemic status would seem to be a step in the right direction, albeit not one others are willing to follow, as is demonstrated by a recent study in which no distinction was made between patients with type I and type II diabetes mellitus, no information was given about the timing of treatment relative to the time of measurements, and, in the absence of any statement to the contrary, one can only assume the investigation was carried out under conditions in which glycaemic control was not achieved.

Similar considerations arise in other groups of patients on chronic drug treatment. For example, it is almost impossible to study untreated hypertensive patients because drug therapy is usually initiated by their general practitioners, so the question arises, how long before any investigation should drug treatment be withdrawn? This question bears not only on the pharmacokinetics of the drug concerned, but also on the functional consequences of treatment. If receptor sensitization or desensitization has occurred as a result of drug treatment, the time course of reversion of these effects may differ from the time course of elimination of the drug from the body. If vascular remodelling and regression of cardiac hypertrophy have been achieved, the persistence of these effects following drug withdrawal may be substantial. How, then, can one argue that withdrawal of drug treatment, 1 week before any clinical study is sufficient to achieve a condition that is equivalent to the untreated state?

Comparable, but possibly more complex, problems probably pertain to patients with disorders such as Parkinson's disease who have been receiving long-term treatment with L-dopa. There may be sustained central effects (in receptors, neurotransmitter systems, and compensatory mechanisms) following withdrawal of treatment, and the time course of these is unknown. Furthermore, as in the insulin-dependent diabetic patient, the treatment itself may be responsible for some of the disorders present; thus we do not know what effects long-term treatment with L-dopa or insulin have independent of the diseases in which they are used. These are scientific problems and the points raised need to be balanced against the important ethical question as to whether or not it is justifiable to withdraw treatment.

In the context of diabetes mellitus, ideas about the biology of insulin and its involvement in a variety of physiological processes are changing rapidly. It is not known if the acute cardiovascular effects of insulin (e.g. Scott *et al.* 1988*a*) are direct or indirect. Euglycaemic hyperinsulinaemia, for example, increases muscle sympathetic nerve activity but, simultaneously, causes forearm vasodilatation. Forearm vasodilatation under the same conditions in normal subjects had been reported by Scott *et al.* (1988*a*). However, they also showed that forearm vasoconstrictor responses to lower body negative pressure were maintained in normal subjects, whereas in type I diabetes mellitus they were impaired. Such observations raise questions regarding relationships between efferent nerve activity and effector response, the involvement of endothelial factors (particularly endothelin and nitric oxide), and the acute and chronic interactions between insulin and these systems. It is likely such factors are not only of importance in diseases such as diabetes mellitus, but also in hypertension where insulin resistance may be of pathophysiological significance.

Bearing these points in mind, we must consider also the precise reasons for making the measurements. Clinically, it is important to know the patient's physiological status under daily circumstances. Thus, measurements should be carried out, ideally under both laboratory and 'field' conditions, the former serving as objective assessments that can be compared at intervals to indicate clinical progression. A systematic comparison of these two sets of data might provide valuable information.

What measurements to make?

In the early days of a new area of study, workers often adhere to measurements that are readily made and/or those with which they are familiar.

With the passage of time, it is appreciated that more subtle approaches are needed. Progress is dependent on reconsideration of 'fixed' views and development of new techniques. However, the latter must also be examined critically as highly intricate and technically complex studies may be at the expense of experimental rigour. It is a truism that more data are obtained the more measurements one makes, but few investigators consider what the measurements mean. Certainly, there is the tacit assumption, on the part of many, that the measurement means the same under all conditions. Sinus arrhythmia can be quantitated precisely, but it does not follow that reduction in sinus arrhythmia is due to the same problem under all conditions. For example, reduced thoracic compliance, sinoatrial dysfunction, afferent neuropathy, cerebral damage, efferent neuropathy, and circulating antibodies to muscarinic receptors could all give rise to reduced sinus arrhythmia. The welter of papers describing 'new' tests of cardiovascular function based on spectral analysis of heart rate variability do not distinguish between such possibilities. The technique of analysis may be new, but the subsequent interpretation of the data still depends on an understanding of basic physiology and additional information about the physiology of the particular subject in question; this is usually not available.

Important disparities between our understanding of cardiovascular physiology and the interpretation of responses to clinical tests are not uncommon. An 'abnormal' response to a particular intervention is not, necessarily, a sign of pathophysiology. An example is in the patterns of cardiovascular response to lower body negative pressure or manipulation of carotid sinus pressure in young trained subjects compared to untrained controls. It has been reported that the young, trained subjects show impaired cardiovascular regulation, but it should be noted that diametrically opposite results have been obtained also.

Considering such contradictions it is reasonable to ask whether or not our approach to the understanding of cardiovascular reflexes is correct. In normal man it has been argued that exposure to minimal levels of lower body negative pressure reduces central venous pressure, but without change in systolic, diastolic, or mean systemic arterial blood pressure, or arterial dP/dt. However, this intervention elicits significant forearm vasoconstriction with little increase in splanchnic vascular resistance, and no tachycardia. Exposure to high levels of lower body negative pressure, sufficient to reduce central venous and systemic arterial blood pressure causes forearm and splanchnic vasoconstriction.

On the basis of observations such as these, it has been claimed that the forearm vasoconstriction seen during exposure to low levels of lower body negative pressure is due, solely, to unloading of cardiopulmonary baroreceptors. However, for this to be a tenable hypothesis something unexplained must be happening, since, if exposure to low levels of lower body negative pressure does not decrease cardiac output, then systemic arterial pressure should go *up*, due to the vasoconstriction in the forearms. The absence of a pressor response to low levels of lower body negative pressure could be due to concurrent vasodilatation in another vascular bed (besides the splanchnic region), but this effect would have to be precisely matched to cancel the vasoconstriction in the forearms, and it is not at all clear how this could be achieved without the mediation of systemic arterial baroreceptors. Furthermore, if exposure to low levels of lower body negative pressure does reduce stroke volume, then this change must be offset *exactly* by the increase in forearm vascular resistance to prevent change in those features of systemic arterial pressure to which carotid sinus baroreceptors are sensitive. This seems most unlikely since the afferent system considered to be responsible for the reflex adjustment of forearm vascular resistance (i.e. cardiopulmonary receptors) are not exposed to what appears to be the controlled variable (i.e. some feature(s) of carotid sinus transmural pressure or flow; Bennett 1987).

The resolution of this anomaly comes from two sets of observations. First, baroreceptor afferent fibres are sensitive to changes in flow, in the absence of changes in pressure or strain, and, second, in a patient with sinoaortic denervation, exposure to lower body negative pressure at −10 mm Hg caused falls in both central venous and systemic arterial blood pressures (Aksamit *et al.* 1987). Since there was a marked increase in muscle sympathetic nerve activity during lower body negative pressure and since sinoaortic afferent pathways were interrupted, it was clear that cardiopulmonary afferent systems were probably responsible for modulating sympathetic efferent outflow. However, it was equally clear that, in the absence of sinoaortic afferent systems, unloading of cardiopulmonary afferents was not capable of preventing hypotension (Aksamit *et al.* 1987). Therefore, the most likely explanation of the absence of changes in arterial blood pressure in normal subjects exposed to minimal levels of lower body negative pressure is that cardiopulmonary and arterial baroreceptors act in concert to effect the necessary adjustments in regional vascular conductances. In spite of what appear to us to be very persuasive observations, many still persist in reiterating the dogma regarding baroreflexes in man.

Another point of note in the context of human baroreflex mechanisms is that the lack of calf, relative to forearm, vasoconstriction in response to lower body negative pressure is associated with *similar* changes in muscle sympathetic nerve activity in the two limbs. Thus, differential involvement of endothelial factors in the two vascular beds is worth considering as an explanation for their disparate behaviour. The sensing of changes in carotid sinus flow by the associated afferent systems also may be modulated by the endothelium (through the mediation of cyclo-oxygenase products and endothelin). Acute effects of inhibition of endothelial cell nitric oxide production on baroreflex mechanisms have, not however, been detected.

To assess properly the integrity of autonomic reflex mechanisms it is thus necessary to be able to quantitate each component of the system, i.e. afferent input, central transmission, efferent output, and effector responsiveness (which includes membrane receptor number and affinity and all those events that represent 'postreceptor coupling'). The latter assertion is not too far-fetched since there is much evidence for marked changes in myocardial receptors in animals with experimentally induced diabetes mellitus, yet these have not been investigated in diabetic patients.

At present, despite the number of readily performed measurements which are routinely made, the use of this information is questionable unless it enables specific clinical intervention, as for postural hypotension and cardiac rhythm disorders such as tachycardia. Given the multifactorial nature of many of the disturbances it is often unjustifiable to extrapolate from one system to another (e.g. reduced sinus arrhythmia does not provide evidence of an organic lesion underlying diabetic impotence or of a widespread parasympathetic lesion). It is, therefore, incumbent upon those who assess 'autonomic function' to consider why they do it, given that the simple repetition of a procedure may not advance knowledge about the mechanisms involved, or the nature of the longitudinal changes, especially if the measurements are made under uncontrolled conditions. Furthermore, one should be aware that the numerical value of variables such as baroreflex sensitivity differ depending on the way in which the test is performed.

The following sections are written with the intention of highlighting areas that would benefit from increased research effort. We have chosen examples from the field of diabetes mellitus to make points of general note.

Autonomic dysfunction

Autonomic dysfunction may be due to afferent, central, or efferent 'disorders'. These may result from anything from irreversible neuronal degeneration to reversible, acute neuronal dysfunction attributable to metabolic disturbance. It is possible, indeed likely, that a combination of disorders may be present but, for convenience, the problems will be considered individually. Except where stated, the studies quoted have not been done under controlled conditions of the sort described above.

Afferent disorders

The cause(s) of these (as with all other neuronal disorders) is unresolved. Factors such as neuronal hypoxia, impaired axonal transport, and membrane dysfunction are being mooted. Several factors other than, or in addition to, neuronal disorders could contribute to afferent dysfunction (Fig. 20.1).

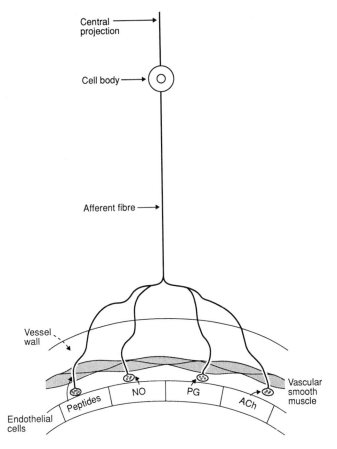

Fig. 20.1. Diagrammatic representation of the functional relationships between vascular afferent neuronal systems and elements in the blood vessel wall. Apart from physical factors, such as stretching of the afferent terminals, several endothelial-derived molecules are now known to influence afferent neuronal signalling. These include peptides (such as endothelin-1), nitric oxide (NO), prostanoids (PG), and molecules such as acetylcholine (ACh).

It is not possible routinely to assess cardiovascular afferent integrity independent of other mechanisms in man, and the relevant physiological experiments have not been done in experimental animals. However, Fagius *et al.* (1985) examined the responses of normal subjects to anaesthesia of the glossopharyngeal and vagal nerves (to achieve cessation of afferent inflows independent of manipulation of sensory terminals). This manoeuvre induced hypertension and tachycardia, associated with intense muscle sympathetic activity, i.e. changes similar to those seen in the Guillain–Barré syndrome. Although hypertension and tachycardia are common in diabetes mellitus, for example, they are not associated with increased muscle sympathetic activity, and it has been suggested this might argue against an afferent disorder (Fagius 1985). However, if selective afferent dysfunction develops, other afferent or central processes may readjust or other dysfunctions may occur concurrently. Examples that may be analogous to the changes in the former category are baroreceptor deafferentation or cardiac denervation, which do not produce sustained elevations in systemic arterial blood pressure or vasopressin release in experimental animals.

There have been no studies involving electrical stimulation of the carotid sinus nerve or examining responses to carotid sinus suction in diabetic patients, but these would not provide information about afferent function independent of central or efferent mechanisms.

There is some evidence for a relatively selective impairment of afferent input from peripheral chemoreceptors in patients with diabetes mellitus, since hypoxic ventilatory drive may be abnormal when hypercapnic drive is not. However, it is difficult to control for the relative strengths of these two stimuli. Other afferent systems such as thermoreceptors that may influence cardiovascular function have been shown to be defective in diabetics, but these studies have not excluded the possibility of impaired central mechanisms.

One approach to investigating the integrity of afferent systems independently of central process would be to challenge with a chemical stimulus that produced an axon reflex. Afferent fibres in the skin, when stimulated with capsaicin, release neuropeptides (including substance P and calcitonin gene-related peptide (CGRP)) and there is an accompanying 'flare'. It has been shown that diabetic patients may have an impaired microvascular hyperaemic response to skin trauma, and it is possible that this is due to loss of capsaicin-sensitive afferent fibres. However, in rats made diabetic with streptozotocin, diminished capsaicin-mediated plasma extravasation is not associated with reduced skin content of substance P. Thus, the phenomenon may be further complicated by changes in microvascular permeability which also occur in diabetic patients. Recent observations by Boolell and Tooke (1990) in patients with uncomplicated type I diabetes mellitus indicate the presence of reduced cutaneous hyperaemia to injections of substance P, but not to capsaicin, consistent with a selective decrease in vascular reactivity to substance P. The extent to which changes in endothelial cell nitric oxide production might have contributed to the abnormal responses to substance P has not been examined.

The afferent fibres sensitive to capsaicin are dependent on nerve growth factor, and hence may be impaired by insulin antibodies and/or deficiency of nerve growth factor, as seen in rats with streptozotocin-induced diabetes mellitus (Hellweg and Hartung 1990). Furthermore, in experimental animals treatment with capsaicin produces changes in cardiovascular control mechanisms remarkably similar to those seen in diabetic animals. Finally, it is intriguing that capsaicin is a particularly potent stimulus for eliciting

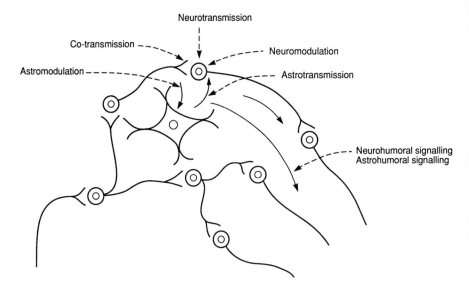

Fig. 20.2. Diagrammatic representation of factors involved in processing of information within the central nervous system. In addition to rapid neuronal neuro-transmission processes and the influence on them of co-transmitters and neuro-modulators, there is the possibility of paracrine or neurohumoral processes being involved in the relatively slower mechanisms. Furthermore, there is now evidence for dynamic interactions between astrocytes and neurons and hence the theoretical possibility that what we have called astrotransmission, astromodulation, and astro-humoral signalling may be important components of central integrative function.

'gustatory sweating' and the latter may occur in response to stimuli, such as chocolate, in diabetic patients.

Central disorders

As with afferent systems it is now clear that central processing may involve more than traditional synaptic transmission. These mechanisms include neuromodulation, trophic changes, astrocytic activity, and the role of extracellular humoral factors in central information processing which must all be considered (Fig. 20.2).

It is not routinely possible to monitor non-invasively central events (such as evoked potentials) associated specifically with processing of cardiovascular information in man, and we know of no such data in animals. However, there is electrophysiological evidence that central pathways subserving auditory function may be abnormal in diabetic patients, but further controlled studies are required.

As alluded to above, major questions regarding hypothalamic sensitivity and other possibilities, such as the involvement of insulin and/or glucagon and/or vasopressin in disorders of central cardiovascular regulation in diabetes mellitus, have barely been considered, let alone investigated. However, in a recent study hypoglycaemic unawareness and inadequate hypoglycaemic counterregulation showed no causal relationship to autonomic neuropathy (as assessed by traditional tests), and this was interpreted as suggestive of reduced responsiveness of a central glucoregulatory centre to hypoglycaemia.

Efferent disorders

Our understanding of factors that can impinge on efferent function has expanded greatly in recent times (Fig. 20.3).

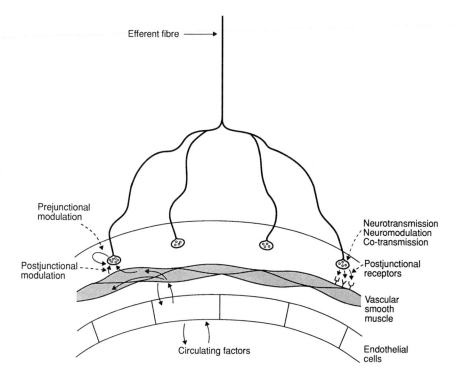

Fig. 20.3. Diagrammatic representation of the relationship between efferent vasomotor nerve terminals and elements within the vascular wall. As in other systems it is now evident that neuroeffector transmission is subject to pre- and postjunctional modulation by various factors including transmitters and co-transmitters (e.g. peptides, purines). Moreover, physical and circulating factors interact with endothelial cells to promote release of agents (nitric oxide, endothelin-1, prostanoids) that influence the underlying vascular smooth muscle and, possibly, the associated nerve terminals.

Neuronal dysfunction

While information on preganglionic efferent activity may be gained by monitoring the changes in postganglionic muscle or skin sympathetic activity (Fagius 1985) in response to edrophonium, this has not yet been done. At a more peripheral level, there have been few systematic comparative studies of effector responses to different manoeuvres under different conditions. This is partly to do with the nature of the measurement, since, generally, those experimental investigations directed towards understanding pathophysiological processes are more invasive than clinical 'bedside tests'. However, the understandable inclination to keep invasive measurements to a minimum probably accounts for the current confusion regarding the relations between peripheral blood flow, muscle sympathetic activity, and catecholamine release (as indices of sympathetic efferent activity). In this context, peripheral blood flow usually refers to forearm or calf blood flow (but see Scott *et al.* 1987, 1988*b*), although there is evidence for differential blood flow responses in these two limbs in response to the same stimulus (see Chapter 5). This is an intriguing observation, since baroreceptor-mediated modulation of muscle sympathetic activity is directed equally to the two limbs. A linear relationship between forearm venous plasma noradrenaline concentrations and muscle sympathetic activity in the leg during drug-induced changes in blood pressure is claimed (Eckberg *et al.* 1988), but the physiological meaning of this impressive correlation needs some reconsideration.

First, the drugs used to elicit changes in muscle sympathetic activity (secondary to changes in systemic arterial pressure) may themselves affect perfusion in the forearm and leg (possibly differentially) and hence may influence catecholamine extraction at those sites (Chang *et al.* 1986). Eckberg *et al.* (1988) have acknowledged this problem and stated 'we do not know if the excellent correlation we found between sympathetic activity and neurotransmitter concentrations would have been significantly different if we had corrected our measurements for concomitant changes in forearm flow'. However, Eckberg *et al.* (1988) failed to emphasize that, even in their studies, muscle sympathetic nerve activity and plasma concentrations of noradrenaline and neuropeptide Y during infusion of phenylephrine showed no significant associations.

Second, the differential flow changes in the two limbs in response to a specific stimulus would be likely to lead to differential changes in venous plasma catecholamine concentrations at those sites. The relationship between leg and forearm venous plasma catecholamines in response to specific stimuli has yet to be delineated. Nevertheless, there is the important observation that the flow changes (reflecting the summation of all the various inputs) may be different in the two limbs. If the changes in sympathetic efferent outflow are the same in the arm and leg in response to any particular manoeuvre then it is possible that differences in the distribution of postjunctional receptor types and/or release of local vasodilator substances may account for the differential flow responses. Whatever the explanation, the problems mentioned are real, and the claim that muscle sympathetic nerve activity correlates well with venous plasma noradrenaline levels does not mean the latter is a reliable *index* of the former, presumably because of the complex series of events whereby noradrenaline released from periadventitial nerves gains access to the plasma (Bennett and Gardiner 1988).

The view that forearm venous catecholamine concentration is a good index of sympathetic efferent outflow to the forearm vascular beds also needs to be examined critically. Catecholamines in antecubital vein plasma may arrive from the arterial inflow and/or from sympathetic nerves in the forearm. Measurements of arterial and venous concentrations simultaneously with blood flow would permit calculation of a 'spillover' rate (Chang *et al.* 1986), but this does not take account of the bidirectional flux of catecholamines that may be occurring. For example, if the forearm removed all the inflowing noradrenaline, but release of noradrenaline in the forearm (due to efferent vasomotor activity) added a similar amount, the apparent spillover rate would be zero (Jie 1986), and one might infer there was no noradrenergic 'tone'. The proper calculation of regional noradrenaline release rate requires the simultaneous measurement of noradrenaline extraction by the tissue, ideally using radiolabelled noradrenaline. However, administering the latter by constant infusion produces problems with recirculation, while bolus administration requires assumptions to be made regarding the disposition of the radiolabelled marker in the non-steady state. Furthermore, it is now apparent that estimation of extraction by use of trace amounts of ^{3}H-noradrenaline may not give an accurate answer as the effluent radioactivity may not all be associated with noradrenaline. The definitive experiment, i.e. simultaneous measurement of forearm and calf flows, muscle sympathetic activity, and regional noradrenaline release rates at rest and following physiological manoeuvres that load or unload arterial and/or cardiopulmonary baroreceptors, has, understandably, yet to be done!

In the light of these problems, the observations of Eckberg *et al.* (1986) are of interest. They studied 10, unselected, young (20–36 years), insulin-dependent, diabetic patients with no symptoms or signs of autonomic neuropathy, and compared them with 12, age-matched, non-diabetic subjects. They measured forearm venous plasma noradrenaline levels and R–R interval variability under resting conditions, and during changes of arterial blood pressure elicited by infusions of nitroprusside or phenylephrine. The latter manoeuvres produced complex changes in forearm plasma noradrenaline levels in the non-diabetic subjects, but had little effect on the group mean values in the diabetic patients. However, there were marked interindividual differences in the latter. Nevertheless, Eckberg *et al.* (1986) felt their results in diabetic patients signified 'profound disturbances of sympathetic control' with 'no credible evidence that sympathetic outflow was modulated by changes of arterial pressure'. Two points need to be made here.

1. Since the patients were asymptomatic, it would have to be argued that the abnormality detected by Eckberg *et al.* (1986) was confined to the forearm (and, possibly, other vascular beds not involved in orthostatic reflexes).

2. Patients similar to those in the studies by Eckberg *et al.* (1986) show competent forearm vasoconstriction in response to manoeuvres such as lower body negative pressure (Scott *et al.* 1988*a*). Hence, antecubital venous plasma noradrenaline levels in such subjects may not reflect end-organ responses.

It is possible there are abnormalities of postjunctional adrenoceptors (see below) or endothelial cell function in the diabetic forearm that may influence any relation between vasoconstriction and venous noradrenaline concentration, but it is not unlikely that a different answer to that arrived at by Eckberg *et al.* (1986) would be obtained if the definitive experiment described above was carried out in his patients with diabetes mellitus.

The earlier findings indicating disorders of catecholamine biosynthesis (such as in apparent noradrenaline secretion rate and integrated noradrenaline excretion rate) in diabetic patients with impaired cardiovascular control also need to be re-examined in the light of the more sophisticated approaches described above. However, it is of interest that postural hypotension in some diabetic patients is not associated with signs of a hyperdopaminergic state, since the vasodilator effects of dopamine have been thought to explain the effectiveness of treatment with metoclopramide in diabetic postural hypotension (see below).

One of the many difficulties concerning cardiovascular studies in man (or animals) relates to the different receptor sites that the catecholamines may act upon to influence regional flows. The effects of local arterial infusions of agonists and antagonists on forearm blood flow have been examined (Jie 1986). In normal subjects, there appear to be postjunctional α_1- and α_2-adrenoceptors capable of mediating vasoconstriction. There is marked hyperaemia seen with yohimbine (an α_2-antagonist) indicating an important contribution of postjunctional α_2-adrenoceptors to the maintenance of resting vascular tone, but this response is markedly inhibited by β-adrenoceptor antagonism suggesting that it might be due to active vasodilatation. A similar phenomenon occurs in conscious rats and cautions against simplistic explanations. The important experiment of assessing the forearm vascular responses to release of endogenous noradrenaline in the presence of an antagonist of the vasodilator β_2-adrenoceptors, and delineating the influences of selective α_1- and α_2-adrenoceptor antagonists on these responses remains to be done, as does the experiment demonstrating a role of dopamine receptors in peripheral vascular control. Needless to say, these are even more virginal territories in patients with disorders such as diabetes mellitus.

Given the current uncertainty about the physiological role (if any) of pre- or postjunctional vascular α_2-adrenoceptors in normal man, and the lack of any evidence that adrenoceptors on non-vascular tissues are 'models' of vascular adrenoceptors, one can only be entertained by the gazelle-like conceptual leaps involved in relating decreased α_2-adrenoceptors on platelet membranes to vascular abnormalities of orthostatic hypotension in diabetes mellitus (Abraham *et al.* 1986).

Hormonal abnormalities: vasopressin

A role for vasopressin (ADH) in cardiovascular regulation has been widely debated (e.g. Bennett and Gardiner 1986; Gardiner and Bennett 1987*a*) and, in the context of diabetes mellitus, ADH takes on an intriguing aspect since its release is normally influenced by extracellular fluid osmolality (which may be abnormal in diabetic patients) and ADH may exert important influences on hepatic metabolism and haemostasis. A particularly important point in regard to the osmoreceptor control of ADH in diabetic patients concerns the possibility that glucose could act as a stimulus for thirst and vasopressin release if its normal lack of effectiveness in this regard were due to an insulin-dependent uptake into osmoreceptor cells. Although infusion of hypertonic glucose does not stimulate ADH release in either normal subjects or diabetic patients, it has been pointed out the latter were not insulin-deficient at the time of the measurements. Indeed, it has been claimed that acute insulin deficiency increases ADH secretion by sensitizing the osmoreceptors to stimulation by hyperglycaemia in patients with insulin-dependent diabetes mellitus. However, more recent work indicates that the earlier studies may have suffered from inappropriate data analysis (Durr *et al.* 1990).

Infusion of hypertonic saline increases ADH in control subjects and in patients with diabetes mellitus, but the changes in cardiovascular variables under those conditions indicate that the results do not fit readily into the dogma regarding ADH and baroreflex mechanisms (see Bennett and Gardiner 1986). However, a greater responsiveness of ADH release to orthostatic stimuli in diabetic patients without postural hypotension and a greater postural fall in blood pressure in diabetic patients showing diminished ADH release indicates that the hormone may play an overt role in cardiovascular regulation when other systems are impaired, but, presumably, only if vascular sensitivity to ADH is not diminished. This proposition appears to be supported by the finding that patients with type II diabetes mellitus and orthostatic hypotension showed marked exacerbation of the postural fall in blood pressure following administration of a V_1-receptor antagonist (Saad *et al.* 1988). However, it is unlikely this effect was due to antagonism of the vasoconstrictor effects of ADH because the effect occurred about 1 h after orthostasis and ambulation. Saad *et al.* (1988) suggested, therefore, that these results were consistent with the V_1-receptor antagonist inhibiting effects of ADH on baroreflex and/or central mechanisms involved in blood pressure control. Previously, we had argued there was little evidence that ADH showed any unique interaction with baroreflex mechanisms in man (Bennett and Gardiner 1986; Gardiner and Bennett 1987), although the opposite view was maintained by Ebert *et al.* (1986) and Goldsmith (1987). However, it is notable that these authors have recently adopted our viewpoint, and now consider that endogenous ADH does not alter baroreflex function in man (Ebert *et al.* 1990; Goldsmith and Simon 1990).

One further confounding factor is the ability of ADH to activate vasodilator mechanisms (see Bennett and Gardiner 1986), and it is of interest that this effect may be due to the involvement of cyclo-oxygenase products and/or nitric oxide, possibly produced by endothelial cells. In spite of these controversies, the findings that, in patients with diabetes mellitus, ADH release in response to haemodynamic stimuli can be impaired when that in response to osmotic stimuli is not may provide evidence of selective baroreceptor afferent dysfunction.

In summary, there is little direct information regarding the cardiovascular influences of ADH in patients with diabetes mellitus, but it may be we know more than we know we know! For example, based on the proposition that excessive dopamine secretion could, by its vasodilator effects, cause orthostatic hypotension, it was found that treatment with metoclopramide (a dopamine antagonist) facilitated vasoconstriction and hence opposed diabetic orthostatic hypotension. However, this action of metoclopramide may have been due to augmented ADH release, consistent with its ability to stimulate basal release of ADH particularly in diabetic patients. The cardiovascular sequelae of possible interactions between metoclopramide and other ADH-releasing mechanisms (insulin, hypoglycaemia, neuroglycopenia) in normal subjects and diabetic patients await investigation.

Hormonal abnormalities: atrial natriuretic peptide

Plasma atrial natriuretic peptide (ANP) levels are elevated in patients with diabetes mellitus. This makes assessment of cardiovascular function even more difficult since ANP can attenuate sympathetic reflexes in normal subjects. As yet, there have been no studies concerned with the putative physiological effects of ANP on autonomic function in patients with diabetes mellitus.

Hormonal abnormalities: renin–angiotensin system

Plasma renin levels are reduced in diabetics with hypertension and neuropathy. Several factors, including plasma volume expansion, juxtaglomerular cell damage, and abnormal renin synthesis, and/or release, could account for such observations. However, in patients with uncontrolled diabetic ketoacidosis, plasma renin activity may be increased due to hypovolaemia. Little is known about local tissue renin–angiotensin systems in diabetes mellitus, but it is feasible that these show abnormalities (Franken *et al.* 1990) that could have important consequences for cardiovascular function.

Angiotensin-converting enzyme (ACE) inhibitors are reputedly particularly beneficial in the treatment of hypertension associated with diabetes mellitus, since they may retard the progression of diabetic nephropathy and improve glucoregulation. If local tissue renin–angiotensin systems are involved in the development of microvascular complications (Franken *et al.* 1990), it is feasible that ACE inhibitors might ameliorate these problems. However, the inhibition of bradykinin catabolism by ACE inhibitors could exacerbate hypotension under these circumstances.

One area of particular interest currently is the putative interaction between the sulphydryl-containing ACE inhibitors, such as captopril, and superoxide radicals that inactivate endothelium-derived nitric oxide. If disorders of endothelial cell function in diabetes mellitus cause diminished production of nitric oxide (and hence attenuation of its vasodilator, anti-aggregatory, and antimitogenic effects; see Moncada and Higgs 1990) these problems might be alleviated by reducing the availability of superoxide radicals.

Hormonal abnormalities: islet-associated polypeptide

There is much discussion about the possible involvement of islet-associated polypeptide (IAPP) in the aetiology of diabetes mellitus and its role in the complications of this disease. It is notable that IAPP shows marked structural homology with CGRP, and that both peptides are vasoactive, having similar regional haemodynamic profiles (Gardiner *et al.* 1991*a*). Even more intriguing is the finding that the peptide fragment, human α-CGRP [8–37], inhibits the cardiovascular effects of human α-CGRP and of IAPP (Gardiner *et al.* 1990, 1991*a*), and that the cardiovascular effects of intact human α-CGRP involve nitric oxide-mediated mechanisms, but only in some vascular beds (Gardiner *et al.* 1991*b*). It remains to be determined if peptides such as IAPP and CGRP are involved in cardiovascular pathophysiology in patients with diabetes mellitus and if peptide fragments, such as human α-CGRP [8–37], may be used therapeutically.

Endothelial factors

Another area that must receive serious attention in future work is the effect of endothelial cell function on cardiovascular regulation. It is clear already that there are important, acute and trophic effects of insulin on endothelial cell biology. Thus disorders of endothelial cell function could be involved in a variety of cardiovascular abnormalities in diabetes mellitus. Patients with this disease may have markedly elevated plasma endothelin-1 levels (Takahashi *et al.* 1990), which may be due to hypersecretion from endothelial cells. However, it does not follow that endothelin-1 exerts its expected effects on the heart and vascular system under these circumstances since, in experimental diabetes mellitus, there is evidence of reduction in the numbers of myocardial receptors for endothelin-1.

One possible explanation for increased plasma levels of endothelin-1 in diabetes mellitus is diminished endothelial cell nitric oxide production, as the latter normally inhibits endothelin secretion. To understand such putative interactions we are investigating factors influencing cardiovascular status in rats with streptozotocin-induced diabetes mellitus. Under resting conditions these animals have renal and mesenteric vasodilatation but a hindquarters vasoconstriction (Kiff et al. 1991a). The renal and mesenteric vasodilatation are not suppressed by human α-CGRP [8–37], or octreotide. However, administration of N^G-nitro-L-arginine methyl ester (L-NAME) to inhibit endothelial cell nitric oxide production causes greater vasoconstriction in the renal and mesenteric vascular beds in diabetic than in control animals. Hence, it is feasible that abnormal nitric oxide production is implicated in the resting vasodilatations in these regional vascular beds. The reverse, however, seems to be the case in the hindquarters vascular bed, since vasoconstrictor responses to L-NAME are impaired at that site in diabetic animals (Kiff et al. 1991a). We have also found that vasodilator responses to different agonists are differentially impaired in different vascular beds in diabetic animals (Kiff et al. 1991b). These studies are ongoing and clearly much has to be learned.

Conclusions

Although the mass of new information is overwhelming we are beginning to appreciate the subtle aspects of in vivo cardiovascular physiology and the remarkable ways in which normal integration is achieved at different levels. Thus, it is becoming clear that factors such as insulin, angiotensin II, neuropeptides, endothelin, and nitric oxide interrelate locally to control, acutely, cardiovascular function and, chronically, to effect appropriate adjustments in tissue maintenance, interactions between blood and endothelial surfaces, immune status, and angiogenesis, among other factors. While agents such as insulin may appear to have a pivotal role in several aspects of these control mechanisms, it is feasible that we will discover that those factors listed above (and others besides) will turn out to be important intermediaries. For example, it is becoming clear that nitric oxide acts as a critical signal in endothelial cells, vascular smooth muscle, the heart, liver, kidneys, brain, blood cells, etc. (Moncada and Higgs 1990). Hence, the likelihood that it is involved in insulin's action in vivo seems inevitable. Considerations such as these are not confined to the control of cardiovascular function, or to disorders such as diabetes mellitus, but are likely to impinge on all body systems under normal and various pathological conditions. Viewed from this angle it is apparent that what appears as a single disease or disorder could come about in a variety of different ways. Profiling of the disorder could thus lead to individually tailored therapy that was appropriately targetted.

Epilogue

Recent developments highlight the complexities of effector systems, particularly with regard to postreceptor signal transduction. These findings re-emphasize the need for systematic assessment of effector integrity in circumstances where tests of autonomic function are employed. In the context of cardiovascular mechanisms it should be noted that, although systemic injections of direct pressor agents, such as noradrenaline, or indirect pressor agents, such as tyramine, may indicate the presence of abnormalities, they do not localize or define them. Ideally, as a first step, comparisons of the effects of intraarterial injections of adrenoceptor-selective agonists and tyramine should be made, as should responses to vasodilators in the absence and presence of agents that influence nitric oxide synthesis. Furthermore, such investigations ought to be performed in the forearm and in the calf, at least, to take into account the known regional differences.

Assessment of cardiac effector function is even less straightforward, but some of the newer *in vivo* tomographic imaging techniques (using ^{125}I-meta-iodobenzylguadine, for example) may help. Although the 'isoprenaline test' is widely used as a means of assessing cardiac β-adrenoceptor integrity, the responses to this test are complex, involving withdrawal of vagal tone, probably due to changes in regional blood flows consequent upon isoprenaline-induced vasodilatation (Bennett and Gardiner 1988). Clearly, it would be helpful if β_1-adrenoceptor selective agonists were available for use in man, so the complications of secondary effects on the heart due to β_2-adrenoceptor-mediated changes in haemodynamics could be avoided. However, even if we had such agents it is unlikely that their administration would give a clearer picture of cardiac adrenoceptor function, since their administration to elicit tachycardia would inevitably change flow patterns through the carotid sinus and, as mentioned already, such changes could have substantial effects on carotid sinus afferent signalling.

Similar difficulties arise when one considers ways in which cardiac muscarinic receptor function could be assessed *in vivo*. Although one might entertain the theoretical possibility of carrying out investigations in the presence of ganglion blocking drugs to avoid the problems mentioned above, such an intervention causes hypotension and tends to increase ADH release and activate the renin–angiotensin system and thereby changes baseline status. This last point is a recurrent problem in any comparative study where there are differences, in the resting state, between control and abnormal subjects, since it is arguable how best to express responses to interventions.

On balance, from a physiological viewpoint, we judge it would be logical first to assess effector function (as far as that is possible). If effector function is impaired then, clearly, abnormal responses to tests of reflex integrity might occur for that reason rather than being due to problems with autonomic neuronal activity. However, it would be very interesting to know if one could elicit 'normal' reflex responses under conditions in which effector function could be shown to be impaired. If so, it would indicate adaptation of the system (possibly by utilization of the synergistic effects of neuropeptides or cotransmitters), analogous to the situation in patients with congenital absence of dopamine β-hydroxylase activity who show no obvious behavioural signs of the deficiency of central noradrenaline (see Chapter 38).

We would advocate the use of tests concerned specifically with regional functions. Thus, it is not adequate these days to consider the forearm as a representative of the vasculature generally. In normal subjects there may be differences in the behaviour of calf and forearm vascular beds (see Chapter 5), independent of muscle sympathetic nerve activity, and, under several conditions, sympathetic efferent outflow to different effectors changes differentially. Thus, one cannot infer, from constrained observations, the aetiology of a disorder that may affect different organ systems disparately.

Another aspect of pathophysiological processes that must be borne in mind when carrying out clinical assessments is that of compensatory changes for some primary disturbance and the extent of redundancy in normal physiological systems. It is very rare that a particular dysfunction gives rise to an obvious, uncompensated abnormality and it is feasible that what appears abnormal is a compensatory event for some underlying disorder. Furthermore, evidence is now accruing that some compensatory mechanisms seen in disease states may be peculiar to that condition, i.e. not expressed in normal individuals. An example of this is the occurrence of novel cardiac enzymes capable of generating angiotensin II in patients with congestive heart failure. Even more intriguing is the recent finding that in various inflammatory conditions there may be *de novo* synthesis of nitric oxide synthetase in tissues not usually expressing this enzyme. Hence, in the future, it is feasible that the investigation of 'autonomic failure' will have to take into account molecular pathology. However, the ultimate arbiter of the clinical relevance of molecular pathology must be the demonstration of functional consequences and, ideally, the ability to influence the latter through an understanding of that molecular pathology.

References

Abrahm, D. R., Hollingworth, P. J., Smith, C. B., Jim, L., Zucker, L. B., Sobotka, P. A., and Vinik, A. I. (1986). Decreased α_2-adrenergic receptors on platelet membranes from diabetic patients with autonomic neuropathy and postural hypotension. *J. clin. Endocrinol. Metab.* **63**, 906–12.

Aksamit, T. R., Floras, J. S., Victor, R. G., and Aylward, P. E. (1987). Paroxysmal hypertension due to sinoaortic baroreceptor denervation in humans. *Hypertension* **9**, 309–14.

Bennett, T. (1987). Cardiovascular responses to central hypovalemia in man: physiology and pathophysiology. *Physiologist* **30**, S143–6.

Bennett, T. and Gardiner, S. M. (1986). Influence of exogenous vasopressin on baroreflex mechanisms. *Clin. Sci.* **70**, 307–15.

Bennett, T. and Gardiner, S. M. (1988). Physiological aspects of the aging cardiovascular system. *J. cardiovasc. Pharmacol.* **12** (suppl. 8), S1–10.

Boolell, M. and Tooke, J. E. (1990). The skin hyperaemic response to local injection of substance P and capsaicin in diabetes mellitus. *Diabet. Med.* **7**, 898–901.

Chang, P. C., van der Krogt, J. A., Vermey, P., and van Brummelen, P. (1986). Norepinephrine removal and release in the forearm of healthy subjects. *Hypertension* **8**, 801–9.

Durr, J. A., Hoffman, W. H., Hensen, J., Sklar, A. H., Gammal, T. E., and Steinhart, C. M. (1990). Osmoregulation of vasopressin in diabetic ketoacidosis. *Am. J. Physiol.* **259**, E723–8.

Ebert, T. J., Cowley, A. W., and Skelton, M. (1986). Vasopressin reduces cardiac function and augments cardiopulmonary baroreflex resistance increases in man. *J. clin. Invest.* **77**, 1136–42.

Ebert, T. J., Skelton, M., and Cowley, A. W. (1990). Arginine vasopressin does not alter baroreflex function in humans. *Circulation* **82** (suppl. III), III634.

Eckberg, D. L., Harkins, S. W., Fritsch, J. M., Musgrave, G. W., and Gardner, D. F. (1986). Baroreflex control of plasma norepinephrine and heart period in healthy subjects and diabetic patients. *J. clin. Invest.* **78**, 366–74.

Eckberg, D. L., Rea, R. F., Andersson, O. K., Hedner, T., Pernow, J., Lundberg, J. M., and Wallin, B. G. (1988). Baroreflex modulation of sympathetic activity and sympathetic neurotransmitters in humans. *Acta physiol. scand.* **133**, 221–31.

Fagius, J. (1985). Autonomic neurophysiology in long-term diabetes. *Clin. Physiol.* **5** (suppl. 5), 74–8.

Fagius, J., Wallin, B. G., Sundlöf, G., Nerhed, C., and Englesson, S. (1985). Sympathetic outflow in man after anaesthesia of the glossopharyngeal and vagus nerves. *Brain* **108**, 423–38.

Franken, A. A. M., Derkx, F. H. M., Man in't Veld, A. J., Hop, W. C. J., van Rens, G. H., Peperkamp, E., de Jong, P. J. V. M., and Schalekamp, M. A. D. H. (1990). High plasma prorenin in diabetes mellitus and its correlation with some complications. *J. clin. Endocrinol. Metab.* **71**, 1008–15.

Gardiner, S. M. and Bennett, T. (1987). Influence of endogenous vasopressin on baroreflex mechanisms. *Brain Res. Rev.* **11**, 317–34.

Gardiner, S. M., Compton, A. M., Kemp, P. A., Bennett, T., Bose, C., Foulkes, R., and Hughes, B. (1990). Antagonistic effect of human α-CGRP [8–37] on the *in vivo* regional haemodynamic action of human α-CGRP. *Biochem. biophys. Res. Commun.* **171**, 938–43.

Gardiner, S. M., Compton, A. M., Kemp, P. A., Bennett, T., Bose, C., Foulkes, R., and Hughes, B. (1991a). Antagonistic effect of human α-calcitonin gene-related peptide [8–37] on the regional haemodynamic actions of rat islet amyloid polypeptide in conscious, Long Evans rats. *Diabetes* **40**, 948–51.

Gardiner, S. M., Compton, A. M., Kemp, P. A., Bennett, T., Foulkes, R., and Hughes, B. (1991b). Haemodynamic effects of human α-calcitonin gene-related peptide following administration of endothelin-1 or N^G-nitro-L-arginine methyl ester in conscious rats. *Br. J. Pharmacol.* **103**, 1256–62.

Goldsmith, S. R. (1987). Vasopressin as vasopressor. *Am. J. Med.* **82**, 1213–19.

Goldsmith, S. R. and Simon, A. B. (1990). Physiologic arginine vasopressin levels do not suppress sympathetic activity in normal humans. *Circulation* **82** (suppl. III), III634.

Hellweg, R. and Hartung, H.-D. (1990). Endogenous levels of nerve growth factor (NGF) are altered in experimental diabetes mellitus: a possible role for NGF in the pathogenesis of diabetic neuropathy. *J. neurosci. Res.* **26**, 258–67.

Jie, K. (1986). Characterization and (patho)-physiology of vascular α-adrenoceptors: studies in the forearm. Unpublished MD thesis, Leiden.

Kiff, R. J., Gardiner, S. M., Compton, A. M., and Bennett, T. (1991*a*). The effects of endothelin-1 and N^G-nitro-L-arginine methyl ester on regional haemodynamics in conscious, Wistar rats with streptozotocin-induced diabetes mellitus. *Br. J. Pharmacol.* **103**, 1321–6.

Kiff, R. J., Gardiner, S. M., Compton, A. M., and Bennett, T. (1991*b*). Selective impairment of hindquarters vasodilator responses to bradykinin in conscious, Wistar rats with streptozotocin-induced diabetes mellitus. *Br. J. Pharmacol.* **103**, 1357–62.

Moncada, S. and Higgs, E. A. (1990). *Nitric oxide from L-arginine: a bioregulatory system*. Excerpta Medica, Amsterdam.

Saad, C. I., Ribiero, A. B., Zanella, M. J., Mulinari, R. A., Gavras, I., and Gavras, H. (1988). The role of vasopressin in blood pressure maintenance in diabetic orthostatic hypotension. *Hypertension* **11** (suppl. I), I217–1.

Scott, A. R., Bennett, T., and Macdonald, I. A. (1987). Diabetes mellitus and thermoregulation. *Can. J. Physiol. Pharmacol.* **65**, 1365–76.

Scott, A. R., Bennett, T., and Macdonald, I. A. (1988*a*). Effects of hyperinsulinaemia on the cardiovascular responses to graded hypovolaemia in normal and diabetic subjects. *Clin. Sci.* **75**, 85–92.

Scott, A. R, Macdonald, I. A., Bennett, T., and Tattersall, R. B. (1988*b*). Abnormal thermoregulation in diabetic autonomic neuropathy. *Diabetes* **37**, 961–8.

Takahashi, K., Ghatei, M. A., Lam, H.-C., O'Halloran, D. J., and Bloom, S. R. (1990). Elevated plasma endothelin in patients with diabetes mellitus. *Diabetologia* **33**, 306–10.

21. Testing of sweating

Phillip A. Low and R. D. Fealey

Introduction

Sudomotor function depends on the integrity of the sympathetic neural pathways, the eccrine sweat gland, and the skin. Assuming that the latter two components are normal, sudomotor function can be used as an index of sympathetic sudomotor function. Four tests, the thermoregulatory sweat test (TST), the quantitative sudomotor axon reflex test (Q-SART), the sweat imprint test, and the peripheral autonomic skin potential (PASP) recordings are in relatively common use and will be described in some detail.

The thermoregulatory sweat test

TST provides a sweat stimulus via raised blood and mean skin temperature. The efferent sympathetic response is mediated by preganglionic centres including the hypothalamus, bulbospinal pathways, the intermediolateral cell columns, and white rami. Postganglionic paths include the sympathetic chain and postganglionic sudomotor nerves to the sweat glands.

The TST done in the Mayo Thermoregulatory Laboratory is a modification of Guttmann's quinizarin sweat test. Unclothed subjects lie supine on a cart and exposed body surface (exclusive of eyes, nose, mouth, and genitalia) is covered with an indicator powder mixture (alizarine red, sodium carbonate, and cornstarch; Low *et al.* 1975; Fealey *et al.* 1989). Subjects are totally enclosed in the sweat cabinet for 30–45 min (air temperature 44–50 °C; relative humidity 40–50 per cent) and skin temperature is maintained between 39 and 40 °C via overhead infra-red heaters. The oral temperature must rise to at least 38.0 °C or by 1.0 °C, whichever yields the highest temperature. The mean temperature rise for our patients and controls is 1.5 °C. The patient's sweat distribution is photographed and an accurate digitized image is created on a standard anatomic drawing. The areas of anhidrosis are determined directly by planimetry (LASICO, model 1252M, resolution = 0.005 cm^2) and the percentage of anterior body surface anhidrosis (TST%) is the total measured area of anhidrosis divided by the area of the anatomic figure multiplied by 100. Normal sweat distributions and TST% have been published (Fealey *et al.* 1989).

Thermoregulatory sweating abnormalities
in pure autonomic failure (PAF) and multiple system
atrophy with autonomic failure (MSA; Shy–Drager syndrome)

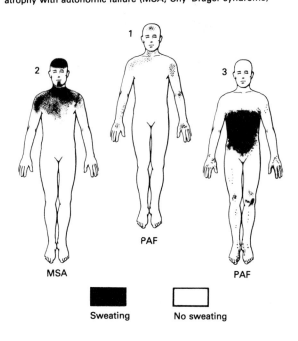

Fig. 21.1. Thermoregulatory sweat test results showing characteristic anhidrosis in MSA and PAF. (Taken with permission from Cohen *et al.* (1987).)

Widespread anhidrosis is characteristic of multiple system atrophy (MSA) and pure autonomic failure (PAF) (Bannister *et al.* 1967; Fealey *et al.* 1985). Cohen *et al.* (1987) found median values of body surface anhidrosis (TST%) of 91 and 97 per cent for PAF and MSA patients, respectively, and representative sweat distributions are shown in Fig. 21.1.

Most recently, we have shown that the severity of clinical autonomic failure in patients with extrapyramidal and cerebellar system disorders regressed significantly with the TST% (Sandroni *et al.* 1991). The orthostatic blood pressure decrement and TST% were found to have a near identical rank order of severity by disease category, being milder for Parkinson's disease and progressive supranuclear palsy and severe for MSA. The TST% has a high degree of correlation with the clinical severity of diabetic autonomic neuropathy ($p = 0.0004$; Fealey *et al.* 1989). The thermoregulatory sweat test has the distinct capacity to monitor the course of both pre- and postganglionic sudomotor failure in individual patients (Fig. 21.2).

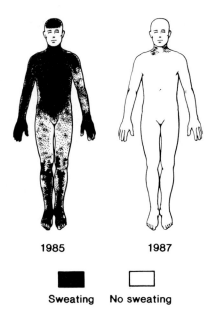

Fig. 21.2. Progressive sweat loss in a patient with an L-dopa responsive, extrapyramidal disorder and mild orthostatic hypotension in 1985 and
severe MSA unresponsive to L-dopa with disabling autonomic failure by
1987.

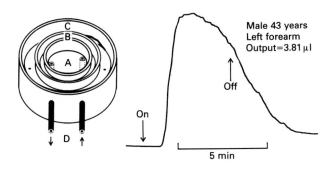

Fig. 21.3. Multicompartmental sweat cell (left) and evoked sweat response
(right). The capsule is strapped on to skin, and acetylcholine (compartment C)
is iontophoresed using a constant current generator with the anode connected
to compartment C. Axon reflex evoked sweat response in compartment A is
evaporated off by a stream of nitrogen at a controlled flow rate and quantitated
dynamically by a sudorometer. Compartment B and associated ridges prevent
diffusion and leakage of acetylcholine. (Taken with permission from Low
(1986).)

The quantitative sudomotor axon reflex test

In this test, the stimulus is applied via one compartment (C, Fig. 21.3) and the evoked sweat response recorded from a nearby compartment (A, Fig. 21.3) using a sudorometer. The stimulus is acetylcholine, iontophoresed using a constant current generator. Acetylcholine binds to nicotinic receptors of the postganglionic sympathetic sudomotor axon to activate a nerve impulse. This travels antidromically to a branch point and then orthodromically to release acetylcholine at the nerve terminal. The released acetylcholine binds to muscarinic (M_3) receptors (Torres *et al.* 1991) to evoke a sweat response. The multicompartmental sweat cell consists of a central recording compartment (A, Fig. 21.3) 1 cm in diameter surrounded by an air gap (B, Fig. 21.3), 1.5 mm wide, separating the recording compartment from a circular stimulus moat 4 mm wide (C, Fig. 21.3) that is filled with 10 per cent acetylcholine via a cannula (E, Fig. 21.3) and any residual air exits via a second cannula. Nitrogen is passed through a gas inlet and outlet (D, Fig. 21.3). Acetylcholine is iontophoresed using a constant current generator. Anodal current is passed via the anodal electrode connected to the stimulus well. The cathode is a 4×6 cm rectangular lead strip wrapped in flannel and soaked in isotonic saline. Sweat droplets in compartment A are evaporated off by a nitrogen stream of constant flow, and humidity and the sweat output are quantitated by a sudorometer and dynamically recorded.

Under controlled conditions Q-SART provides a reproducible, sensitive, and accurate measurement of postganglionic sudomotor function (Low *et al.* 1983, 1986). There are now several recognized abnormal Q-SART patterns. The response may be: (1) normal; (2) reduced; (3) absent; (4) excessive; (5) persistent. Short latencies are common with patterns 4 and 5. Pattern 5, consisting of a pattern of persistent sweat activity, where the sweat response fails to turn off when the stimulus ceases, is often seen in mildly damaged peripheral nerves, and may be associated with reduced latencies. An ultrashort latency is often seen in patients with painful neuropathies and other peripheral pain states. They are probably due to enhanced somatosympathetic reflexes, with the afferent component mediated by the polymodal C nociceptor.

Q-SART has been used to monitor the progress of sympathetic sudomotor function in the peripheral neuropathies and in treatment trials. For instance, we are into the fifth year of a prevalence study of autonomic function in a population-based study of neuropathy including autonomic function in diabetes in Rochester, Minnesota, USA. We have used this method to monitor the efficacy of treatment with 3,4-diaminopyridine in the Lambert–Eaton myasthenic syndrome (McEvoy *et al.* 1989), with aldose reductase inhibitors in diabetic neuropathy, with plasma exchange in chronic inflammatory polyradiculoneuropathy, and with capsaicin in painful neuropathies. It is useful, in conjuction with the thermoregulatory sweat test, in defining the site of the lesion in patients with sweating impairment. The technique has been used to study the effects of ageing (Low *et al.* 1990), MSA and PAF (Cohen *et al.* 1987), amyotrophic lateral sclerosis, and reflex sympathetic dystrophy.

The silastic imprint method

An alternative quantitative method to sudorometry is the sweat imprint method. Kennedy *et al.* (1984) published a detailed quantitative study in which they measured the number and sizes of sweat droplets using a silastic imprint method. They stimulated sweating by iontophoresis of pilocarpine, a muscarinic agonist. Pilocarpine binds to the muscarinic receptor, presumably M_3, on the eccrine sweat gland to evoke a sweat response. They obtained a sweat imprint from the stimulated sweat glands. The silastic impression material (Elasticon, Kerr Co, Romulus, MI) is spread over the stimulated surface and, upon hardening, each sweat droplet leaves an imprint of characteristic size and shape. The sweat imprint can then be analysed by computer morphometry in which the image is magnified and the number and size of sweat droplets determined and a sweat histogram constructed. The method appears to reliably detect sweat gland failure in diabetic neuropathy (Kennedy *et al.* 1984). The evoked sweat response continues to be active for more than 2 h following stimulation in contrast to the Q-SART which turns off within 5–10 min (Low *et al.* 1983). Similar recordings can be performed for the indirect response.

We recently found that patients with mild neuropathy have enlarged direct and indirect droplet sizes (Kihara *et al.* 1989). Whether the increase in size is due to multi-innervation, or receptor alterations is currently not known. The density and total area of sweating within the C (directly stimulated) and A (axon-reflex mediated) compartments are, in general, lower for diabetics. The diameter distribution was different for males and females in that males had an overrepresentation of large droplets for both direct and axon-reflex responses. Comparing diabetics with control subjects, diabetics had an overrepresentation of large-diameter droplets in both the direct and axon-reflex compartments (Kihara *et al.* 1989).

Peripheral autonomic surface potentials (PASP)

The skin potential change recorded in response to somatosympathetic activation requires the intactness of sympathetic pathways and functioning sweat glands. It probably requires the synchronized activation of eccrine sweat glands. In normal humans, recordings are usually symmetrical and larger in the upper extremity than the lower. The latency of the response is more constant than the amplitude or morphology, which depends on the resistance of the skin. Sourek (1965) obtained estimated conduction velocities of 1.5 and

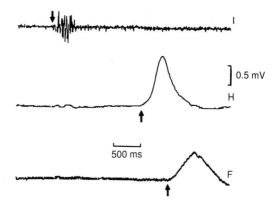

Fig. 21.4. PASP recorded simultaneously in the hand (H) and foot (F) of a control subject following a deep inspiration (I). Uppermost tracing is a diagram of the electromyographic activity. Upward arrows indicate the onset of the response. (Taken with permission from Shahani *et al.* (1984).)

0.8 m/s for upper and lower extremities, respectively. He obtained recordings from different sites on the same limb and divided the distance between electrodes by the latency changes. The response may be evoked as a reflex by emotionally or physically painful stimuli or by direct nerve stimulation.

Following peripheral nerve section, PASP can no longer be obtained in the affected dermatome and there is usually associated hypothermia and anhidrosis. Following sympathectomy, skin potentials are also lost, but only temporarily, returning in 4–6 months, probably related to the propensity of sympathetic postganglionic fibres to regenerate.

Recordings of skin resistance (galvanic skin response) and potential differ in the mode of stimulation (spontaneous or evoked) and in the mode of recording (Low 1984). Recordings to detect sympathetic sudomotor deficit in the peripheral and central autonomic neuropathies have also become popular (Shahani *et al.* 1984). The recording electrodes are commonly electrode pairs 1 cm in diameter applied to the dorsal and ventral surfaces of the foot, the hand, or thighs. The stimulus might be an inspiratory gasp (Fig. 21.4), a cough, a loud noise, an electric shock, or a stroke of the skin. Indeed, any form of somatic stimulation or psychic stress may evoke a response. The most effective stimuli activate type II–III afferents. The sources of the skin potential are the sweat gland and the epidermis. The major advantage of the method is its simplicity so that it can be used in any electromyographic laboratory. The disadvantages are its variability and the tendency of the responses to habituate. Skin potential abnormalities have been found in some patients with diabetic neuropathy (Knezevic and Bajada 1985). In patients with severe neuropathy the test correlates well with Q-SART (Maselli *et al.* 1989).

The neural pathway of this reflex has been surmised based on known neurological lesions. The medial and basal frontal lobe and medial temporal lobe are probably involved in the transmission of this somatosympathetic reflex, and in the cervical and thoracic cord the pathways are considered to be deeply seated in the dorsal part of the anterolateral quadrant and are mostly crossed (Sourek 1965). Crossing is thought to occur mainly between T2 and T6. The final common pathway is the preganglionic autonomic neuron from the intermediolateral column and the postganglionic neuron from the paravertebral ganglia.

Comparison of methods of measuring sudomotor activity

The sudomotor tests are best considered as complementary to one another. The silastic imprint method is the only one that provides an evaluation of the single sweat gland and its morphometric analysis generates a sweat histogram, while the Q-SART recording provides a dynamic quantitation of sweat output. The two can be combined to evaluate the dynamic function of sweat gland units. The principles of the two methods are quite different. The silastic method depends on the function of directly stimulated sweat glands (the denervated gland losing its sudomotor response), whereas the Q-SART depends on the integrity of the axon reflex rather than sweat gland function. Perhaps because of the longer pathway tested in Q-SART (sympathetic C $\rightarrow$ branch point $\rightarrow$ sympathetic C) this test detects sudomotor failure before the silastic imprint method. The second major advantage is its dynamic sudorometry so that one is able, for instance, to determine if there is persistent sweat activity or to study somatosympathetic reflexes.

The TST is a straightforward simple test that provides important information on the distribution of sweat activity. Because of the sampling problems inherent in quantitative tests such as the silastic imprint and Q-SART recordings (which record from small areas of skin), TST provides important complementary information. Diabetic neuropathy appears to be characterized by multifocal nerve involvement so that the patient with, for example, diabetic thoracic radiculopathy may have a diagnostic thermo-regulatory sweat test pattern but may lack distal anhidrosis (and have a normal silastic or Q-SART recording). TST and Q-SART in combination can be used to define the site of the lesion causing anhidrosis (pre- versus postganglionic).

The PASP recording is dynamic but subject to great variability because it readily habituates and is a function of many factors. It has an evolving role in the electromyographic laboratory but is unsuitable for clinical trials.

References

Bannister, R., Ardill, L., and Fentem, P. (1967). Defective autonomic control of blood vessels in idiopathic orthostatic hypotension. *Brain* **90**, 725–46.

Cohen, J., Low, P. A., Fealey, R. D., Sheps, S., and Jiang, N-S. (1987). Somatic and autonomic function in progressive autonomic failure and multiple system atrophy. *Ann. Neurol.* **22**, 692–9.

Fealey, R. D., Schirger, A., and Thomas, J. E., (1985). Orthostatic hypotension. In *Clinical medicine*, Vol. 7 (ed. J. A. Spittell Jr), pp. 1–12. Harper and Row, Philadelphia.

Fealey, R. D., Low, P. A., and Thomas, J. E. (1989) Thermoregulatory sweating abnormalities in diabetes mellitus. *Mayo Clinic Proc.* **64**, 617–28.

Kennedy, W. R., Sakuta, M., Sutherland, D., and Goetz, F. C. (1984). Quantitation of the sweating deficit in diabetes mellitus. *Ann. Neurol.* **15**, 482–8.

Kihara, M., Opfer-Gehrking, T. L., and Low, P. A. (1989). Comparison of directly stimulated with axon reflex-mediated sudomotor responses in human subjects. *Ann. Neurol.* **26**, 169A.

Knezevic, W. and Bajada, S. (1985). Peripheral autonomic surface potential. A quantitative technique for recording sympathetic conduction in man. *J. neurol. Sci.* **67**, 239–51.

Low, P. A. (1984). Quantitation of autonomic function. In *Peripheral neuropathy* (2nd edn) (ed. P. J. Dyck, P. K. Thomas, E. H. Lambert, R. Bunge), pp. 1139–66. Saunders, Philadelphia.

Low, P. A. (1986). Sudomotor function and dysfunction. In *Diseases of the nervous system* (ed. A. K. Asbury, G. M. McKhann, and W. I. McDonald), pp. 596–605. Saunders, Philadelphia.

Low, P. A., Walsh, J. C., Huang, C. Y., and McLeod, J. G. (1975). The sympathetic nervous system in diabetic neuropathy. A clinical and pathological study. *Brain* **98**, 341–56.

Low, P. A., Caskey, P. E., Tuck, R. R., Fealey, R. D., and Dyck, P. J. (1983). Quantitative sudomotor axon reflex test in normal and neuropathic subjects. *Ann. Neurol.* **14**, 573–80.

Low, P. A., Zimmerman, B. R., and Dyck, P. J. (1986). Comparison of distal sympathetic with vagal function in diabetic neuropathy. *Muscle Nerve* **9**, 592–6.

Low, P. A., Opfer-Gehrking, T. L., Proper, C. J., and Zimmerman, I. (1990). The effect of aging on cardiac autonomic and postganglionic sudomotor function. *Muscle Nerve* **13**, 152–7.

Maselli, R. A., Jaspan, J. B., Soliven, B. C., Green, A. J., Spire, J-P., and Arnason, B. G. W. (1989). Comparison of sympathetic skin response with quantitative sudomotor axon reflex test in diabetic neuropathy. *Muscle Nerve* **12**, 420–3.

McEvoy, K. M., Windebank, A. J., Daube, J. R., and Low, P. A. (1989). 3,4-diaminopyridine in the treatment of Lambert–Eaton myasthenic syndrome. *New Engl. J. Med.* **321**, 1567–71

Sandroni, P., Ahlskog, E. J., Fealey, R. D., and Low, P. A. (1991). Autonomic involvement in extrapyramidal and cerebellar system disorders. *Clin. autonom. Res.* **1**, 147–55.

Shahani, B. T., Halperin, J. J., Boulu, P., and Cohen, J. (1984). Sympathetic skin response—a method of assessing unmyelinated axon dysfunction in peripheral neuropathies. *J. Neurol. Neurosurg. Psychiat.* **47**, 536–42.

Sourek, K. (1965). The nervous control of skin potentials in man. *Rozpravy Ceskoslovenske Akademie Ved Roenik (Prague)* **75**, 1–97.

Torres, N. E., Zollman, P. J., and Low, P. A. (1991). Characterization of muscarinic receptor subtype of rat eccrine sweat gland by autoradiography. *Brain Res.* **550**, 129–32.

22. Pupil function: tests and disorders

Shirley A. Smith

Introduction

This chapter describes how to assess pupil function and its involvement in a number of autonomic disorders. Ocular parasympathetic deficits are seen most commonly in Adie's syndrome. Increased parasympathetic activity resulting from central disinhibition occurs in Argyll Robertson pupils and narcolepsy. Sympathetic deficits give the classical ptosis and miosis of Horner's syndrome, whereas sympathetic overactivity causes large pupils in oculosympathetic spasm. Pupils are involved in the generalized disorders of pure autonomic failure and diabetic autonomic neuropathy. First, the anatomy and physiology which underlies normal pupil function is described.

Pupillary constriction

Contraction of the circular smooth muscle fibres of the sphincter pupillae constricts the pupil during the reflex responses to light and near vision. Both reflexes involve activation of parasympathetic preganglionic neurons whose cell bodies lie in the Edinger–Westphal nuclei, a pair of slim columns of small cells situated dorsorostrally to the main mass of the oculomotor nuclear complex in the anterior midbrain. These preganglionic neurons pass uncrossed in the superficial part of the third cranial nerve to synapse in the ciliary ganglion which lies about 10 mm in front of the superior orbital fissure in the loose fatty tissue at the orbital apex. This ganglion contains cell bodies of the postganglionic parasympathetic fibres whose axons travel forward to the ciliary muscle and iris sphincter via the short ciliary nerves which penetrate the eyeball at its posterior pole. Fibres subserving pupillary constriction comprise only 3 per cent of the parasympathetic outflow from the ciliary ganglion; the majority subserve accommodation, in accordance with the relatively greater bulk of the ciliary compared with the sphincter muscle.

The course of the light reflex pathway from the retina to the sphincter is illustrated in Fig. 22.1. Afferent impulses for visual perception and pupillary constriction diverge in the posterior (central) third of the optic tracts. The

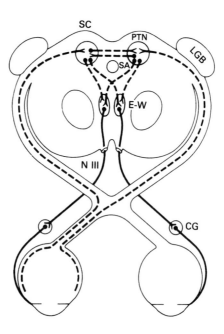

Fig. 22.1. The light reflex pathway from the retina to the iris sphincter. SC, superior colliculus; PTN, pretectal nucleus; LGB, lateral geniculate body; SA, Sylvian aqueduct; E–W, Edinger–Westphal nucleus; N III, oculomotor (third) nerve; CG, ciliary ganglion. (Taken with permission from Alexandridis (1985).)

visual fibres relay in the lateral geniculate bodies, whereas the pupillary fibres leave the optical tracts and synapse in the pretectal nuclei in the midbrain. Fibres from these nuclei carry the pupillomotor impulses to Edinger–Westphal nuclei of both sides. In man this crossing, together with the preceding one at the optic chiasm, is essentially symmetrical. Thus, illumination of only one eye produces reflex constriction of both pupils of approximately equal magnitude.

During fixation on a near object, the pupil constricts in association with accommodation produced by ciliary muscle contraction and convergence elicited by contraction of the medial rectus muscles. The light and near pupillary reflexes share a common neuronal path only from the Edinger–Westphal nucleus onward. Prior to that, the near reflex pathway descends from the occipital cortex bypassing the pretectal nucleus on its way to the Edinger–Westphal nucleus. As the fibres approach the nucleus they are probably situated more ventrolaterally than the light reflex fibres because they are often spared in patients in whom pineal or collicular tumours have abolished the light reflex by pressure from the dorsal side (Lowenstein and Loewenfeld 1969).

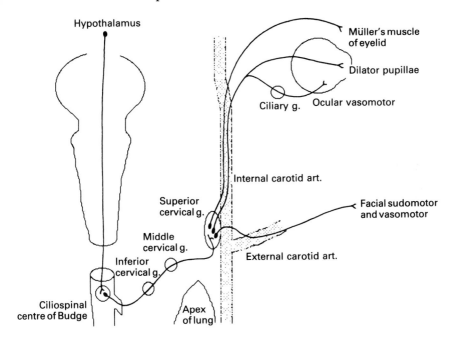

Fig. 22.2.   The sympathetic pathway subserving pupillary dilatation.

The postganglionic nerves release acetylcholine to activate muscarinic receptors on the sphincter pupillae. Some muscarinic receptors are present on the dilator which may relax the radial smooth muscle fibres during pupil constriction.

Pupillary dilatation

Dilatation of the pupil in darkness and during arousal is elicited by two mechanisms: central inhibition of the Edinger–Westphal nucleus and activation of the peripheral sympathetic innervation of the radial smooth muscle fibres of the dilator pupillae. The central inhibition is said to be via sympathetic fibres from the posterior hypothalamus to the oculomotor nucleus (Lowenstein and Loewenfeld 1950).

The peripheral sympathetic pathway comprises three parts (Fig. 22.2). The first neuron arises in the hypothalamus where connections from higher centres, including the cortex, influence sympathetic control of the pupil. From the hypothalamus the fibres descend uncrossed through the brainstem to the ciliospinal centre of Budge in the intermediolateral columns at the level of the last cervical and the first two thoracic segments. This centre contains the cell bodies of the preganglionic neurons which form the second stage of the pathway. Their axons leave the cord by the ventral roots of the first two thoracic segments and enter the cervical sympathetic trunk. They traverse the inferior and middle cervical ganglia before reaching the superior cervical ganglion near the bifurcation of the internal and external carotid arteries. Since these preganglionic axons pass close to the apex of the lung, the sympathetic pathway to the pupil may be interrupted by malignancy in this area arising from pulmonary or breast tissue. Within the superior cervical ganglion they synapse with the cell bodies of the postganglionic nerves which form the third stage of the pathway. Fibres which subserve pupillary dilatation, movement of the eyelids via Muller's (smooth) muscle, and local vasomotor function leave the ganglion and follow the course of the internal carotid arteries into the cranium. The pupillary fibres join the fifth (trigeminal) nerve and approach the orbit in its ophthalmic branch, entering via the superior orbital fissure. They continue in its nasociliary division and enter the eye in the long ciliary nerves. In man, some of the sympathetic fibres to the pupil may traverse, but do not synapse in, the ciliary ganglion.

The postganglionic nerves release noradrenaline on to α-adrenoceptors on the dilator pupillae. A small number of β-adrenoceptors are present on the sphincter which relax these circular fibres during pupillary dilatation. As with the cholinergic reciprocal innervation, there is no indication that these are of physiological significance and they do not mediate a change of pupil size during glaucoma treatment with β-adrenoceptor blocking drugs.

Pupillometric methods

There is a wide range of techniques available. Television systems, though expensive, enable dynamic parameters to be measured. Photographic methods are useful for accurate measurement of static pupil size. For all types of pupillometry, the subjects should fix on a distant target to avoid accommodative effort and the room should be quiet with stable, reproducible, and preferably variable background lighting.

Television pupillometry

These systems can be monocular or binocular. The eyes are illuminated with infra-red light so that pupils can be measured in darkness. The infra-red sensitive television cameras scan the front of the eye and the image is analysed to provide a measure of either vertical pupil diameter or pupil area. Light stimulation is provided from a bright source to one or both eyes at a length, frequency, and brightness all of which can be varied over a wide range. Light reflexes are usually elicited with open-loop stimulation, i.e. the stimulus light is too small to be reduced in size by a constricting pupil. The pupillometric output can be both analogue for chart display and digital for direct computer analysis.

Photographic methods

Any camera that can provide a clear magnified image of the front of the eye will suffice. Infra-red illumination will allow the eye to be viewed in darkness, and infra-red sensitive film can be used for darkness diameter measurement. However, light reflex latencies are in excess of 0.2 s, so that conventional flash light photographs can be taken even in darkness before the pupil starts to constrict. Close-up Polaroid photography gives instant results that are convenient clinically. Monocular photography allows for greater magnification and thus accuracy, but for measuring drug effects on pupil size it is better to photograph both pupils together.

Physiological pupil function tests

Darkness diameter

The size of the healthy pupil at rest in darkness is determined by the amount of central inhibition of the parasympathetic outflow and the level of peripheral sympathetic drive. It is age-dependent, being small in infancy but gradually increasing to a peak diameter in adolescence (Miller 1985). Thereafter, it decreases linearly at about 0.4 mm per decade. Presumably, changing levels of supranuclear inhibition and decreasing sympathetic tone contribute to this decline in adults.

An age-related normal range must be used to identify abnormality in darkness pupil size, such as that in Table 22.1 which was constructed from a healthy population of 163 subjects aged 16 to 92 years (Smith and Dewhirst 1986). A convenient way of expressing pupil size is the pupil diameter per cent (PD%: Table 22.1). This represents the amount of iris taken up by the dilated pupil and is calculated as the ratio of the pupil to the iris diameter. It is dependent only on age, which accounts for 48 per cent of the total variance, and is independent of the image magnification.

Measuring pupil size in darkness allows for universal applicability of such a normal range as darkness, unlike a light environment, can be reproduced consistently. The range shown was obtained using monocular Polaroid photography, and the results agreed well with those from television pupillometry (Smith and Smith 1983a) and infra-red photography in a larger population (Miller 1985). Darkness pupil diameter is a highly reproducible measure with coefficients of variation averaging 3 per cent.

Table 22.1. Age-related normal range for pupil diameter in darkness expressed as the absolute measure and as a percentage of iris diameter (PD%). Values shown are the 2.5, 50, and 97.5 percentiles which define the lower, mean, and upper limits of normal

Age range (year)	Mean (year)	Pupil diameter (mm)			PD%		
		Lower	Expected	Upper	Lower	Expected	Upper
15–19	17	6.0	7.4	8.8	52.0	63.3	74.6
20–24	22	5.8	7.2	8.6	50.5	61.8	73.1
25–29	27	5.6	7.0	8.4	49.0	60.3	71.5
30–34	32	5.4	6.8	8.2	47.5	58.8	70.0
35–39	37	5.2	6.6	8.0	46.0	57.3	68.5
40–44	42	5.0	6.4	7.8	44.5	55.8	67.0
45–49	47	4.8	6.2	7.6	43.0	54.3	65.5
50–54	52	4.6	6.0	7.4	41.5	52.7	64.0
55–59	57	4.4	5.8	7.2	40.0	51.2	62.5
60–64	62	4.2	5.6	7.0	38.5	49.7	61.0
65–69	67	4.0	5.4	6.8	37.0	48.2	59.5
70–74	72	3.8	5.2	6.6	35.4	46.7	58.0

Near reflex

When a subject changes fixation from far to near there is a miosis which accompanies the accommodation and convergence. The three functions are associated but are not dependent on each other, and focal electrical stimulation in the oculomotor nucleus and the third nerve have been shown in animal studies to elicit each function independently. The time course and amplitude of the pupillary near reflex can be measured with television pupillometry. The amplitude of the miosis increases with the amount of accommodative effort. It is a less useful test of parasympathetic integrity than the light reflex, because the stimulus is subjective. An absent near reflex indicates either parasympathetic dysfunction or a lack of accommodative effort by the subject. However, it is a useful sign when found to be greater than the light reflex, as such 'light–near dissociation' is an important diagnostic sign in some autonomic neuropathies.

Light reflex amplitude and dynamics

Normal reflex responses to light depend on intact parasympathetic innervation and sensitivity to light. Thus, light reflexes are reduced if retinal pathology or optic nerve lesions have reduced visual perception. However, a patient blind from a lesion to the lateral geniculate nucleus or beyond will retain intact light reflexes. If the efferent side of the light reflex is to be tested independently, visual perception threshold should be measured first so that

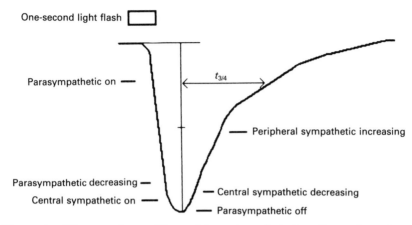

Fig. 22.3. Diagram of a pupillographic tracing of a light reflex to show the $t_{3/4}$ measure of redilatation time. The presumed activity of the autonomic system in shaping the reflex is indicated.

any afferent defects can be quantified and light intensity adjusted accordingly.

Measurement of static pupil size in the light can be made photographically to indicate parasympathetic integrity. More comprehensive information is obtained from continuous measurement of response to short-duration light stimuli in background darkness. Smooth light reflex profiles can be obtained by standard averaging techniques as illustrated in Fig. 22.3. The amplitude of the reflex from its starting darkness diameter to its peak is a measure of the parasympathetic response. This is attenuated first by central inhibition of the Edinger–Westphal nuclei via probable adrenergic inputs from the hypothalamus, then by peripheral sympathetic activation of the iris dilator.

Reflex amplitude is not affected by age directly, but it is reduced in pupils which are small in darkness due to age or sympathetic neuropathy. This is a mechanical restriction, whereby a small pupil has limited scope for further constriction (Smith and Smith 1983b).

Analysis of the averaged reflex provides data on latency, time to peak constriction, and the maximum velocities of constriction and dilatation. All these kinetic parameters are strongly dependent on amplitude, so that small reflexes have prolonged latencies, reduced times to peak, and slower maximum velocities of constriction and dilatation. These dynamic variables thus also reflect parasympathetic events, and are generally less reproducible than amplitude as pupillary measures.

Hippus

When pupils from healthy subjects are stimulated with continuous bright light they constrict initially, then redilate partially as the eye adapts to the

Table 22.2. Normal range for the $t_{3/4}$ redilatation time. Values shown are the 2.5, 50, and 97.5 percentiles which define the lower, mean, and upper limits of normal

Reflex amplitude (mm)	$t_{3/4}$ (s)		
	Lower	Expected	Upper
1.0	0.00	1.46	3.07
1.2	0.04	1.62	3.20
1.4	0.23	1.79	3.34
1.6	0.42	1.95	3.49
1.8	0.60	2.12	3.63
2.0	0.78	2.28	3.79
2.2	0.95	2.45	3.94
2.4	1.12	2.61	4.11
2.6	1.29	2.78	4.27
2.8	1.44	2.94	4.45
3.0	1.60	3.11	4.62
3.2	1.74	3.28	4.81
3.4	1.89	3.44	4.99
3.6	2.03	3.61	5.18

stimulus. Pupil size oscillates slowly as the redilatation ensues, a phenomenon known as hippus (Lowenstein and Loewenfeld 1969). This pupillary unrest is always synchronous in the two eyes and is therefore likely to be central in origin. The oscillations can be measured by Fourier frequency analysis, which separates them into their component sinusoidal wavelengths. Hippus comprises mostly low-frequency waves of less than 0.2 Hz.

Redilatation time

The recovery from a light reflex is shown in Fig. 22.3. Initially, the pupil dilates rapidly as the parasympathetic drive finishes and it is during this phase that the pupil reaches its maximum dilatation velocity. Thereafter, the peripheral sympathetic widens the pupil more slowly, and studies with adrenoceptor antagonists have shown that the time to three-quarter dilatation ($t_{3/4}$) accurately reflects this sympathetic activity (Smith and Smith 1990). A healthy population was studied to define a normal range for $t_{3/4}$ using television pupillometry. Bright lights elicited large reflexes in the dark-adapted state. Starting diameter and age had little influence, but $t_{3/4}$ time increased proportionally with amplitude (Table 22.2). Times that exceed the 97.5 percentile indicate a significant redilatation lag. This is a sensitive indicator of peripheral sympathetic dysfunction if reflex averaging is used to improve reproducibility.

A photographic method can be used to identify dilatation lag in patients with unilateral Horner's syndrome, where there is a normal pupil available for comparison (Thompson 1977*b*). Binocular photographs are taken at 5 and at 15 s after turning the room lights out. If there is more anisocoria in the 5-s photograph than in the 15-s one, the subject has a relative dilatation lag. The 5-s photograph corresponds approximately to the $t_{3/4}$ time.

Psychosensory dilatation

When a subject is aroused, alarmed, or afraid the pupils dilate. Central inhibition of the parasympathetic outflow, peripheral sympathetic drive, and circulating adrenaline may all contribute. The binocular dilatation can be measured with television pupillometry in background light to a stimulus such as a loud noise. This test has limited reproducibility.

Pupil cycle time

Another method of testing pupillary parasympathetic function is the pupil cycle time (Martyn and Ewing 1986). The test was first described as a means of quantifying afferent pupillary defects in optic neuritis. Regular oscillations of the pupil are induced by focusing a narrow beam of light on the pupil margin using a slit lamp. The constricting pupil interrupts the light beam, removing the stimulus and thereby dilating the pupil enabling the light to restimulate the retina ('closed loop stimulation'). The mean time is calculated from 100 cycles with a stop watch. It has been found to increase with increasing age. The pupil cycle time is lengthened by parasympathetic, but not sympathetic, drug blockade. It does not differentiate between afferent and efferent pupillary defects, and pupils in a proportion of patients cannot be made to cycle.

Pharmacological pupil function tests

These are a useful supplement to clinical and physiological signs. However pupillary responses to drugs show wide inter- and intraindividual variability. There is poor bioavailability from eyedrops because of low and variable corneal penetration. Dark eyes are more resistant to drug effects due to a thicker iris stroma reducing access to the smooth muscle. Many drugs are absorbed by melanin pigment, which will reduce bioavailability in dark eyes more than in light eyes which have less melanin.

Sources of variability should be minimized where possible. Binocular measurement can eliminate arousal effects, which affect the pupils equally. The effects of drugs on the pupil are often long-lasting, and at least 48 h should elapse between repeated drug tests. Systemic drugs with pupillary effects should be discontinued temporarily if possible. Ideally, dilutions of drugs should be made up freshly in a buffered diluent at room temperature to avoid lacrimation from stinging drops. Two drops should be given at 1 m apart to ensure effective dosing. Experiments with miotics are best performed in darkness, whereas mydriatics need stable background light to increase the available range of pupillary movement. Pupils should be measured several times post-instillation so that peak responses can be identified. Between-subject variation should be defined in healthy controls so that normal ranges can be constructed (Smith and Smith 1983a; Cremer et al. 1990).

Denervation supersensitivity

An important principle utilized in drug tests is that of denervation super-sensitivity. An organ deprived of its innervation becomes more sensitive to the transmitter normally released from those nerves. This 'up-regulation' is thought to be mediated by an increase in the number and activity of the receptors on the end-organ. The increased sensitivity extends to other agonists active at those receptors. It is a general principle applying to denervated voluntary muscle, glands, postsynaptic nerve cell bodies, and smooth muscle. It occurs not only with complete lesions to the postganglionic nerve, but also to a lesser degree with partial lesions, lesions more proximal in the nerve pathway, and even with functional, not anatomical, deficits. It is now understood to be one end of a regulatory spectrum, the other end of which is the decreased sensitivity or 'down-regulation' that follows excessive excitation as, for example, after treatment with high doses of miotic drugs.

Cholinergic tests

A large pupil with poor light and near reflexes may be caused by a parasympathetic deficit, local iris sphincter trauma, or cholinolytic mydriatic treatment. The former can be usefully differentiated from the latter two with a muscarinic agonist. The denervated pupil will show a supersensitive miosis, whereas the damaged or atropinized pupil will not constrict. If only one pupil is large, binocular responses to a weak concentration of the agonist should be measured to establish a relative supersensitivity. If both pupils are large, one eye should be treated and the drug effect taken as the difference in anisocoria before and after miosis. The response can then only be judged as supersensitive if data is available from matched healthy controls.

   Pilocarpine, an alkaloid with good corneal penetration that is resistant to cholinesterase destruction, is often used to test for sphincter supersensitivity. Thompson (1977a) recommends pilocarpine 0.125 per cent, which usually gives a small miosis in a healthy pupil. He studied patients with Adie's pupils having unilateral postganglionic parasympathetic denervation and found that

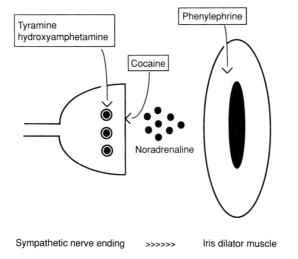

Fig. 22.4. Diagram to show the site of action of drugs used in the diagnosis of sympathetic dysfunction. Phenylephrine excites receptors on the dilator muscle, cocaine blocks the uptake of noradrenaline into the terminal, and tyramine and hydroxyamphetamine release noradrenaline from the terminal.

80 per cent of affected pupils constricted 0.2 mm more than the fellow eyes. Peak effects occur at approximately 1 h after instillation.

A supersensitive response indicates dysfunction anywhere from the midbrain to the nerve endings in the iris sphincter (Ponsford *et al.* 1982; Jacobson, 1990). The response to pilocarpine is age-dependent and control studies in healthy pupils should be included when investigating binocular parasympathetic neuropathies.

Sympathetic tests

There is a wider range of drug tests for sympathetic deficits (Fig. 22.4). Phenylephrine and cocaine are used to establish whether a small pupil is caused by sympathetic dysfunction, and hydroxyamphetamine or tyramine can help to locate the lesion.

Phenylephrine is an α-adrenoceptor agonist which is used to test for supersensitivity caused by a lesion anywhere along the three stages of the peripheral sympathetic pathway. Phenylephrine 2 per cent causes a small mydriasis in young adults, which increases markedly with age (Table 22.3). It is thus again important to use age-matched controls when testing binocular conditions which do not have a normal pupil available for comparison.

Cocaine (4–10 per cent) dilates the normal pupil by blocking re-uptake of noradrenaline, which then accumulates at the adrenoceptors. A lesion anywhere in the pathway will reduce the mydriasis, since there is less

Table 22.3. Age-related normal ranges for 2 per cent phenylephrine and 0.5 per cent hydroxyamphetamine drug tests. Values shown are the 2.5, 50, and 97.5 percentiles which define the lower, mean, and upper limits of normal

Age range (year)	Mean (year)	Phenylephrine mydriasis (mm)			Hydroxyamphetamine mydriasis (mm)		
		Lower	Expected	Upper	Lower	Expected	Upper
15–19	17	—	0.2	1.6	0.25	1.6	2.9
20–24	22	—	0.4	1.8	0.3	1.7	3.0
25–29	27	—	0.6	2.0	0.4	1.7	3.05
30–34	32	—	0.85	2.2	0.5	1.8	3.1
35–39	37	—	1.1	2.4	0.55	1.9	3.2
40–44	42	—	1.3	2.6	0.6	1.9	3.2
45–49	47	0.2	1.5	2.8	0.7	2.0	3.3
50–54	52	0.4	1.7	3.0	0.75	2.05	3.4
55–59	57	0.6	1.9	3.25	0.8	2.1	3.4
60–64	62	0.8	2.1	3.5	0.9	2.2	3.5
65–69	67	1.0	2.4	3.7	0.9	2.25	3.6
70–74	72	1.2	2.6	3.9	1.0	2.3	3.6

transmitter being released. Cocaine thus gives the same information as phenylephrine, the former showing a reduction and the latter an increase in mydriatic response in pupillary sympathetic dysfunction.

Hydroxyamphetamine (0.5 or 1 per cent) and tyramine (2–5 per cent) dilate the pupil by first entering the nerve endings from where they displace noradrenaline from its storage sites. If the postganglionic sympathetic nerve is damaged, these agents will cause less mydriasis as there will be less transmitter to release. Neither agent has any significant direct action at the receptors. If the lesion is preganglionic or central in origin, these agents will give a normal or slightly enhanced mydriasis, as decentralized nerves have increased stores of transmitter which will then act on supersensitive receptors. The response to hydroxyamphetamine 0.5 per cent is weakly age-dependent (Table 22.3).

Pupillary disorders

Tonic pupils

Lesions to the postganglionic parasympathetic innervation give 'tonic' pupils, i.e. the constrictions to light and near are slow and inextensive. Acutely, there may be complete internal ophthalmoplegia but reinnervation often restores some function. A variety of inflammatory, infective, malignant, or traumatic conditions can cause tonic pupils by damaging the ciliary ganglion or the short ciliary nerves. They are, however, seen most commonly in Adie's syndrome.

Adie's syndrome

This is a benign condition in which the idiopathic ciliary ganglion pathology is associated with loss of deep tendon reflexes. Usually, a patient with Adie's syndrome of recent onset presents with accommodative paresis and has one large pupil with poor or absent light reflexes. Further examination shows segmental iris sphincter palsy, denervation supersensitivity to topical pilocarpine, and deep tendon areflexia of the upper and lower extremities. Corneal sensation may be reduced from involvement of sensory nerves, some of which pass through the ciliary ganglion to join the ophthalmic division of the trigeminal nerve.

Many cases of Adie's pupils are investigated in the clinic some time after the initial onset of symptoms when the affected pupil is in fact smaller than the normal one. An Adie's pupil only remains larger than its fellow for about 2–6 months (Thompson 1977a). Thereafter, aberrant regeneration of fibres subserving accommodation, which are far in excess of those subserving pupil constriction, causes innervation of the affected sections of the sphincter pupillae (Loewenfeld and Thompson 1981). The neuronal drive associated with ciliary muscle function then constricts the pupil via its aberrant nerves to give a small pupil. This also results in a 'light–near dissociation' with pupillary constriction to near exceeding that to light, though both reflexes are abnormally slow. The initial accommodative difficulties resolve as the ciliary muscle reinnervates. The pupils at this stage may be difficult to distinguish from spastic miotic pupils (Argyll Robertson pupils, see next section) caused by midbrain lesions anterior to the oculomotor nucleus. The differential diagnosis may be made on the presence of segmental sphincter palsy and denervation supersensitivity (as in Adie's pupils) and the nature of the pupillary near reflex response which is slow in Adie's but brisk in Argyll Robertson's syndrome.

Adie's syndrome is a progressive condition with loss of the light reaction in further segments of the sphincter, further loss of the deep tendon reflexes, and eventual second eye involvement. This has led to the suggestion that a slow virus may be the cause of Adie's syndrome although immunological studies have, as yet, proved inconclusive.

There is clear histological evidence of loss of ganglion cells from the ciliary ganglia which explains the ocular signs. The cause of the progressive areflexia is less clear. However, post-mortem evidence has indicated that there is degeneration in the dorsal columns of the spinal cord, notably in the fasciculus gracilis and the fasciculus cuneatus.

There is recent evidence from patients with longstanding Adie's syndrome that sweating deficits are much more common than previously supposed (Bacon and Smith 1988). Thus the separately classified Ross's syndrome, defined as Adie's syndrome with segmental hypohidrosis, may be part of the same disorder. These and other workers (Hope-Ross *et al.* 1990) have also reported that some Adie's patients have impaired cold pressor responses and reduced Valsalva responses, although the vasomotor sympathetic deficit was not enough to cause postural hypotension. One can speculate that the spinal cord pathology cited above could involve the efferent sympathetic pathway. Thus, although the symptoms of Adie's that trouble the patient are exclusively ocular, it appears that there is often a much wider neurological involvement.

Argyll Robertson pupils

Pupillary dysfunction occurs in some conditions from disinhibition of the Edinger–Westphal nuclei which results in spastically miotic pupils. Such is the case in Argyll Robertson pupils of neurosyphilis, now a clinical rarity but still of considerable theoretical interest.

In the Argyll Robertson syndrome the pupils are small and light reflexes are reduced or absent, whereas the pupillary constriction to near is well preserved. The pupil signs are usually bilateral and may be associated with tabes dorsalis and general paresis although vision is not impaired. The pupillary abnormalities are thought to be due to pathology close to and slightly anterior to the oculomotor nucleus in the midbrain (Lowenstein and Loewenfeld 1969). Such a lesion would destroy the terminal branches of both the crossed and the uncrossed pretectal fibres subserving the light reflex, but would spare the more ventrally situated supranuclear pathways for the near vision reaction. Other inhibitory inputs from higher brain centres would also be interrupted thereby disinhibiting the parasympathetic motor nuclei. Marked, diffuse damage around the Sylvian aqueduct and the posterior portion of the third ventricle has been found post-mortem, which could explain the pupillary signs. The pupils are often irregular and tonic, which is thought to be due to postganglionic parasympathetic function in addition to the central pathology.

Narcolepsy

Other situations in which there is a small pupil due to central disinhibition are fatigue, sleep (physiological or drug-induced), and narcolepsy. This is a condition of chronic hypersomnia for which pupillography can be a valuable diagnostic tool (Yoss *et al.* 1969). Responses to light and near are normal, but measurement in darkness reveals abnormally small pupils which show large spontaneous oscillations in diameter reflecting the sleepiness that

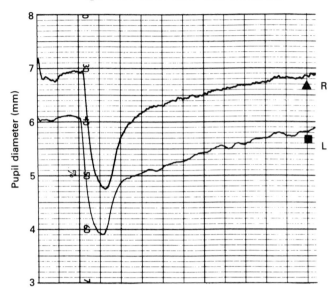

Fig. 22.5. Pupillograph from a patient with a left-sided Horner's syndrome obtained with infra-red television pupillometry. The right (R) and left (L) traces are separated on the time axis (1 vertical bar = 1 s) for convenience.

characterizes this condition. These 'fatigue waves' are of much larger amplitude and slower frequency than hippus. Treatment with amphetamines, which usually give an excellent clinical response, reverses these pupillary abnormalities which represent one end of the spectrum of arousal effects on pupil size.

Small pupils are a characteristic sign of narcotic addiction. A central parasympathetic disinhibition is accompanied by a smaller local miotic action, probably involving an inhibition of transmitter release from sympathetic terminals in the iris dilator (Ghodse *et al.* 1986).

Horner's syndrome

In this condition, sympathetic dysfunction leads to small pupils which have normal reflex constriction to light and near. This miosis is usually accompanied by ptosis and, in cases of preganglionic lesions, by sweating deficits of the face and neck. There is sometimes an apparent, not a real, enophthalmos due to the narrowing of the palpebral fissure caused by denervation of Mullers smooth muscles of the eyelids. Horner's syndrome results from partial or complete interruption of the sympathetic pathway in any of its three parts. Patients with damage to the first neuron may have had a medullary infarction or have cervical cord disease. Second neuron lesions can occur when a lung or breast malignancy has spread to the thoracic outlet, or when surgery or trauma to the neck has involved the sympathetic nerves. Causes of postganglionic lesions include vascular headache syndromes, intraoral or retroparotid trauma, internal carotid artery pathology, and tumours of the middle cranial fossa or the cavernous sinus.

The pupillary behaviour in Horner's syndrome is illustrated in Fig. 22.5. This pupillographic record from a 62-year-old patient with cluster headaches shows a left-sided Horner's pupil. Compared with the normal right pupil, the affected one has a small darkness diameter, normal constriction to light, and a redilatation lag. The $t_{3/4}$ time in the affected pupil was 6.4 s considerably prolonged in comparison with the 3.1 s measured in the fellow eye. Drug tests in postganglionic Horner's pupils show reduced mydriasis to cocaine and tyramine, and an enhanced response to phenylephrine.

A painful Horner's syndrome characterized by unilateral headache or facial pain in the distribution of the first division of the trigeminal nerve is termed Raeder's syndrome (Grimson and Thompson 1980). Some patients with Raeder's syndrome have multiple cranial nerve involvement and require thorough investigation for possible tumours or aneurysms involving the internal carotid artery. Other patients with Raeder's syndrome without multiple cranial nerve involvement have a benign condition such as cluster headache.

In cluster headache the unilateral pain is very severe, lasts up to 2 h, and may occur several times daily during the cluster period which lasts for several weeks or months. Patients with cluster headache may show signs of sympathetic hyperactivity during attacks on the side affected by pain which include lacrimation, nasal stuffiness, conjunctival hyperaemia, and hyperhidrosis. Between attacks, there is sometimes reduced forehead sweating on heating and a relative miosis with drug tests suggestive of a partial Horner's syndrome (Salvesen et al. 1987). Grimson and Thompson (1980) state that 5–22 per cent of patients with cluster headache have clinically evident Horner's syndrome. Presumably the position of the postganglionic fibres in the plexus surrounding the internal carotid artery renders them susceptible to irritation during attacks and ultimately to permanent damage.

Congenital Horner's syndrome, which is rarer than the acquired syndrome, is accompanied by heterochromia iridis since an intact noradrenaline synthetic pathway is required for melanin synthesis. Loss of pigment in acquired Horner's syndrome occurs rarely.

Oculosympathetic spasm

Irritation of sympathetic nerves anywhere from the brainstem to the iris dilator can cause intermittent ipsilateral mydriasis, sometimes associated with hyperhidrosis. Clinically, it is not difficult to distinguish from parasympathetic dysfunction as light and near reflexes are intact. This irritation can be associated with Horner's syndrome as in cluster headache described above. Other causes are cervical cord disease, lung malignancy, and carotid artery trauma.

One type of oculosympathetic spasm dilates just a section of the pupil to give peaked or 'tadpole' pupils. Episodes last about a minute, may occur several times a day, are unilateral and benign, and resolve with no neurological or systemic sequelae apart from a mild Horner's syndrome in some cases.

Pure autonomic failure (PAF) and multiple system atrophy (MSA)

In our clinical experience (Smith and Smith, unpublished observations), patients with PAF have the pupillary signs of Horner's syndrome, unlike patients with MSA and AF in whom the only consistent abnormality is larger than normal darkness diameters. It is possible, however, that these mydriatic pupils may result from the systemic drug therapy. In the last edition of Bannister this book reported that the most common abnormality in patients with AF associated with MSA or Parkinson's disease is cholinergic super-sensitivity to topical methacholine (see also Chapter 28). More work is needed before these observations can be ascribed to a parasympathetic deficit.

Diabetic autonomic neuropathy

Small pupils for age are a characteristic sign in this condition (Smith *et al.* 1978; Hreidarsson 1982). There is evidence that sympathetic dysfunction is partly responsible. However the size is sometimes smaller than that seen in Horner's syndrome in non-diabetics and it usually affects both pupils equally, implying that central control mechanisms may be damaged. There is also evidence for parasympathetic dysfunction but, as small pupils with normal light reflexes are found to be much more common than large pupils with reduced reflexes, it appears that the sympathetic pupillary innervation is the more susceptible in diabetes. Histological studies of irides from diabetic patients removed during cataract surgery have confirmed that loss of nerve terminals occurs mostly from the dilator pupillae (Ishikawa *et al.* 1985).

Significant associations between small pupils and a wide range of diabetic complications have been recorded: cardiovascular autonomic dysfunction (Smith and Smith 1983*a*), peripheral sensory loss (Smith *et al.* 1978; Hreidarsson 1982), retinopathy (Hayashi and Ishikawa 1979), and nephropathy (Hreidarsson 1982). Patients are more likely to have small pupils if their hyperglycaemia has been of a marked degree and duration (Smith and Smith 1983*a*; Hreidarsson 1982).

Redilatation lag occurs in diabetic miosis. Figure 22.6 shows redilatation in two healthy non-diabetic subjects and one diabetic with autonomic neuropathy. The diabetic patient has small pupils in darkness which constrict well to light but are slow to redilate. The $t_{3/4}$ times are 6 and 6.5 s in the

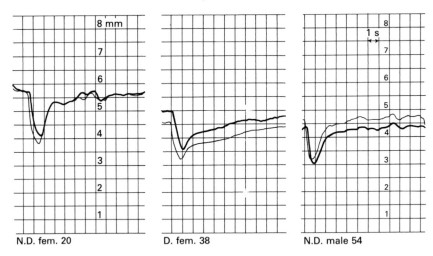

Fig. 22.6. Pupillographs from a non-diabetic (N.D.) 20-year-old female, a diabetic (D.) 38-year-old female with autonomic neuropathy, and a non-diabetic 54-year-old male subject. The bolder line indicates the right pupil, and the responses from the two pupils are separated on the time axis (1 vertical bar = 1 s) for convenience. For each subject, measurements were made in darkness interrupted by a single 1-s light flash. The diameter scale in mm is shown on the left graph. Note the bilateral redilatation lag and absent hippus in the diabetic patient.

right and left eyes, respectively, which are significantly prolonged for this 1.4 mm reflex size (Table 22.2).

The mydriatic response to directly acting sympathomimetic agents is exaggerated in patients with diabetic autonomic neuropathy suggesting that there is denervation supersensitivity as in Horner's syndrome (Hayashi and Ishikawa 1979; Smith and Smith 1983a). However, the response to hydroxy-amphetamine does not differ significantly from normal, from which one can conclude that postganglionic nerve function is essentially normal. It would be surprising if a multifactorial disorder such as diabetes caused dysfunction at one specific point in the pathway. More probably the sympathetic deficit results from a composite of mildly reduced function throughout.

The finding that small diabetic pupils dilate well to sympathomimetics shows that damage to the muscle itself is not responsible for the limited movement in darkness. In severe diabetic eye disease rubeosis iridis and glaucoma will eventually limit pupillary movements but the evidence available shows that muscle function in most patients is remarkably well preserved.

Diabetics with neuropathy show reduced hippus (Fig. 22.6), which indicates that central pupillary control may be affected.

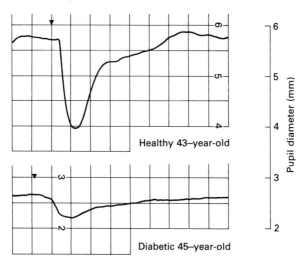

Fig. 22.7. Pupillographic record from a diabetic patient with marked autonomic neuropathy (lower trace). A normal light reflex from an age-matched healthy subject (upper trace) is shown for comparison. The pupil of the diabetic patient failed to dilate in the dark, and constricted poorly to a bright 1-s light flash (▼).

Light reflex amplitude is reduced in diabetic autonomic neuropathy (Smith and Smith 1983*b*; Hreidarsson and Gundersen 1985). This reduction is usually only seen in pupils which are already small from sympathetic dysfunction. Figure 22.7 shows a pupil recording from a patient with severe autonomic neuropathy. Pupil size remained almost the same despite a change in illumination from darkness to bright flash stimulation. Myopathy was not responsible for the limited mobility since drugs were effective in changing pupil size, nor was an afferent defect reducing reflex response since visual perception was intact. Presumably the iris was essentially denervated in both autonomic branches.

It is difficult to establish genuine reductions in reflex amplitude in pupils that start small due to sympathetic dysfunction. However Smith and Smith (1983*b*) found that light reflexes in diabetic miosis were significantly smaller than in non-diabetic senile miosis. It is likely that the additional reduction in diabetics is due to parasympathetic dysfunction. The supersensitive response to cholinomimetic drugs (Hayashi and Ishikawa 1979) supports this hypothesis.

Reversal of chronic hyperglycaemia does not appear to improve autonomic function. The St Thomas's Diabetic Study Group (1986) reported a prospective trial of a 2-year improvement in glycaemic control in 20 insulin-treated diabetic patients with established autonomic dysfunction. There was no reversal of the neuropathy and, in fact, two pupillary and three cardiovascular tests indicated a significant deterioration which exceeded that explicable by ageing.

Drug effects on the pupil

Many drugs, given locally or systemically, affect pupil size and may thus complicate the diagnosis of neurological disease. Glaucoma may be treated with eyedrops that constrict the pupil, as with pilocarpine, or dilate the pupil, as with adrenaline. Certain mydriatic agents such as cyclopentolate used to enable fundal inspection can dilate the pupil for several days after a single application. Many insecticides contain powerful anticholinesterase agents which may give pinpoint pupils if the eyes have been contaminated.

Patients taking tricyclic antidepressant drugs will have large pupils as these drugs are muscarinic antagonists. Drugs used to treat Parkinson's disease, particularly the anticholinergic agents such as procyclidine, may cause mydriasis. Arteriolar vasodilator agents used to treat hypertension will dilate the pupil by α-adrenoceptor blockade. Patients using or abusing opiates will have small pupils. Many sedative drugs will constrict the pupils in association with the sleepiness.

Acknowledgements

I would like to thank Professor Stephen Smith for his invaluable contributions to this manuscript.

References

Alexandridis, E. (1985). *The pupil*. Springer-Verlag, New York.
Bacon, P. J. and Smith, S. E. (1988) Adie's syndrome. *Ophthalmic Dialogue*, no. 3.
Cremer, S. A., Thompson, H. S., Digre, K. B., and Kardon, R. H. (1990). Hydroxyamphetamine mydriasis in normal subjects. *Am. J. Ophthalmol.* **110**, 66–70.
Ghodse, A. H., Bewley, T. H., Kearney, M. K., and Smith, S. E. (1986). Mydriatic response to topical naloxone in opiate abusers. *Br. J. Psychiat.* **148**, 44–6.
Grimson, B. S. and Thompson, H. S. (1980). Raeder's syndrome. A clinical review. *Survey Ophthalmol.* **24**, 199–210.
Hayashi, M. and Ishikawa, S. (1979). Pharmacology of pupillary responses in diabetics-correlative study of the responses and grade of retinopathy. *Jap. J. Ophthalmol.* **23**, 65–72.
Hope-Ross, H., Buchanan T. A. S., Archer, D. B., and Allen, J. A. (1990). Autonomic function in Holmes–Adie syndrome. *Eye* **4**, 607–12.
Hreidarsson, A. B. (1982). Pupil size in insulin-dependent diabetes. *Diabetes* **31**, 442–8.
Hreidarsson, A. B. and Gundersen, H. J. G. (1985). The pupillary response to light in Type I (insulin-dependent) diabetes. *Diabetologia* **28**, 815–21.

Ishikawa, S., Bensaoula, T., Uga, S., and Mukono, K. (1985) Electron microscopic study of iris nerves and muscles in diabetes. *Ophthalmologica* **191**, 172–83.

Jacobson, D. M. (1990). Pupillary responses to dilute pilocarpine in preganglionic 3rd nerve disorders. *Neurology* **40**, 804–8.

Loewenfeld, I. E. and Thompson, H. S. (1981). Mechanism of tonic pupil. *Ann. Neurol.* **10**, 275–6.

Lowenstein, O. and Loewenfeld, I. E. (1950). Mutual role of sympathetic and parasympathetic in shaping of the pupillary reflex to light. Pupillographic studies. *Arch. Neurol. Psych.* **64**, 341–77.

Lowenstein, O. and Loewenfeld, I. E. (1969). The pupil. In *The eye*, Vol. 3 (ed. H. Davson) pp. 255–337. Academic Press, New York.

Martyn, C. N. and Ewing, D. J. (1986). Pupil cycle time: a simple way of measuring an autonomic reflex. *J. Neurol. Neurosurg. Psychiat.* **49**, 771–4.

Miller, N. R. (1985). The autonomic nervous system: pupillary function, accommodation and lacrimination. In *Walsh and Hoyt's clinical neuro-ophthalmology*, (4th edn), Vol. 2, (ed. N. R. Miller), pp. 385–556. Williams & Wilkins, Baltimore.

Ponsford, J. R., Bannister, R., and Paul E. A. (1982). Methacholine pupillary responses in third nerve palsy and Adie's syndrome. *Brain* **105**, 583–97.

Salvesen, R., Bogucki, A., Wysocka-Bakowska, M. M., Antonaci, F., Fredricksen, T. A., and Sjaastad, O. (1987). Cluster headache pathogenesis: a pupillometric study. *Cephalalgia* **7**, 273–84.

Smith, S. A. and Dewhirst, R. R. (1986). A simple diagnostic test for pupillary abnormality in diabetic autonomic neuropathy. *Diabetic Med.* **3**, 38–41.

Smith, S. A. and Smith, S. E. (1983a). Evidence for a neuropathic aetiology in the small pupil of diabetes mellitus. *Br. J. Ophthalmol.* **67**, 89–93.

Smith, S. A. and Smith, S. E. (1983b). Reduced pupillary light reflexes in diabetic autonomic neuropathy. *Diabetologia* **24**, 330–332.

Smith, S. A. and Smith, S. E. (1990). The quantitative estimation of pupillary dilatation in Horner's syndrome. In *Sympathicus und Auge* (ed. A. Huber), pp. 152–65. Enke, Stuttgart.

Smith, S. E., Smith, S. A., Brown, P. M., Fox, C., and Sonksen, P. H. (1978). Pupillary signs in diabetic autonomic neuropathy. *Br. med. J.* **2**, 924–7.

St Thomas's Diabetic Study Group (1986). Failure of improved glycaemic control to reverse diabetic autonomic neuropathy. *Diabetic Med.* **3**, 330–4.

Thompson, H. S. (1977a). Adie's syndrome: some new observations. *Trans. Am. ophthalmol. Soc.* **75**, 587–626.

Thompson, H. S. (1977b). Diagnosing Horner's syndrome. *Trans. Am. Acad. Ophthalmol. Otolaryngol.* **83**, 840–2.

Yoss, R. E., Moyer, N. J., and Ogle, K. N. (1969). The pupillogram and narcolepsy. *Neurology* **19**, 921–8.

23. The assessment of sleep disturbance in autonomic failure

Sudhansu Chokroverty

Introduction

The autonomic nervous system (ANS) is intimately involved in the control of sleep and breathing. The nucleus of the tractus solitarius (NTS) in the medulla orchestrates the central autonomic network by its ascending and descending projections. The NTS also contains the lower brainstem hypnogenic and central respiratory neurons. Dysfunction of the ANS thus may have serious impact on human sleep and respiration during sleep. Furthermore, sleep has a profound effect on the functions of the ANS. It is, therefore, logical to expect sleep disorder and respiratory dysfunction during sleep in patients with autonomic failure. Sleep and breathing disturbances in conditions associated with autonomic failure should be easy to understand when one also remembers that the peripheral respiratory receptors and central respiratory and lower brainstem hypnogenic neurons are intimately linked by the ANS. This chapter is concerned with an assessment of sleep and respiratory disturbances in autonomic failure including the influence of the ANS on cardiac rhythm during sleep. A basic familiarity with the stages of sleep, the control of breathing, and the interrelationship between the central autonomic network and the neuronal network controlling breathing and sleep–wake states is a prerequisite to an understanding of sleep and breathing dysfunction in autonomic failure.

Central autonomic network

Over the past 15 years a central circuitry of the autonomic network has been identified (Loewy and Spyer 1990). The NTS in the medulla is the single most important structure of the autonomic network in the brainstem. The NTS receives afferents from the cardiovascular and the respiratory systems for autonomic control of cardiac rhythm, circulation, and respiration. Lower brainstem hypnogenic neurons are also located in the NTS. The NTS has ascending projections to the supramedullary including the hypothalamic

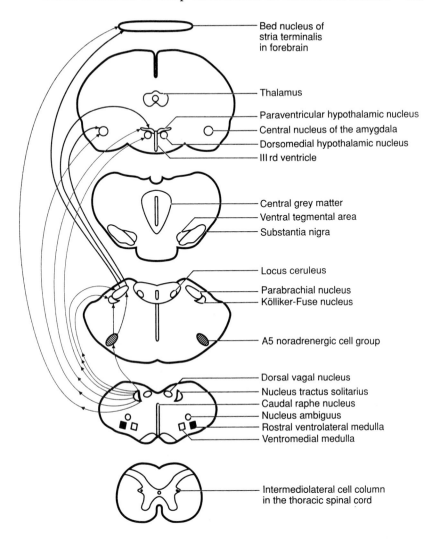

Fig. 23.1. Central autonomic network: ascending projections (schematic). (Modified from Loewy and Spyer (1990); reproduced with permission from Chokroverty (1991) and the American Academy of Neurology.)

and limbic regions and descending projections to ventral medulla which also sends efferents to intermediolateral neurons of the spinal cord (Loewy and Spyer 1990). Many of the ascending and descending projections (Figs 23.1 and 23.2) are reciprocal in nature. Through its connections in the dorsal and ventral medulla the NTS directly influences the inputs to the vagal (the dorsal nucleus of the vagus and the nucleus ambiguus) and sympathetic preganglionic neurons in the spinal cord. The NTS thus orchestrates the central autonomic

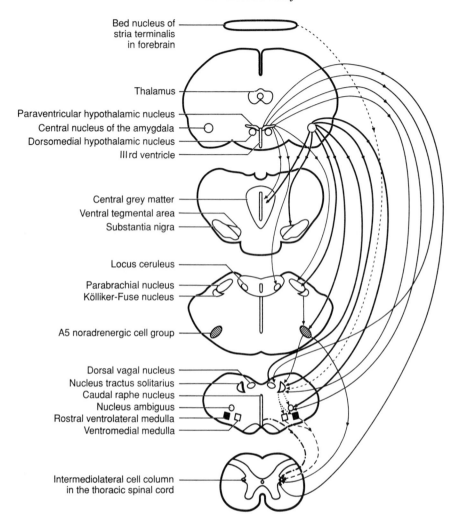

Fig. 23.2. Central autonomic network: descending projections (schematic). (Modified from Loewy and Spyer (1990); reproduced with permission from Chokroverty (1991) and the American Academy of Neurology.)

network for autonomic control of the vital cardiorespiratory functions during sleep.

An overview of sleep

Based on the electroencephalographic (EEG), behavioural, and physiological observations two types of sleep have been recognized (Chokroverty 1986,

1990): non-REM or slow wave sleep comprising 75–80 per cent and REM or paradoxical sleep comprising 20–25 per cent of sleep time in adults. EEG criteria establish four stages of non-REM sleep: stages I–IV. In normal individuals the REM sleep begins 60–90 min after sleep onset and recurs in a cyclic manner every 90 min throughout the night. REM sleep is divided into tonic and phasic stages (Chokroverty 1986) based on EEG, electro-myographic (EMG), and eye movements criteria.

Based on the ablation and stimulation experiments, single-unit recordings, and pathological findings, it is believed that non-REM or synchronized sleep results from a combination of two factors (Chokroverty 1986, 1990): inhibition of the ascending reticular activating system and activation of the hypnogenic neurons in the anterior hypothalamus and the preoptic region as well as the NTS in the dorsomedial medulla. The original concept of a reciprocal interactive model for REM sleep generation has recently been revised (Chokroverty 1990). The recent theory suggests that there are anatomically distributed and neurochemically interpenetrated REM 'on' and REM 'off' cells in the brainstem. The interaction and oscillation between the cholinergic REM-promoting and aminergic REM-inhibiting neurons generate the REM–non-REM cycle.

Control of breathing during sleep and wakefulness

The anatomical relationship suggests a close functional interdependence between the central autonomic network and the respiratory and hypnogenic neurons. Two separate and independent controlling systems are responsible for breathing (Chokroverty 1986, 1990): the metabolic or automatic system and a voluntary or behavioural system. Both voluntary and metabolic systems operate during wakefulness but respiration during sleep depends upon the inherent rhythmicity of the automatic respiratory control system located in the medulla. These two controlling systems are complimented by a third system, the reticular arousal system exerting a tonic influence on the brainstem respiratory neurons (McNicholas et al. 1983).

Upper brainstem respiratory neurons located (Cherniack and Longobardo 1986) in the rostral pons in the region of parabrachial and Kölliker–Fuse nuclei (pneumotaxic centre), and in the dorsolateral region of the lower pons (apneustic centre) influence the automatic respiratory neurons. The medullary (automatic) respiratory neurons consist of two principal groups (Cherniack and Longobardo 1986; Chokroverty 1986, 1990): the dorsal respiratory group located in the NTS responsible predominantly but not exclusively for inspiration and the ventral respiratory group located in the region of the nucleus ambiguus and retroambigualis responsible for both inspiration and expiration (Fig. 23.3). These respiratory premotor neurons send axons which decussate below the obex and descend in the reticulospinal tracts in the

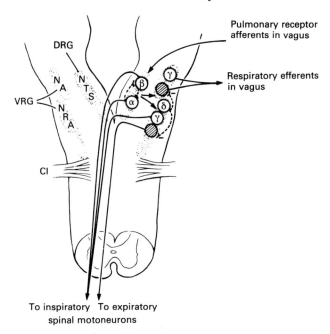

Fig. 23.3. Medullary respiratory neurons, cell types, and interconnections are shown schematically. DRG, Dorsal respiratory group; VRG, ventral respiratory group; NTS, nucleus tractus solitarius; NA, nucleus ambiguus: NRA, nucleus retroambigualis; CI, first cervical dorsal root; subscripts α, β, γ, δ, inspiratory cell subtype designations. The DRG located in the ventrolateral NTS is the site where vagal sensory information is first incorporated into a respiratory motor response. The DRG drives the VRG and some spinal inspiratory motoneurons. The VRG is composed of NA and NRA. Vagal respiratory motoneurons arise from NA. Axons from NRA project to some spinal inspiratory and probably all spinal expiratory motoneurons. Inspiratory cells are indicated by open circles, and expiratory by hatched circles. Dashed lines indicate some of the hypothesized intramedullary neural interconnections. (Taken with permission from Berger *et al.* (1977).)

ventrolateral spinal cord to synapse with spinal respiratory motor neurons innervating the various respiratory muscles. Respiratory rhythmogenesis depends upon tonic inputs from the peripheral and central structures converging on the medullary neurons (Cherniack and Longobardo 1986; Chokroverty 1986, 1990). Figure 23.4 shows schematically the effects of various brainstem and vagal transections on the ventilatory patterns.

The voluntary breathing system originating in the cerebral cortex (forebrain and limbic system) controls respiration during wakefulness in addition to participating in non-respiratory functions (Chokroverty 1986, 1990). The system descends partly to the automatic medullary controlling system and

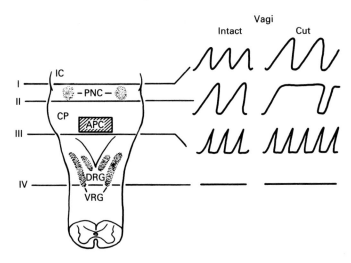

Fig. 23.4. Schematic representation of effects of various brainstem and vagal transections on the ventilatory pattern of the anaesthetized animal. IC, Inferior colliculus; PNC, pneumotaxic centre; CP, cerebellar peduncle; APC, apneustic centre; DRG, dorsal respiratory group; VRG, ventral respiratory group. On the left is a representation of the dorsal surface of the lower brainstem and, on the right, a representation of tidal volume with inspiration upwards. Transection I, just rostral to the PNC, does not affect normal breathing, but, in combination with vagotomy, slow deep breathing results. Transection II, isolating the PNC from the lower brainstem, causes slow deep breathing with the vagi intact, and either apneusis (sustained inspiration) or apneustic breathing (rhythmic respiration with marked increase in inspiratory time) when the vagi are cut. Transection III, isolating structures rostral to the medulla, results in most cases in a regular gasping breathing that is generally not affected by vagotomy. Transection IV, at the medullospinal junction, results in respiratory arrest. (Taken with permission from Berger *et al.* (1977).)

integrates in part there but mostly descends with the corticobulbar and corticospinal tracts to the spinal respiratory motor neurons where the fibres finally integrate with the reticulospinal fibres originating from the automatic medullary respiratory neurons.

The control of respiration during non-REM sleep in normal individuals is entirely dependent upon the automatic control system (Phillipson and Bowes 1986). The ventilation, tidal volume, and respiratory rate decrease in non-REM sleep. Ventilatory responses to hypercapnoea and hypoxia are attenuated during non-REM sleep in normal individuals. These findings suggest decreased sensitivity of the central chemoreceptors subserving medullary respiratory neurons. In REM sleep respiration is rapid and erratic; tonic and phasic activities in the intercostal and upper airway muscles decrease while phasic activity is maintained in the diaphragm but the tonic activity in diaphragm is reduced (Phillipson and Bowes 1986). There is some uncertainty about the ventilatory responses to CO_2 and hypoxia in REM sleep (Phillipson and Bowes 1986). Compared with the responses during non-REM sleep the hypercapnoeic and hypoxic ventilatory responses in the adult human are reduced during REM sleep. The voluntary respiratory control system may be active during some part of REM sleep. Thus, in normal individuals, respiration is vulnerable during sleep; mild respiratory irregularities and pauses may occur in normals, but in disease states these may assume a pathological significance.

Sleep and respiratory disturbances in autonomic failure

The best known condition with autonomic failure in which sleep and respiratory disturbances have been reported and well described is the Shy–Drager syndrome or multiple system atrophy with autonomic failure (MSA). Familial dysautonomia, a recessively inherited disease with autonomic failure, is also known to be associated with disturbances of breathing and sleep. A large number of neurological and general medical disorders are associated with prominent secondary autonomic failure. In many neurological conditions sleep and respiratory disturbances are secondary to the structural lesions involving the central hypnogenic or respiratory neurons.

In this section an assessment of sleep and respiratory disturbances in the Shy–Drager syndrome, familial dysautonomia, and diabetic autonomic neuropathy will be discussed. Following this, a description of sleep-induced autonomic changes in the cardiovascular functions and how these changes may affect cardiac rhythm will be given.

Primary autonomic failure

Multiple system atrophy (Shy–Drager syndrome)

Since the original description by Shy and Drager (1960) of a neurodegenerative disorder characterized by autonomic failure and multiple system atrophy there have been numerous reports (Bannister *et al.* 1967, 1981; Chokroverty *et al.* 1969; Bannister and Oppenheimer 1972; Chokroverty 1986, 1990) of the condition which has generally come to be known as the Shy–Drager syndrome or multiple system atrophy with autonomic failure. Patients with this syndrome frequently manifest sleep and respiratory disturbances. Further clinical details are given in Chapter 28. In the later stages of the illness a variety of respiratory and sleep disturbances add to the progressive disability. Occasionally, respiratory dysfunction, particularly dysrhythmic breathing in wakefulness becoming worse in sleep, manifests in the initial stage of the illness. In the final stage there is progressive autonomic and somatic dysfunction compounded by respiratory failure. The ventilatory disturbances now may be present both in wakefulness and sleep.

The sleep disturbances in this syndrome as documented by polysomnographic study may comprise the following (Wooten 1989): a reduction of total sleep time, REM, and slow-wave sleep with increased sleep latency; and an increased number of awakenings during sleep.

The clinical manifestations resulting from respiratory dysfunction may consist of daytime hypersomnolence, early morning headache, daytime fatigue, severe disturbance of nocturnal sleep, intellectual deterioration, pulmonary hypertension, cor pulmonale, congestive cardiac failure, and occasionally cardiac arrhythmias.

The spectrum of respiratory dysrhythmias in MSA may be summarized as follows (Chokroverty 1986, 1990):

(1) central, upper-airway obstructive and mixed apnoeas associated with oxygen desaturation during non-REM stages I and II and REM sleep;

(2) irregular rate, rhythm, and amplitude of respiration with and without oxygen desaturation becoming worse in sleep (dysrhythmic breathing);

(3) transient occlusion of the upper airway or transient uncoupling of the intercostal and diaphragmatic muscle activities;

(4) prolonged periods of central apnoea accompanied by mild oxygen desaturation in relaxed wakefulness;

(5) Cheyne–Stokes pattern and Cheyne–Stokes variant (hypopnoea substitutes apnoea) pattern of breathing becoming worse in sleep;

(6) periodic breathing in the erect posture accompanied by postural fall of blood pressure;

(7) inspiratory gasps and apnoeustic-like breathing;

(8) nocturnal stridor;

(9) transient sudden respiratory arrest.

Figure 23.5 schematically shows the various breathing patterns.

To be significant an apnoea or hypopnoea should be at least 10 s in duration and the patient should have at least 30 periods of apnoea–hypopnoea during 7 h of all-night sleep or an apnoea–hypopnoea index (number of apnoea–hypopnoea per hour of sleep) of at least 5 (Chokroverty 1986). Three types of apnoeas may be recognized (Chokroverty 1986, 1990):

(1) central apnoea, characterized by the suppression of diaphragmatic and intercostal muscle activity and absence of air exchange through the nose and mouth;

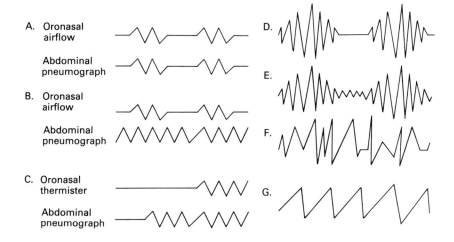

Fig. 23.5. Different respiratory patterns in MSA are shown schematically. A, central apnoea; B, upper-airway obstructive apnoea; C, mixed apnoea; D, Cheyne–Stokes breathing; E, Cheyne–Stokes variant pattern; F, dysrhythmic breathing; G, apneustic breathing.

(2) upper-airway obstructive apnoea manifested by an absence of air exchange detected by the oronasal thermistors but persistence of the diaphragmatic and intercostal muscle activities;

(3) mixed apnoea manifested by an initial period of central apnoea followed by a period of upper-airway obstructive apnoea before resumption of regular breathing.

Bannister and Oppenheimer (1972) initially reported periodic inspiratory gasps resembling apnoeustic breathing in two patients with this syndrome; they did not, however, perform polysomnographic or respiratory recordings to confirm these findings.

Lockwood (1976) described a 54-year-old man with the syndrome who had cluster breathing with periods of apnoea of up to 20 s duration during wakefulness and of up to 40 s during sleep. The patient died of a sudden respiratory arrest at night. The pathological findings showed widespread diffuse lesions typical of MSA in addition to gliosis in the pontomedullary reticular formation.

Laryngeal abductor paralysis giving rise to laryngeal stridor and excessive snoring during sleep has been described in cases of MSA by Bannister *et al.* (1967, 1981), Israel and Marino (1977), Williams *et al.* (1979), and Munschauer *et al.* (1990). The nocturnal stridor can be inspiratory, expiratory, or both. This stridor may give rise to a striking noise which may be likened to a 'donkey braying'.

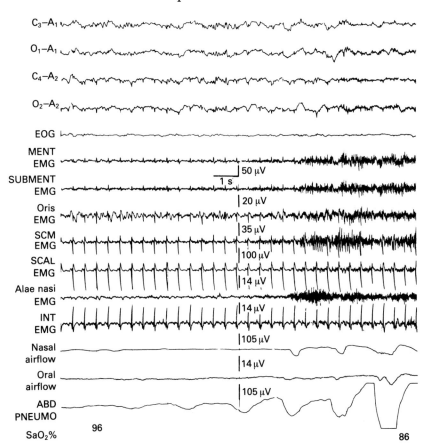

Fig. 23.6. Polygraphic recordings in a patient with MSA showing EEG (top four channels), vertical electrooculogram (EOG), EMG of mentalis (MENT), submental, oris, sternocleidomastoideus (SCM), scalenus anticus (SCAL), alae nasi and intercostal (INT) muscles, nasal and oral airflow, abdominal pneumogram (ABD PNEUMO), and oxygen saturation (SaO$_2$%). The patient has mixed apnoea (only a portion of the episode is shown) associated with oxygen desaturation during stage II non-REM sleep.

Briskin *et al.* (1978) and Guilleminault *et al.* (1981) described patients with this syndrome who had predominantly upper-airway obstructive apnoea during sleep on polygraphic study. Sleep scoring showed very little non-REM sleep stages III and IV and almost total absence of REM sleep.

McNicholas *et al.* (1983) described patients with MSA in whom hypoxic and hypercapnoeic ventilatory responses were impaired suggesting a defect in the metabolic control system. The most striking abnormality, however, was an irregular pattern of breathing during sleep on overnight polysomnographic study. These findings suggested a defect in the automatic respiratory rhythm generator in the brainstem.

Chokroverty *et al.* (1978) described four patients with MSA who had periodic central apnoea in the erect position. In one patient hypercapnoeic ventilatory response in the supine position was impaired and the post-mortem findings in the same patient of neuronal loss and astrocytosis in the pontine tegmentum suggested involvement of the respiratory neurons in the brainstem.

Recently, the author and colleagues (Chokroverty 1990) have studied another 10 patients with MSA showing a variety of respiratory disturbances consisting of central apnoea, including Cheyne–Stokes or Cheyne–Stokes variant breathing and upper-airway obstructive and mixed apnoeas accompanied by oxygen desaturation, predominantly during non-REM sleep stages I and II and REM sleep (Fig. 23.6). Heart rate variation during apnoeic–eupnoeic cycles was not seen in these patients indicating cardiac autonomic denervation. Other abnormalities included episodes of central apnoeas during relaxed wakefulness as if the respiratory centre 'forgot' to breathe, inspiratory gasps, and dysrhythmic breathing. All-night polysomnographic studies in two patients revealed marked reduction of non-REM sleep stages III and IV and REM sleep, increased awakenings after sleep onset, snoring, excessive body movements, and frequent arousal responses in the EEG accompanied by mild to moderate oxygen desaturation. Impaired hypercapnoeic ventilatory response and mouth occlusion pressure response in one patient suggested impairment of the metabolic respiratory system while normal hypercapnoeic and hypoxic ventilatory responses in another patient in the presence of an abnormal respiratory pattern resembled that noted by Lockwood (1976) indicating that the chemoreceptor control and respiratory pattern generator are probably subserved by different populations of neurons with selective vulnerability of these neurons in MSA. The finding that in eight of 10 patients dysrhythmic breathing occurred mostly during sleep and in four patients also during wakefulness implied that this type of respiratory disturbance is very common in MSA. These observations are in agreement with the suggestion of McNicholas *et al.* (1983) that such findings imply an impaired respiratory pattern generator in these patients.

Munschauer *et al.* (1990) studied respiration during sleep in seven patients with MSA whose respiratory disturbances included inspiratory gasping during wakefulness or stridor and upper-airway obstruction during sleep, and greater coefficients of variability in respiratory rate, tidal volume, and inspiratory flow rate than in controls. Post-mortem examination in four patients confirmed the diagnosis of MSA. Three patients showed marked neuronal loss in the region of the pontine tegmentum and medullary reticular formation including neurons around the nucleus tractus solitarius.

The suggested pathogenetic mechanisms for respiratory dysrhythmia in MSA include:

(1) direct involvement of the medullary respiratory neurons;

(2) involvement of the arousal system (ascending reticular activating system) and severe compromise of the wakefulness stimulus;

(3) involvement of the respiratory and the non-respiratory motor neurons in the brainstem, e.g. affection of the nucleus ambiguus and hypoglossal nucleus causing laryngeal abductor paresis and pharyngeal and genio-glossal weakness causing upper-airway obstructive apnoea;

(4) involvement of the respiratory motor neurons (anterior horn cells) in the cervical and thoracic spinal cord, thereby reducing impulse traffic along the phrenic and intercostal nerves to the diaphragm and intercostal muscles. If there is differential affection between the upper airway motor neurons and spinal respiratory motor neurons, there may be obstructive and mixed apnoeas;

(5) interference with the forebrain, midbrain, and pontine inputs to the medullary respiratory neurons causing dysrhythmic and apnoeustic breathing;

(6) involvement of the direct projections from the hypothalamus and central nucleus of amygdala to the respiratory neurons in the NTS and nucleus ambiguus;

(7) involvement of the vagal afferents from the lower and upper airway receptors may reduce the input to the central respiratory neurons causing respiratory dysrhythmia;

(8) sympathetic denervation of the nasal mucosa causing increased nasal resistance may promote upper-airways obstructive apnoea;

(9) finally, discrete neurochemical alterations in MSA may interfere with normal regulation of breathing.

Familial dysautonomia

This condition is a recessively inherited disorder confined to the Jewish population and presenting in childhood. The clinical manifestations comprise autonomic, neuromuscular, cardiovascular, skeletal, renal, and respiratory abnormalities. They characteristically show absence of the fungiform papillae of the tongue. Other features include defective lacrimation and sweating, vasomotor instability, fluctuation of blood pressure (postural hypotension and paroxysmal hypertension), relative insensitivity to pain, and absent muscle stretch reflexes. Most patients have a mild respiratory and sleep disorder associated with both central and obstructive sleep apnoeas (Gadoth *et al.* 1983). The sleep abnormalities may be summarized as follows (Gadoth *et al.* 1983; Wooten 1989): increased arousals and awakenings; prolonged sleep onset; prolonged REM sleep onset but reduced total REM sleep time; apnoeas during sleep and absent or impaired cardiac responses to sleep apnoea. The patients with familial dysautonomia often show severe breath-holding spells due to defective responses of central respiratory neurons to changes in $PaCO_2$ (partial pressure of CO_2 in the arterial blood).

Guilleminault et al. (1981) and McNicholas et al. (1983) found an irregular pattern of breathing in patients with familial dysautonomia similar to that noted in Shy–Drager syndrome. Oesophageal reflux during sleep causing frequent awakenings was noted in one patient by Guilleminault et al. (1981).

Secondary autonomic failure (those associated with other medical and neurological disorders)

Diabetic autonomic neuropathy

Autonomic neuropathies have been described in many neurological and medical disorders. However, the sleep and respiratory functions have not been studied well in most of these conditions. In diabetic polyneuropathies, however, there have been reports of disturbances of sleep and respiration.

Rees et al. (1981) studied eight diabetic patients with autonomic neuropathy and eight without autonomic neuropathy. They monitored their respiration during sleep using magnetometer and thermistors. In three patients with autonomic neuropathy 30 or more apnoeic episodes per night (two patients with mainly central and one with predominantly obstructive) were noted. The authors concluded that such episodes may be responsible for the cardiorespiratory arrest reported in such patients. There were no sleep-related respiratory disturbances in patients without autonomic neuropathy.

Guilleminault et al. (1981) also studied four patients with juvenile diabetes mellitus and autonomic neuropathy. In two patients they found obstructive sleep apnoea syndrome with autonomic failure along with clear dissociation ('decoupling') between heart rate and respiratory response. Bursts of central apnoeas were noted in one diabetic patient. They also found respiratory irregularities in one patient associated with oesophageal reflux during sleep causing frequent awakenings.

Autonomic nervous system, sleep, and cardiac dysrhythmias

There are a number of changes in the autonomic functions during sleep affecting particularly the cardiovascular and the respiratory systems (Loewy and Spyer 1990). The neural regulation of the heart predominantly involves the sympathetic and parasympathetic divisions of the ANS but to an extent involves the whole CNS axis. The limbic–hypothalamic region by controlling the central autonomic network (Loewy and Spyer 1990) affects cardiac rhythm. Sympathetic preganglionic neurons in the intermediolateral column of the spinal cord and the parasympathetic preganglionic neurons in the nucleus ambiguus and dorsal motor nucleus of the vagus along with the extensive connections with the central autonomic network and the peripheral afferent inputs to the central autonomic network control the cardiovascular regulation in wakefulness and sleep (Loewy and Spyer 1990). Based on animal experiments and human studies it is known that heart rate slows during non-REM sleep due to tonic increase in parasympathetic activity. There is further slowing of the heart rate during REM sleep due to combination of two factors: persistence of parasympathetic predominance and an additional decrease of sympathetic activity. Similarly, the blood pressure falls during non-REM with further fall during REM sleep due to same mechanisms. Blood pressure and heart rate are unstable during phasic REM due to phasic inhibition of the vagus and phasic activation of sympathetic tone resulting from changes in the brainstem neural activity. The reduction in cardiovascular haemodynamic activities in normal sleep, involving the heart rate, peripheral vascular resistance, blood pressure, blood flow, and cardiac output, becomes critical in patients with cardiopulmonary diseases (e.g. ischaemic heart disease, congestive cardiac failure, pulmonary emphysema, and chronic obstructive pulmonary disease).

Sleep and cardiac arrhythmias

Several studies have been obtained in normal individuals using Holter monitoring to understand the effect of sleep on cardiac rhythm (Parish and Shepard 1990). The most frequent nocturnal dysrhythmia is sinus arrhythmia which is noted in 50 per cent of young individuals (see Parish and Shepard 1990). One-third of them had sinus pauses lasting from 1.8 to 2 s and in another 6 per cent there were episodes of atrioventricular block. In young healthy adults sinus arrest has been noted lasting up to 9 s during REM sleep without associated apnoeas or significant oxygen desaturation (see Parish and Shepard 1990).

Although human studies revealed contradictory results about the effect of sleep on ventricular arrhythmia, the majority (Verrier and Kirby 1988) showed an anti-arrhythmic effect of sleep on ventricular premature beats. There are also several reports of ventricular arrhythmias occurring during arousal from sleep. A classic example was a 14-year-old girl who was awakened from sleep by a loud auditory stimulation with ventricular tachyarrhythmia (see Verrier and Kirby 1988). This was thought to be due to an increase of sympathetic activity as the episodes could be prevented by propranolol, a β-blocker.

In patients with ischaemic heart disease, 24-h Holter monitoring may reveal several different electrocardiographic changes during sleep: ST segment depression and T-wave inversion. Nocturnal cardiac ischaemia associated with ST segment depression or elevation has been noted in some middle-aged men and also in postmenopausal women during sleep.

Sleep and sudden cardiac death

Muller *et al.* (1987) analysed the time of sudden cardiac death in 2203 individuals dying out of the hospital in 1983. There was low incidence during the night and high incidence from 7 to 11 a.m. This pattern is similar to the incidence of non-fatal myocardial infarction and episodes of myocardial ischaemia which are more likely to occur in the morning. One suggestion is that the sudden cardiac death may result from a primary arrhythmic event. It is known that in the morning there is increased sympathetic activity which may increase myocardial electrical instability giving rise to fatal arrhythmia.

Cardiac arrhythmias and obstructive sleep apnoea syndrome

Several varieties of cardiac dysrhythmias are noted in patients with obstructive sleep apnoea syndrome (Parish and Shepard 1990). These arrhythmias are determined by the changes in autonomic nervous system. The most common is bradytachyarrhythmia alternating during apnoea and immediately after termination of apnoea. The other dysrhythmias consist of the following: sinus bradycardia with less than 30 beats/min; sinus pauses lasting for 2 to 13 s; second degree heart block; and ventricular ectopic beats including complex and multifocal ectopic beats and ventricular tachycardia. There is a clear relationship between the level of oxygen saturation (SaO_2) and premature ventricular complex and sleep apnoea syndrome. Patients with SaO_2 below 60 per cent are the most vulnerable.

Laboratory diagnosis of sleep and respiratory dysfunction in autonomic failure

The diagnosis of the primary and secondary autonomic failure is based on a combination of clinical manifestations, documentation of autonomic dysfunction, and exclusion of other causes of dysautonomia and somatic neurological diseases. The computerized tomography (CT) brain scan, magnetic resonance imaging, positron emission tomography using fluorodopa, electromyographic (EMG) and nerve conduction study, cerebral spinal fluid examination, and routine EEG in addition to special autonomic function studies may be necessary to establish the diagnosis. Once the diagnosis of MSA or other secondary autonomic failure is made, further studies are necessary in patients suspected of sleep and respiratory dysrhythmia to diagnose and treat the specific disturbance. A thorough history and physical examination including orolaryngological examination to detect laryngeal and oropharyngeal muscle weakness should precede the special studies described.

Polysomnographic study

For the assessment of sleep and respiratory dysfunction in autonomic failure it is important to obtain a complete polysomnographic study. To assess the severity of the sleep and respiratory disturbances and to fully understand the structure of sleep all night recordings should be obtained. The study should include simultaneous recordings of multiple channels of EEG, EMG of orofacial muscles, electrocardiogram, electrooculogram, respiratory recordings, and continuous oxygen saturation by an oximeter. Respiration can be monitored by oronasal thermistors to detect airflow and by use of an abdominal pneumograph or inductive plethysmograph (Respitrace).

The importance of studying the sleep architecture is that sleep may accentuate respiratory abnormalities and respiratory dysfunction may affect sleep structure adversely (Chokroverty 1986); both these factors may alter the long-term course of the illness. One may also obtain 24-h ambulatory recording of sleep and breathing to assess the circadian variation of sleep and breathing.

Multiple sleep latency test

This is an objective test for assessment of daytime pathological sleepiness (Carskadon *et al.* 1986). This test may help in assessing the severity of daytime hypersomnolence and for monitoring the effect of treatment. In this recording four or five daytime tests at 2-h intervals, each time lasting for 20 min, are obtained. The patients are encouraged to remain awake in between the recordings and the recording must follow a standardized protocol (Carskadon *et al.* 1986) to validate the results of the tests adequately. Sleep onset latency and sleep onset REM are noted. Sleep onset latency of 5 min or less is indicative of pathological sleepiness.

Pulmonary function tests

In order to exclude intrinsic bronchopulmonary disease contributing to respiratory dysfunction in autonomic failure, one should obtain measurements of spirometry, lung volumes, pulmonary diffusing capacity, and blood gases. One should also measure the maximum static inspiratory and expiratory pressures. These are more important than the dynamic measurements in detecting respiratory muscle weakness. To measure the chemical control of breathing, hypercapnoeic or hypoxic ventilatory and mouth occlusion pressure ($P_{0.1}$) responses, with or without load, should be studied (Phillipson and Bowes 1986). Mouth occlusion pressure reflects central respiratory drive and inspiratory muscle strength independent of pulmonary mechanical factors. These measurements may be impaired in patients with dysfunction of the metabolic respiratory control system.

EMG of respiratory muscles

Electrical activity of the respiratory and upper airway including genioglossus and laryngeal muscles may be obtained to assess ventilatory activity and upper airway muscle tone. Laryngeal EMG is important in patients suspected of laryngeal paresis.

Electrocardiogram (ECG)

ECG recording is essential in patients with suspected cardiac dysrhythmia or in those at high risk for developing such arrhythmias. Continuous monitoring of ECG by Holter monitoring for one or more days is required. This will give an indication about the circadian variation of the heart rate as well as the circadian influence on the cardiac dysrhythmias.

Treatment of sleep-related respiratory dysfunction

In the absence of an adequate understanding of the pathogenesis and a lack of a definite aetiological agent causing MSA, treatment remains unsatisfactory and consists of symptomatic measures only. Similarly, the pathogenesis of sleep-related respiratory dysfunction in MSA is not clearly understood; therefore, the treatment remains difficult. Repeated hypoxaemias during sleep are potentially harmful not only to the immediate health of the patient but also to the long-term course of the illness. It is, therefore, important to diagnose and assess the type of respiratory dysrhythmia and take appropriate measures to ameliorate the disability.

General measures

The patients must avoid alcohol and sedative–hypnotic drugs which may further depress the respiratory centre. The role of alcohol and sedative–hypnotic drugs in disrupting the sleep architecture and in increasing the frequency and duration of sleep apnoeas is well established but the mechanism is not known. These agents may selectively depress genioglossal muscle activity thus promoting upper-airway obstructive apnoea.

Pharmacological treatment

This should ideally be directed towards the search for agents which will change the respiratory centre motor output selectively to stimulate the upper airway muscles to overcome the hypotonia of the genioglossal and other upper airway muscles and so prevent central and obstructive apnoeas. By correcting these apnoeas these agents might then improve the sleep architecture. However, no such selective and ideal agents have yet been found. Protriptyline, a non-sedating tricyclic antidepressant, and medroxyprogesterone acetate have been used with some success in patients with mild-to-moderate obstructive sleep apnoea. Acetazolamide has been used to treat central apnoea in MSA. One must, however, be cautious because of the danger of increasing orthostatic hypotension resulting from diuresis and natriuresis. Unfortunately, these pharmacological agents have not been very helpful in patients with MSA because the natural history of the illness shows relentless progression despite treatment.

Continuous positive airway pressure (CPAP)

CPAP treatment delivered through the nose has been the most significant recent development in the treatment of patients with obstructive sleep apnoea syndrome. This treatment may be tried in patients with MSA showing predominantly obstructive or mixed sleep apnoea. One should use the lowest pressure which will be effective in decreasing the number and duration of apnoeic events. If nasal CPAP shows a good response during polysomno-graphic study in the laboratory then this treatment may be considered in patients with moderate-to-severe obstructive or mixed sleep apnoea. There are several types of home CPAP units available for this purpose. In patients with obstructive sleep apnoea following CPAP treatment there is dramatic improvement in apnoea–hypnoea index along with amelioration of daytime hypersomnolence and correction of oxygen desaturation. It should, however, be noted that the polysomnographic study will show REM rebound with increased REM density and reduction of REM latency along with marked increase of slow wave sleep. The long-term effect of CPAP treatment in the usual patients of obstructive sleep apnoea syndrome is probably beneficial but cannot be definitely stated without prolonged follow-up and the mechanism of its action is not definitely known. Patients with MSA showing obstructive sleep apnoea syndrome may show temporary improvement following the nasal CPAP treatment but as stated above, the natural history of the disease is one of relentless progression and, therefore, the benefit appears transient.

Tracheostomy

This remains the only effective treatment used as an emergency measure in patients with severe respiratory dysfunction accompanied by marked hypoxaemia and cyanosis and in patients with sudden respiratory arrest after resuscitation by intubation. Tracheostomy is also the only form of treatment used successfully in patients with severe laryngeal stridor due to laryngeal abductor paralysis. An attempt should be made to wean a patient from a tracheostomy but the weaning procedure may be difficult in patients with MSA because of the progressive course of the illness.

Despite considerable advances in our understanding of MSA and the sleep and respiratory disturbances observed in this illness an effective therapy for the respiratory dysrhythmias continues to elude us. In autonomic failure other than MSA causing sleep and respiratory disturbances similar lines of treatment may be tried.

Acknowledgement

The author wishes to thank Lena DiMauro for typing the manuscript.

References

Bannister, R. and Oppenheimer, D. R. (1972). Degenerative disease of the nervous system associated with autonomic failure. *Brain* **95**, 457–74.

Bannister, R., Ardill, L., and Fentem, P. (1967). Defective autonomic control of blood vessels in idiopathic orthostatic hypotension. *Brain* **90**, 725–46.

Bannister, R., Gibson, W., Michaels, L., and Oppenheimer, D. R. (1981). Laryngeal abductor paralysis in multiple system atrophy. *Brain* **104**, 351–68.

Berger, A. J., Mitchell, R. A., and Severinghaus, J. N. (1977). Regulation of respiration. *New Engl. J. Med.* **297**, 138–43.

Briskin, J. G., Lehrman, K. L., and Guilleminault, C. (1978). Shy–Drager syndrome and sleep apnea. In *Sleep apnea syndromes* (ed. C. Guilleminault and W. C. Dement), pp. 316–22. Alan R. Liss, New York.

Carskadon, M. A., Dement, W. C., Mitler, M., *et al.* (1986). Guidelines for the multiple sleep latency test (MSLT): A standard measure of sleepiness. *Sleep* **9**, 519–24.

Cherniack, N. S. and Longobardo, G. S. (1986). Abnormalities in respiratory rhythm. In *Handbook of physiology*, Section 3. *The respiratory system*, Vol. II, Part 2 (ed. A. F. Fishman, N. S. Cherniack, and J. G. Widdicombe), pp. 729–49. American Physiological Society, Bethesda, Maryland.

Chokroverty, S. (1986). Sleep and breathing in neurological disorders. In *Breathing disorders of sleep* (ed. N. H. Edelman and T. V. Santiago), pp. 225–64. Churchill Livingstone, New York.

Chokroverty, S. (1990). The spectrum of ventilatory disturbances in movement disorders. In *Movement disorders* (ed. S. Chokroverty), pp. 365–92. PMA Publishing Corp, Costa Mesa, California.

Chockroverty, S. (1991). Functional anatomy of the autonomic nervous system: autonomic dysfunction and disorders of the CNS. In *Correlative neuroanatomy and neuropathology for the clinical neurologist*. American Academy of Neurology Course No. 144. American Academy of Neurology, Minneapolis.

Chokroverty, S., Barron, K. D., Katz, F. M., Del Greco, F., and Sharp, J. T. (1969). The syndrome of primary orthostatic hypotension. *Brain* **92**, 743–68.

Chokroverty, S., Sharp, J. T., and Barron, K. D. (1978). Periodic respiration in erect posture in Shy–Drager syndrome. *J. Neurol. Neurosurg. Psychiat.* **41**, 980–6.

Gadoth, N., Sokol, J., and Lavie, P. (1983). Sleep structure and nocturnal disordered breathing in familial dysautonomia. *J. neurol. Sci.* **60**, 117–25.

Guilleminault, C., Briskin, J. G., Greenfield, M. S., and Silvestri, R. (1981). The impact of autonomic nervous system dysfunction on breathing during sleep. *Sleep* **4**, 263–78.

Israel, R. H. and Marino, J. M. (1977). Upper airway obstruction in the Shy–Drager syndrome. *Ann. Neurol.* **2**, 83.

Lockwood, A. H. (1976). Shy–Drager syndrome with abnormal respirations and antidiuretic hormone release. *Arch. Neurol.* **33**, 292–5.

Loewy, A. D. and Spyer, K. M. (1990). *Central regulation of autonomic functions.* Oxford University Press, Oxford.

McNicholas, W. T., Rutherford, R., Grossman, R., Moldofsky, H., Zamel, N., and Phillipson, E. A. (1983). Abnormal respiratory pattern generation during sleep in patients with autonomic dysfunction. *Am. Rev. resp. Dis.* **128**, 429–33.

Muller, J. E., Ludmer, P. L., Willich, S. N., Tofler, G. H., Aylmer, G., Klangos, I., and Stone, P. H. (1987). Circadian variation in the frequency of sudden cardiac death. *Circulation* **75**, 131–8.

Munschauer, F. E., Loh, L., Bannister, R., and Newsom-Davis, J. (1990). Abnormal respiration and sudden death during sleep in multiple system atrophy with autonomic failure. *Neurology* **40**, 677–9.

Parish, J. M. and Shepard, J. W., Jr., (1990). Cardiovascular effects of sleep disorders. *Chest* **97**, 1220–6.

Phillipson, E. A. and Bowes, G. (1986). Control of breathing during sleep. In *Handbook of physiology*, Section 3. *The respiratory system*, Vol. II, Part 2 (ed. A. F. Fishman, N. S. Cherniack, and J. G. Widdicombe), pp. 649–89. American Physiological Society, Bethesda, Maryland.

Rees, P. J., Cochrane, G. M., Prior, J. G., and Clark, T. J. H. (1981). Sleep apnoea in diabetic patients with autonomic neuropathy. *J. roy. Soc. Med.* **74**, 192–5.

Shy, G. M. and Drager, G. A. (1960). A neurological syndrome associated with orthostatic hypotension. *Arch. Neurol., Chicago* **2**, 511–27.

Verrier, R. L. and Kirby, D. A., (1988). Sleep and cardiac arrhythmias. *Ann. NY Acad. Sci.* **533**, 238–51.

Williams, A., Hanson, D., and Calne, D. B. (1979). Vocal cord paralysis in the Shy–Drager syndrome. *J. Neurol. Neurosurg. Psychiat.* **42**, 151–3.

Wooten, V. (1989). Medical causes of insomnia. In *Principles and practice of sleep medicine* (ed. M. H. Kryger, T. Roth, and W. C. Dement), pp. 456–75. W. B. Saunders, Philadelphia.

24. Investigation and treatment of bladder and sexual dysfunction in diseases affecting the autonomic nervous system

Christopher D. Betts and Clare J. Fowler

Introduction

The lower urinary tract and genitalia are largely innervated by autonomic fibres and, consequently, disturbances of micturition, continence, and sexual function are common in patients with diseases of the autonomic nervous system. In some cases it may be difficult to differentiate between symptoms due to autonomic dysfunction and symptoms caused by local pathological processes and it is in these circumstances that urodynamic and neurophysiological studies may prove helpful. Since there is no treatment to restore the autonomic supply to the bladder and genitalia, the management of urinary and sexual dysfunction arising from autonomic failure is essentially symptomatic; many of the methods now available are highly effective.

Methods of investigation

Urodynamic studies

Urodynamic studies include various tests devised to investigate the storage and emptying function of the lower urinary tract. The tests range from simple charting of the voided volumes over a 24-h period, to complex studies involving the simultaneous recording of intravesical pressure, intra-abdominal pressure, urinary flow rate, and sphincter electromyographic (EMG) activity. Although of value in providing descriptive information about the pathophysiological behaviour of the bladder, urodynamic studies are of limited value in neurological localization.

Uroflowmetry and postmicturition studies

Measurement of the urinary flow rate and the postmicturition residual are useful initial screening tests. Portable flow meters, suitable for use both in

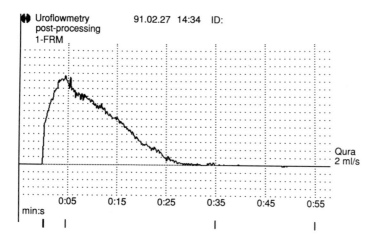

Fig. 24.1. Normal uroflowmetry. Qura is the urinary flow rate. The maximum flow rate is 22 ml/s and the trace is smooth indicating an uninterrupted urine flow.

the out-patient department and on hospital wards are now available. These provide a graphic trace (Fig. 24.1) of the urinary flow, and most devices are also able to give values for maximum flow rate, voided volume, and the time taken to complete micturition. After voiding, the residual urine can be measured either by passing a catheter or by ultrasonic examination of the bladder.

Urinary flow rates can only be properly assessed if the patient voids a reasonable volume of at least 150 ml. Nomograms, adjusted for age, sex, and voided volume, can be used to interpret the result. If the patient voids with a normal flow rate and the residual is less than 50 ml, a significant abnormality of the innervation of the bladder is unlikely.

Filling cystometry

This test involves the measurement of detrusor pressure during bladder filling. It is most useful in the investigation of patients with symptoms of urgency and frequency or incontinence. Total intravesical pressure is monitored by a small catheter (1 mm diameter) passed into the bladder catheter alongside a larger Nelaton catheter (3 mm diameter), which is used to fill the bladder at a controlled rate. Rectal pressure, which provides a measure of intraabdominal pressure, is recorded by means of another fine catheter inserted into the rectum. The urodynamic machine calculates the detrusor pressure by subtraction of the rectal pressure from the total intravesical pressure. Normally, during filling there is only a small rise in the detrusor pressure which occurs when the bladder is nearly full (Fig. 24.2).

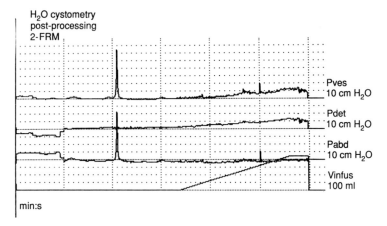

H₂O cystometry
post-processing
2-FRM

Pves
10 cm H₂O

Pdet
10 cm H₂O

Pabd
10 cm H₂O

Vinfus
100 ml

min:s

Fig. 24.2. Filling cystometry (normal). The bottom trace (Vinfus) shows the volume infused. Pdet, the detrusor pressure is derived by subtracting the intra-abdominal pressure (Pabd) from the measured intravesical pressure (Pves). The abrupt rises in pressure (large spike, small spike) are the result of the subject coughing. That Pdet did not rise shows there was good subtraction between Pves and Pabd. On filling to 450 ml the detrusor pressure rise does not exceed 15 cm H₂O.

Abnormal detrusor contractions may be recorded during filling cystometry (Fig. 24.3). If they occur in patients not known to have a disease or injury involving the nervous system, this type of inappropriate activity has been termed detrusor instability. In patients with a known neurological lesion, uncontrolled contractions of the bladder are called *detrusor hyperreflexia* (Abrams *et al.* 1988). The urinary symptoms reported by patients with detrusor hyperreflexia include frequency, urgency, and urge incontinence. Loss of the parasympathetic supply to the detrusor will result in an underactive detrusor (hyporeflexia) and filling cystometry may demonstrate a bladder that holds unusually large volumes.

Voiding cystometry

Pressure/flow studies during micturition are useful in the investigation of patients with varying degrees of urinary retention and difficulty in voiding. The detrusor pressure sustained during voiding is recorded together with the urinary flow rate. These studies allow the distinction to be made between a failure of detrusor contraction and obstruction causing low flow. An abnormality of the parasympathetic innervation to the bladder will result in weak, poorly sustained detrusor contractions during attempts to void (Fig. 24.4). Voiding urodynamic studies may show a reduced urinary flow rate, low voiding detrusor pressure, and a high postmicturition residual volume.

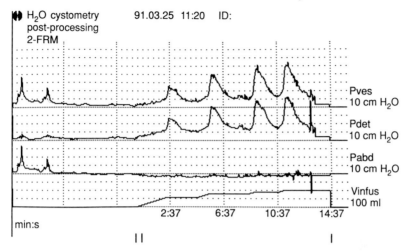

Fig. 24.3. Filling cystometry showing hyperreflexia. Unlike the detrusor pressure in the normal bladder which does not exceed 15 cm H_2O on filling (see Fig. 24.2), these traces were from a patient with a hyperreflexic bladder. Involuntary rises of pressure occur after filling with 100 ml, which become increasingly stronger with further filling. Abbreviations as in Fig. 24.2.

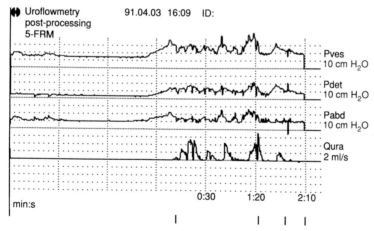

Fig. 24.4. Voiding cystometry (parasympathetic failure). Qura is the urinary flow rate. With impaired detrusor contractility due to parasympathetic failure, voiding is facilitated by abdominal straining. The result is a poor, interrupted urine flow (compare Qura bottom trace with Fig. 24.1).

The striated muscle of the external urethral sphincter is tonically active and cessation of electrical activity of the muscle is normally the first recordable event that heralds the onset of micturition. Recordings of the EMG activity of the sphincter during voiding studies may demonstrate a failure of relaxation during detrusor contraction, known as *detrusor sphincter dyssynergia*. This neurological abnormality implies there is a spinal lesion interrupting the bulbospinal pathway to the sacral cord.

If fluoroscopy is used during filling and voiding studies, the investigation is known as a *videocystometrogram*. In addition to detrusor pressure measurements, it provides information about the appearance of the bladder and outflow tract. This is of particular value in the assessment of bladder neck competence.

Neurophysiology

At present there is no neurophysiological method of investigating the autonomic nerve supply to the bladder and genital organs. The neurophysiological tests most often employed in the investigation of pelvic floor disorders include measurement of the latency of the cortical evoked potential following stimulation of the dorsal nerve of the penis/clitoris, measurement of the latency of the bulbocavernosus reflex, and EMG examination of the striated, external urethral sphincter. Although these tests only examine the somatic innervation of the lower urinary tract, combining the neurophysiological results with the results of urodynamic studies may lead to a better understanding of the nature of an underlying neurological lesion affecting the innervation of the urogenital tract.

Electromyography of the urethral sphincter can be carried out as part of the urodynamic study, in which case the examiner is concerned mainly with the relationship between sphincter activity and detrusor contraction. Alternatively, urethral sphincter EMG can be performed as a separate neurophysiological study, using a coaxial needle electrode, so that the integrity of the innervation of the sphincter striated muscle is examined. Using a trigger and delay line individual motor units can be captured and their duration and amplitude measured.

Measurements of sacral reflex latencies and cortical evoked responses have been advocated, but these techniques are usually more appropriate for the investigation of lesions affecting the somatic rather than autonomic nervous systems.

Erectile dysfunction

Physiology

An increase in the blood flow to the corpora is essential for normal penile erection. This is thought to result from relaxation of the corporeal and arteriolar smooth muscle under the control of the autonomic nervous system. Penile erection is primarily controlled by parasympathetic fibres but sympathetic erector pathways are known to exist within the hypogastric nerves. Erectile difficulties can result from abnormalities of the innervation or vascular supply to the penis, but psychological factors may also be important and in some patients a combination of disorders may be operating.

Investigation

The introduction of intracorporeal injections of vasoactive substances as effective medical treatment has transformed management such that investigations to make the distinction between neurogenic and psychogenic erectile dysfunction are of less importance and nocturnal penile tumescence studies have been largely abandoned. The response to an intracorporeal injection of papaverine is of great value in the investigation of the cause of erectile dysfunction: an adequate response indicates the problem must be either neurogenic or psychogenic, whereas repeated failure to develop an erection suggests a vascular pathology, such as inadequate arterial inflow or abnormal venous outflow.

Investigation of the blood supply to the corpora by measurement of the penile brachial index has been superseded by the more accurate technique of colour duplex ultrasonography (Lue *et al*. 1985). Arteriography of the iliac vessels and selective internal pudendal arteriography may be employed to diagnose disease of the larger vessels and appropriate vascular surgery or percutaneous angioplasty may improve the blood flow. Infusion cavernoso-graphy and cavernometry, combined with intracorporeal papaverine, is used to diagnose 'venous leaks' which may be the cause of impotence in some patients. Although these apparently abnormal veins draining the corpora may be ligated, the overall results of surgery are somewhat disappointing.

Treatment

Intermittent catheterization

Incomplete bladder emptying resulting from a disturbance of the parasympathetic innervation of the detrusor is best managed by intermittent catheterization. Introduced for the treatment of urinary dysfunction in patients with spinal injuries, the techique has since revolutionized the management of patients with urinary dysfunction resulting from many different neurological diseases.

Intermittent cateheterization was initially performed in an aseptic manner only by medical staff, but Lapides *et al*. (1974) demonstrated that a clean rather than a sterile technique was equally safe. In order to achieve complete emptying of the bladder, clean intermittent self-catheterization is now practised by a large number of patients with neurological disorders. In general, the greatest symptomatic improvement can be expected in those patients with large residual volumes and good storage function. In our experience, patients with residuals consistently more than 100 ml are most likely to benefit from intermittent catheterization. Patients with significant residual volumes and detrusor hyperreflexia will only gain maximum symptomatic improvement from intermittent catheterization if the hyper-reflexia is controlled with anticholinergic medication.

A specialist nurse or continence advisor is the most suitable person to instruct the patient and, if necessary, their carer in the technique of intermittent catheterization. In general, female patients find the procedure more difficult and at first usually require a mirror to help locate the urethral meatus. Most patients performing clean intermittent self-catheterization will void a variable amount before passing the catheter but, after commencing anticholinergic medication, effective voiding may be so reduced that the patient relies entirely on intermittent catheterization. Surprisingly, this is often more acceptable since it enables the patient to regain control over bladder function. Frequency of catheterization will be best determined by the patient. Initially the patient should be advised to perform the procedure three or four times a day, ensuring the residuals are kept lower than 500 ml. Asymptomatic bacteriuria is not an uncommon finding in those using intermittent catheterization but serious urinary tract infection is fortunately rare.

Anticholinergics

Detrusor hyperreflexia is commonly managed by drugs with anticholinergic properties. Propantheline (15–30 mg four times a day) is of value in the treatment of detrusor hyperreflexia but the side-effects of this and other anti-cholinergics are well known and include a dry mouth, impaired accommodation, and constipation, which limit their usefulness. Oxybutinin (2.5 mg three times a day) has been shown to be beneficial and more effective than propantheline for the treatment of detrusor hyperreflexia in patients with MS (Gajewski and Awad 1986). In addition to its anticholinergic effects, oxybutinin is a smooth muscle relaxant. Drugs with anticholinergic action may result in poor bladder emptying and residual volumes should be checked after commencing treatment.

Impotence and intracorporeal injection therapy

Patients should be counselled before commencing treatment and many benefit from an explanation of the sexual difficulties in relation to their illness. Partners also should be counselled and, once a couple have been told about the various forms of treatment, some may decide to develop sexual relations not based on intercourse. At present, men wishing to proceed with medical intervention will be offered intracorporeal injection therapy. The partners of men with poor hand function, may have to give the injection.

Intracorporeal injection of papaverine for the treatment of impotence was first described by Virag (1982) and the use of phentolamine for the same purpose was first reported by Brindley (1983). Papaverine has a direct relaxant effect on smooth muscle and is currently the most commonly used vasoactive substance for the treatment of impotence. Phentolamine produces vasodilatation through α-adrenergic blockade and it may be used alone but is more often given in combination with papaverine. Bruising and local discomfort are not uncommon; fibrosis involving the corpora is a more worrying but unusual complication. Systemic side-effects, such as hypotension, may occasionally occur after a large-dose papaverine injection.

Injection therapy is particularly effective in patients with neurogenic erectile failure, such as multiple sclerosis, and, in general, only small doses of papaverine are required (Kirkeby *et al.* 1988). Patients with neurogenic impotence are particularly prone to develop episodes of prolonged erection following these injections. Erections persisting for more than 4 h require reversal and this is achieved by aspiration of the corpora. If this fails then aspiration is used in combination with the intracorporeal injection of the α-adrenergic agent, metaraminol or adrenaline. Careful initial titration to determine the smallest amount of papaverine required should help reduce the risk of a patient developing a prolonged erection. In our experience of using this treatment in 60 men with various neurological disorders, 11 episodes of prolonged erection requiring reversal have occurred. These have always been easily reversed with the measures outlined above, no serious complications have occurred, and surgery has never been required.

Prostaglandin E1 has recently been suggested as an alternative agent for intracorporeal therapy. It is an endogenous substance which is rapidly metabolized, conveying two advantages over papaverine and phentolamine: (1) priapism is a very uncommon complication even in patients with neurogenic impotence; and (2) no systemic side-effects have been reported. However, penile discomfort following injection can be troublesome and the long-term effects of injection therapy with this substance are unknown.

Prostheses

If intracorporeal injection therapy fails or is unsuitable, some patients may consider implantation of a penile prosthesis. The prostheses available include the malleable and inflatable varieties. The malleable types are reliable but since the penis remains semirigid, concealment can be a problem. The inflatable types have the advantage of only being rigid at the time of intercourse but they are a great deal more expensive.

Ejaculatory disturbance

Little is known about the neurophysiology of ejaculation in man but it is thought to be under sympathetic control. Sympathetic fibres control the emission of semen from the seminal vesicles and the closure of the bladder neck at the time of ejaculation. The sympathetic fibres that innervate the smooth muscle of the bladder neck, vas deferens, seminal vesicles, and prostate fibres arise from the anterior roots of T10–L2 and pass through the hypogastric plexus. In congenital dopamine β-hydroxylase (DBH) deficiency (see Chapter 38), which is characterized by a deficiency of noradrenaline, patients are capable of an erection but ejaculation is difficult to achieve or absent. This can be reversed by selectively replacing noradrenaline, emphasizing the role of the α-adrenergic system in control of this function. The pelvic floor muscles that contract in a rhythmic manner during ejaculation are innervated by somatic fibres from the pudendal nerve.

Retrograde ejaculation occurs when there is emission of semen into the prostatic urethra and, at the time of ejaculation, the bladder neck fails to close so that semen is forced back into the bladder. This is a common occurrence after transurethral prostatectomy and operations on the bladder neck. Retrograde ejaculation may also result from disorders affecting the sympathetic innervation of the muscle in the region of the bladder neck. Lumbar sympathectomy and retroperitoneal lymph node dissection are known to cause retrograde ejaculation by interruption of the sympathetic supply to the bladder neck. Retrograde ejaculation is also a recognized complication of diabetic autonomic neuropathy (see Chapter 37).

Although injection of papaverine will usually result in an adequate erection, it is unlikely to have any beneficial effect on ejaculatory failure. Drugs in various doses taken 1–2 h before intercourse that have been advocated as improving ejaculatory function and orgasm include desimpramine, yohimbine, and the α-sympathomimetic, ephedrine. Semen can be obtained by electro-ejaculation, but this technique is used only for purposes of fertilization and has no role in improving the quality of sexual intercourse.

Autonomic failure with multiple system atrophy

Urinary and sexual symptoms are a pronounced feature of patients with autonomic failure (AF) and multiple system atrophy (MSA) (commonly now referred to for simplicity as MSA), as was recognized by Shy and Drager (1960) in their original report. In men, impotence is frequently the first symptom of the disease. In a retrospective review of the sexual symptoms in 24 male patients with definite multiple system atrophy, 14 patients recalled impotence as being the first symptom of the disease (Beck, in preparation). The early urinary symptoms include urgency and frequency of micturition and patients may also complain of a reduced urinary stream. These symptoms are also typical of the much commoner condition of prostatic hypertrophy and male patients with MSA have not infrequently undergone transurethral resection of the prostate for what was thought to be bladder outflow obstruction, without benefit. Incontinence associated with marked urgency of micturition develops as the disease progresses but some patients suffer predominantly from stress urinary incontinence. Women may also undergo

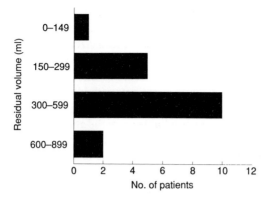

Fig. 24.5.   Measurement of the postmicturition residual volume in 18 patients with autonomic failure with multiple system atrophy.

surgery for stress incontinence before the underlying neurological disorder is appreciated.

As the strength of the detrusor contractions during voiding diminishes, the bladder fails to empty and large postmicturition residual urine volumes develop (Fig. 24.5). Upper urinary tract complications are rare, possibly because the residual urine remains at a low pressure as a consequence of the abnormal detrusor innervation.

Urodynamic studies have shown detrusor hyperreflexia in the early stages of the disease, but later the urinary dysfunction is characterized by high residual volumes (Berger *et al.* 1990). The bladder becomes 'atonic', and the strength of the hyperreflexic detrusor contractions diminishes. Voiding becomes intermittent, incomplete, and is achieved mainly by abdominal straining. Videocystometrography often demonstrates a widely patent and incompetent bladder neck (Kirby *et al.* 1986). These changes in urodynamic patterns are reflected by alterations in urinary symptoms with progress of the disease.

Detrusor hyperreflexia in MSA may result from the degeneration of areas in the midbrain and basal ganglia that are important in the control of micturition (Kirby *et al.* 1986). The atonic bladder seen in the later stages of the disease is more readily explained as being due to the progressive degeneration of the interomediolateral co umns of the cord and the loss of cells from preganglionic neurons of the thoracolumbar and sacral spinal segments. The urethral and anal sphincters are innervated by motoneurons whose cell bodies lie in Onuf's nucleus in the ventral horn of the spinal cord at S2, S3, and S4, which also undergo selective degeneration.

In AF with MSA pathological studies have shown selective loss of cells from Onuf's nucleus (Sung *et al.* 1978) and this is reflected in EMG abnormalities of the urethral and anal sphincters. Motor units recorded from the anal (Sakuta *et al.* 1978) and urethral sphincter (Kirby *et al.* 1986) are of increased duration and amplitude, changes consistent with denervation and reinnervation. Sphincter EMG with measurement of the mean duration of 10 motor units now forms the basis of a test used to detect the pathological changes in Onuf's nucleus which occur in MSA. Sphincter EMG analysis can be used to distinguish between patients with idiopathic Parkinson's disease and patients with MSA who present with atypical parkinsonism (Eardley *et al.* 1989; Fig. 24.6). The test is reliable since the abnormalities are so extreme. However, the EMG changes of reinnervtion are not specific and results from women who have had multiple deliveries or patients who have undergone pelvic surgery must be interpreted with caution. Denervation of the urethral sphincter from loss of anterior horn cells in Onuf's nucleus may account for the difference in the severity of urinary incontinence in patients with MSA and idiopathic Parkinson's disease.

Treatment of the urinary dysfunction in patients with MSA can be effective until the very late stages of the disease: initially, detrusor hyperreflexia is the predominant abnormality and, if there is no significant residual,

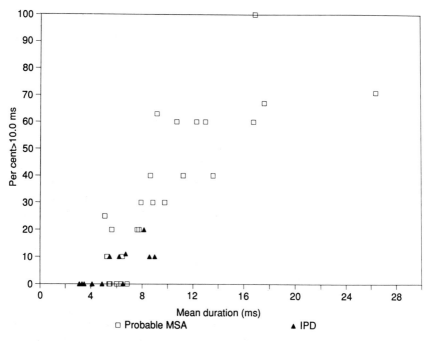

Fig. 24.6. In each patient, 10 motor units from the urethral sphincter were captured and measured. The mean duration and percentage of those longer than 10.0 ms were plotted as shown. The square symbols represent 26 patients with probable multiple system atrophy. The black triangles represent 13 patients with idiopathic Parkinson's Disease (IPD). (From Eardley *et al.* (1989).)

anticholinergic medication alone is helpful. Patients with MSA often develop large residual volumes in the later stages of the disease, volumes in excess of 300 ml are not unusual (see Fig. 24.5). Intermittent catheterization should be instituted if there is a significant residual. If the patient or carer is unable to do intermittent catheterization, it may be necessary to resort to an indwelling catheter as a means of managing intractable incontinence. Desmopressin (DDAVP) nasal spray administered at night is valuable in reducing nocturia and nocturnal enuresis.

In contrast to impotence resulting from other neurological conditions such as multiple sclerosis, men with MSA require large doses of papaverine. Our experience has shown that these patients nearly always require 80 mg of papaverine and 2 mg of phentolamine. The need for large papaverine doses seems related to the severity of hypotension at the time of the injection (Beck, in preparation). The combination of abnormal corporeal innervation and poor arterial inflow may make impotence in MSA relatively resistant to treatment with vasoactive substances.

Parkinson's disease

Urinary symptoms can be as marked in Parkinson's disease but the nature of the bladder dysfunction in this disorder is very different from that in MSA (Berger et al. 1990). Frequency and urgency of micturition are common urinary symptoms in patients with idiopathic Parkinson's disease and, although urge incontinence may occur, the continuous leakage from stress incontinence that is so troublesome in MSA is not a feature of idiopathic Parkinson's disease.

In animal studies, the basal ganglia have been shown to exert an inhibitory effect upon the bladder (Lewin et al. 1967). Loss of this central inhibition may explain the high incidence of detrusor hyperreflexia in patients with idiopathic Parkinson's disease. Studies have been performed to examine the relationship between detrusor hyperreflexia and the effect of antiparkinsonian drugs underwent cystometric studies in both 'on' and 'off' states. Although differences between the cystometrograms were found, the changes were unpredictable (Fitzmaurice et al. 1986), and the role of the basal ganglia in the control of micturition seems more complicated than simple inhibition of detrusor activity. The effects of subcutaneous apomorphine on voiding function of patients with idiopathic Parkinson's disease and urinary symptoms have been investigated (Christmas et al. 1988). Following apomorphine injections flow rates were shown to increase and residual volumes decreased. It has been proposed that there is a failure of relaxation of the urethral sphincter in patients with Parkinson's disease and, in men, apomorphine injections may be helpful in deciding whether urinary symptoms are due to prostatic enlargement or Parkinson's disease.

The urethral sphincter in patients with Parkinson's disease has been studied electromyographically and the motor units were found to be indistinguishable from those of age-matched controls. This contrasts with the highly abnormal sphincter EMG findings in the majority of patients with MSA (see Fig. 24.6).

Although there have been several reports concerning hypersexual behaviour and L-dopa therapy in patients with Parkinson's disease, there have been few studies of sexual dysfunction. In a recent questionnaire survey of patients and their partners, Brown *et al.* (1990) found a high level of sexual dysfunction, particularly in couples in which the affected partner was the man. Erectile difficulties and premature ejaculation were common. An association between idiopathic Parkinson's disease and impotence has not previously been widely recognized and the reasons for this are unclear. Patients with Parkinson's disease are often elderly and erectile difficulties may have been regarded as secondary to an ageing process or, perhaps, as resulting from psychological factors associated with a chronically disabling disease.

Bladder dysfunction resulting from spinal cord pathology

Bladder dysfunction resulting from spinal cord pathology such as injury, demyelination, or neoplastic changes, causes a severe disruption of bladder function. This is because of interruption to efferent and afferent spinal pathways which pass between the pontine micturition centre and the sacral spinal cord and which, in health, maintain the bladder as a low-pressure compliant storage organ during filling, and which co-ordinate the relaxation of the striated muscle of the urethral sphincter, preceding a detrusor contraction, during voiding. The result is that the bladder becomes hyperreflexic, emptying as a result of insuppressible contractions after partial filling. A further problem is that the bladder may not empty completely, due to a combination of poorly sustained detrusor contractions and detrusor sphincter dyssynergia. Effective management for many patients, particularly those less severely disabled, can be achieved by the same combination of oral anticholinergic medication and use of intermittent self-catheterization as advocated in the treatment of bladder symptoms in MSA. Such patients should be kept under review and if ureteric reflux and upper tract dilatation occur, surgical intervention may be necessary.

Distal autonomic neuropathy

There have now been at least 15 reports of distal autonomic neuropathy affecting both the sympathetic and parasympathetic systems. The term pandysautonomia has been applied to the disorder but, if only the parasympathetic system is involved, then the condition is known as cholinergic dysautonomia. Painful urinary retention usually occurs in both conditions. Additional urological symptoms include erectile failure and, in the variant that involves the sympathetic nerves, impairment of ejaculation.

Kirby reported urodynamic findings in two patients with these two variants of distal autonomic neuropathy (Kirby *et al*. 1985). Bladder sensation was apparently normal in both patients. Filling cystometry demonstrated interesting differences: in cholinergic dysautonomia the intravesical pressure remained low in response to bladder filling but in pandysautonomia there was a steady rise in pressure throughout filling indicating a loss of the normal bladder compliance. It was proposed that the poor bladder compliance found in pandysautonomia resulted from the loss of β-adrenergically mediated detrusor inhibition. The competence of the bladder neck was investigated by videocystometrography and in cholinergic dysautonomia the bladder neck was found to be closed and competent, whereas in pandysautonomia the bladder neck was wide open. These findings are in keeping with previous studies which indicate that contraction of the detrusor in the region of the bladder neck is mediated by sympathetic fibres.

Diabetes mellitus

Diabetic cystopathy

Cystopathy was once considered a rare complicaton of diabetes but the greater use of techniques for studying bladder function has shown this to be incorrect. The condition is mostly asymptomatic and discovered incidentally. The exact prevalence of the disorder is uncertain but has been estimated as occurring in between 44 to 87 per cent of cases (McCulloch *et al*. 1980).

The condition develops gradually over several years, with progressive loss of bladder sensation and impairment of bladder emptying, eventually culminating in chronic low-pressure urinary retention. Urodynamic studies demonstrate impaired detrusor contractility, a reduction in the urinary flow rate, an increase in postmicturition residual volumes, and reduction in bladder sensation (Blaivas 1988). The sequence of pathophysiological events that result in diabetic neurocystopathy are uncertain but it seems likely that there is involvement of both the vesical sensory afferent fibres causing a reduced awareness of bladder filling and involvement of parasympathetic efferent fibres to the detrusor, decreasing the ability of the bladder to empty. The density of acetylcholinesterase positive staining nerves in the bladder wall has been shown to be reduced in diabetics as compared with controls (Faerman *et al*. 1973). The bladder neck, which is principally innervated by sympathetic fibres, is competent in most cases of diabetic cystopathy, suggesting that, as in the cardiovascular system, sympathetic denervation is probably a late phenomenon.

Asymptomatic diabetics with cystopathy should be made aware of their disorder since, having lost their normal desire to micturate, they may void infrequently. They should be advised to void at regular intervals and before going to bed at night. Symptomatic patients are best managed by clean intermittent self-catheterization.

Sexual dysfunction in diabetes

Diabetes is one of the commonest causes of erectile failure and, compared to the mostly asymptomatic condition of diabetic cystopathy, it is a problem for which many diabetics may seek help. Occasionally impotence may be the presenting symptom of diabetes. The incidence of erectile failure in diabetic patients has been estimated at being between 25 and 59 per cent (Fairburn et al. 1982). Affected by this problem the diabetic usually complains of a gradually progressive loss of rigidity of erection over some months until there is complete failure. This is not initially accompanied by loss of libido but decrease in sexual interest sometimes follows in reaction to the erectile problem.

Several processes are thought to contribute to the high prevalence of erectile problems of diabetics. These include large vessel disease, micro-angiopathy, and autonomic neuropathy as well as psychological factors. Diabetic patients are prone to an accelerated form of atherosclerosis and the association between large vessel disease and impotence is well recognized (Leriche's syndrome). Observing the response to an intracorporeal injection of papaverine may provide some indication of the cause of the erectile difficulties. If a rigid erection develops following a small dose of papaverine then the cause is either neurological or psychological and the vascular supply is most likely to be normal.

Although a relationship between diabetic autonomic neuropathy and impotence has long been recognized, there is still no direct means of testing the autonomic nerves that innervate the corpora. Histological study of tissue from diabetic patients has shown morphological abnormalities of the autonomic fibres of the corpora cavernosa (Faerman et al. 1974). In vitro studies of the corporeal smooth muscle from impotent diabetic patients have demonstrated impaired muscle relaxation in response to autonomic nerve stimulation and also after administration of acetylcholine (Saenz de Tejada et al. 1989).

Prolongation of the bulbocavernosus reflex is sometimes cited as evidence of relevant peripheral neuropathy in diabetic patients with impotence. Although several studies examining the latency of the bulbocavernosus reflex in diabetics with erectile failure have shown a prolongation of mean latency in diabetics compared with control subjects, many series include a number of diabetic patients in whom other evidence points to a neurogenic basis for their disorder and yet the bulbocavernosus reflex latency is within normal limits (Fowler *et al.* 1988). The test is therefore insufficiently sensitive to be a useful investigation of individual patients. The explanation for this lies in the pathways tested by this reflex since it is a reflex mediated by larger myelinated somatic fibres which are of limited importance in the physiology of erection. Penile erection is mediated by small myelinated and unmyelinated autonomic fibres which have conduction velocities of less than 2 m/s. Cutaneous thermal sensations are conducted by small-diameter fibres and measurements of thermal thresholds can provide evidence of a neuropathy involving the smaller classes of nerve fibre. Thermal sensitivity tested on the dorsum of the penis (Robinson *et al.* 1987) and on the sole of the feet (Fowler *et al.* 1988) was found to be abnormal in all diabetics with impotence.

Diabetic patients may complain of a failure of ejaculation despite normal orgasm (Greene and Kelalis 1968). In these patients an autonomic neuropathy is thought to affect the sympathetic innervation to the genital tract and either ejaculation occurs in a retrograde manner or there may be a failure of emission from the seminal vesicles. If retrograde ejaculation is suspected then the urine passed after ejaculation may appear cloudy and microscopic examination may reveal spermatozoa.

References

Abrams, P., Blaivas, J. G., Stanton, S. L., and Andersen, J. T. (1988). The standardisation of terminology of lower urinary tract function. *Scand. J. Urol. Nephrol.* Suppl. **114**, 5–19.

Berger, Y., Salinas, J. N., and Blaivas, J. G. (1990). Urodynamic differentiation of Parkinson disease and the Shy–Drager syndrome. *Neurourol. Urodynam.* **9**, 117–21.

Blaivas, J. G. (1988). Neurologic dysfunctions. In *Neurourology and urodynamics: principles and practice* (ed. S. Yalla *et al.*), pp. 343–57. Macmillan, New York.

Brindley, G. S. (1983). Cavernosal alpha-blockade: a new technique for investigating and treating erectile impotence. *Br. J. Psychiat.* **143**, 332.

Brown, R. G., Jahanshahi, M., Quinn, N., and Marsden, C. D. (1990). Sexual function in patients with Parkinson's disease and their partners. *J. Neurol. Neurosurg. Psychiat.* **53**, 480–6.

Christmas, T. J., Kempster, P. A., Chapple, C. R., Frankel, J. P., Lees, A. J., Stern, G. M., and Milroy, E. J. M. (1988). Role of subcutaneous apomorphine in Parkinsonian voiding dysfunction. *Lancet* **ii**, 1451–3.

Eardley, I., Quinn, N. P., Fowler, C. J., Kirby, R. S., Parkhouse, H. F., Marsden, C. D., and Bannister, R. (1989). The value of urethral sphincter electromyography in the differential diagnosis of parkinsonism. *Br. J. Urol.* **64**, 360–2.

Faerman, I., Glocer, L., Celener, D., Jadzinsky, M., Fox, D., Maler, M., and Alvarez, E. (1973). Autonomic nervous system and diabetes. Histological and histochemical study of the autonomic nerve fibres of the urinary bladder in diabetic patients. *Diabetes* **22**, 225–37.

Faerman, I., Glocer, L., Celener, D., Fox, D., Jadinsky, M., and Rapaport, M. (1974). Impotence and diabetes. Histological studies of the autonomic nervous fibers of the corpora cavernosa in impotent diabetic males. *Diabetes* **23**, 971–6.

Fairburn, C. G., Wu, F. C. W., McCulloch, D. K., Borsey, D. Q., Ewing, D. J., Clarke, B. F., and Bancroft, J. H. J. (1982). The clinical features of diabetic impotence: a preliminary study. *Br. J. Psychiat.* **140**, 447–52.

Fitzmaurice, H., Fowler, C. J., Rickards, D., Kirby, R. S., Quinn, N. P., Marsden, C. D., Milroy, E. J. G., and Turner-Warwick, R. T. (1986). Micturition disturbance in Parkinson's disease. *Br. J. Urol.* **577**, 652–6.

Fowler, C. J., Ali, Z., Kirby, R. S., and Pryor, J. P. (1988). The value of testing for unmyelinated fibre, sensory neuropathy in diabetic impotence *Br. J. Urol.* **61**, 63–7.

Gajewski, J. B. and Awad, S. A. (1986). Oxybutinin versus probantheline in patients with multiple sclerosis and detrusor hyperreflexia. *J. Urol.* **135**, 966–8.

Greene, F. L. and Kelalis, P. P. (1968). Retrograde ejaculation of semen due to diabetic neuropathy. *J. Urol.* **98**, 693–6.

Kirby, R., Fowler, C. J., Gosling, J. A., and Bannister, R. (1985). Bladder dysfunction in distal autonomic neuropathy of acute onset. *J. Neurol. Neurosurg. Psychiat.* **48**, 762–7.

Kirby, R., Fowler, C. J., Gosling, J., and Bannister, R. (1986). Urethro-vesical dysfunction in progressive autonomic failure with multiple system atrophy. *J. Neurol. Neurosurg. Psychiat.* **49**, 554–62.

Kirkeby, H. J., Poulsen, E. U., Petersen, T., and Dorup, J. (1988). Erectile dysfunction in multiple sclerosis. *Neurology* **38**, 1366–71.

Lapides, J., Diokno, A. C., Lowe, B. S., and Kalish, M. D. (1974). Follow up on unsterile, intermittent self-cathertization. *J. Urol.* **111**, 184–7.

Lewin, R. J., Dillard, G. V., and Porter, R. W. (1967). Extrapyramidal inhibition of the urinary bladder. *Brain Res.* **4**, 301–7.

Lue, T. F., Hricak, H., Marich, K. W., and Tanagho, E. A. (1985). Vasculogenic impotence evaluated by high resolution ultrasonography and pulsed doppler spectrum analysis. *Radiology* **155**, 777–81.

McCulloch, D. K., Campbell, I. W., Wu, F. C., Prescott, R. J., and Clarke, B. F. (1980). The prevalence of diabetic impotence. *Diabetologia* **18**, 279–83.

Robinson, L. Q., Woodcock, J. P., and Stephenson, T. P. (1987). Results of investigation of impotence in patients with overt or probable neuropathy. *Br. J. Urol.* **60**, 583–7.

Saenz de Tejada, I., Goldstein, I., Azadzoi, K., Krane, R. J., and Cohen, R. A. (1989). Impaired neurogenic and endothelium-mediated relaxation of penile smooth muscle from diabetic men with impotence. *New Engl. J. Med.* **320** (16), 1025–34.

Sakuta, M. S., Nakanishi, T., and Toyakuru, M. (1978). Anal muscle electromyograms differ in amyotrophic lateral sclerosis and the Shy–Drager syndrome. *Neurology* **28**, 1289–93.

Shy, G. M. and Drager, G. A. (1960). A neurological syndrome associated with orthostatic hypotension. *Arch. Neurol.* **2**, 511–27.

Sung, J. H., Mastri, A. R., and Segal, E. (1978). Pathology of the Shy–Drager syndrome. *J. Neuropathol. exp. Neurol.* **38**, 253–68.

Virag, R. (1982). Intracavernous injection of papaverine for erectile failure. *Lancet* **ii**, 938.

25. Skin axon-reflex vasodilatation—mechanisms, testing, and implications in autonomic disorders

Praveen Anand

Introduction

The response to injury and inflammation in skin includes a local vasodilatation mediated by sensory nerve fibres. This chapter describes the nature of this vasodilatation and considers its relationship to autonomic failure.

In 1910, Bruce demonstrated that the reddening which followed the instillation of mustard oil into the conjunctiva was mediated locally by sensory fibres. The reddening response was preserved after the sensory nerves were divided acutely, but abolished if they were allowed to degenerate, or were anaesthetized. He postulated that this reddening resulted from an 'axon reflex': impulses travelling up a terminal branch of a sensory nerve fibre spread down other terminal branches of the same axon to blood vessels, producing dilatation. In 1919, Breslauer described the same phenomenon in skin. This skin axon-reflex flare (or vasodilatation) was one component of the 'triple response' of Lewis (for historical references see Lewis 1927).

Lewis observed that various skin stimuli—mechanical, electrical, thermal, chemical—all produced a similar triad of responses. 'The full reaction to stroking, namely, the local vasodilatation, the flare, and eventually local oedema, constitutes what I shall henceforth call the triple response.' (Lewis 1927) Lewis noted that the first component of the triple response, the local red reaction to a firm stroke, was 'a primary and local dilatation of the minute vessels of the skin'; the second component, or flare was 'a widespread diltation of the neighbouring strong arterioles brought about entirely through a local nervous reflex'; the third component, or wheal, was a local 'increased permeability of the vessel wall'. The red reaction and wheal were independent of the skin innervation.

Nerve stimulation studies suggested that the axon-reflex flare was produced by unmyelinated primary afferent fibres, the C fibres (Celander and Folkow 1953), with a possible contribution from small myelinated fibres (Lynn 1988).

Stimulation of sensory fibres was also shown to increase microvascular permeability in skin, a phenomenon termed 'neurogenic plasma extravasation' (Jansco 1960).

This chapter is divided into two parts. In the first part, the mechanisms of the skin axon-reflex flare and the methods of its measurement are described. In the second part, studies of skin flares in syndromes of autonomic failure are reviewed, and the role of skin flares in the diagnosis and treatment of these conditions is discussed.

Mechanisms of skin axon-reflex vasodilatation

The classical studies of Bruce and Lewis established the basis of axon reflex vasodilatation (Lewis 1927). The presence of the skin flare indicated the integrity of the dorsal root ganglion cell body and its peripheral axon. Bonney (1954) used axon-reflex vasodilatation to distinguish whether in brachial plexus injuries the lesion was peripheral or proximal to the dorsal root ganglion; the flare response was preserved in the latter and was associated with a poor prognosis for recovery of function.

A model of axon-reflex vasodilatation

A model of the mechanisms of skin axon-reflex vasodilatation is illustrated in Fig. 25.1. There is increasing evidence in support of this model, which is reviewed in brief.

The axon-reflex flare follows skin stimulation, including intradermal injection of histamine (Lewis 1927) and other neuroeffector agents such as the neuropeptides, substance P, calcitonin gene-related peptide (CGRP), somatostatin, vasoactive intestinal polypeptide (VIP), neurotensin, encephalin, and endothelin (Hagermark *et al.* 1978; Anand *et al.* 1983*a*; Anand 1984). Injection of these neuroeffector substances causes a triple response, and itch. It is likely that neuropeptides, in pharmacological doses, release histamine from mast cells at the injection site and that histamine in turn activates sensory nerve terminals to cause axon-reflex vasodilatation following release from terminal branches of one or more peptides or adenosine triphosphate (ATP) (Hagermark *et al.* 1978; Anand *et al.* 1983*a*). The released substances also lead to further histamine release, which activates other sensory terminals, and hence a cascade develops with spread of flare.

In support of the proposed mechanism, substance P, somatostatin, and VIP release histamine from the perfused rat hindquarter, and histamine is released from human skin by substance P (Barnes *et al.* 1986). Antihistamines reduce flare and itch induced by histamine and substance P; local histamine depletion by compound 48/80 abolishes flares caused by subsequent injection of substance P and compound 48/80, but not histamine (Hagermark *et al.* 1978).

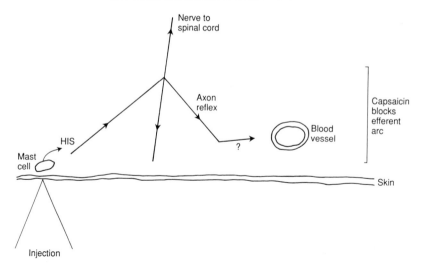

Fig. 25.1.   A diagram to show the possible mechanisms involved in the wheal and flare response: repeated topical capsaicin application blocks the efferent arc. HIS, histamine.

The mechanism of coupling of unmyelinated fibres in the spread of flare deserves further study (Lynn 1988).

It is important to distinguish between the pharmacological effects of injected substances and the physiological neuroeffector substances which are released from afferent terminals to induce vasodilatation. For example, neurotensin can induce wheal and flare in human skin, but neurotensin has not been detected in the sensory innervation of human skin. The neuropeptide candidates present in normal or injured sensory fibres that could mediate flare responses include substance P, CGRP, somatostatin, and VIP (Hagermark *et al.* 1978; Anand 1984).

Visceral afferent fibres also mediate neurogenic vasodilatation, although this is difficult to test in man.

Capsaicin studies

Capsaicin, the active ingredient of chilli peppers, has a selective action on unmyelinated and small myelinated afferent fibres, and has been a useful tool in investigating the mechanisms of the human skin axon flare response (Bernstein *et al.* 1981; Anand *et al.* 1983*a*). Topical skin application of capsaicin produces erythralgia. The initial effect is erythema (flare) at the site of application, and a burning sensation, which is similar to the effect of eating spicy food on the oral cavity. The erythralgia is exacerbated by gentle pressure, with temporal and spatial summation, and relieved by

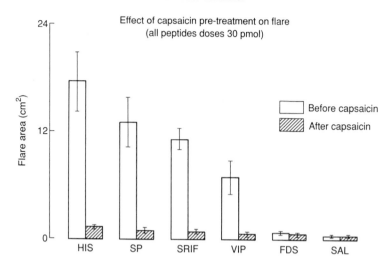

Fig. 25.2. Area of flare in cm² (mean values) in vehicle pre-treated (open columns) and capsaicin pre-treated (closed columns) skin. All peptides: 30 pmol; histamine mg/ml, 0.03 ml; *n* = 4; vertical lines show SEM. HIS, histamine; SP, substance P; SRIF, somatostatin; VIP, vasoactive intestinal polypeptide; FDS, freeze-drying solution; SAL, saline. (Reprinted with permission from Anand *et al.* (1983*a*).)

application of cold stimuli. However, repeated topical application of capsaicin produces local desensitization of skin to chemogenic noxious agents (Jansco 1960) and inhibits the skin flares induced by a number of agents (Fig. 25.2; Bernstein *et al.* 1981; Anand *et al.* 1983*a*). The skin flare responses recover over 3 to 4 weeks.

Capsaicin may deplete sensory nerve terminals of peptides, thus abolishing the axon reflex flare. It may also damage the nerve terminals, or terminal receptors. The wheal is unaffected by capsaicin pre-treatment, and is presumably caused by the direct action of released histamine and possibly other neuroeffector agents on capillary permeability at the site of the injection. Thus capsaicin pre-treatment of skin results in responses similar to those described in denervated human skin to intradermally injected histamine (Lewis 1927), substance P, CGRP, somatostatin, and VIP (Anand 1984).

It is likely that there is constant physiological release of peptides and other neuroeffective agents from cutaneous sensory nerve terminals, leading in turn to histamine release, and that this process is enhanced by skin stimuli. This phenomenon occurs at a low firing frequency of unmyelinated fibres, below the threshold for sensation, thus being in effect a 'local autonomic function', and it also occurs at higher frequencies associated with sensation. In support of the idea of constant physiological release of neuropeptides from nerve terminals in skin is the finding that, following capsaicin treatment of newborn rats, which leads to irreversible degeneration of unmyelinated fibres, there is a permanent increase in skin concentrations of histamine.

The acute effect of capsaicin in producing and enhancing skin flares, and the slow recovery of skin flares in capsaicin pre-treated skin, suggests that topical capsaicin acts in human skin in two ways. It acts acutely on nerve terminals to enhance release of neuropeptides causing depletion (and then blocking C-fibre conduction), and chronically to inhibit the repletion of the terminals by neuropeptides. Capsaicin application on nerve trunks in rats leads to loss of synthesis and axonal transport of substance P in sensory fibres (Anand *et al.* 1990), probably by producing axonal transport blockade at the site of application, and preventing the retrograde transport of nerve growth factor. Nerve growth factor is necessary for the production of substance P and CGRP in the dorsal root ganglia of adult rats.

Opioid action and skin flares

Opiates release histamine from mast cells in skin (Feldberg and Paton 1951), and this may account for the itch experienced by some subjects after intravenous injection of opiates. Opioids may also act directly on sensory fibres. A study of the role of opioids in human skin provided further support for the model presented above (Anand 1984). Morphine, leuencephalin, and met-encephalin produced weak dose-dependent triple responses when injected in human skin. Topical application of encephalin in aqueous cream produced itch and erythema and markedly enhanced skin flares but not wheals on subsequent injection of histamine. It is likely that opioids prime the flare mechanism and amplify the cascade response triggered by skin stimuli.

Sympathetic activity and skin flares

Sympathetic activity influences skin flares (Hornyak *et al.* 1990; Wallin 1990). Sympathetic impulses to skin reduce axon-reflex responses, by vasoconstrictor action which counters axon-reflex vasodilatation.

Measuring skin flares

The effect of sympathetic drive on skin flares emphasizes the need to perform flare tests on relaxed, acclimatized subjects in a defined thermoneutral ambience with age-matched controls. In adults, skin flares and sensory neuropeptide levels decrease with age. The studies should be performed at the same time of day, as there is a diurnal variation of flare response. The subjects should not be taking any drugs, such as histamines, which affect the flare response.

The skin may be stimulated by a number of different methods, including intradermal injection of histamine and neuropeptides (see Anand *et al.* 1983*a*), the electrophoresis of acetylcholine, which activates unmyelinated afferents directly via nicotinic receptors (see Parkhouse and Le Quesne 1988a), and electrically by means of a surface electrode (see Hornyak et al. 1990). The use of capsaicin is limited for the reasons discussed above, including conduction block and desensitization on repeated testing.

Histamine acid phosphate (1 mg/ml) or neuropeptides may be injected intradermally with a 0.4 mm diameter needle in a fixed volume of up to 0.03 ml. Neuropeptides must be stored and reconstituted in a manner that prevents losses by degradation and adsorption: they may be stored at $-20\,°C$ in freeze dried aliquots prepared in a solution consisting of lactose (140 mmol/ml), bovine serum albumin (40 μmol/ml), L-cysteine hydrochloride (6 mmol/ml), and aprotinin (8×10^5 kIU/l). The peptides and freeze-drying solution (for control injections) must be reconstituted immediately before injection, and the pH of both solutions should be between 6.5 and 7.0.

Acetylcholine (10 per cent) may be electrophoresed for 5 min with a 1 mA current from the outer ring of a capsule with two concentric chambers, the flare response being measured with a Doppler probe at the centre of the capsule: the method has been described in detail (Parkhouse and Le Quesne 1988a). This method of stimulation is reproducible and atraumatic.

Electrical skin stimulation may be performed with an Ag/AgCl surface cathode, 10 mm in diameter, with a series of stimuli (0.2–1 ms, 15–40 mA) in trains of 4, 8, and 16 square-wave pulses (2 Hz) from a stimulator with a constant-current unit. The probe to measure skin blood flow may be placed 6–8 mm from the stimulated area.

The flare response may be measured by marking its maximal borders and calculating the surface area (see Anand et al. 1983a), which limits the test to non-hairy, non-digital, lightly pigmented skin; by measuring rise in skin temperature, although the temperature rise is not linear to blood flow; or laser Doppler flowmetry (see Parkhouse and Le Quesne 1988a). The laser Doppler flowmeter gives values which indicate relative changes in the flux of red blood cells and hence changes in the superficial skin blood flow: it provides a sensitive and versatile quantitative method. The output of the flowmeter in mV is traced on a chart recorder.

Skin axon-reflex vasodilatation and autonomic failure

Theoretical considerations

In what way may skin flares, mediated by somatic primary sensory neurons, be linked to autonomic failure?

Skin blood flow is regulated by both central sympathetic and local sensory reflex mechanisms. As sympathetic activity may influence skin flares, changes in skin flares, tested in appropriate conditions, may indicate the nature of the sympathetic dysfunction.

Skin flare tests provide evidence of dysfunction of unmyelinated sensory fibres in peripheral neuropathies, including diabetes, leprosy, and familial dysautonomia (Riley–Day syndrome), which may primarily affect small fibres of the autonomic and sensory nervous system. The loss of fibres in peripheral nerves in familial dysautonomia is not restricted to unmyelinated fibres, but their depletion is consistent with the impairment of pain and temperature sensation, and loss of skin axon flares is helpful in diagnosis (Smith and Dancis 1963). Abnormalities of axon-reflex vasodilatation may also be correlated with pathological consequences. In a study of the non-neurogenic red reaction and axon flares in longstanding diabetic patients, the development of foot complications correlated with diminution of flares and pain sensation (Parkhouse and Le Quesne 1988b). Further quantitative studies of flares and sensory neuropeptides in the evolution of diabetic neuropathy are indicated.

Nerve growth factor (NGF) is a requirement for survival of developing sympathetic and sensory fibres, which have in common the ability to take up NGF from target tissue and retrogradely transport it to the cell body. In adult rats sympathetic fibres still require NGF for survival, but sensory fibres require it only for expression of their neuropeptides, substance P and CGRP, which mediate skin flare responses. Abnormalities of these common factors may thus affect sympathetic and sensory fibres, including skin flare responses. A role for NGF in diabetic neuropathy is discussed below. A new syndrome of autonomic failure with loss of adrenergic sympathetic function and reduced skin flares, described below, may be attributed to NGF deprivation in late development.

There is competition between sensory and sympathetic fibres for NGF, which is produced by the target organ (see Kessler et al. 1983; Anand 1986). Sympathectomy results in increased sensory neuropeptides in nerve fibres of the iris and ciliary body, and this increase has been linked to the increased inflammatory response of the sympathectomized eye to injury. The increased substance P and CGRP in sensory fibres in inflammatory arthritis (Lembeck and Gamse 1982) may result from increased NGF synthesis mediated by factors released by invading macrophages, including interleukin-1. In contrast, neuropeptide levels are decreased in wound healing (Senapati et al. 1986), presumably because of decreased uptake and retrograde transport of NGF by injured nerve endings. Changes in neurogenic vasodilatation and extravasation may contribute to the pathology of the above conditions.

Sympathetic and sensory fibres may express the same neuroeffector agent. For example, VIP is present in postganglionic sympathetic fibres that innervate sweat glands and skeletal muscle blood vessels, and in somatic sensory fibres, particularly after injury (Anand et al. 1990). There is considerable evidence that neuropeptides are selective markers of unmyelinated afferent fibres that mediate flares and of autonomic pathways (Anand *et al.* 1983*b*; Anand and Bloom 1984*b*); neuropeptide dysfunction may therefore affect both systems.

Skin flares in multiple system atrophy

In a study of neuropeptides in the post-mortem spinal cords of patients with multiple system atrophy (MSA), it was discovered that there was a marked depletion of substance P, substance K, and CGRP in dorsal regions, including the dorsal columns (Anand *et al.* 1987). None of the cases studied had clinical evidence of somatic sensory neuropathy. As this suggested loss of neuropeptides that mediate skin flares in MSA, a study was made of skin flares in this condition. Histamine-induced skin flare responses in thoracic and forearm skin were found to be intact in patients with MSA (Anand *et al.* 1987). It was considered that the neuropeptide depletion may occur exclusively in visceral afferents, or that there is much redundancy in the system (Anand *et al.* 1987). Further studies of sensory neuropeptides and visceral axon reflexes in MSA and pure autonomic failure are necessary to distinguish between these possibilities. It has been postulated that defects of neurotrophic agent synthesis, including peptides, may be responsible for the 'chain' pattern of cell loss in degenerative syndromes of autonomic failure.

Reduced skin flare in a new syndrome of autonomic failure

A new syndrome of autonomic failure has been described with loss of sympathetic adrenergic function and skin sensory neuropeptides (Anand *et al.* 1991). A 30-year-old woman presented with longstanding symptoms of dizziness and weakness on exercise. Clinical examination revealed a marked postural fall in blood pressure and small pupils. Autonomic tests indicated selective impairment of adrenergic sympathetic function, with undetectable plasma noradrenaline, adrenaline, dopamine, and dopamine-beta-hydroxylase. Sweat tests were normal. Skin testing with intradermal histamine showed normal wheal but diminished flare responses: the flare was less than half the area of control flares.

Skin biopsy showed loss of sensory neuropeptides, substance P and CGRP, which may mediate skin flares, and of tyrosine hydroxylase and neuropeptide Y, which mark adrenergic sympathetic fibres. In contrast, cholinergic sympathetic fibres to sweat glands containing VIP were normal. Sural nerve biopsy showed marked loss of unmyelinated fibres.

As this constellation of losses may be produced by NGF deprivation in rats, it was proposed that this new syndrome may be explained by loss of the trophic action of NGF. An initial study of NGF in the patient's tissues is in accord with this explanation.

It has been proposed that NGF loss may be the cause of certain sensory and autonomic neuropathies, including the Riley–Day syndrome, but there is little support for these suggestions. The structural β-NGF gene is not abnormal in the Riley–Day syndrome. Retrograde axonal transport of NGF has been shown to be impaired in streptozotocin-diabetic rats, but lack of NGF cannot be the sole cause of diabetic autonomic neuropathy as it is not restricted to sympathetic adrenergic dysfunction. However, reduced NGF may influence the pattern of diabetic neuropathy, by predisposing unmyelinated sympathetic and sensory fibres to dysfunction. A consequent decrease of sensory neuropeptide expression may account for the reduced skin flares in diabetics, which may also result from the loss of unmyelinated fibres.

Further studies of skin flares and neurotrophic factors are likely to provide insight into the causation of sensory and autonomic syndromes. The imminent prospect of a number of human neurotrophic factors for clinical use holds much promise in the treatment of these conditions. Skin flares will play an important role in monitoring the progress of such treatments.

References

Anand, P. (1984). The role of neuropeptides in the pathophysiology of the peripheral nervous system. MD thesis, Cambridge University.

Anand, P. (1986). Postsympathectomy pain and sensory neuropeptides. *Lancet* i, 512.

Anand, P. and Bloom, S. R. (1984). Neuropeptides are selective markers of spinal cord autonomic pathways. *Trends Neurosci.* 7, 267–8.

Anand, P., Bloom, S. R., and McGregor, G. P. (1983a). Topical capsaicin pretreatment inhibits axon reflex vasodilatation caused by somatostatin and VIP in human skin. *Br. J. Pharmacol.* 78, 665–9.

Anand, P., Gibson, S. J., McGregor, G. P., Blank, M. A., Bacarese-Hamilton, A. J., Polak, J. M., and Bloom, S. R. (1983b). A VIP-containing system concentrated in the lumbosacral region of human spinal cord. *Nature* 305, 143–5.

Anand, P., Bannister, R., McGregor, G. P., Ghatei, M. A., Mulderry, P. K., and Bloom, S. R. (1987). Marked depletion of dorsal spinal cord substance P and calcitonin gene-related peptide with intact skin flare responses in multiple system atrophy. *J. Neurol. Neurosurg. Psychiat.* 51, 192–6.

Anand, P., Gibson, S. J., Scaravilli, F., Blank, M. A., McGregor, G. P., Appenzeller, O., Dhital, K., Polak, J. M., and Bloom, S. R. (1990). Studies of VIP expression in injured peripheral neurons using capsaicin, sympathectomy and mf mutant rats. *Neurosci. Lett.* 118, 61–6.

Anand, P, Rudge, P., Mathias, C. J., Ghatei, M. A., Springall, D., Naher-Noe, M., Sharief, M., Misra, V. P., Polak, J. M., Bloom, S. R., and Thomas, P. K. (1991). A new syndrome of autonomic failure with loss of postganglionic adrenergic sympathetic function and sensory neuropeptides. *Lancet* 337, 1253–4.

Barnes, P. J., Brown, M. J., Dollery, C. T., Fuller, R. W., Heavey, D. J., and Ind, P. W. (1986). Histamine is released from skin by substance P but does not act as the final vasodilator in the axon reflex. *Br. J. Pharmacol.* 88, 741–5.

Bernstein, J. E., Swift, R. M., Soltani, K., and Lorincz, A. L. (1981). Inhibition of axon reflex vasodilatation by topically applied capsaicin. *J. Invest. Dermatol.* **76**, 394–5.

Bonney, G. (1954). The value of axon responses in determining the site of lesion in traction injuries of the brachial plexus. *Brain* **77**, 588–609.

Celander, O. and Folkow, B. (1953). The nature and distribution of afferent fibres provided with the axon reflex arrangement. *Acta physiol. scand.* **29**, 359–70.

Feldberg, W. and Paton, W. D. M. (1951). Release of histamine from the skin and muscle in the cat by opium alkaloids and other histamine liberators. *J. Physiol.* **114**, 490–509.

Hagermark, O., Hökfelt, T., and Pernow, B. (1978). Flare and itch induced by substance P in human skin. *J. Invest. Dermatol.* **71**, 233–5.

Hornyak, M. E., Naver, H. K., Rydenhag, B., and Wallin, B. G. (1990). Sympathetic activity influences the vascular axon reflex in the skin. *Acta physiol. scand.* **139**, 77–84.

Jansco, N. (1960). The role of nerve terminals in the mechanism of inflammatory reaction. *Bull. Millard Filmore Hosp., Buffalo, NY* **7**, 53–77.

Kessler, J. A., Bell, W. O., and Black, I. B. (1983). Interaction between the sympathetic and sensory innervation of the iris. *J. Neurosci* **3**, 1301–7.

Lembeck, F. and Gamse, R. (1982). Substance P in peripheral sensory processes. In *Substance P in the nervous system*, Ciba Foundation Symposium, no. 91, (ed. R. Porter and M. O'Connor) pp. 35–40. Pitman Medical, London.

Lewis, T. (1927). *Blood vessels of the human skin and their responses*. Shaw, London.

Lynn, B. (1988). Neurogenic inflammation. *Skin Pharmacol.* **1**, 217–24.

Parkhouse, N. and Le Quesne, P. M. (1988*a*). Quantitative objective assessment of peripheral nociceptive C fibre function. *J. Neurol. Neurosurg. Psychiat.* **51**, 28–34.

Parkhouse, N. and Le Quesne, P. M. (1988*b*). Impaired neurogenic vascular response in patients with diabetes and neuropathic foot lesions. *New Engl. J. Med.* **318**, 1306–9.

Senapti, A., Anand, P., McGregor, G. P., Ghatei, M. A., Thompson, R. P. H., and Bloom, S. R. (1986). Depletion of neuropeptides during wound healing in rat skin. *Neurosci. Lett.* **71**, 101–5.

Smith, A. A. and Dancis, J. (1963). Response to intradermal histamine in familial dysautonomia—a diagnostic test. *J. Paediat.* **63**, 889–94.

Wallin, B. (1990). Neural control of human skin blood flow. *J. autonom. nerv. Syst.* **30** (suppl.), S185–90.

26. Postcibal hypotension in autonomic disorders

Christopher J. Mathias and Roger Bannister

Introduction

In normal subjects, food ingestion results in a number of hormonal, neural, and regional haemodynamic changes. A variety of pancreatic and gastro-intestinal peptides are released. Some of these may affect the cardiovascular system either directly, or indirectly through modulation of autonomic nervous activity. There is a marked increase in splanchnic blood flow, but systemic blood pressure remains virtually unchanged in normal subjects, presumably because activation of the sympathetic nervous system, together with release of vasoactive hormones, results in appropriate readjustment.

In patients with disturbances of autonomic function, ingestion of food may substantially lower blood pressure. Postcibal hypotension as a clinical problem, was first reported by Seyer-Hansen (1977) in a 65-year-old man with autonomic failure and parkinsonism, who suffered from severe dizziness and visual disturbance during almost every meal and in whom hypotension could be provoked by oral glucose. A group of patients with autonomic dysfunction were studied by Robertson *et al.* (1981) who confirmed a profound fall in both systolic and diastolic blood pressure after food ingestion. In these studies, the patients were seated and it was unclear to what degree the upright posture contributed to the hypotension. Our own interest in postcibal hypotension was triggered in 1982, when a patient complained of considerable worsening of posturally induced dizziness after breakfast, which lowered her pressure to levels of 80/50 mm Hg even in the supine position for 3 h (see Fig. 26.1).

From our own observations and those of others, it was clear that postcibal hypotension could be a major clinical problem in some patients with autonomic failure. To embark on rational approaches of intervention and management it was necessary to determine the mechanisms responsible, with an emphasis on the haemodynamic and biochemical basis of postprandial hypotension, and which specific components of the meal may be responsible. In this chapter we concentrate on the pathophysiological basis of postcibal hypotension in primary autonomic failure. No attempt will be made initially to separate responses within the two major subgroups, pure autonomic failure (PAF)

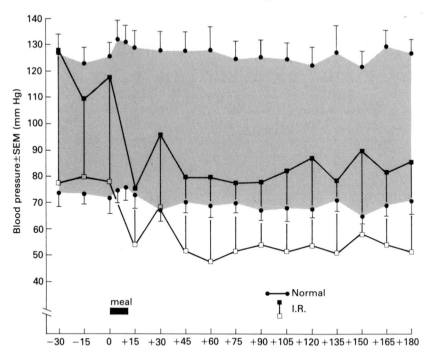

Fig. 26.1. Supine systolic and diastolic blood pressure before and after a standard meal in a group of normal subjects (stippled area, with ± SEM bars) and in a patient with autonomic failure (I.R.). Blood pressure does not change in the normal subjects after a meal. In the patient, there is a rapid fall in blood pressure to levels around 80/50 mm Hg which remain low in the supine position over the 3-h observation period.

and multiple system atrophy (MSA); recent work emphasizing differences between them, however, will be discussed later. Brief descriptions are also provided of responses to food in other patients with autonomic dysfunction and those who, despite not having an autonomic disorder, may be at risk from the effects of food ingestion.

Haemodynamic changes to food ingestion

In normal subjects, food ingestion in either the seated or the supine position usually causes minimal or no change in blood pressure. In normal subjects given a standard meal (450 kcal, containing carbohydrate, protein, and fat) in the supine position, there is a rise in heart rate together with an elevation in stroke volume and cardiac output (Mathias *et al.* 1989*a*). Forearm blood flow falls with an elevation in forearm vascular resistance. There are no

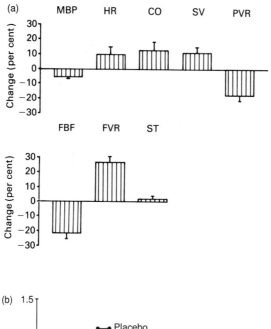

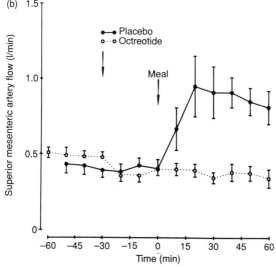

Fig. 26.2. (a) Maximum percentage change in mean blood pressure (MBP), heart rate (HR), cardiac output (CO), stroke volume (SV), calculated peripheral vascular resistance (PVR), forearm muscle blood flow (FBF), calculated forearm vascular resistance (FVR), and skin temperature to the index finger (ST) in six normal subjects in the first hour after food ingestion. Vertical bars indicate ± SEM. (b) Superior mesenteric artery blood flow in normal subjects before and after a balanced liquid meal, when given either saline placebo (continuous line, filled circles) or 50 μg of Octreotide (dotted line, open circles), both subcutaneously. (From Kooner *et al.* (1989).)

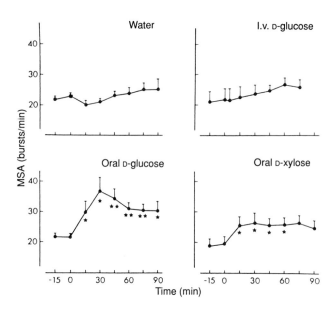

Fig. 26.3. Muscle nerve sympathetic activity (MSA) expressed as the number of bursts per minute in normal subjects after ingestion of either 300 ml of water orally, D-glucose (0.35 g/kg body weight i.v.), 100 g of D-glucose, 75.8 g of D-xylose orally. *, $p < 0.05$; **, $p < 0.01$. (Modified from Berne *et al.* (1989).)

changes in the cutaneous circulation. There is a fall in calculated peripheral vascular resistance (Fig. 26.2(a)), presumably because of a large increase in splanchnic blood flow, as has been demonstrated by non-invasive measurements of a major splanchnic vessel, the superior mesenteric artery (Fig. 26.2(b)). Plasma noradrenaline levels rise, suggesting an increase in overall sympathetic nervous activity. There are no changes in plasma adrenaline levels. Plasma renin activity levels double. Measurement of sympathetic nerve activity by microneurographic techniques indicate a rise after ingestion of a nutrient such as glucose (Berne *et al.* 1989; Fig. 26.3). It appears that the nervous and endocrine systems, among others, exert multiple adjustments which result in the maintenance of blood pressure in normal man.

In patients with autonomic failure, however, even in the supine position, there is a substantial fall in blood pressure which occurs within 10 to 15 min of ingestion and reaches its nadir within 60 min (Fig. 26.4). There are often modest or no changes in heart rate, particularly if there is associated cardiac parasympathetic denervation. Superior mesenteric artery blood flow rises to an extent similar to that in normal subjects, but there are no changes in blood flow to the skin and forearm vasculature, and no increase in cardiac output, indicating that appropriate haemodynamic adjustments are not being exerted

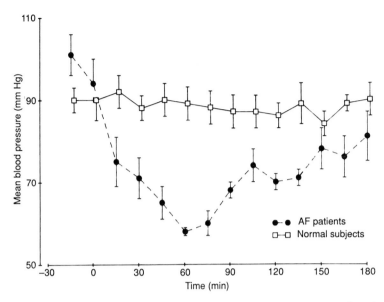

Fig. 26.4. Percentage change in mean blood pressure in a group of patients with chronic autonomic failure (dashed line, filled circles) and in normal subjects (continuous line, open squares) before and after food ingestion at times 0. The bars indicate means ± SEM. (From Mathias *et al.* (1989*a*).)

to counteract the splanchnic vasodilatation (Mathias *et al.* 1989*a*; Kooner *et al.* 1990). Plasma noradrenaline and adrenaline levels remain unchanged, consistent with the inability of these patients to activate the sympathetic nervous system. Postural change after food ingestion often results in a fall in blood pressure to even lower levels and has the potential to markedly enhance symptoms of impaired cerebral perfusion (Mathias *et al.* 1991).

Gastrointestinal motility

The gut is richly innervated by autonomic nerves and patients with autonomic failure often have impaired motility of the large bowel, mainly causing constipation but with occasional diarrhoea. The possibility of 'dumping' has been considered, as in many patients there is evidence of cardiac vagal denervation, which may have also involved the upper gut. In the classical 'dumping syndrome', which is known to occur after gastric drainage procedures and truncal vagotomy, patients suffer from weakness, sweating, tachycardia, palpitations, and occasionally a modest fall in blood pressure soon after food ingestion, especially if this contains a high carbohydrate load. In this 'early' dumping syndrome, there is rapid entry of an hyperosmotic (often carbohydrate) load into the jejunum, causing fluid absorption within

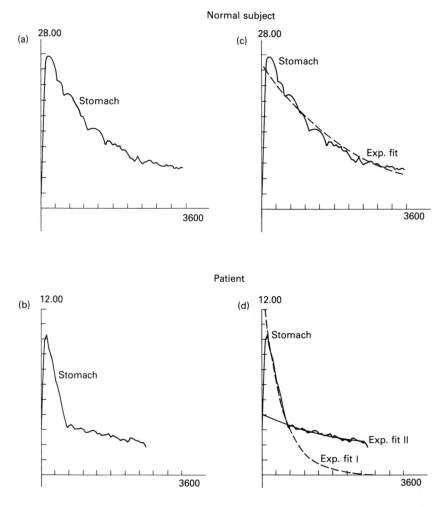

Fig. 26.5. Gastric emptying curves in (a) and (c) a normal subject and in (b) and (d) a patient with chronic autonomic failure. Integrated counts are indicated on the vertical axis and time in seconds on the horizontal axis. A computer exponential (Exp) fit is indicted on the right. In the autonomic failure patient there is rapid emptying initially (Exp. fit I) with a later slower phase (Exp. fit II).

the gut, thus reducing plasma volume and raising the haematocrit. This normally would be opposed by an increase in sympathetic activity. In the autonomic failure patients there are no changes in plasma osmolality or the haematocrit after food, making it less likely that fluid translocation into the gut, either as a result of osmotic changes or for other reasons, results in a contraction in plasma volume as in the early dumping syndrome (Mathias *et al.* 1989*a*).

To determine if increased gastric emptying is related to postcibal hypotension, studies have been performed using a technetium-labelled meal with the patient in the sitting position, with quantification of gastric emptying by gamma scintillation scanning. In many of the patients there was an increase in emptying, along with postprandial hypotension (Fig. 26.5). In some, however, the rate of emptying was normal while in two others (one with amyloidosis) gastric emptying was delayed but they still developed marked postprandial hypotension. It seemed unlikely, therefore, that increased gastric emptying is a major factor accounting for postprandial hypotension.

Food components

Ingestion of a largely solid balanced meal causes a similar fall in blood pressure when compared with the effects of an isocaloric, balanced liquid meal in autonomic failure. A series of further studies using different food components, which were isocaloric, isovolumic, and, wherever possible, isotonic, indicates major differences between the hypotensive effects of different food components (Fig. 26.6). After glucose, the hypotension is similar to that observed after a balanced meal. Lipid, however, has slower, smaller, and less sustained hypotensive effects while an elemental protein meal causes virtually no change in blood pressure.

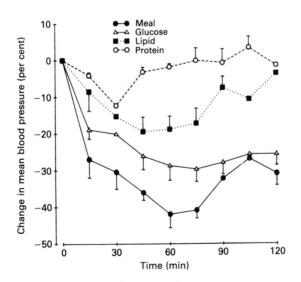

Fig. 26.6. Percentage change in mean blood pressure in six patients with chronic autonomic failure given either a standard meal or an isocaloric and isovolumic solution of carbohydrate (glucose, 1 g/kg body weight), lipid (prosperol 0.95 mg/kg), or protein (maxipro, 1 g/kg) alone orally. Vertical bars indicate ± SEM. (Taken with permission from Mathias *et al.* (1987).)

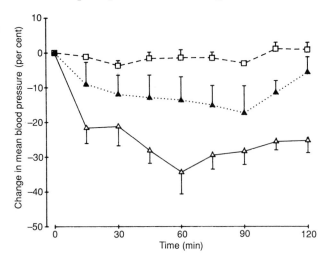

Fig. 26.7. Percentage change in mean blood pressure in eight normal subjects after oral glucose (dashed line, open squares) and in six chronic autonomic failure patients after glucose (continuous line, open triangle) and xylose (dotted line, filled triangles). Results are means ± SEM as vertical bars. The difference between the fall in blood pressure after glucose and xylose in the autonomic failure patients, calculated as the area under the curve, is highly significant ($p < 0.01$). (From Mathias *et al.* (1989*b*).)

The hypotensive effects of oral glucose are not related to its hyperosmolality, as in the same patients an isocaloric, isosmotic, and isovolumic solution of the inert carbohydrate, xylose, causes much smaller falls in blood pressure (Fig. 26.7). The effects of glucose are not related to its increasing plasma concentration, as intravenous infusion of glucose, often causing even higher plasma levels, do not lower blood pressure to the same extent as after oral glucose.

Pancreatic/gut hormones and their effects

Food ingestion causes release of pancreatic and gastrointestinal hormones, some of which are released into the circulation to exert distant effects, while others may act locally. A number were measured in both normal subjects and in autonomic failure patients before and after food ingestion. Changes in plasma levels of gastrin, vasoactive intestinal polypeptide, somatostatin, and cholecystokinin-8 are similar in both groups (Mathias *et al.* 1989). Enteroglucagon, pancreatic polypeptide, and neurotensin levels rise to a greater extent in the autonomic failure patients (Fig. 26.8). The first two do not have vasodilatory or negative cardiac inotropic effects and are unlikely to contribute to the hypotension. Neurotensin, however, has potential

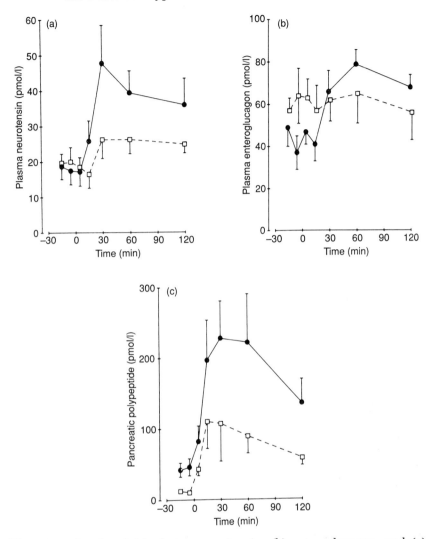

Fig. 26.8. Levels of (a) plasma neurotensin, (b) enteroglucagon, and (c) pancreatic polypeptide in patients with chronic autonomic failure (continuous line, filled circles) and in normal subjects (dashed line, open squares) before and after food ingestion at time 0. The vertical bars are ± SEM. (From Mathias *et al.* (1989*b*).)

vasodilatatory effects. The haemodynamic studies indicated that it was unlikely that this occurred because of its systemic effects. One of the peptides which rose during food ingestion and may have contributed was insulin. Evidence both from our laboratory and others indicates that insulin can lower blood pressure substantially in autonomic failure, even in the absence of changes

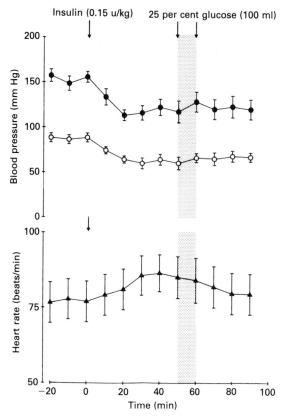

Fig. 26.9. Systolic (filled circles) and diastolic (open circles) blood pressure and heart rate in five patients with chronic autonomic failure before and after intravenous insulin. Both systolic and diastolic blood pressure fall within 10 min. Hypoglycaemia occurred at around 30 minutes and did not result in a further fall in blood pressure. Blood pressure remained low even after reversal of hypoglycaemia with 25 per cent glucose infused over 10 min. (From Mathias *et al.* (1987).)

in blood glucose (Brown *et al.* 1986; Mathias *et al.* 1987). Bolus intravenous insulin (0.15 units/kg) causes hypotension (Fig. 26.9) without dilatation in forearm muscle or cutaneous vascular beds. When administered with an euglycaemic clamp, blood pressure falls (Bannister *et al.* 1987; Brown *et al.* 1989), but independently of changes in blood glucose and without changes in cardiac output and forearm or skin blood flow, thus favouring an effect on a large vascular bed such as the splanchnic circulation (Bannister *et al.* 1987). In normal subjects, insulin does not lower blood pressure, but increases sympathetic nerve activity (measured by microneurography) and elevates plasma noradrenaline levels (Fagius *et al.* 1986); these changes occur even in

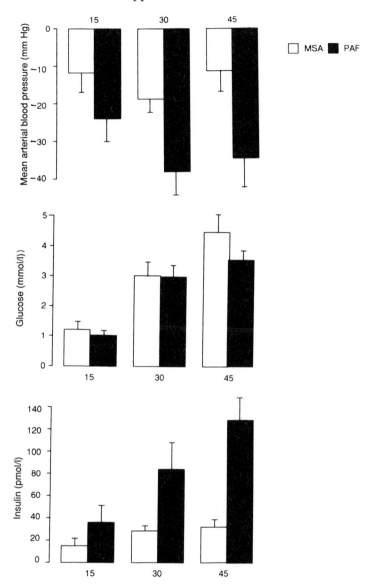

Fig. 26.10. Fall in mean blood pressure in patients with multiple system atrophy (open histograms, MSA) and patients with pure autonomic failure (filled histograms, PAF) at intervals of 15, 30, and 45 min after a balanced liquid meal ingested in the supine position. The middle panel indicates the changes in plasma glucose and the lower panel in plasma insulin at similar time points. In PAF there is a greater fall in blood pressure than in MSA. The rise in plasma glucose levels appear similar while the rise in plasma insulin levels are considerably greater in PAF.

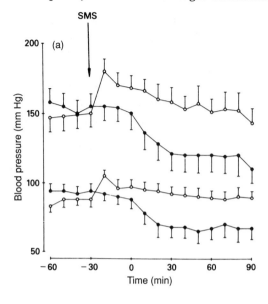

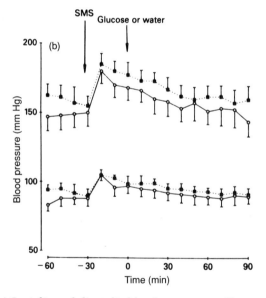

Fig. 26.11. (a) Systolic and diastolic blood pressure and heart rate in patients with chronic autonomic failure on two occasions when given oral glucose at time 0 with pre-treatment at −30 min with either Octreotide (SMS 201–995) 50 μg (open circles) or saline placebo (filled circles) both subcutaneously. (b) Systolic and diastolic blood pressure in patients with chronic autonomic failure given Octreotide (SMS 201–995) 50 μg subcutaneously at −30 min followed at 0 min by either oral glucose (open circles) or an equivalent amount of water (filled squares) (From Raimbach *et al.* (1989).)

adrenalectomized patients, excluding a role for the adrenal medulla. It is likely that, in our patients, insulin causes splanchnic vasodilatation and this lowers blood pressure as there is no compensatory increase in sympathetic nerve activity as is normally seen. This is consistent with the ability of insulin to lower blood pressure in diabetics with autonomic neuropathy (Page and Watkins 1976). Recent observations indicate that patients with PAF have a greater degree of postprandial hypotension than those with MSA (Fig. 26.10). Plasma glucose levels before and after a meal are similar in both groups. Although basal insulin levels are similar, there is a greater rise in postmeal insulin levels in PAF which may account for their greater degree of postprandial hypotension (Armstrong and Mathias 1991).

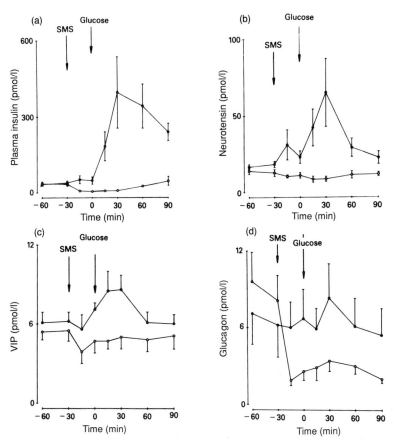

Fig. 26.12. Changes in plasma levels of (a) insulin, (b) neurotensin, (c) vasoactive intestinal polypeptide (VIP), and (d) glucagon in patients with chronic autonomic failure after placebo (filled circles) or Octreotide (SMS 201–995) (open circles), given at –30 min followed by oral glucose at 0 min. Results are means ± SEM. (From Raimbach *et al.* (1989).)

The somatostatin analogue octreotide (SMS 201–995) in normal subjects is effective in preventing the pancreatic and gut hormone responses to various stimuli, including food ingestion. An initial report indicated that somatostatin infusion could prevent postprandial hypotension in secondary autonomic neuropathy (Hoeldtke *et al.* 1985). Subcutaneous octreotide causes an initial but transient elevation in blood pressure which occurs only in autonomic failure patients and not in normal man. It is effective in preventing both glucose- and food-induced hypotension in autonomic failure (Fig. 26.11) (Raimbach *et al.* 1989). It prevents the rise in insulin, neurotensin, and a range of other hormones in response to food (Fig. 26.12), but has no effect on cardiac output or peripheral muscle or skin blood flow, suggesting that it prevents postprandial hypotension largely by exerting its effects on the splanchnic vasculature. This has been recently confirmed by non-invasive measurement of superior mesenteric artery blood flow, which is unchanged after octreotide, in contrast to the placebo phase when it rises markedly after a liquid meal (Kooner *et al.* 1990). This emphasizes the role of the splanchnic circulation and of vasodilatatory gut hormones in postprandial hypotension.

Management of postcibal hypotension

A better understanding of the pathophysiological mechanisms and increased therapeutic possibilities are helping to limit the problems caused by postcibal hypotension (Table 26.1). Advice is of importance and this concerns the quality, quantity, and frequency of meals. Carbohydrate increases vulnerability to postural hypotension and small meals at regular intervals may be helpful. After large meals it is necessary to ensure that patients do not stand or walk about. The vasodilatatory effects of alcohol are likely to enhance hypotension and should be avoided.

Table 26.1.   Some of the therapeutic approaches used to prevent or reduce postprandial hypotension

Advice

Small meals, more frequently
Less carbohydrate
Avoid alcohol
Rest after meals

Drugs

Indomethacin
Caffeine
Octreotide

A variety of drugs have been used. In the initial studies of Robertson *et al.* (1981), single doses of propranolol, diphenyhydramine, cimetidine, and indomethacin were evaluated. Propranolol (40 mg orally) had no beneficial effect and may even have worsened postcibal hypotension. The H_1 antihistaminic, diphenhydramine, and the H_2 blocker, cimetidine, had no effect, making it unlikely that histamine played a role in the responses. The hypotensive response to food was attenuated by indomethacin (50 mg orally), suggesting that vasodilatatory prostaglandins or arachidonic acid metabolites may be responsible. Long-term studies in postcibal hypotension have not been reported with indomethacin. It, however, has the potential to induce gastrointestinal erosions and bleeding.

A promising approach appeared to be the use of caffeine, which in normal subjects raises blood pressure by stimulating the sympathetic or renin–angiotensin system. It was initially reported to be highly effective in preventing postprandial hypotension in autonomic failure (Onrot *et al.* 1985). This occurred independently of stimulation of the sympathetic or renin–angiotensin systems and a postulated mechanism was blockade of vasodilatatory adenosine receptors. Our experience with caffeine has, however, not been favourable (Armstrong *et al.* 1990). When administered to patients with PAF and MSA in single doses of 250 and 500 mg and also on a regular basis, there was neither objective nor subjective evidence of benefit. Whether patients with incomplete autonomic lesions (in whom the residual sympathetic or renin–angiotensin systems may be stimulated) are likely to benefit remains to be elucidated.

An effective drug in preventing postprandial hypotension in primary and certain forms of secondary autonomic failure is the somatostatin analogue, octreotide (Fig. 26.13). This was first used by Hoeldtke *et al.* (1986) and is a synthetic, long-acting peptide release inhibitor. It has disadvantages which include its subcutaneous administration and local discomfort because of its low pH; it may also induce diarrhoea especially after a fatty meal, and its longer-term side effects, although well charted in various endocrine conditions, are unclear in autonomic failure. The availability of oral analogues will be a major step forward in the management of this distressing condition.

Effects of food in other groups of patients with autonomic dysfunction

Patients on ganglionic blockers and following splanchnic denervation

The hypotensive effect of food appears to have been first recorded by Smirk (1953) in hypertensive patients after the ganglionic blocker, pentolinium. He observed a fall in pressure in the lying, sitting, and standing position after

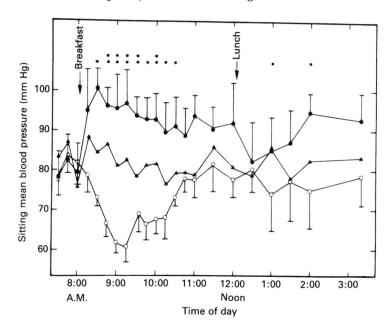

Fig. 26.13.   Sitting mean blood pressure after breakfast and lunch in six patients with autonomic failure of different aetiology, when given placebo (open circle) or two different doses of the somatostatin analogue SMS 201–995 (filled circles, 0.4 µg/kg and filled triangles, 0.2 µg/kg). For comparisons of drug and placebo, single asterisks signify $p < 0.05$ and double asterisks $p < 0.001$. SEM for low doses of drug are omitted for clarity. (Taken with permission from Hoeldtke *et al.* (1986).)

lunch. Whether postprandial hypotension occurs after other antihypertensive sympatholytic drugs known to cause postural hypotension, such as reserpine, debrisoquine, guanethidine, and bethanidine, is not clearly documented.

Insulin, when given to normal subjects after a ganglionic blocker (hexamethonium), lowers blood pressure (di Salvo *et al.* 1956). Insulin-induced hypotension has been recorded in patients after splanchnic denervation from T7 to L3 inclusive, performed for the relief of severe hypertension (French and Kilpatrick 1955). It is likely that, in both groups, splanchnic vasodilatation not accompanied by appropriate compensatory sympathetic nervous activity was responsible for the fall in blood pressure.

Diabetes mellitus (see Chapter 37)

Insulin lowers blood pressure in diabetics with autonomic neuropathy and baroreceptor abnormalities and can provoke or enhance postural hypotension (Miles and Hayter 1968; Page and Watkins 1976). In postprandial hypotension in diabetics with autonomic neuropathy, it has been difficult to separate the effects of food itself from that of insulin. The former is likely to have hypotensive effects, in keeping with the suggestion that factors in addition to insulin are also important in causing hypotension.

The elderly (see Chapter 44)

Postprandial hypotension is now recognized as occurring in a significant number of the elderly, especially in patients over the age of 80 (Lipschitz *et al.* 1983; Fig. 26.14). Food predominantly lowers systolic blood pressure but there are additional falls in diastolic pressure. It is unclear whether this is related to partial autonomic failure associated with the elderly, or to a combination of other factors including impairment of hormonal responses,

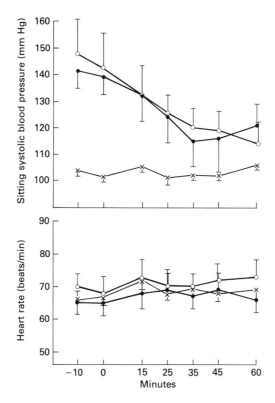

Fig. 26.14.   Sitting systolic blood pressure and heart rate before and after food ingestion. The upper panel shows mean systolic blood pressure (± SEM) at intervals before and after the start of a meal (0 time) in elderly subjects with (filled circles) and without (open circles) syncope. Data from 11 young normal subjects (×) is included. The lower panel shows the mean heart rate taken at the same time. (Taken with permission from Lipschitz *et al.* (1983).)

baroreceptor activity, and target organ function including cardiac function. A range of studies indicates that some of the mechanisms responsible in autonomic failure are similar in the elderly; so also are some of the therapeutic endeavours, which include the administration of caffeine (Lenders *et al.* 1988) and octreotide (Jansen *et al.* 1989).

Tabes dorsalis with an afferent lesion

We have studied one patient with tabes dorsalis who had, on detailed autonomic testing, evidence of an afferent baroreceptor lesion without impairment of central and peripheral sympathetic pathways. He had pronounced hypotension after food, suggesting that the lesion, which probably also involved afferents from the gut, blocked the normal activation of corrective reflexes and thus contributed to the fall in blood pressure after food.

Tetraplegia (see Chapter 43)

Patients with complete cervical spinal cord transection cannot activate sympathetic activity in response to agents with vasodilatatory properties. Exogenous insulin also lowers blood pressure in tetraplegics (Mathias *et al.* 1979), but the fall appears smaller than in autonomic failure, although no direct comparison has been performed. In these patients, using a similar protocol to those with autonomic failure, ingestion of either food or glucose causes only modest changes in systolic and diastolic blood pressure with a rise in heart rate in the supine position. The reason for the difference is unclear but it could include the ability of the intact vagus to increase heart rate and cardiac output and thus partially buffer the fall in blood pressure. Although plasma noradrenaline levels did not change after food, these measurements were made in forearm venous blood and would not have detected more localized activation of spinal reflexes induced by stimulation of intestinal afferents, as described in spinal animals (Stein and Weaver 1988). The precise reasons, however, remain unclear.

Dopamine β-hydroxylase deficiency (see Chapter 38)

These patients are unable to synthesize either noradrenaline or adrenaline and have severe postural hypotension with selective sympathetic adrenergic failure. Food ingestion does not lower their blood pressure, unlike patients with pure autonomic failure (Mathias *et al.* 1990). They differ in their ability to release dopamine and presumably other vasoactive chemicals from otherwise intact sympathetic nerve endings. Whether their ability to release dopamine, (which could affect the heart and vasculature), or other vasoconstrictors, (such as neuropeptide Y and adenosine triphosphate) from nerve terminals, accounts for their resistance to postprandial hypotension remains to be resolved.

Patients with cerebrovascular and coronary artery disease

These patients do not necessarily have an autonomic deficit, but when on vasoactive drugs they may be prone, because of their regional vascular deficits, to the potentially deleterious effects induced by food ingestion. In the presence of carotid artery stenosis an even modest fall in blood pressure may critically impair cerebral perfusion, resulting in a transient ischaemic attack or a stroke. In coronary artery disease, the increased cardiac workload following food ingestion may contribute to angina pectoris and possibly to myocardial infarction. This relationship was documented in the original description by Heberden in 1772, who noted that exercise, particularly after food, exacerbated angina. Whether there are differences in the efficacy of anti-anginal drugs in preventing postprandial exacerbations of angina is unclear; β-adrenergic blockers may be more effective if they prevent sympathetically mediated cardiac work. If, however, vasoconstrictor neuropeptides such as neuropeptide Y play an important intracoronary role, vasodilators like nifedipine may counteract food induced myocardial ischaemia more effectively.

References

Armstrong, E. and Mathias, C. J. (1991). The effects of the somatostatin analogue, Octreotide, on postural hypotension, before and after food ingestion, in primary autonomic failure. *Clin. autonom. Res.* 1, 135–40.

Armstrong, E., Watson, L., Hardman, T. C., Bannister, R., and Mathias, C. J. (1990). Effect of oral caffeine on post-prandial and postural hypotension in chronic autonomic failure. *J. autonom. nerv. Syst.* 31, 174–5.

Bannister, R., Da Costa, D. F., Kooner, J. S., Macdonald, I. A., and Mathias, C. J. (1987). Insulin induced hypotension in autonomic failure in euglycaemia in man. *J. Physiol.* 382, 36P.

Berne, C., Fagius, J., and Niklasson, F. (1989). Sympathetic response to oral carbohydrate administration. Evidence from micro-electrode recordings. *J. clin. Invest.* 84, 1403–9.

Brown, R. T., Polinsky, R. J., Lee, G. K., and Deeter, J. A. (1986). Insulin-induced hypotension and neurogenic orthostatic hypotension. *Neurology* 36, 1402–6.

Brown, R. T., Polinsky, R. J., and Bancom, C. E. (1989). Euglycemic insulin-induced hypotension in autonomic failure. *Clin. Neuropharmacol.* 12, 227–31.

di Salvo, R. J., Bloom, W. L., Brost, A. A., Ferguson, W. F., and Ferris, E. B. (1956). A comparison of the metabolic and circulatory effects of epinephrine, norepinephrine and insulin hypoglycaemia with observations on the influence of autonomic blocking agents. *J. clin. Invest.* 35, 568–77.

Fagius, J., Niklasson, F., and Berne, C. (1986). Sympathetic outflow in human muscle nerves increases during hypoglycaemia. *Diabetes* 35, 1124–9.

French, E. B. and Kilpatrick, R. (1955). The role of adrenaline in hypoglycemic reactions in man. *Clin. Sci.* **14**, 639–51.

Heberden, W. (1772). Some account of a disorder of the breast. *Medical Transactions* (published by the College of Physicians in London) **2**, 59–67.

Hoeldtke, R. D., O'Dorisio, T. M., and Boden, G. (1985). Prevention of post prandial hypotension with somatostatin. *Ann. intern. Med.* **103**, 889–90.

Hoeldtke, R. D., O'Dorisio, T. M., and Boden, G. (1986). Treatment of autonomic neuropathy with a somatostatin analogue, SMS 201–995. *Lancet* ii, 602–5.

Jansen, R. W. M. M., Peeters, T. L., Lenders, J. W. M., van Lier, H. J. J., V'tlaar, A., and Hoefnagels, W. H. L. (1989). Somatostatin analogue Octreotide (SMS 201–995) prevents the decrease in blood pressure after oral glucose loading in the elderly. *J. clin. Endocrinol. Metab.* **68**, 752–5.

Kooner, J. S., Peart, W. S., and Mathias, C. J. (1989). The peptide release inhibitor Octreotide (SMS 201–995), prevents the haemodynamic changes following food ingestion in normal human subjects. *Quart. J. exp. Physiol.* **74**, 569–72.

Kooner, J. S., Armstrong, E., Bannister, R., Peart, W. S., and Mathias, C. J. (1990). Octreotide (SMS 201–995) prevents superior mesentric artery vasodilatation and post-prandial hypotension in human autonomic failure. *Br J. clin. Pharmacol.* **29**, 154P.

Lenders, J. W. M., Morre, H. L. C., Smitz, P., and Thien, Th. (1988). The effects of caffeine on the post-prandial fall of blood pressure in the elderly. *Age Ageing* **17**, 236–40.

Lipschitz, L. A., Nyquist, R. H., Wei, J. Y., and Rowe, J. W. (1983). Postprandial reduction in blood pressure in the elderly. *New Engl. J. Med.* **309**, 81–3.

Mathias, C. J., Frankel, H. S., Turner, R. C., and Christensen, N. J. (1979). Physiological responses to insulin hypoglycaemia in spinal man. *Paraplegia* **17**, 319–26.

Mathias, C. J., Da Costa, D. F., Fosbraey, P., Christensen, N. J., and Bannister, R. (1987). Hypotensive and sedative effects of insulin in autonomic failure. *Br. med. J.* **295**, 161–3.

Mathias, C. J., Da Costa, D. F., Fosbraey, P., McIntosh, C., and Bannister, R. (1988). Factors contributing to food induced hypotension in patients with autonomic dysfunction. In *Vasodilatation: vascular smooth muscle, peptides, autonomic nerves and endothelium* (ed. P. M. Vanhoutte), pp. 351–6. Raven Press, New York.

Mathias, C. J., Da Costa, D. F., Fosbraey, P., Bannister, R., Wood, S. M., Bloom, S. R., and Christensen, N. J. (1989a). Cardiovascular, biochemical and hormonal changes during food induced hypotension in chronic autonomic failure. *J. neurol. Sci.* **94**, 255–69.

Mathias, C. J., Da Costa, D. F., McIntosh, C. M., Fosbraey, P., Bannister, R., Wood, S. M., Bloom, S. R., and Christensen, N. J. (1989b). Differential blood pressure and hormonal effects after glucose and xylose ingestion in chronic autonomic failure. *Clin. Sci.* **77**, 85–92.

Mathias, C. J., Bannister, R., Cortelli, P., Heslop, K., Polak, J. M., Raimbach, S., Springall, D. R., and Watson, L. (1990). Clinical, autonomic and therapeutic observations in two siblings with postural hypotension and sympathetic failure due to an inability to synthesise noradrenaline from dopamine because of a deficiency of dopamine beta hydroxylase. *Quart. J. Med.*, NS 75, **278**, 617–33.

Mathias, C. J., Holly, E., Armstrong, E., Shareef, M., and Bannister, R. (1991). The influence of food on postural hypotension in three groups with chronic autonomic failure—clinical and therapeutic implications. *J. Neurol. Neurosurg. Psychiat.* **54**, 726–30.

Miles, D. W. and Hayter, C. J. (1968). The effects of intravenous insulin on the circulatory responses to tilting in normal and diabetic subjects with special reference to baroreceptor reflex block and atypical hypoglycaemic reactions. *Clin. Sci.* **34**, 419–30.

Onrot, J., Goldberg, M. R., Biaggioni, I., Hollister, A. S., Kincaid, D., and Robertson, D. (1985). Haemodynamic and humoral effects of caffeine in autonomic failure. Therapeutic implications for post-prandial hypotension. *New Engl. J. Med.* **313**, 549–54.

Page, M. N. and Watkins, P. J. (1976). Provocation of postural hypotension by insulin in diabetic autonomic neuropathy. *Diabetes* **25**, 90–5.

Raimbach, S. J., Cortelli, P., Kooner, J. S., Bannister, R., Bloom, S. R., and Mathias, C. J. (1989). Prevention of glucose-induced hypotension by the somatostatin analogue Octreotide (SMS 201–995) in chronic autonomic failure—haemodynamic and hormonal changes. *Clin. Sci.* **77**, 623–8.

Robertson, D., Wade, D., and Robertson, R. M. (1981). Post-prandial alterations in cardiovascular haemodynamics in autonomic dysfunction states. *Am. J. Cardiol.* **48**, 1048–52.

Seyer-Hanson, K. (1977). Post-prandial hypotension. *Br. med. J.* **2**, 1262.

Smirk, F. M. (1953). Action of a new methonium compound in arterial hypotension, M & B 205A. *Lancet* **i**, 457.

Stein, R. B. and Weaver, L. C. (1988). Multi- and single-fibre mesenteric and renal sympathetic responses to chemical stimulation of intestinal receptors in cats. *J. Physiol., London* **396**, 155–72.

27. Autonomic dysfunction and the gut

David L. Wingate

Introduction

It has been estimated that up to 50 per cent of the patients seen by gastroenterologists are diagnosed as suffering from functional disorders, that is, they manifest subjective symptoms (pain, nausea, etc.) or objective disorders of function (vomiting, constipation, diarrhoea, etc.) for which no organic cause can be identified. On the eve of the twenty-first century, this might be regarded as a somewhat lamentable state of affairs, but it is attributable to, among other things, the considerable difficulties encountered by physiologists and clinicians in studying function and dysfunction in a system which is both extensive and inaccessible, with a variable morphology that obstructs the technology of imaging, and with a range in time base of function that varies between seconds (the transit of material through the oesophagus) and days (the residence of material in the colon).

In the last two decades there has been much progress in unravelling the complexities of the neural control of the gut. The sympathetic and parasympathetic divisions of the autonomic nervous system (ANS) that innervate the digestive tract (Fig. 27.1) have long been well recognized, and it has been generally agreed that the parasympathetic innervation is primarily excitatory, while the sympathetic system is generally inhibitory. Study of these two classical divisions of the ANS as defined by Langley did not, however, lead to the insights into the nature of the control mechanisms of the gut that might have been predicted, and it has now become apparent that this was due to the neglect of the third, or 'enteric', division that was also postulated by Langley. This division of the autonomic system is peculiar to the digestive tract as its name implies, and it consists of the intrinsic nerve plexuses of the gut, principally the myenteric plexus (Auerbach's plexus) and the submucous plexus (Meissner's plexus), that invest the entire digestive tube from oesophagus to anorectum (Fig. 27.2). These plexi are now known collectively as the 'enteric nervous system' (ENS). This separation between ANS (sympathetic and parasympathetic) and ENS (enteric) may at first be baffling to the reader who might have followed Langley in regarding all of these as no more than different divisions of the same system, but it makes

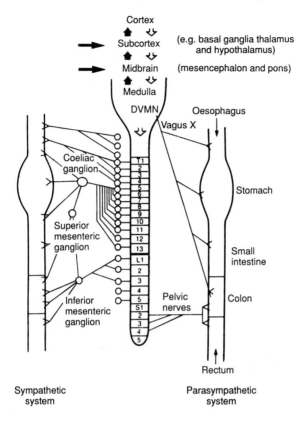

Fig. 27.1. The sympathetic (left) and parasympathetic (right) innervation of the digestive tract. The third—or enteric (see text)—division of the autonomic innervation is not included.

sense, as will become apparent later in this chapter, to draw a clear distinction between the autonomic nerves that are *intrinsic* to the gut (ENS), and those that are *extrinsic* (ANS). Neurons of the ENS do not synapse at any point with those of the central nervous system (CNS).

Understanding the contemporary view of autonomic dysfunction is impossible without some knowledge of the recent insights into digestive neurophysiology. These have been derived, for the most part, from the study of the motor activity of the digestive tract. Just as skeletal motor physiology was advanced by Sherrington and his colleagues in their studies of the reflex activity of the spinal cord, so has study of the movements of the bowel begun to reveal the underlying control mechanisms by which they are governed. 'Gastrointestinal motility' as a subject for study was flourishing at the beginning of the twentieth century, under the impetus of the fluoroscopic studies of Walter Cannon and the study of the peristaltic reflex by Bayliss

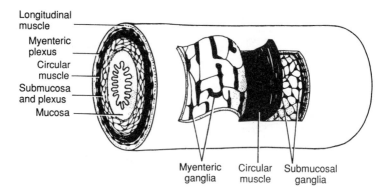

Longitudinal muscle
Myenteric plexus
Circular muscle
Submucosa and plexus
Mucosa

Myenteric ganglia   Circular muscle   Submucosal ganglia

Fig. 27.2. The location of the intrinsic nerve plexuses of the gut, with the longitudinal muscle peeled back to display the myenteric plexus and the circular muscle peeled back to display the submucosal plexus. In this drawing, the magnification has been distorted to display the reticular arrangement of the connectives and ganglia; these are invisible to the naked eye in a dissected specimen.

and Starling, but, for no very clear reason, interest flagged and, until the last quarter of this century, gastrointestinal physiologists were much more concerned with the mechanisms of mucosal absorption and exocrine secretion. The resurgence of interest in this field was partly fuelled by the technical advances in peptide assay and immunofluorescence, which revealed large numbers of hitherto unidentified 'gut hormones', and the subsequent and rather slower realisation that these peptides are neither confined to the gut nor are they conventional humorally acting substances, but are, for the most part, neurotransmitters and neuromodulators that exist in the central nervous system and also in other parts of the autonomic nervous system.

Control mechanisms of gastrointestinal motor activity

The effector system

The marked differences between the control of skeletal muscle and that of gastrointestinal smooth muscle reflect the differences in the physiology of the muscle. Gastrointestinal smooth muscle is, like myocardium, syncytial in organization and shares the same property of spontaneous rhythmic electrical depolarization. There is one important difference between gut and heart muscle. Myocardial fibres contract with each wave of depolarization, and the only way in which extrinsic control of myocardial function can be exercised is by changes in the frequency of depolarization. In the gut, however, contraction with each wave of depolarization is facultative rather than obligatory; each depolarizing wave represents an opportunity for contraction, but this may not be realized, depending upon the magnitude of the depolarizing event. In the gut, there is very little variation in the rate of depolarization, these rates being specific to the species and the region of the gut. For example, the rate of depolarization, or *basic electrical rhythm* is 3/min in the human stomach and 5/min in the canine stomach, while the corresponding rates are 11/min and 17/min in the duodenum of the respective species. These frequencies are governed by dominant pace-making sites in the orad portions of the viscera—the gastric fundus and the first part of the duodenum. Control of contractile activity is not directed at these pace-making sites, but directly upon the smooth muscle fibres throughout the gut, and the mechanism of control is the modulation at every point in the bowel of the magnitude of depolarization. Denervated gut exhibits continuous spontaneous rhythmic contractile activity, whereas *in situ* contraction is relatively infrequent and organized into specific patterns of activity; consequently, it follows that the main function of the control system is the *inhibition* of spontaneous rhythmic contractile activity.

The paradigm of this inhibitory activity is the co-ordinated movements that constitute peristalsis (Fig. 27.3). It was Bayliss and Starling who first recognized that peristaltic propulsion was accomplished by a repetitive aboral

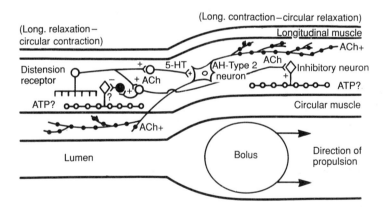

Fig. 27.3. The neuronal circuitry of the peristaltic reflex. This schematic diagram illustrates the minimal circuitry that would be required to operate the peristaltic reflex on the basis of existing experimental evidence; the actual circuitry is likely to be more complex, with the involvement of other neurotransmitters and neuromodulators. A key element in this scheme is the operation of inhibitory cholinergic neurons to produce the circular muscle relaxation that is required to accommodate the advancing bolus. It has been suggested that such circuitry is replicated over and over again along the length of the bowel in order to effect the smooth transit of material. Ach, acetylcholine; ATP, adenosine triphosphate; 5-HT, 5-hydroxytryptamine.

sequence of relaxation of the bowel caudad to a bolus of material within its lumen and contraction orad to the bolus, and they also demonstrated experimentally that the control of peristalsis was a property of the intrinsic innervation of the bowel. For many years, it was believed that the control of peristalsis was the *only* function of the intrinsic innervation, since no other control functions could be identified.

The hierarchy of control

There appears to be a hierarchy of neural control of gut motor activity which is illustrated in Fig. 27.4. At the lowest level is the smooth muscle mass itself. All the motor innervation of the smooth muscle is provided by ENS neurons, but sensory information is transmitted not only to the ENS, but via the sympathetic and parasympathetic system to the CNS. There appears to be a division of sensory modalities between parasympathetic and sympathetic afferents; the latter appears to be chiefly concerned with the mediation of pain, while the former relays information about luminal content, and about the movements of the gut wall to the brainstem. Motor activity is not directly

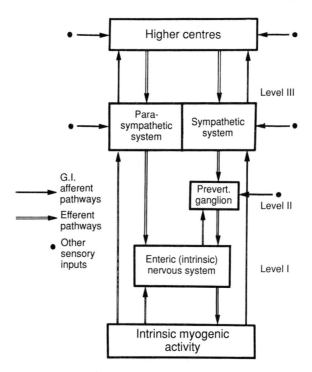

Fig. 27.4. The hierarchy of control of gastrointestinal (G. I.) motor activity showing the principal efferent (motor) and afferent (sensory) links between the levels of control.

controlled by the CNS since autonomic efferent neurons do not directly innervate muscle fibres but terminate within the enteric nervous system. Disregarding the physiological evidence of ENS autonomy, it is clear from morphological considerations alone that the autonomic efferent system is too sparse to provide direct innervation of effector cells in the gut. It is now known that probably about 90 per cent of the fibres in the vagus nerve are afferent; reliable estimates suggest that this gives a total of about 5000 neurons. This contrasts with an estimated population in the ENS of approximately 50 000 000–100 000 000 neurons.

The prevertebral ganglia serve to provide rapid communication between remote parts of the bowel. Transmission of information along the ENS is relatively slow because the neurons appears to be short and this route of transmission involves multiple synaptic transmission. Even if such direct communication is possible, transmission along the ENS between the distal colon and the proximal small bowel might involve 50 or more synapses, whereas transmission via the inferior and superior mesenteric ganglia will require three synapses at the most. Whether the prevertebral ganglia have any regulatory functions remains to be determined.

The hierarchy that is illustrated is based on morphological and electro-physiological evidence, but does not provide information about the relative contributions of the different levels of control to the regulation of gut function. This knowledge, which is crucial to an understanding of autonomic dysfunction, has been provided by the study of the periodic activity of the bowel.

Periodic gastrointestinal motor activity

In 1969 Joseph Szurszewski published a study on the periodic nature of canine gastrointestinal motor activity in the chronic fasted dog that caught the attention of gastrointestinal physiologists, and which acted as the catalyst for the study of this phenomenon. He showed that fasting motor activity is characterized by brief bursts of intense contractile activity recurring every 90 min; these bursts appeared to migrate slowly from stomach to terminal ileum over a period of approximately 90 min. Since gastrointestinal motor activity is organized in this way in all mammalian species so far studied (except the cat) and also in birds, it would have been surprising if this had never been noticed before. In fact, it had been clearly described at the beginning of the twentieth century by W. N. Boldyreff, working in the laboratory of I. P. Pavlov, and had excited considerable interest, but within a decade this interest had become so dissipated that research into this field was abandoned (for historical background, see Wingate 1981). Szurszewski considerably advanced knowledge by showing that motor activity is not only periodic but migratory, and he named this phenomenon the 'migrating myoelectric complex' as it was detected by electromyography; the same phenomenon can

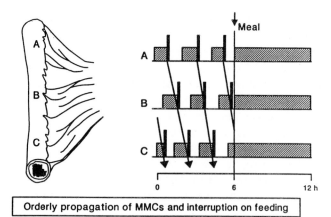

Orderly propagation of MMCs and interruption on feeding

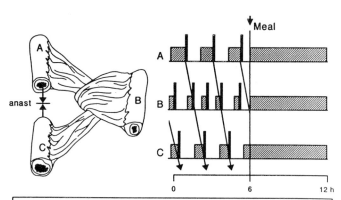

Asynchronous periodic activity in segment, interrupted on feeding

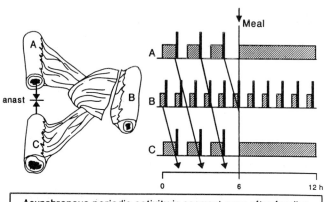

Asynchronous periodic activity in segment even after feeding

be detected by prolonged recording of muscle contractions of intraluminal pressure change when it is known as the 'migrating motor complex' and both are conveniently abbreviated to the identical acronym—MMC. Subsequently, Code and Marlett (1975) showed that periodic activity is arrested at all levels of the small bowel on feeding and returns only when the phase of digestion and absorption is completed. Within a short time, Vantrappen *et al.* (1977) confirmed the migratory nature of human periodic motor activity and this signalled the start of a dichotomy in subsequent research as physiologists laboured to elucidate the control mechanisms governing the MMC while clinicians sought to define the changes of the MMC in human disease.

Szurzewski's work was published at a time when gut function was considered to be dominated by 'gut hormones', and periodic motor activity was attributed to periodic changes in the plasma level of the peptide, motilin; subsequently it has seemed more likely that peaks of motilin release are an epiphenomenon associated with the regular contractile phase ('phase III', 'activity front') of the MMC as it traverses the proximal duodenum. It has now become clear that periodic activity is an expression of the activity of the ENS, the enteric division of the autonomic nervous system. The elegant

---

Fig. 27.5. Summary of the evidence for the role of the ANS and ENS in periodic motor activity, based on evidence in animals with innervated and denervated Thiry–Vella bowel segments. (Above) A length of bowel *in situ* with three segments (A, B, C,) in continuity. In this preparation, it is assumed that both ENS and ANS are intact. Motor activity in each segment is summarized on the right. In the first 6 hours of fasting, normal periodic activity migrates through the segments in sequence and is interrupted on feeding. Thus, *in the itact bowel, periodic activity is propagated in an orderly manner and is interrupted at all levels on feeding.*

(Centre) The middle segment (B) has been prepared as a Thiry–Vella segment with an intact neurovascular pedicle: segments A and C have been anastomosed in continuity. Consequently the extrinsic innervation (ANS) is intact, but the continuity of the intrinsic innervation (ENS) is interrupted. Periodic activity is present at all levels during fasting, but MMCs in B are synchronous with those in A and C. On feeding, periodic activity is interrupted at all levels, even though nutrient will bypass B. Thus, (1) *the continuity of the NES is a condition for the sequential synchrony of MMCs*; (2) *the effect of feeding is not mediated by luminal contact with nutrient.*

(Below) In this model, the neurovascular pedicle of B has been severed, and an alternative blood supply provided (autotransplantation). Thus ANS innervation of the segment is interrupted, and the only innervation in B is provided by intrinsic neurons. B now exhibits synchronous MMC activity that is not interrupted on feeding. Thus, (1) *periodic activity is a motor programme that resides within the intrinsic innervation (ENS) of the bowel*; (2) *the extrinsic innervation (ANS) is required to convey the stimulus of feeding to the ENS to operate the motor programme appropriate to the digestion and transport of food along the bowel.*

experiments from a number of laboratories on which this conclusion is based are summarized schematically in Fig. 27.5 and more fully described in a review by Sarna (1985). As shown, these experiments are based on techniques of functional isolation of bowel segments and rely upon the fact that, after a period of healing, there is functional union of the intrinsic innervation across an anastomosis (Galligan *et al.* 1989) even though there is no electrical continuity between the muscle.

The ENS as the 'gut brain'

The experimental evidence points unequivocally to the conclusion that the ENS provides not only the motor neurons for the muscle, but also the control circuitry that contains the programmes of motor activity that are appropriate to the physiological state of the organism. To this extent, the ENS has the functional characteristics of a brain (Wood 1984) in that it acquires sensory information and, on the basis of this sensory information, implements stereotypic programmes of motor activity that are co-ordinated along the length of the gut. These stereotypic programmes of gut activity may be regarded as analogous to the stereotypic programmes of locomotor activity that are resident within the CNS; they have a similar ontogeny and are only fully expressed in the postnatal infant (Bisset *et al.* 1988).

The ANS provides connections between the CNS and the ENS. The afferent pathways ensure that the CNS receives information on the events occurring within the bowel, while the efferent pathways permit CNS modulation of ENS-programmed motor activity. Physiologically, this modulation is evident in the changes in motor activity seen during sleep (Kumar *et al.* 1989) and mental stress (Valori *et al.* 1986). The vagus nerve and the dorsal motor complex in the medulla function as a vagovagal pathway essential for the transmission of information from vagal receptors in the gut wall to the ENS; as might be predicted from the experimental data summarized in Fig. 27.5, vagotomy impairs the motor response of the bowel to food (Thompson *et al.* 1982).

It is noteworthy that both the CNS and the ENS lapse into a periodic biorhythm in the absence of exogenous stimulation; in the ENS this is represented by the MMC biorhythm during fasting and in the CNS by the REM/non-REM biorhythm during sleep. This has led to suggestions that the MMC biorhythm may be centrally modulated (Finch *et al.* 1982), but recent evidence (Kumar *et al.* 1990) suggests that, although the biorhythms may be interactive, they are independently generated. This functional homology can be added to other homologies between the ENS and the CNS such as the presence of glial cells, a common population of neuropeptides, and a dense synaptic neuropil.

The physiological purpose of periodic activity in both systems remains a matter for speculation. While it has been suggested that periodic activity may be important in the prevention of bacterial overgrowth in the human bowel, since overgrowth has been reported in the presence of impaired periodic activity (Vantrappen *et al.* 1977; Kellow *et al.* 1990*a*), this is unlikely to be a general biological function since motor activity in the ruminant bowel, which is normally colonized by bacteria, is also periodic.

Autonomic dysfunction

Clinical presentation

Thus far in this chapter, autonomic control has been considered in terms of gut motility. It would be wrong to conclude from this that the autonomic nervous system does not modulate other gut functions, and there is good evidence for the autonomic control of secretion, absorption, and blood flow. However, in terms of autonomic pathophysiology, changes in these other functions have not been clearly demonstrated in autonomic disturbances, whereas changes in motor activity as a consequence of autonomic pathology have been documented in a number of conditions and have been shown to produce significant deficits in function.

It is not always appreciated that intestinal transit is an active process; as exemplified in the condition of paralytic ileus, without propulsion there is no movement. In general, autonomic dysfunction results in the delay or the arrest of transit through the bowel. Since this resembles intestinal obstruction due to mechanical obstruction, as occurs with tumour or volvulus, it is known as 'pseudo-obstruction'. In its most florid form the clinical picture often so closely resembles mechanical obstruction that patients are submitted to laparotomy in an attempt to relieve a mechanical obstruction which does not, in fact, exist.

The full clinical picture of intestinal obstruction is a comparatively infrequent outcome of autonomic dysfunction, but lesser degrees of autonomic dysfunction can be viewed as, in terms of function, relative pseudo-obstruction. The clinical presentation of complete or relative pseudo-obstruction varies according to the region affected.

Oesophagus
   Dysphagia and regurgitation
   Retention of food within the oesophagus
   Aspiration pneumonia

Stomach
   Epigastric fullness and bloating
   Vomiting

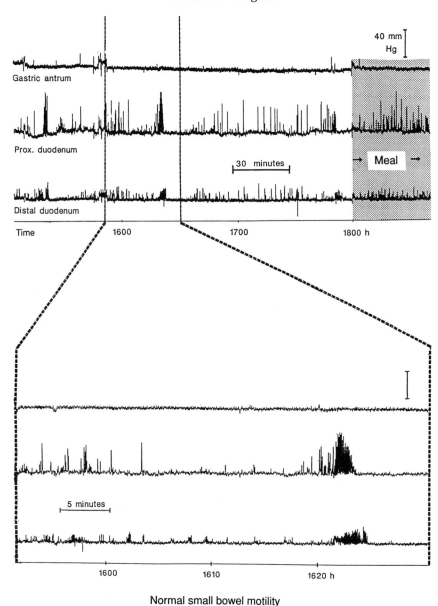

Normal small bowel motility

Fig. 27.6. Normal duodenal periodic activity. This manometric recording shows (upper panel) three MMC cycles, with the bursts of regular contractions that characterize the 'activity front' (Phase III) being visible in the two lower traces at the beginning of the recording, 1 hour later, and again just before a meal is given. After the meal, the onset of frequent irregular contractions can be seen. One cycle of the MMC is shown on an expanded time base (lower panel) and

Small bowel

Distension
Colic
Constipation
Diarrhoea secondary to bacterial overgrowth
Malnutrition secondary to bacterial overgrowth

Large bowel

Distension
Colic
Constipation
'Spurious diarrhoea'

ANS or ENS?

The role of the intrinsic innervation (ENS) in the direct control of motor function and of the parasympathetic and sympathetic innervation (ANS) in the modulation of ENS-programmed motor activity has been described above. Determining which of the two divisions of the autonomic system is responsible for the functional deficit in autonomic dysfunction is not easy. There are several reasons for this. First, there is the difficulty by characterizing the functional deficit itself in other than the crudest terms such as the documentation in the delay of the transit of a marker substance between defined points; with the exception of the oesophagus, techniques of studying motility still remain within the research domain, and agreement as to what constitutes a motor abnormality is by no means universal. Second, even when abnormal patterns of motor activity or transit have been clearly defined, neuropathological confirmation of the site of a lesion is usually lacking; tissue is rarely available for histological study and, even when it is, tengential sections that are required to display the intrinsic innervation are rarely cut, and stains that will demonstrate neural structures are not often used.

The most useful classification of pseudo-obstructive syndromes that can be achieved at the present time is into *primary* and *secondary disorders* (Christensen *et al.* 1990). Primary pseudo-obstruction refers to disease confined to the bowel wall that is not associated with disease elsewhere and is not due to exogenous factors such as toxins or pathogens; it may be neuropathic, myopathic, or both. Primary neuropathic pseudo-obstruction involves only the ENS, and it is in the diagnosis of intrinsic neuropathies that the phenomenon of periodic activity is diagnostically valuable. The

---

Fig. 27.6. *(continued)* this shows the Phase II activity migrating aborally between the two intraduodenal pressure sensors.

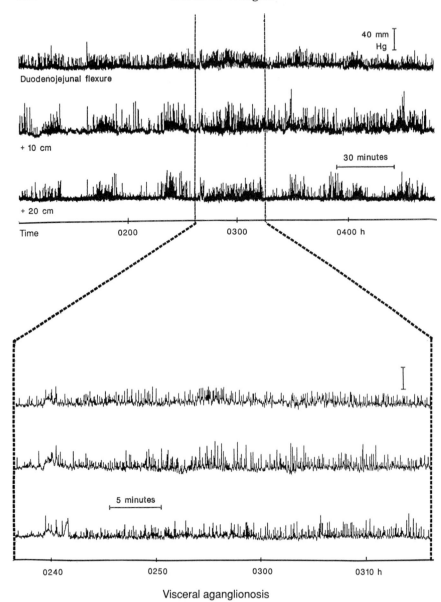

Fig. 27.7. Nocturnal manometric recording of jejunal motor activity in a sleeping patient suffering from acquired visceral aganglionosis (chronic idiopathic intestinal pseudo-obstruction). In the upper panel, it will be seen that contractions are frequent in all three sectors, and the motor quiescence which normally dominates nocturnal recording is absent. Even though there are periods of more intense contractile activity that, in the compressed record (upper panel), suggest MMC activity, expansion of the time base (lower panel) reveals that these

presence of normal periodic activity provides evidence of the relative integrity of the ENS (Fig. 27.6); conversely, absence of normal MMCs is strongly suggestive of ENS dysfunction (Fig. 27.7).

Neuropathy of the enteric nervous system: primary pseudo-obstruction

Intrinsic neuropathy presents with manifestations of pseudo-obstruction as outlined above, and may be confirmed by manometric studies showing that MMC activity is absent. The technique of manometry is important because of the variability of the human MMC, particularly during the waking state. Stanghellini et al. (1987) used a manometric protocol, in which the recording of fasting motility was confined to 3 h, and suggested that absence of MMCs during this time was diagnostic of pseudo-obstruction. Studies on healthy subjects have shown, however, that intervals between MMCs may exceed 3 h in healthy subjects (Thompson et al. 1980), and longer recordings are required to discriminate between different patterns of small bowel motility (Summers et al. 1983). Ideally minimally invasive techniques for prolonged manometry that allow subjects to sleep normally during the recording period are required for the clear discrimination of abnormal periodic activity (Kellow et al. 1990a, b). The technology for such recordings is not yet generally available, although this will undoubtedly change. An ingenious alternative to prolonged manometry to test ENS integrity is to use balloon distension to determine the presence or absence of the peristaltic reflex (Kendall et al. 1987). Imaging may be used to define the functional alteration in transit (Greydanus et al. 1990) but, while this is non-invasive, it lacks specificity as a diagnostic technique.

Neuropathy of the enteric nervous system: secondary pseudo-obstruction

Secondary pseudo-obstruction refers to syndromes that are associated with disease outside the bowel or due to exogenous agents. Some of these mimic primary pseudo-obstruction since only the intrinsic innervation is affected in the bowel.

Fig. 27.7. *(continued)*   contractions although frequent are not regular, and there is no evidence of the propagated regular burst of contractions that are present in normal periodic activity (cf. Fig. 27.6). This patient was well until the age of 33, when she developed achalasia of the cardia. A year later she developed increasingly severe constipation culminating in recurrent episodes of subacute intestinal obstruction. Histology of the bowel showed an almost complete absence of intrinsic neurons with replacement of the plexuses by glial cells, analogous to the cortical changes seen in dementia. After resection of much of the small bowel and colon with ileorectal anastomosis, the patient survives but requires home parenteral nutrition.

Chagas' disease

The parasite *T. cruzii* is a blood-borne infection carried by an insect vector, and is seen only in endemic areas, of which Brazil is the primary locus. The neuropathic mechanism is due to a chance affinity of the antibody to the parasite for enteric nerves; it is the resulting binding of the antibody rather than the parasite itself that causes the neuronal degeneration. Because the disease is associated with poor living standards and hence scarce medical resources, there have been few functional studies of the disorder, but it appears to affect primarily the oesophagus and colon, resulting in mega-oesophagus and megacolon. It is estimated that there are about 10 000 000 patients in Brazil suffering from the disease.

Paraneoplastic syndromes

Degeneration of the enteric nervous system resulting in pseudo-obstruction has been reported as a neuropathy associated with carcinoma of the lung (Chinn and Schuffler 1988).

Parkinson's disease

Bowel dysfunction in Parkinson's disease is common. It has been attributed—and may often be due—to the unwanted side-effects of drugs, but Loewy bodies have been reported as being presented in the colon and oesophagus in Parkinson's disease. There has been no systematic study of the dysfunction, but isolated studies (Wingate, unpublished observations) suggest a change resembling pseudo-obstruction.

Neuropathy of the extrinsic
(parasympathetic and sympathetic) innervation

Because of the relative autonomy of the ENS, neuropathy confined to the extrinsic innervation is poorly characterized in terms of altered function. Only in the case of diabetes mellitus does there seem to be any reasonably clear definition of the syndrome and, even in this disease, there are questions that remain to be answered. In disorders of the extrinsic innervation, studies of motor function tend to show deviations from normal patterns which are, as in diabetes, quantitative rather than qualitative.

Diabetic neuropathy

The common gastrointestinal manifestation of diabetic autonomic neuropathy is *diabetic gastroparesis*. The defect is due to severe diminution or abolition of contractile activity, and this is manifested in several ways. Impaired gastric motility following food results in gastric emptying that is very slow, with prolonged retention of food in the stomach. Vomiting is therefore a frequent concomitant. Gastroparesis is more common in insulin-dependent diabetics, but its true incidence is unknown; evidence of impaired function on testing is very much more frequent than are symptoms due to the deficit (Ewing and Clarke 1986). Since it is the phase III contractions of the fasting MMC that are responsible for the gastric emptying of indigestible solids and such contractile activity is impaired or absent in the diabetic stomach, solids may be retained and only emptied by vomiting. The syndrome is associated with poor diabetic control, almost certainly due to the difficulty of knowing when ingested carbohydrate will actually be delivered to the small intestine, and this constitutes a vicious circle which can be broken, in some patients, by improving both gastric function and thus also the control of blood sugar. It is thought that it is likely to be involved, since diabetic gastroparesis resembled the gastroparesis that can be induced after vagotomy. Recent work suggests that erythromycin is effective in the management of the problem, and this is because erythromycin binds to motilin receptors in the gut.

Diabetic diarrhoea is an even more uncommon complication of diabetes. It is associated with bacterial overgrowth, and abnormalities of small bowel motility have been reported (Dooley *et al.* 1988) but there are few data on the subject.

Porphyria

Symptoms of gastrointestinal dysfunction occur in acute intermittent porphyria, presumed to be due to autonomic neuropathy; one study has shown abnormal gastrointestinal motility (Gorchein *et al.* 1982).

Primary autonomic failure

Gastrointestinal dysfunction in this condition is thought to be due to neuropathy of the extrinsic innervation.

The irritable bowel syndrome

The irritable bowel syndrome (IBS) is a common affliction characterized by irregular defecation with associated abdominal pain, bloating, stool mucus, and fatigue. It is not generally thought of as an autonomic disturbance, and the exact nature of the syndrome remains unknown; indeed, its existence as a disease entity remains a matter of debate. Autonomic involvement appears to be both motor and sensory. Intermittent motor abnormalities in the form of regular clusters of contractions have been reported in IBS (Thompson *et al.* 1979; Kellow and Phillips 1987; Kellow *et al.* 1990*b*), and these dysrhythmias may be associated with abdominal discomfort. In healthy subjects, controlled psychological stress diminishes the incidence of MMCs (Valori *et al.* 1986); equivalent stressors in IBS patients have an even greater effect on MMCs, but will also evoke the clustered contractions (Kumar and Wingate 1985). It is tempting to regard IBS as a variant of pseudo-obstruction, but the motility changes differ in one major respect from mild pseudo-obstruction in that, during sleep, motility appears to be normal (Kellow *et al.* 1990*b*).

IBS is an entity characterized by symptoms of discomfort, and this appears to be due to visceral hypersensitivity (Whitehead *et al.* 1990). Many if not most workers would consider that it is premature, in the current confused state of knowledge on this topic, to characterize IBS as an autonomic dysfunction, but it does seem probable that autonomic dysfunction is at least a major component of the syndrome.

Conclusion

The subject of autonomic dysfunction in the gut remains to be fully elucidated; progress is dependent upon collaboration between physiologists, gastroenterologists, neurologists, and morphologists which is not easily arranged. Among gastroenterologists and neurologists alike the neurology of the gut is not a topic that has attracted much attention. However, our improved understanding of enteric neurophysiology has provided a stimulus for renewed efforts in this direction, and it is to be hoped that the response will be appropriate. With half of all gastroenterology patients suffering from symptoms of organ dysfunction that remain to be adequately explained or treated, the clinical rewards might be considerable.

References

Bisset, W. M., Watt, J. B., Rivers, R. P., and Milla, P. J. (1988). Ontogeny of fasting small intestinal motor activity in the human infant. *Gut* **29**, 483–8.

Chinn, S. and Schuffler, M. D. (1988). Paraneoplastic visceral neuropathy as a cause of severe gastrointestinal dysfunction. *Gastroenterology* **95**, 1279–86.

Christensen, J., Dent, J., Malagelada, J.-R., and Wingate, D. L. (1990). Pseudo-obstruction. *Gastroenterol. Int.* **3**, 107–19.

Code, C. F. and Marlett, J. A. (1975). The interdigestive myoelectric complex of the stomach and small bowel of dogs. *J. Physiol., London* **246**, 298–309.

Dooley, C. P., el Newihi, H. M., Zeidler, A., and Valenzuela, J. E. (1988). Abnormalities of the migrating motor complex in diabetics with autonomic neuropathy and diarrhoea. *Scand. J. Gastroenterol.* **23**, 217–23.

Ewing, D. J. and Clarke, B. F. (1986). Diabetic autonomic neuropathy: present insights and future prospects. *Diabetes Care* **9**, 648–65.

Finch, P. M., Ingram, D. M., Henstridge, J. D., and Catchpole, B. N. (1982). Relationship of fasting gastroduodenal motility to the sleep cycle. *Gastroenterology* **83**, 605–12.

Galligan, J. J., Furness, J. B., and Costa, M. (1989). Migration of the myoelectric complex after interruption of the myenteric plexus: intestinal transection and regeneration of enteric nerves in the guinea pig. *Gastroenterology* **97**, 1135–46.

Gorchein, A., Valori, R. M., Wingate, D. L., and Bloom, S. R. (1982). Abnormal proximal gut motility in acute intermittent porphyria: a neuropathic model. *Gastroenterology* **82**, 1070.

Greydanus, M. P., Camilleri, M., Colemont, L. J., Phillips, S. F., Brown, M. L., and Thomforde, G. M. (1990). Ileocolonic transfer of solid chyme in small intestinal neuropathies and myopathies. *Gastroenterology* **99**, 158–64.

Kellow, J. E. and Phillips, S. F. (1987). Altered small bowel motility is correlated with symptoms in irritable bowel syndrome. *Gastroenterology* **92**, 1885–93.

Kellow, J. E., Gill, R. C., Wingate, D. L., and Calam, J. E. (1990a). Small bowel motor activity and bacterial overgrowth. *J. gastrointest. Motility* **2**, 180–3.

Kellow, J. E., Gill, R. C., and Wingate, D. L. (1990b). Prolonged ambulant recordings of small bowel motility demonstrate abnormalities in the irritable bowel syndrome. *Gastroenterology* **98**, 1208–18.

Kendall, G. P., Thompson, D. G., and Day, S. J. (1987). Motor responses of the small intestine to intraluminal distension in normal volunteers and a patient with visceral neuropathy. *Gut* **28**, 714–20.

Kumar, D. and Wingate, D. L. (1985). The irritable bowel syndrome: a paroxysmal motor disorder. *Lancet* **ii**, 973–7.

Kumar, D., Soffer, E. E., Wingate, D. L., Mridha, K., Britto, J., and Das-gupta, A. (1989). Modulation of the duration of human postprandial activity by sleep. *Am. J. Physiol.* **256**, G851–5.

Kumar, D., Idzikowski, C., Wingate, D. L., Soffer, E. E., Thompson, P. D., and Siderfin, C. (1990). Relationship between the enteric migrating motor complex and the sleep cycle. *Am. J. Physiol.* **259**, G983–90.

Sarna, S. K. (1985). Cyclic motor activity: migrating motor complex. *Gastroenterology* **89**, 894–913.

Stanghellini, V., Camilleri, M., and Malagelada, J.-R. (1987). Chronic idiopathic intestinal pseudo-obstruction: clinical and intestinal findings. *Gut* **28**, 5–12.

Summers, R. W., Anuras, S., and Green, J. (1983). Jejunal manometry patterns in health, partial intestinal obstruction and pseudoobstruction. *Gastroenterology* **85**, 1290–300.

Szurszewski, J. H. (1969). A migrating electric complex of the canine small intestine. *Am. J. Physiol.* **217**, 1757–63.

Thompson, D. G., Laidlaw, J. M., and Wingate, D. L. (1979). Abnormal small bowel motility demonstrated by radiotelemetry in a patient with irritable colon. *Lancet* **ii**, 321–3.

Thompson, D. G., Wingate, D. L., Archer, L., Benson, M. J., Green, W. J., and Hardy, R. J. (1980). Normal patterns of human upper small bowel motor activity recorded by prolonged radiotelemetry. *Gut* **21**, 500–6.

Thompson, D. G., Ritchie, H. D., and Wingate, D. L. (1982). Patterns of small intestinal motility in duodenal ulcer patients before and following vagotomy. *Gut* **23**, 517–23.

Valori, R. M., Kumar, D., and Wingate, D. L. (1986). Effects of different types of stress and of 'prokinetic' drugs on the control of the fasting motor complex in humans. *Gastroenterology* **90**, 1890–900.

Vantrappen, G., Janssens, J., Hellemans, J., and Ghoos, Y. (1977). The interdigestive motor complex of normal subjects and patients with bacterial overgrowth of the small intestine. *J. clin. Invest.* **59**, 1158–66.

Whitehead, W. E., Holtkotter, B., Enck, P., Hoelzl, R., Holmes, K. D., Anthony, J., Shabsin, S. H., and Schuster, M. M. (1990). Tolerance for rectosigmoid distention in the irritable bowel syndrome. *Gastroenterology* **98**, 1187–92.

Wingate, D. L. (1981). Backwards and forwards with the migrating motor complex. *Dig. Dis. Sci.* **26**, 641–66.

Wood, J. D. (1984). Enteric neurophysiology. *Am. J. Physiol.* **247**, G585–98.

PART IV

Primary autonomic failure—clinical and pathological studies in pure autonomic failure and multiple system atrophy

28. Clinical features and investigation of the primary autonomic failure syndromes

Roger Bannister and Christopher J. Mathias

Classification

The clinical classification of primary autonomic failure adopted in this book (see Chapter 1) is as follows.

1. Patients with pure autonomic failure (PAF), without associated neurological disorders, formerly known as 'idiopathic orthostatic hypotension'.

2. Patients with autonomic failure (AF) and multiple system atrophy (MSA). MSA is a group of central neurological degenerations, often but not always including parkinsonism (Bannister and Oppenheimer 1972). The combination of AF and MSA was known as the Shy–Drager syndrome (Shy and Drager 1960). For brevity, in this book the use of the acronym MSA can be taken to mean MSA associated with AF. MSA in the form of striatonigral degeneration (SND) may occasionally occur without the symptoms of autonomic failure in life (Fearnley and Lees 1990).

3. Patients with autonomic failure (AF) associated with Parkinson's disease (PD).

Of these three disorders MSA is the most common. Hughes *et al.* (in press), summarizing the results from the Parkinson's Disease Brain Bank at the Institute of Neurology, London (see p. 579) found that seven of the first 100 cases, supposed in life by the referring physicians to have PD, in fact had striatonigral degeneration, that is, MSA. This means that MSA may have a prevalence rate as high as 10 per 100 000 by comparison with the prevalence rate of 100–150 per 100 000 for PD. PAF is much less common than MSA and AF with PD rarer still.

Clinical features of primary autonomic failure

The clinical features of autonomic failure can be described separately from the neurological features which are characteristic of MSA or PD.

The particular autonomic functions affected differ in degree from patient to patient but are remarkably similar in all three groups. The patients are usually middle-aged or elderly and, in MSA, males are affected more often than females. In men impotence and loss of libido are commonly the first symptoms. Patients living in hot climates may complain of inability to sweat which could lead to hyperpyrexia and collapse in the tropics but rarely causes problems in temperate countries. The most dramatic symptom, however, and the commonest reason for seeking medical advice, is postural dizziness, or even fainting, on standing erect, especially in the morning or after meals or exercise.

One curious symptom of autonomic failure, which presumably reflects a phase of denervation supersensitivity, is that in some patients, over a few weeks or months, an autonomic function may appear hyperactive before failure occurs. This may in particular be noted in salivation or sweating and in sexual function in the male in which more frequent spontaneous erection may precede erectile failure.

Postural hypotension

The postural attacks may be 'drop' attacks resembling sudden brainstem vascular dysfunction, but more commonly there is a gradual fading of the consciousness over half a minute or so while the patient is standing or walking. A neckache radiating to the occipital region of the skull and to the shoulders often precedes actual loss of consciousness. The neckache may be due to ischaemia in continuously contracting postural muscles in the neck and back but the mechanism of this very common and virtually unique symptom of postural hypotension is unknown.

Occasionally, patients may complain of other symptoms suggesting muscle ischaemia. For example, some have described the classical symptoms of angina on exercise and others have described leg symptoms which have features suggestive of 'claudication' affecting the cauda equina. Perhaps surprisingly, despite a very low systolic blood pressure of under 60 mm Hg during exercise at the time anginal symptoms occur, the electrocardiogram usually fails to show T-wave inversion or other signs of ischaemia.

In the postural hypotensive attacks, usually after a visual disturbance or sensation of dizziness, the patient may then fall slowly to his knees; experience teaches him that, after lying flat, recovery and loss of all symptoms, including the neckache, will occur within a few minutes. The recovery from such transient neurological symptoms is usually complete and occlusive cerebrovascular incidents are rare, possibly because many patients, after years of postural hypotension, have not only preserved but enhanced compensatory cerebral autoregulation (Thomas and Bannister 1980). The attacks of loss of consciousness also differ from normal fainting in that the patient usually does not sweat, and there is no vagally induced bradycardia (see Chapter 39).

Symptoms are strikingly worse in the mornings and also after meals, in hot weather, and after exercise, all of which cause an unfavourable redistribution of blood volume. The disease is likely to be progressive for several years before significant incapacity occurs because autonomic compensatory mechanisms postpone overt failure. A few patients, if treated by bed rest for hypotensive symptoms, develop persistent recumbent hypertension, mainly due to loss of baroreflexes, of such severity that they may develop papilloedema with retinal haemorrhages.

Visual disturbances

Sometimes there are transient visual disturbances, scotomata, hallucinations, or tunnel vision, suggesting occipital-lobe ischaemia. The symptoms of visual disturbance may be particularly striking in some patients with autonomic failure. One observant patient was able to classify the disturbances into three kinds. First, there was a disturbance of primary colours, but particularly yellow and red, in which they became brilliant, and secondary colours, or pastel shades, appeared non-existent. Second, objects might appear in a photonegative form, that is dark shades being light and the light shades being dark, mostly in various shades of green. Finally, if he did not lie down promptly and had developed a severe neckache and one of the previous disturbances of vision had been present for several minutes, he would then find that his central vision was blurred. On closing his eyes he would see a very clear oval orange or yellow shape filling the whole of the central field with a dark background outside it and in the very centre what appeared to be an irregularly shaped black hole. Once this particular disturbance had occurred it might take some 30 min to subside completely.

On occasion patients describe visual disturbances accompanied by neck and even lumbar aching, brought on by physical exertion while standing, particularly after a meal. The effects of arm exercise, such as washing up after meals or using an ironing board, appear, under conditions of critically reduced systolic blood pressure, to imitate the effects of the subclavian steal syndrome. This is similar to the visual disturbances described by Ross Russell and Page (1983) in patients with critical underperfusion of the brain and retina with extensive occlusive disease of the extracranial arteries. In patients with autonomic failure, however, such symptoms are relatively benign and patients quickly learn to use them as a warning sign that they must lie down quickly to restore an adequate perfusion pressure.

Defective sweating

Defective sweating (Fig. 28.1) causes the risk of hyperpyrexia and collapse in hot climates. The testing of thermoregulatory sweating is described in Chapter 21.

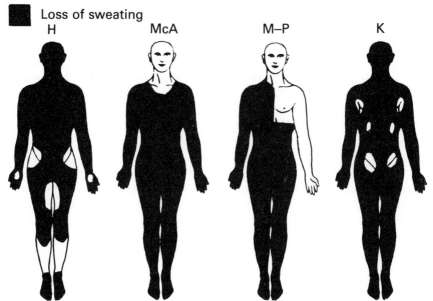

Fig. 28.1.   Sweating response to 1°C rise in central body temperature in four patients with autonomic failure. (Taken with permission from Bannister *et al.* (1967).)

Sexual function

Sexual function in the male is lost early. Failure of erection occurs first, though occasionally after an initial period with excessive erections, and later is followed by disturbance of ejaculation consistent with progressive parasympathetic and then sympathetic failure. As discussed in Chapter 24, complex techniques using pharmacological agents or electrical stimulation may enable some sexual function to be achieved for a time.

Bowel function

Bowel control is sometimes affected, with constipation, intermittent diarrhoea, or rectal incontinence as symptoms. A few cases of MSA with predominant bowel disturbance and cholinergic dysfunction (including salivation) have been described (Khurana *et al.* 1980). A marked disturbance of bowel function with a predominance of diarrhoea and faecal incontinence suggests the possibility of amyloid.

Clinical features of multiple system atrophy

Three principal forms of motor disturbance occur in MSA: (1) striatonigral degeneration; (2) olivopontocerebellar atrophy; (3) pyramidal lesions.

Striatonigral degeneration (SND)

This term was first used by Adams *et al.* (1964) to describe patients with a parkinsonian syndrome with special pathological distinguishing features (see Chapter 30). Often the disorder was clinically indistinguishable from PD and, with hindsight, these patients, especially if autonomic defects had been looked for and found, could now be classified as having MSA. In this disease there is a predominance of rigidity without much tremor, associated with progressive loss of facial expression and limb akinesis. The limbs show rigidity on examination, without the classical 'cog wheel' or 'lead pipe' rigidity of PD. Facial expression is often less affected than in PD. The patient has difficulty in standing, walking, or turning and has difficulty in feeding himself. Salivation is reduced. As a result of akinesis the speech becomes faint and slurred. The patient's gait becomes slow and clumsy, superficially resembling PD, with an attitude of stooping and often extreme forward cervical flexion which makes forward gaze difficult.

Olivopontocerebellar atrophy (OPCA)

In this form of MSA, not included in Shy and Drager's original clinical description of only two cases, there is a prominent disturbance of gait with truncal ataxia which frequently makes it impossible for the patient to stand without support. In addition, marked slurring of speech occurs with irregularity of speed of diction. There may also be a mild or moderate intention tremor affecting the arms and legs. This form of MSA is to be distinguished from familial OPCA in which the associated clinical features may include optic atrophy, retinitis pigmentosa, chorea, cataracts, and areflexia (Harding 1981).

Pyramidal lesion

In either of these forms of degeneration there may be a pyramidal increase in tone, together with impaired rapid hand and foot movements and exaggerated deep-tendon jerks and bilateral extensor plantar responses. It is, of course, difficult to detect a pyramidal disturbance of tone in the presence of the extrapyramidal disturbance. Primitive reflexes such as the palmomental reflex may also be present.

Other clinical features in multiple system atrophy

Muscle wasting and neuropathy

Progressive muscle wasting not infrequently occurs (see Chapter 29C) though this is not as marked as in motor neuron disease. Fasciculation occurs rarely but on electromyographic examination there is usually some evidence of denervation with little evidence of any abnormality of peripheral nerve motor conduction. Rarely in PAF and uncommonly in MSA there is clinical and electrophysiological evidence of a mild distal sensorimotor neuropathy with the report of a mild reduction of myelinated fibre density on sural nerve biopsy (Cohen *et al.* 1987).

Intellectual state

Dementia is no more common than might be expected on the basis of chance in patients of this age group. It is surprising to observe preserved intellectual function in a patient who is almost totally incapacitated in terms of motor control, orthostatic blood pressure regulation, and bladder disturbance. This is, of course, in striking contrast to the neuronal degeneration of presenile dementia (Alzheimer's disease) in which the predominant degeneration affects cortical cholinergic neurons. It is also in contrast to the intellectual impairment which is a feature of many cases of PD.

Affect

There is no evidence of a mood defect when allowance is made for the considerable disability of patients with AF and MSA (Robertson and Bannister, unpublished observations). This is surprising in view of the hypothesis that central catecholamine function plays a part in the preservation of normal mood and that patients with depression can be helped by augmenting central noradrenergic function.

Sensory function

In two cases out of a personal series of more than 150 patients with AF and MSA, there was sensory loss in the legs, confirmed by loss of sural sensory action potentials in one and by post-mortem studies in the other (Bannister and Oppenheimer 1972).

Pupils

Abnormalities recorded in patients with MSA include Horner's syndrome, alternating anisocoria, and abnormal pupillary responses to drugs. Ponsford, Paul, and Bannister (unpublished observations) studied 16 patients with AF and MSA and compared them with patients with PD and age-matched controls. There was alternating anisocoria in five patients. This was variable and different from the alternating resting anisocoria which was noted in a single case of acute pandysautonomia. It was concluded that in MSA the disturbance was due to a central lesion rather than to unilateral hypersensitivity to cholinergic drugs on one side and to adrenergic drugs on the contralateral side. Alternating anisocoria differs from the variable but consistently lateralized anisocoria in the patients with pandysautonomia and the pupillotonia of the Holmes–Adie syndrome which reflects the different hypersensitivity of the two pupils to circulating cholinergic drugs.

In more than half the patients with MSA or PD with or without AF, there was an abnormal and excessive constrictor response to methacholine. The degree of constriction in the more sensitive pupils was in the same range as in the Holmes–Adie syndrome. More than half of the patients with AF, whether PAF or AF associated with MSA or PD, showed an abnormal sensitivity.

Ocular movements

There is frequently restriction of conjugate ocular movements in advanced MSA but this is usually an upward rather than a downward restriction and is less severe than in progressive supranuclear palsy (PSP), in which the ocular movement disorder dominates the clinical picture. Nuchal rigidity and striatonigral features in PSP, superficially resembling MSA, may make the differential diagnosis difficult at an early stage. In due course the ocular movement disorder of PSP becomes more apparent and this, with the lack of autonomic symptoms and signs, will distinguish it from MSA.

Detailed testing of ocular movements by Dr T. J. Anderson of the National Hospital, London (personal communication) has shown that only a minority of patients with probable MSA have normal eye movements. Often the findings are similar to those of idiopathic PD, with hypometria of saccades, particularly upwards saccades. Prominent slowing of saccades is not normally seen and suggests familial OPCA or PSP. A supranuclear gaze paresis, seldom severe and usually affecting vertical more than horizontal gaze, is present in up to 20 per cent of cases. Cerebellar eye signs—particularly gaze-evoked nystagmus, saccadic dysmetria, and poor smooth pursuit and vestibulo-ocular response suppression—are often present in patients with other features of cerebellar dysfunction, but may be found in the absence of cerebellar ataxia or limb dysmetria. Down-beat nystagmus (DBN) is present in up to a third of probable cases of MSA. In a minority of these, the DBN is noted in the head upright (i.e. sitting) position, but in most it is only elicited on positioning the patient with the head hanging (Dix–Hallpike or Barany manoeuvre) and may be of relatively short duration.

Disturbances of breathing

Rhythm and depth control (see Chapter 23)
The disturbance of breathing may occur during the day with involuntary inspiratory gasps (Bannister *et al.* 1967) or 'cluster' breathing, apparently

normal breathing interspersed with regular apnoeic periods lasting about 20 s (Lockwood 1976), which appear to have a central origin. At night the patients may develop the sleep apnoea syndrome. The sleep apnoea may be 'central' with cessation of respiratory motor activity or 'obstructive' in which there is a disturbance of the pharyngeal and laryngeal muscles. There is, in addition, evidence of an alteration of CO_2 sensitivity in patients with AF probably due to the brainstem lesion. The patient of Guilleminault et al. (1977) with AF and MSA also had a reduced amount of rapid eye movement (REM) sleep and had disturbed non-REM sleep. This study showed that pulmonary arterial pressure rose progressively during sleep in direct association with each apnoeic episode and related hypoxaemia and hypocapnia, but without the extreme bradycardia which occurred in the REM sleep of patients who did not have autonomic failure.

Laryngeal function (see Chapter 23)

At night, stridor with consequent hypoxia may secondarily cause disturbances of brainstem function and apnoea. The laryngeal stridor is due to a bilateral defect of the laryngeal abductors (Williams et al. 1979; Guindi et al. 1980) with changes of denervation on laryngeal electromyography (Guindi et al. 1981). At post-mortem an atrophy of the posterior cricoarytenoid muscles was found, due to an unusual form of denervation (Bannister et al. 1981). In the only case in which the laryngeal nerve was studied at post mortem there appeared to be a reduced number of nerve fibres, although the nucleus ambiguus, thought to be the nucleus from which neurons innervating the laryngeal abductors arise, failed to show any selective neuronal loss. Once stridor and apnoea occur, tracheostomy cannot be long delayed. It is justified because such patients may manage well for several years before other symptoms become troublesome or incapacitating. However, sudden death during sleep remains a frequent cause of death in MSA (Munschauer et al. 1990).

Urinary bladder function

Bladder symptoms are a combination of urgency, frequency, and nocturia due to uninhibited detrusor activity, or incontinence due to sphincter weakness, or, later, overflow incontinence due to an atonic bladder. During attempted evacuation there may be a weak or interrupted stream or incomplete evacuation, with residual urine. At its most severe there may be a complete inability to urinate. In MSA there may be various combinations of upper and lower motor neuron lesions affecting the detrusor and internal and external sphincter muscles.

As described in Chapter 24, the degeneration of sacral autonomic neurons (Onuf's nucleus) leads to the loss of both autonomic and somatic efferents as the nucleus has a status intermediate between ordinary somatic motorneurons and autonomic neurons. The anal and urethral sphincter impairment results from the loss of both innervations. Incontinence, usually without retention, is the result. There is, in addition, detrusor instability with lack of the capacity to initiate micturition in MSA, which is probably the result of a lesion of the pontine centre for micturition. Very occasionally, reduction of the outflow resistance can be achieved surgically, although routine operations based on the common belief that the patient may have prostatism almost always make these patients worse. An appropriate operation, however, may postpone the need for the use of surgical drainage in the male. Ureteric sphincter implants are now available. In younger females with good co-ordination, intermittent self-catheterization may sometimes be an acceptable management instead of continuous drainage or the use of incontinence pads.

Biochemical investigation

The most useful investigation is the measurement of plasma noradrenaline, taken under standard resting conditions, which is in the normal range in MSA but low in PAF. In neither disorder does the level rise on tilting or standing, because of the blockage of baroreceptor pathways (see Chapter 17). The low levels also help to separate the rare syndrome of dopamine β-hydroxylase deficiency (see Chapter 38) which may not at first appear to differ from PAF and MSA, apart from its earlier age of onset.

Other investigations in multiple system atrophy
(see also Chapter 29)

Computerized tomography (CT) scanning

With the modern CT scan the enlargement of the cisterna ambiens associated with brainstem atrophy in MSA is visible along with atrophy of the pons and cerebral peduncles. In OPCA, atrophy of the vermis and cerebellar cortex is visible (Savoiardo et al. 1983; Huang and Plaitakis 1984).

Magnetic resonance imaging

The putaminal changes which are unique to multiple system atrophy can be identified by T_1 weighted magnetic resonance imaging (MRI) (Pastakia et al. 1987). Brown et al. 1987 found that MRI changes ranked with the severity of the rigidity but not the other parkinsonian features of tremor or bradykinesia. The advances in MRI have increased the precision of diagnosis of MSA. Figure 28.2 shows MRI scans of patients with MSA and PAF.

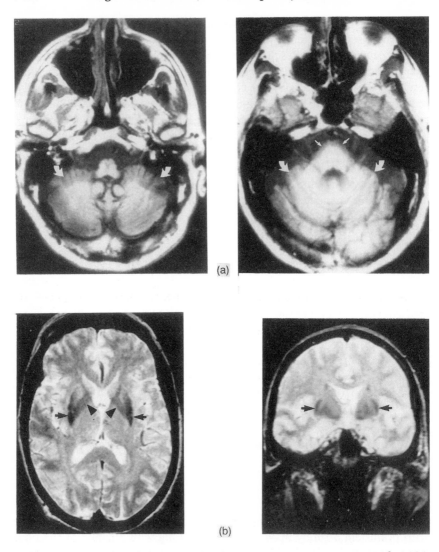

Fig. 28.2. (a) MRI axial T_1-weighted images, in two patients with MSA showing cerebellar hemispheric atrophy (curved arrows); the belly of the pons (small arrows) is flattened and atrophic. (b) Axial (on left) and coronal (on right) MRI T_2-weighted images in a patient with MSA. There is severe signal hypointensity in the posterolateral putamina (arrows) greater than in the globus pallidus (triangular arrows) (from Fulham *et al.* 1991).

Fulham *et al.* (1991) showed that the commonest MRI finding in MSA, present in 82 per cent of their series, was cerebellar atrophy, which was seen in many patients whose symptoms were parkinsonian rather than cerebellar (see Fig. 28.2(a)). The second commonest finding, present in more than half the patients in their series, was hypodensity in the posterolateral putaminal region, which matches exactly the region of cell loss found pathologically in MSA (Fig. 28.2(b)). In contrast, the MRI scans in patients with PAF were normal. An abnormal MRI scan provides a reliable method of diagnosing MSA even though the neurological signs of parkinsonism or cerebellar atrophy may be slight. Clearly, as with PD, the pathological changes in the brain in MSA may precede by some years the development of recognizable neurological clinical signs. In contrast, a normal MRI scan in a patient with severe orthostatic hypotension but without neurological symptoms strengthens the likelihood of the diagnosis of PAF.

Brainstem auditory evoked potentials in autonomic failure

The usefulness of brainstem auditory evoked responses in providing an easier non-invasive means of assessing the integrity of brainstem function in multiple sclerosis (Prasher and Gibson 1980) led us to investigate its use in patients with AF (Prasher and Bannister 1986). A group of patients with PAF and uncomplicated PD failed to show any abnormality. However, in nearly all patients with MSA there was a disruption of the brainstem responses in the pontomedullary region with delay or reduction of components of the response generated beyond this region (Fig. 28.3). The brainstem auditory evoked potentials, which are now widely available, may be helpful in distinguishing at an early stage the patients developing MSA from the patients with PAF, in whom the prognosis is so much better and the management so much easier. These findings have been confirmed by Vamatsu *et al.* (1987).

Cognitive events-related potentials

Cognitive events-related potentials provide a unique means of separating decision processes from motor involvement. The cerebral potentials are associated with information processing, especially the timing of sensory stimulus discrimination and categorization, together with the reaction time measures. These studies were undertaken in four patients with MSA by D. K. Prasher at the National Hospital Human Movement and Balance Unit (personal communication). They showed normal results by comparison with patients with PD, in whom they were all delayed. These findings are of interest in view of the impression of normal intellectual function in MSA.

Distinction between MSA with striatonigral degeneration (SND) and olivopontocerebellar atrophy (OPCA)

Clearly there are difficulties in distinguishing clinically the degree of SND and OPCA in patients with the features of both. In our experience careful

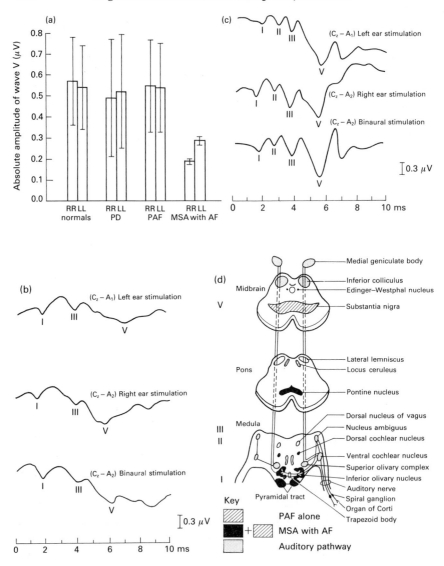

Fig. 28.3. (a) Mean and standard deviation of absolute amplitude of Wave V for the groups tested. PD, Parkinson's disease; PAF, pure autonomic failure; MSA with AF, multiple system atrophy with autonomic failure. Note the major reduction in the mean and variance of the amplitude of Wave V in MSA with AF. (b) Brainstem responses of MSA: bilateral abnormalities more severe on the left. (c) Brainstem responses of PAF: normal in amplitude and latency. (d) This diagram shows sites involved in PAF alone which clearly do not affect the brainstem auditory evoked potential. As these sites, which involve central autonomic control, are also affected in AF with MSA it is necessary to exclude the sites common to both syndromes. Therefore, by subtraction, the remaining

attempts to elicit signs of striatonigral disease and cerebellar disease will usually give a correct diagnosis of MSA as judged by the only real criterion, the ultimate pathological verification. There may be only limited value in striving clinically to separate SND from OPCA though we attempt to do so on the grounds of clinical signs at diagnosis. The association with AF is more frequent with SND than with OPCA but the ultimate pathology usually shows the changes of both MSA and OPCA (Fearnley and Hughes 1990; see also Chapter 30), even though in life one form may predominate at first diagnosis and in the early stages. The association with AF, however, marks out these patients from the other progressive cerebellar syndromes, especially predominantly inherited cases, which have little relationship with SND or AF.

Autonomic failure and Parkinson's disease

The question of whether, and to what degree, autonomic involvement occurs in PD has been discussed for many years. The problem has been confused by the clinical description of supposed minor autonomic disturbances in PD, whose significance is difficult to assess, such as greasy skin or unequal pupils. Autonomic involvement should be defined as a measurable sympathetic or parasympathetic dysfunction, assessed by physiological or biochemical means. If a battery of tests of the kind described in Chapter 14 is undertaken, a few parkinsonian patients have AF according to defined autonomic criteria. The autonomic failure syndrome associated with PD as defined by these tests is rare and much less common than the association of AF with MSA.

Many patients with classical PD do have mild orthostatic hypotension when compared with control groups. There have been reports that resting recumbent levels of plasma noradrenaline in these patients are in a lower range than in normal controls (Turkka 1986). However, such patients do not have the abnormalities of cardiovascular reflex control which are linked with baroreceptor defects and intermediolateral column cell loss which are characteristic of the autonomic failure syndrome. Gross *et al.* (1972) studied 20 patients with moderate PD, wishing to exclude abnormalities which occur with advanced parkinsonism, and compared them with controls. The only abnormality was that on head-up tilt their blood pressures were significantly lower than those of matched controls. There was, therefore, some increased lability of cardiovascular control. The conclusion was drawn that, because the cardiovascular reflexes and Valsalva tests were normal, there may be changes in the midbrain or hypothalamus associated with classical PD

Fig. 28.3. (*continued*)   sites in which degeneration is exclusive to the MSA component of the syndrome may be obtained. The auditory pathways are also shown with the Roman numerals indicating the generator sites of the brainstem potentials.

pathology that affect the input to the autonomic nervous system and that might well be the reason for these relatively mild abnormalities.

The clinical distinction between multiple system atrophy and Parkinson's disease

The differential diagnosis clinically between MSA and PD can sometimes be difficult. There are, however, certain clinical features which should make the clinician suspicious that the true diagnosis is MSA, not PD. Sometimes the patient with parkinsonism with atypical featurees is known by the title 'parkinsonism plus'. We avoid using this term, but, until the diagnosis becomes unequivocal clinically, which is usually within a year or so of presentation, we preface the diagnosis with the word 'probable'. In this group a patient with the diagnosis of probable PD may well become a patient with probable MSA. The clinical features favouring a clinical diagnosis of MSA may be listed.

1. *Marked orthostatic hypotension.* Mild orthostatic hypotension occurs in PD and this effect is exaggerated by the action of levodopa used in its treatment. The hypotension may be worse on standing or after exercise or after food. This distinction, of course, does not apply when the autonomic failure syndrome with severe postural hypotension is associated with PD.

2. *Levodopa unresponsiveness.* It should, however, be remembered that about 15 per cent of patients with MSA show a significant but short-lived improvement in their akinetic-rigid symptoms on levodopa.

3. *Erectile impotence* in males in their forties (see p. 466). This symptom is unlikely to be prominent in PD, though, of course, it will be present if the autonomic failure syndrome is associated with PD.

4. *Urinary symptoms*, usually frequency, urgency, and a poor and intermittent stream (see Chapter 24). The suspicion of MSA arises when urinary symptoms occur in younger males or older males in the absence of prostatic hypertrophy or, in women, in the absence of other causes such as pelvic trauma with multiple births.

5. *Mild pyramidal or cerebellar signs* or involvement of both these symptoms.

6. A parkinsonian syndrome in which *rigidity* and *akinesis* are more marked than tremor.

7. *Nocturnal stridor* which may be inspiratory or expiratory and may be extraordinarily loud, sometimes likened to the braying of a donkey. The recent onset of snoring at night or sudden inspiratory gasps during the day may be a warning of more rapid progression of the disease.

It should be stressed that the diagnosis of MSA can be difficult but can only be based on clinical features and investigation. The most that can be expected is a probable diagnosis which may eventually be confirmed at post-mortem.

The clinical distinction between pure autonomic failure and early multiple system atrophy

There is a second area in which diagnosis can be difficult. The wrong clinical diagnosis of PAF may be made in a patient who is in fact in the earliest stage of developing MSA or, much less commonly, PD. We made this error in a 68-year-old with severe postural hypotension but no other detectable signs of a neurological disorder. We thought she had PAF. We did, however, note that her plasma noradrenaline was in the normal range which should have made us suspicious that she might be developing MSA. In fact, 2 years after her severe orthostatic hypotension had been diagnosed, she developed a tremor of one hand. In the course of the next 18 months she developed all the signs of an akinetic-rigid syndrome with nocturnal stridor requiring a tracheostomy; in other words she had typical MSA. After this experience we have made the plasma noradrenaline value an essential part of the investigation of all our patients.

Clinical course of primary autonomic failure

The clinical progression of patients with pure autonomic failure (PAF) is relatively benign since the hypotensive symptoms can usually be controlled by head-up tilt or fludrocortisone (see Chapter 32) so that life expectancy is only a little reduced and sphincter disturbance may be minimal. Occasionally, patients may survive from diagnosis for more than 20 years, raising the possibility that, in some patients, non-progressive lesions occur. Patients with AF and PD fare less well than patients with uncomplicated PD but again may survive for many years.

Patients with AF and MSA face a distressing progression of their disability, unmitigated by any loss of insight as their intelligence is almost always preserved. They often remain surprisingly cheerful, especially when attempts to help them with various drug regimes are pursued (see Chapter 33). The attempts are entirely justifiable since there is never any single drug regime that can be automatically applied to patients with such a variety of sites and extents of their lesions. But within some 5 years the patients with AF can barely move, due to the extrapyramidal and pyramidal weakness, and have a sphincter disturbance that may be helped but cannot be cured. The preterminal development is often sleep apnoea or stridor (see p. 538).

Death in sleep may be due to stridor or apnoea causing hypoxia and may sometimes be a providential release. The denervation supersensitivity of α- and β-adrenoceptors of the heart may render these patients more liable to cardiac arrhythmias from which they may die, as in patients with diabetic autonomic neuropathy (Page and Watkins 1978).

Despite all the physiological, biochemical, and pharmacological investigations in patients with autonomic failure, it must be stressed that the diagnosis remains a clinical one in individual cases. The final verification of the correctness of the diagnosis lies in the post-mortem examination (see Chapter 30), but, from a practical point of view, the diagnosis in life is important because of the prognostic implications and the consideration of supportive and preventative aspects of care of the patient's acute and other disabilities.

References

Adams, R. D., van Bogaert, L., and van der Eecken, H. (1964). Striato-nigral degeneration. *J. Neuropathol. exp. Neurol.* **23**, 584–608.

Bannister, R. and Oppenheimer, D. R. (1972). Degenerative diseases of the nervous system associated with autonomic failure. *Brain* **95**, 457–74.

Bannister, R., Ardill, L., and Fentem, P. (1967). Defective autonomic control of blood vessels in idiopathic orthostatic hypotension. *Brain* **90**, 725–46.

Bannister, R., Gibson, W., Michaels, L., and Oppenheimer, D. R. (1981). Laryngeal abductor paralysis in multiple system atrophy. *Brain* **104**, 351–68.

Brown, R. T., Polinsky, R. J., DiChiro, G., Pastakia, B., Wener, L., and Simmons, J. T. (1987). MRI in autonomic failure. *J. Neurol. Neurosurg. Psychiat.* **50**, 913–14.

Cohen, J., Low, P., Fealey, R., Sheps, S., and Jiang, N-S. (1987). Somatic and autonomic function in progressive autonomic failure and multiple system atrophy. *Ann. Neurol.* **22**, 692–9.

Fearnley, J. M. and Lees, A. J. (1990). Striatonigral degeneration: a clinico-pathological study. *Brain* **113**, 1823–42.

Fulham, M. J., Dubinsky, R. M., Polinsky, R. J., Brooks, R. A., Brown, R. T., Curras, M. T., *et al.* (1991). Computed tomography, magnetic resonance imaging and positron emission tomography with [^{18}F] fluorodeoxyglucose in multiple system atrophy and pure autonomic failure. *Clin. autonom. Res.* **1**, 27–36.

Gross, M., Bannister, R., and Godwin-Austen, R. (1972). Orthostatic hypotension in Parkinson's disease. *Lancet* **i**, 174–6.

Guilleminault, C., Tilkian, A., Lehrman, K., Forno, L., and Dement, W. C. (1977). Sleep apnoea syndrome: states of sleep and autonomic dysfunction. *J. Neurol. Neurosurg. Psychiat.* **40**, 718–25.

Guindi, G. M., Michaels, M., Bannister, R., and Gibson, W. (1980). Pathology of the intrinsic muscles of the larynx. *Clin. Otolaryngol.* **6**, 101–9.

Guindi, G. M., Bannister, R., Gibson, W., and Payne, J. K. (1981). Laryngeal electromyography in multiple system atrophy with autonomic failure. *J. Neurol. Neurosurg. Psychiatr.* **44**, 49–53.

Harding, A. E. (1981). Idiopathic late onset cerebellar ataxia. A clinical and genetic study of 36 cases. *J. neurol. Sci.* **51**, 259–71.

Huang, Y. O. and Plaitakis, A. (1984). Morphological changes of olivopontocerebellar atrophy in computed tomography and comments on its pathogenesis. *Adv. Neurol.* **41**, 39–85.

Hughes, A. J., Daniel, S. E., Kilford, L., and Lees, A. J. (in press). The accuracy of clinical diagnosis of idiopathic Parkinson's disease: a clinical pathological study of 100 cases. *J. Neurol. Neurosurg Psychiatr.*

Khurana, R. K., Nelson, E., Azzarelli, B., and Garcia, J. H. (1980). Shy–Drager syndrome: diagnosis and treatment of cholinergic dysfunction. *Neurology, Minneapolis* **30**, 805–9.

Lockwood, A. H. (1976). The Shy–Drager syndrome with abnormal respiration and antidiuretic hormone release. *Arch. Neurol., Chicago* **33**, 292–5.

Munschauer, F., Loh, L., Bannister, R., and Newsom Davis, J. (1990). Abnormal respiration and sudden death during sleep in multiple system atrophy with autonomic failure. *Neurology* **40**, 677–9.

Page, M. McB. and Watkins, P. J. (1978). Cardiorespiratory arrest and diabetic autonomic neuropathy. *Lancet* **i**, 14–16.

Pastakia, B., Polinsky, R., DiChiro, G., Simmons, J. T., Brown, R., and Wener, L. (1987). Multiple system atrophy (Shy–Drager syndrome) MR imaging. *Radiology* **159**, 499–502.

Prasher, D. K., and Bannister, R. (1986). Brainstem auditory evoked potentials in patients with multiple system atrophy with progressive autonomic failure (Shy–Drager syndrome). *J. Neurol. Neurosurg. Psychiatr.* **49**, 278–89.

Prasher, D. K. and Gibson, P. R. (1980). Brainstem auditory evoked potentials. A comparative study of monaural vs binaural stimulation in the detection of multiple sclerosis. *J. Clin. Neurophysiol.* **50**, 247–53.

Ross Russell, R. W. and Page, N. G. R. (1983). Critical perfusion of brain and retina. *Brain* **106**, 419–34.

Savoiardo, J. W., Bracchi, M., Passerini, A., Visciani, A., DiDonato, S., and Cocchinni, F. (1983). Computed tomography of olivopontocerebellar atrophy. *Am. J. Neuroradiol.* **4**, 509–12.

Shy, G. M. and Drager, G. A. (1960). A neurological syndrome associated with orthostatic hypotension. *Arch. Neurol., Chicago* **3**, 511–27.

Thomas, D. J. and Bannister, R. (1980). Preservation of autoregulation of cerebral blood flow in autonomic failure. *J. neurol. Sci.* **44**, 205–12.

Turkka, J. (1986). Autonomic dysfunction in Parkinson's disease. *Acta universitatis ouluensis* **D142**, 15–66.

Vamatsu, D., Hamada, J., and Gotoh, F. (1987). Brainstem auditory evoked responses and CT findings in multiple system atrophy. *J. neurol. Sci.* **77**, 161–71.

Williams, A., Hanson, D., and Calne, D. B. (1979). Vocal cord paralysis in the Shy–Drager syndrome. *J. Neurol. Neurosurg. Psychiatr.* **42**, 151–3.

29. Special investigations in multiple system atrophy

A. Positron emission tomography (PET) studies

David J. Brooks

Introduction

Neurodegenerative conditions associated with autonomic failure include pure autonomic failure (PAF), Parkinson's disease (PD), and multiple system atrophy (MSA). The pathologies of PD and MSA are distinct. In PD degeneration of pigmented brainstem nuclei, sympathetic ganglia, and the nucleus accumbens occurs, and Lewy neuronal inclusion bodies are found (Bethlem and den Hartog Jager 1960). MSA is associated with neuronal loss from the striatum, pallidum, pigmented brainstem nuclei, dentate nuclei, and intermediolateral columns of the spinal cord, in the absence of neuronal inclusion bodies (Spokes *et al.* 1979). Those few PAF patients who have come to autopsy have shown degeneration of the intermediolateral columns of the spinal cord similar to that found in MSA, but Lewy bodies have also been reported in the substantia nigra and sympathetic ganglia (Johnson *et al.* 1966; Vanderhaeghen *et al.* 1970). It can be seen, therefore, that the reported pathology of PAF has shown some overlap features with both that of MSA and PD.

Clinically the three syndromes of PAF, PD, and MSA also overlap. All three are associated with autonomic failure, though this is rarely a presenting feature of PD. MSA and PD result in an akinetic-rigid syndrome, and in some MSA patients this shows a good and sustained response to L-dopa. It has been estimated that about 10 per cent of patients confidently diagnosed as having PD on clinical grounds turn out to have MSA at post-mortem (Quinn 1989). A second area of clinical confusion is over whether striatonigral degeneration (SND) and olivopontocerebellar atrophy (OPCA) are distinct syndromes, or whether they comprise part of the spectrum of MSA. At post-mortem, patients clinically diagnosed as SND are frequently found to have subclinical cerebellar, and patients diagnosed as OPCA subclinical striatonigral, degeneration.

Positron emission tomography (PET) provides a means of studying regional cerebral blood flow, metabolism, and neurotransmitter function *in vivo*.

The functional resolution of current commercial PET scanners ranges from 3 to 8 mm. In order to perform PET studies it is necessary to tag suitable biological substrates with a short-lived positron-emitting isotope. ^{15}O ($t_{1/2} = 2$ min) can be used to label $C^{15}O_2$ and $H_2^{15}O$ for blood flow measurements, and $^{15}O_2$ for measurements of regional cerebral oxygen metabolism (rCMRO$_2$). There is no positron-emitting isotope of hydrogen, but ^{18}F ($t_{1/2} = 110$ min) bound covalently to carbon behaves chemically like C–H. The tracer ^{18}F-2-fluoro-2-deoxy-D-glucose (FDG) is a positron-emitting analogue of D-glucose which is transported across the blood–brain barrier by the hexose carrier and trapped as FDG-6-phosphate. As a consequence the regional cerebral distribution of ^{18}F after administration of FDG reflects levels of regional cerebral glucose metabolism (rCMRGlu).

^{11}C ($t_{1/2} = 20$ min) can be used to label many pharmacological agents. ^{11}C-nomifensine and ^{11}C-raclopride are reversible antagonists of presynaptic dopamine re-uptake and postsynaptic dopamine D$_2$ receptors, respectively. ^{18}F-6-fluorodopa (FD) is a PET analogue of L-dopa and is transported into caudate and putamen where it is stored as ^{18}F-dopamine and its metabolites. Striatal FD and ^{11}C-nomifensine uptake thus provide a measure of the functional integrity of nigrostriatal dopaminergic nerve terminals, while striatal ^{11}C-raclopride uptake reflects integrity of the postsynaptic dopaminergic system.

In this chapter the role of PET for examining and contrasting the patterns of disruption of the regional cerebral blood flow (rCBF), metabolism, and the pre- and post-synaptic dopaminergic system in PAF, PD, and MSA will be presented. It will be argued that PET can provide a potential means of distinguishing the functional effects of these conditions where diagnostic doubt still remains. The relationship between SND and OPCA will also be considered and evidence suggesting that they are separate conditions will be presented.

Regional cerebral metabolism

PET measurements of regional cerebral oxygen and glucose metabolism with $^{15}O_2$ and FDG primarily reflect the metabolic activity of synaptic vesicles in nerve terminals. Consequently levels of basal ganglia rCMRO$_2$ and rCMRGlu provide a measure of metabolic activity of afferent projections to those nuclei, and of their interneurons, but do not reflect activity of basal ganglia efferent projections. Regional cerebral blood flow, which is coupled to metabolism, also reflects synaptic activity.

In L-dopa responsive hemiparkinsonian patients, who have early disease, PET shows increased oxygen and glucose metabolism in the lentiform nucleus contralateral to the affected limbs (Brooks and Frackowiak 1989). In primates destruction of the nigra compacta has been shown to cause a selective increase in external pallidal glucose utilization (Crossman 1990). These findings suggest that the nigrostriatal dopaminergic system normally exerts an inhibitory action on striato-external pallidal projections, and this is removed in PD. When PD patients with more longstanding bilateral disease are studied, the blood flow and metabolism of the lentiform nuclei generally lie within normal limits. It is likely, therefore, that the increased lentiform metabolism seen in early PD is a transient phenomenon, adaptive mechanisms or treatment returning this to normal in time.

Levels of cortical metabolism of PD patients correlate with their psychometric performance (Brooks and Frackowiak 1989). Non-demented PD patients have either normal cortical function or mild frontal hypometabolism. Typically, FDG scans of demented PD patients show a cortical pattern of dysfunction similar to that found for patients with Alzheimer's disease, the posterior parietal and temporal areas being most affected. Currently it remains unclear whether these demented PD patients have coincident Alzheimer's disease, or whether their cortical dysfunction is a consequence of the diffuse Lewy body disease that is present in many of these subjects.

De Volder *et al.* (1989) have studied regional cerebral glucose utilization in seven cases of probable SND. All these subjects had a poorly L-dopa responsive akinetic-rigid syndrome, but no evidence of a supranuclear gaze disorder. Two of the patients had additional autonomic failure and cerebellar ataxia and so clinically had MSA. The group of seven SND patients showed mean 46 and 36 per cent reductions in putamen and caudate glucose metabolism, respectively. These findings contrast with PD where striatal metabolism is generally normal. There was also a global 20 per cent decrease in cortical glucose utilization in the SND group, frontal cortex being most severely affected. Cerebellar metabolism was normal in five of the SND patients, but reduced in the two with clinical evidence of ataxia.

Fulham *et al.* (1991) have examined rCMRGlu in seven MSA patients with predominant cerebellar ataxia and autonomic failure and found significantly reduced mean cerebellar and frontal glucose utilization. Mean striatal metabolism was normal in their MSA patients, though only one of these seven had significant rigidity clinically. These workers also scanned eight PAF patients (clinical disease duration 5–26 years) and found normal levels of rCMRGlu. PET may well, therefore, provide a means of determining whether patients presenting with autonomic failure have PAF or MSA, though a prospective study will be necessary to answer this question.

To summarize, patients with MSA show either significant depression of striatal or cerebellar glucose utilization depending on whether an akinetic-rigid or ataxic syndrome predominates clinically. Striatal metabolism is normal in PD and PAF, but non-demented PD and MSA patients may show frontal hypometabolism. PET measurements of rCMRGlu have the potential for distinguishing MSA from PAF and PD where clinical doubt is present.

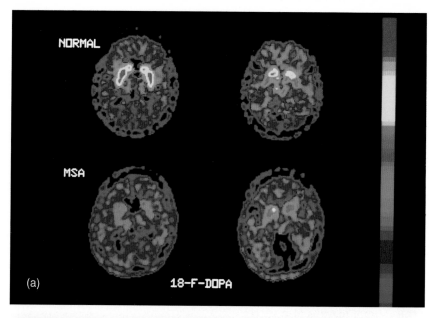

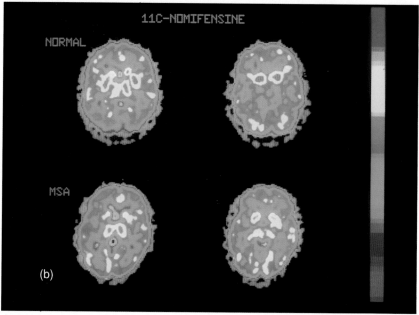

Fig. 29.1.(a) Striatal ^18F-6-fluorodopa (FD) uptake in patient with MSA and normal subject. (b) Striatal uptake of the dopamine re-uptake inhibitor ^11C-nomifensine (NMF) in an MSA patient and a normal subject.

Integrity of the dopaminergic system

Brooks et al. (1990b) studied striatal FD uptake in 10 patients with MSA. All had autonomic failure and a poorly L-dopa responsive akinetic-rigid syndrome, and seven had cerebellar ataxia. Figure 29.1 (a) shows striatal FD uptake in one such MSA patient and a normal control. It can be seen that the MSA patient has uniformly depressed striatal tracer uptake. For the 10 MSA patients mean putamen FD uptake was 41 per cent and caudate 56 per cent of normal. Loss of putamen FD uptake correlated with the degree of disability of these subjects on the Hoehn and Yahr scale, and with their clinical disease duration. A group of eight equivalently disabled L-dopa responsive PD patients showed a similar reduction in putamen FD uptake to the MSA group (38 per cent of normal) but their caudate FD uptake was relatively spared (73 per cent of normal). This differential involvement of caudate FD uptake in MSA and PD is in line with pathological findings in these conditions (Goto et al. 1989). It has been shown that in PD the ventrolateral nigra is targeted, resulting in selective loss of putamen dopamine. In MSA the ventrolateral nigra is also severely involved, but nigral cell loss tends to be more extensive. In a follow-up study involving 18 MSA and 16 PD patients Brooks et al. (1990a) found that loss of caudate FD uptake also correlated with locomotor disability in these conditions.

Figure 29.1 (b) shows striatal uptake of the dopamine re-uptake inhibitor ^{11}C-nomifensine (NMF) in a normal subject and an MSA patient. It can be seen that, as with FD, striatal NMF uptake is severely reduced in both MSA caudate and putamen, but uptake by noradrenergic re-uptake receptors in the thalamus is preserved. Striatal uptake of NMF in groups of MSA and PD patients gave parallel results to that of FD (Salmon et al.1990). Both groups had mean specific:non-specific levels of putamen tracer uptake that were 42 per cent of normal, but, while caudate function was severely affected in MSA (56 per cent of normal), it was again relatively spared in PD (75 per cent of normal). The similar striatal uptake of NMF and FD in MSA and PD confirms that both these tracers provide a measure of functional integrity of the presynaptic dopaminergic striatal nerve terminals. While mean specific putamen FD and NMF uptake is reduced to 40 per cent of normal in both PD and MSA, putamen dopamine levels at post-mortem are far lower (around 10 per cent of normal). It must be remembered, however, that striatal binding of FD and NMF reflects dopa-decarboxylase activity and dopamine re-uptake site integrity, respectively, and not the tyrosine hydroxylase activity which determines endogenous levels of striatal dopamine.

Seven patients with pure autonomic failure of clinical duration 1–12 years also had FD PET (Brooks et al. 1990b). Mean striatal FD uptake for the group was normal, arguing against PAF being a forme fruste of either PD or MSA. One of the seven PAF patients, however, had putamen FD uptake

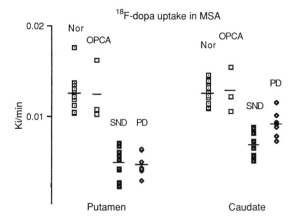

Fig. 29.2. Individual striatal FD influx constants for controls, Parkinson's disease (PD) patients, and MSA patients divided into those with an akinetic-rigid syndrome without ataxia (SND) or cerebellar ataxia without rigidity (OPCA).

reduced $> 2\,SD$ below the normal mean implying that subclinical nigral pathology was present. His autonomic failure had been clinically evident for 7 years without any associated rigidity or ataxia. In the year following PET he developed stridor and died of pneumonia, but, unfortunately, no post-mortem was obtained.

Figure 29.2 shows individual striatal FD influx constants for controls, PD patients, and MSA patients with autonomic failure divided into subgroups with either an akinetic-rigid syndrome without ataxia (SND) or cerebellar ataxia without rigidity (OPCA). It can be seen that none of the three sporadic OPCA cases showed evidence of reduced striatal FD uptake. It has been suggested that OPCA and SND are extremes of a continuous spectrum in MSA. Our finding of normal striatal FD uptake in OPCA, combined with the finding of normal striatal metabolism in the OPCA cases of Fulham *et al.* (1991) and normal cerebellar metabolism in the five SND cases without ataxia of de Volder *et al.* (1989) would support the existence of OPCA and SND as separate conditions on occasion.

Equilibrium striatal:cerebellum ^{11}C-raclopride (RAC) uptake ratios reflect striatal D_2 receptor density (Brooks *et al.* 1991). Table 29.1 shows mean striatal:cerebellum RAC uptake ratios for groups of controls, untreated PD patients, PD patients with fluctuating (on–off) responses to L-dopa, and patients with probable SND. It can be seen that the untreated PD patients had normal or raised levels of striatal D_2 receptors, while those with longstanding disease and a fluctuating response to L-dopa showed a fall in putamen and caudate D_2 binding sites. The poorly L-dopa responsive SND group, four out of eight of whom were on regular treatment at the time of PET, showed significantly reduced putamen and caudate RAC binding.

Table 29.1. Mean striatal:cerebellar ^{11}C-raclopride uptake ratios in PD and SND

	Caudate (mean ± SD)	Putamen (mean ± SD)
Controls (8)	3.78 ± 0.32	3.72 ± 0.36
PD untreated (6)	3.79 ± 0.33	4.24 ± 0.59
PD on–off (5)	2.64 ± 0.48**	3.04 ± 0.52**
SND (10)	3.40 ± 0.28	3.32 ± 0.42*

Student's t test: *$P<0.05$ compared to normal; **$P<0.005$ compared to normal.

These data are in broad agreement with pathological findings; untreated PD patients have been reported to have normal or raised striatal D_2 receptor levels, and PD patients with a fluctuating response to treatment reduced D_2 receptor levels, respectively. Only one study on MSA has been reported; caudate alone was examined and showed reduced D_2 sites (Quik et al. 1979).

To summarize, the majority of PAF patients have an intact nigrostriatal dopaminergic system, arguing against this condition being a variant of PD or MSA in spite of some pathological similarities. PET is capable, however, of detecting subclinical nigral lesions in these patients when present. PD and MSA both show severe loss of putamen FD and NMF uptake, but there is relative sparing of caudate presynaptic dopaminergic function in PD compared to MSA. Striatal D_2 receptors are intact in untreated PD patients and down-regulated in PD patients with a fluctuating response to treatment. SND patients show degeneration of striatal D_2 sites. PET studies of both regional cerebral metabolism and the integrity of the pre- and post-synaptic dopaminergic system provide a potential tool for distinguishing PAF, PD, and MSA patients where clinical uncertainty exists.

B. Biopsy of sympathetic terminals
Roger Bannister

Defective sympathetic reflexes underlie the postural hypotension of autonomic failure (AF) but there remains uncertainty about the precise site of the lesion in the sympathetic pathways. The problem of the site of the lesion is also of clinical importance because the extent of peripheral denervation determines the supersensitivity to pressor drugs which are often used in treatment (Davies et al. 1978). The plasma noradrenaline is low in many cases of autonomic failure and fails to rise on tilting, suggesting a defect of release of noradrenaline from sympathetic vascular endings (Bannister *et al.* 1977; Ziegler *et al.* 1977).

In deltoid muscle from five patients with PAF, Kontos *et al.* (1975) found no catecholamine fluorescence in perivascular nerves. These patients also failed to show any constrictor response in forearm arterioles to intraarterial infusion of tyramine, but were supersensitive to noradrenaline. Rubenstein *et al.* (1978) reported preliminary findings of a similar lack of fluorescence in one case of PAF but found fluorescence in two cases of AF with MSA. Nanda *et al.* (1976) found that in three cases of AF with MSA perivascular catecholamine fluorescence was absent from the palmaris longus and quadriceps biopsies. However, it was present in three other patients, one with AF and MSA and two with apparent PAF. One of the patients with PAF appeared to have a unique defect of noradrenaline release, identified by the lack of response to tyramine but normal catecholamine staining (Nanda *et al.* 1977). The findings suggested failure of noradrenaline release, though noradrenaline synthesis and storage were normal.

We analysed the results of muscle biopsies studied by catecholamine fluorescence and electron microscopy in 10 patients with autonomic failure in whom the defects of cardiovascular reflexes were known (Bannister *et al.* 1981). Six had AF with MSA and four had PAF. The specimens were studied by electron microscopy by Dr R. Eames and special histochemical techniques by Dr R. Crowe (Falk *et al.* 1962; Axelsson *et al.* 1973).

In the control human biopsies and in animal tissues, green varicose fluorescent adrenergic nerve fibres were observed on the adventitial side of the media of arteries (Fig. 29.3 (a), (b)) and veins (diam. 20–200 μm) appeared to be either sparsely innervated or not innervated at all. In most of the arteries autofluorescence was observed in the intima and elastic and collagen fibres. In sections of control tissue examined, more than 85 per cent of the vessels showed some positive fluorescence for catecholamine-containing nerves, whereas in the cases of AF only 2–7 per cent of the arteries and veins (diam. 40–150 μm) were innervated by adrenergic nerves (Fig. 29.3 (c)–(f)). In these vessels, the number of fluorescent nerve bundles observed was approximately 35 per cent of those observed in vessels in the control biopsies. There was no obvious difference in the intensity of fluorescence in the nerves that were observed.

The electron microscopic studies were technically more difficult and insufficient numbers of nerve profiles were available for quantitative analysis. Prolonged searching was necessary to find vessels of a size (100 μm) in which catecholamine fluorescence is normally present and a region where a varicosity was seen in cross-section. In two control biopsies, large granular, small clear, and small granular (adrenergic) vesicles were seen in proportions comparable to those described in other sympathetic nerves (Furness 1973; Burnstock 1975*a,b*) and no preparations showed a scanty population of vesicles such

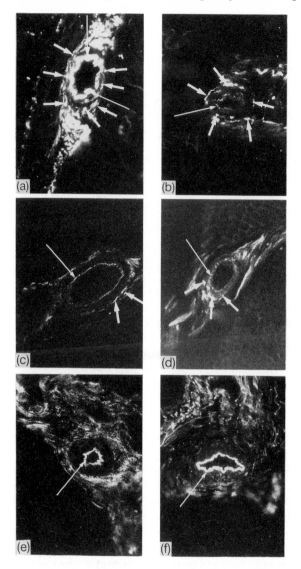

Fig. 29.3. Catecholamine fluorescent nerves associated with blood vessels of human quadriceps muscle. (a) and (b) Control tissue. Note adrenergic nerves on the adventitial side of the media (thick white) of the arteries. Autofluorescence (thin white) can be seen in the intima. Fluorescent micrograph (a) 180 × ; (b) 174 × . (c)–(f) Tissue from patients with autonomic failure. (c) and (d) Note few adrenergic nerves are present on the adventitial–medial border (thick white) of the arteries. Autofluorescence can be seen in the intima (thin white). Fluorescent micrograph. (c) 134 × ; (d) 188 × . (e) and (f) Note lack of adrenergic nerves in the arteries although autofluorescence can be seen, especially in the intima. Fluorescent micrograph. (e) and (f) 134 × . (Taken with permission from Bannister *et al.* (1981).)

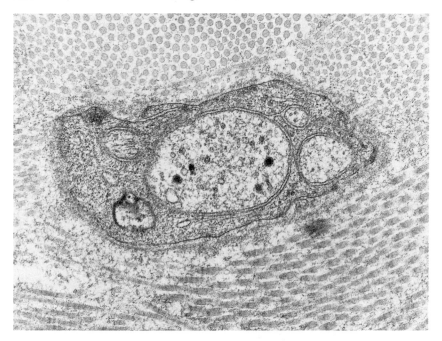

Fig. 29.4. From patient with pure autonomic failure. Electron micrograph showing high-powered views of nerve ending close to blood vessel. The ending shows a marked reduction in the number of vesicles of all three types. 28 500 × ; 5-OHD incubated. (Taken with permission from Bannister *et al.* (1981).

as occurred in the cases of autonomic failure. In one patient with PAF, the sympathetic nerve terminals showed normal general morphology but contained only scanty vesicles, both of the small dense and small clear types (Fig. 29.4). This was the most severe abnormality found. In the case of AF with MSA there were less severe changes although the small dense vesicles were also much reduced in number (Fig. 29.3). In different patients the changes ranged between severe (Fig. 29.4) and moderate (Fig. 29.5). The specimens in the two cases of PAF in which satisfactory electron microscopic material was available were pre-treated with 5-hydroxydopamine but the controls and the three cases of AF with MSA were not so treated. The low number of small dense vesicles in PAF is therefore likely to be significant but the problem of sampling errors makes the study of more patients necessary. Lack of fluorescence cannot, of course, be taken to indicate absence of adrenergic nerves; it may simply mean that noradrenaline levels in intact nerves are below the levels detectable with the formaldehyde method. Despite these problems our results suggest that marked reduction of catecholamine fluorescence is a feature of all moderate or severe cases of AF irrespective of the coexistence of central lesions in MSA which reduce

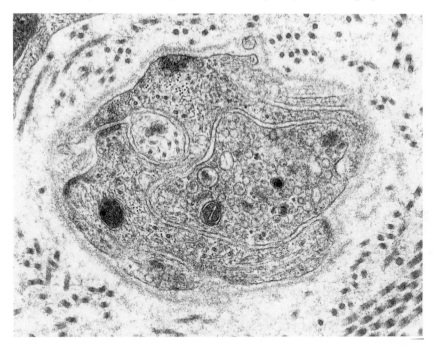

Fig. 29.5.   From a patient with autonomic failure and multiple system atrophy. Electron micrograph showing high-powered view of nerve endings close to small blood vessels. Schwann cell partly enclosing adrenergic axon which contains reduced numbers of vesicles of all three types and a single mitochondrion. 37 500 ×. (Taken with permission from Bannister *et al.* (1981).)

central sympathetic impulse traffic. These results are consistent with the failure of tyramine to release detectable amounts of noradrenaline after an infusion rate which causes a pressor response, in contrast with a 50 per cent rise in plasma noradrenaline in normal subjects (Bannister *et al.* 1979). These observations are also consistent with the fact that small doses of fludro-cortisone, insufficient to increase body weight or plasma volume, increase the sensitivity of vascular receptors to exogenous (intravenous) noradrenaline infusion (Davies *et al.* 1978, 1979). Our results suggest that patients with PAF had more extreme degeneration of adrenergic nerves than patients with AF and MSA but it would be necessary to study a larger number of biopsies to establish this quantitatively, with allowance made for the progression of the disease. Since the catecholamine fluorescence was much reduced, even in the most mildly affected patients, it seems probable that the pathological changes start as soon as or even before symptoms are clinically apparent.

Further types of autonomic failure with specific defects located to the sympathetic terminals have been described. Klein *et al.* (1980), while confirming the lack of perivascular noradrenergic vesicles in three cases of

PAF, described two patients with low levels of circulating noradrenaline but with a hyperadrenergic response to standing, with normal noradrenaline perivascular stores on catecholamine histochemistry and electron microscopy. They proposed a possible blunting of the response of the α-receptor of smooth muscle.

C. Biopsy of muscle

Roger Bannister, Marjorie Ellison, and John Morgan-Hughes

Introduction

Muscle wasting was reported in the original description by Shy and Drager of two cases of the syndrome which now bears their name, autonomic failure with multiple system atrophy. Since then there have been no systematic studies of muscle biopsy changes but a few isolated reports of electromyographic studies and nerve and muscle biopsies. There are several reports of electromyographic signs of degeneration in MSA (Montagna *et al.* 1983). Reports of nerve biopsies in MSA are rare but Toghi *et al.* (1982) found selective loss of small myelinated and unmyelinated fibres in three cases of MSA by comparison with control patients with olivopontocerebellar degeneration without autonomic dysfunction. Galassi *et al.* (1982) described loss of both large and small fibres in a sural–nerve biopsy in a single case of MSA. An anterior tibial muscle biopsy showed chronic neurogenic changes with large fields of atrophic fibres of the same histological type. However, loss of anterior horn cells has been reported in half the neuropathological reports of MSA (see Chapter 30). There is also evidence that, rarely, the muscle wasting in MSA may be part of a mild distal sensorimotor neuropathy (Cohen *et al.* 1987). In the hope of throwing some light on this aspect of the curiously selective degeneration of neurons in MSA, advantage was taken of a previous investigation into the catecholamine fluorescence and electron microscopy of muscle blood vessels (Bannister *et al.* 1981) to study striated muscle, taking advantage of modern histochemical techniques.

Muscle biopsy findings

The biopsies of the quadriceps femoris muscle were examined in 10 patients with MSA, using a battery of histochemical reactions. Fibre diameters were measured with a digitized pit pad on an image analyser. Three patients showed atrophy of type 2a and type 2b fibres, one patient showed selective type 2b atrophy, and in a fifth case the type 1 and type 2b fibres were atrophic (Figs 29.6 and 29.7). The variation in selective fibre-type atrophy could not be

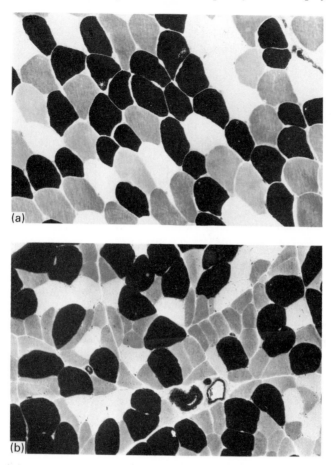

Fig. 29.6. Transverse sections of the vastus lateralis muscle from (a) a normal human control and (b) a patient with MSA stained with the ATPase reaction at pH 4.35. The type 1 fibres are dark, the type 2a fibres are light, and the type 2b fibres are intermediate. Note the presence of type 2a and type 2b muscle-fibre atrophy in the patient.

correlated with the clinical features of the patients nor with their age. The muscle biopsy appearances and fibre-diameter histograms were entirely normal in the remaining five cases, except that one case showed early grouping of the type 1 muscle fibres. Again this patient was not in any other way atypical of the entire group. The morphometric changes were not related to age, as the patients with the selective fibre-type atrophy were generally younger than those with normal fibre diameters.

A biopsy was taken from only one patient with PAF. The patient was a 68-year-old man who had had postural hypotension for 20 years, without

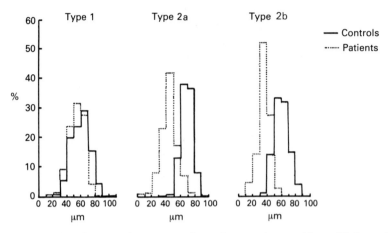

Fig. 29.7. Fibre diameter histograms from three patients with multiple system atrophy to show selective atrophy of the type 2a and type 2b fibres (interrupted line). Three age-matched controls are shown for comparison (continuous lines). Between 400 and 450 muscle fibres were measured in each case.

other significant neurological symptoms or signs apart from impotence. His muscle biopsy was studied by the same histochemical techniques as used for the patients with MSA and there were no abnormalities.

Discussion

The pattern of histochemical muscle fibre responses in human quadriceps is well established (Mahon *et al.* 1984; Dorriguzzi *et al.* 1986). The type of selective fibre atrophy seen in half the patients with MSA is quite abnormal. It is unlike the large-group atrophy or small-group atrophy seen in motor neuron disease, a disease with which, in some clinical respects, it might be thought to have some similarities (Dubowitz 1981; Jennekens 1982). Nor is there a suggestion of type grouping with large clusters of different fibre types adjacent to each other as occurs in regeneration as a result of sprouting. Perhaps a closer parallel is the selective fibre-type atrophy which sometimes occurs in myasthenia gravis (Aström and Adams 1981). Selective fibre atrophy itself is a rather non-specific type of change seen in a range of diverse disease pathologies from steroid or alcoholic myopathy to collagen vascular disease.

It could be argued that in MSA there is a preferential selective involvement of type 2a and 2b neurons by a process that in general seems to spare type 1 neurons and is not associated with sprouting and reinnervation. The morphological appearances of the anterior horn cells giving rise to each type of motor unit are not known. The number of neurons which need to be affected to produce changes of this type may be small, in that up to 1000 muscle fibres in the human quadriceps may be innervated from a single neuron. In MSA the anterior horn cells have not been systematically counted in the same way as intermediolateral column cells and so mild reductions in the number of these cells may have been missed.

References

Aström, K. E. and Adams, R. D. (1981). Pathology of human skeletal muscle. In *Disorders of voluntary muscle* (ed. J. N. Walton), pp. 151–208. Churchill Livingstone, Edinburgh.

Axelsson, S., Bjorklund, A., and Falck, B. (1973). Glyoxylic acid: a new fluorescence method for the histochemical demonstration of biogenic monoamines. *Acta physiol. scand.* **87**, 57–62.

Bannister, R., Sever, P., and Gross, M. (1977). Cardiovascular reflexes and biochemical responses in progressive autonomic failure. *Brain* **100**, 327–44.

Bannister, R., Davies, B., Holly, E., Rosenthal, T., and Sever, P. (1979). Defective cardiovascular reflexes and supersensitivity to sympathomimetic drugs in autonomic failure. *Brain* **102**, 163–76.

Bannister, R., Crowe, R., Eames, R., and Burnstock, G. (1981). Adrenergic innervation in autonomic failure. *Neurology, Minneapolis* **31**, 1501–6.

Bethlem, J. and den Hartog Jager, W. A. (1960). The incidence and characteristics of Lewy bodies in idiopathic paralysis agitans (Parkinson's disease). *J. Neurol. Neurosurg. Psychiatr.* **23**, 74–80.

Brooks, D. J. and Frackowiak, R. S. J. (1989). PET and movement disorders. *J. Neurol. Neurosurg.* **52** (special suppl.), 68–77.

Brooks, D. J., Ibanez, V., Sawle, G. V., Quinn, N., Lees, A. J., Mathias, C. J., Bannister, R., Marsden, C. D., and Frackowiak, R. S. J. (1990a). Differing patterns of striatal ^{18}F-dopa uptake in Parkinson's disease, multiple system atrophy, and progressive supranuclear palsy. *Ann. Neurol.* **28**, 547–55.

Brooks, D. J., Salmon, E. P., Mathias, C. J., Quinn, N., Leenders, K. L., Bannister, R., Marsden, C. D., and Frackowiak, R. S. J. (1990b). The relationship between locomotor disability, autonomic dysfunction, and the integrity of the striatal dopaminergic system in patients with multiple system atrophy, pure autonomic failure, and Parkinson's disease studied with PET. *Brain* **113**, 1539–52.

Brooks, D. J., Ibanez, V., Sawle, G. V., Playford, E. D., Quinn, N., Mathias, C. J., Lees, A. J., Marsden, C. D., Bannister R., and Frackowiak, R. S. J. (1991). Striatal D_2 receptor status in Parkinson's disease, striatonigral degeneration, and progressive supranuclear palsy, measured with ^{11}C-raclopride and PET. *Ann. Neurol.* (In press).

Burnstock, G. (1975a). Innervation of vascular smooth muscle: histochemistry and electron microscopy. In *Physiological and pharmacological control of blood pressure*, IUPS Symposium, October 1974. *Clin. exp. Pharmacol. Physiol.* **Suppl. 2**, 7–20.

Burnstock, G. (1975b). Control of smooth muscle activity in vessels by adrenergic nerves and circulating catecholamines. In *Smooth muscle pharmacology and physiology*. Vol. 50, pp. 251–60. INSERM, Paris.

Cohen, J., Low, P., Fealey, R., Sheps, S., and Jiang, N-S. (1987). Somatic and autonomic function in progressive autonomic failure. *Ann. Neurol.* **22**, 692–9.

Crossman, A. R. (1990). A hypothesis on the pathological mechanisms that underlie levadopa or dopamine agonist induced dyskinesia in Parkinson's disease. Implications for future strategy in treatment. *Movement Disorders* **5**, 100–8.

Davies, B., Bannister, R., and Sever, P. (1978). Pressor amines and monoamine oxidase inhibitors for treatment of postural hypotension in autonomic failure. *Lancet* **i**, 172–5.

Davies, B., Bannister, R., and Sever, P. (1979). The pressor actions of noradrenaline, angiotensin II and saralasin in chronic autonomic failure treated with fludrocortisone. *Br. J. clin. Pharmacol.* **8**, 253–60.

DeVolder, A. G., Francard, J., Laterre, C., Dooms, G., Bol, A., Michel, C., and Goffinet, A. M. (1989). Decreased glucose utilisation in the striatum and frontal lobe in probable striatonigral degeneration. *Ann. Neurol.* **26**, 239–47.

Dorriguzzi, C. P., Palmucci, L., Mongini, T., Leone, M., Gagnor, E., Gagliano, A., and Schiffer, D. (1986). Quantitative analysis of quadriceps muscle biopsy. *J. neurol. Sci.* **72**, 201–9.

Dubowitz, V. (1981). Histochemistry of muscle disease. In *Disorders of voluntary muscle* (ed. J. N. Walton), pp. 261–95. Churchill Livingstone, Edinburgh.

Falk, B., Hillarp, N. A., and Thiem, G. (1962). Fluorescence of catecholamines and related compounds condensed with formaldehyde. *J. Histochem. Cytochem.* **10**, 348–54.

Fulham, M. J., Dubinsky, R. M., Polinsky, R. J., Brooks, R. A., Brown, R. T., Curras, M. T., Baser, S. M., Hallett, M., and Di Chiro, G. (1991). Assessment of multiple system atrophy and pure autonomic failure with CT, MRI, and PET–FDG. *Clin. autonom. Res.* **1**, 27–36.

Furness, J. B. (1973) Arrangement of blood vessels and their relation with adrenergic nerves in the rat mesentery. *J. Anat.* **115**, 437–64.

Galassi, G., Nemni, R., Baraldi, A., Gibertoni, M., and Columbo, A. (1982). Peripheral neuropathy in multiple system atrophy with autonomic failure. *Neurology, NY* **32**, 1116–20.

Goto, S., Hirano, A., and Matsumoto, S. (1989). Subdivisional involvement of nigrostriatal loop in idiopathic Parkinson's disease and striatonigral degeneration. *Ann. Neurol.* **26**, 766–70.

Jennekens, F. G. I. (1982). Muscle histochemistry. In *Skeletal muscle pathology* (ed. F. L. Mastaglia and J. N. Walton), pp. 204–34. Churchill Livingstone, London.

Johnson, R. H., Lee, G. de J., Oppenheimer, D. R., and Spalding, J. M. K. (1966). Autonomic failure with orthostatic hypotension due to intermediolateral column degeneration: a report of two cases with autopsies. *Quart. J. Med.* **35**, 276–92.

Klein, R. L., Baggett, J. McM., Thureson, K. Å., and Langford, H. G. (1980). Idiopathic orthostatic hypotension: circulating noradrenaline and ultrastructure of saphenous vein. *J. autonom. nerv. Syst.* **2**, 205–22.

Kontos, H. A., Richardson, D. W., and Narvell, J. E. (1975). Norepinephrine depletion in idiopathic orthostatic hypotension. *Ann. intern. Med.* **82**, 336–41.

Mahon, M., Toman, A., Willan, P. L. T., and Bagnall, K. M. (1984). Variability of the histochemical and morphometric data from needle biopsy specimens of human quadriceps. *J. neurol. Sci.* **63**, 85–100.

Montagna, P., Martinelli, P., Rizzuto, N., Salviati, A., Rasi, F., and Lugaresi, E. (1983). Amyotrophy in Shy–Drager syndrome. *Acta neurol. belg.* **83**, 142–57.

Nanda, R. N., Boyle, R. C., Gillespie, J. S., Johnson, R. M., and Keogh, H. J. (1976). Adrenergic innervation of peripheral blood vessels in patients with neurogenic orthostatic hypotension. *J. Neuropathol. appl. Neurobiol.* **2**, 49.

Nanda, R. N., Boyle, R. C., Gillespie, J. S., Johnson, R. M., and Keogh, H. J. (1977). Idiopathic orthostatic hypotension from failure of noradrenaline release in a patient with vasomotor innervation. *J. Neurol. Neurosurg. Psychiatr.* **40**, 11–19.

Quik, M., Spokes, E., Mackay, A., and Bannister, R. (1979). Alterations in ³H-spiperone binding in human caudate nucleus, substantia nigra, and frontal cortex in the Shy–Drager syndrome and Parkinson's disease. *J. neurol. Sci.* **43**, 429–37.

Quinn, N. (1989). Multiple system atrophy—the nature of the beast. *J. Neurol. Neurosurg. Psychiatr.* **52** (special suppl.), 78–89.

Rubenstein, A. E., Yahr, M. D., and Mytilineou, C. (1978). Peripheral adrenergic hypersensitivity in orthostatic hypotension: the effects of denervation versus decentralization. *Neurology, Minneapolis* **28**, 376.

Salmon, E. P., Brooks, D. J., Leenders, K. L., Turton, D. R., Hume, S. P., Cremer, J. E., Jones, T., and Frackowiak, R. S. J. (1990). A two-compartment description and kinetic procedure for measuring regional cerebral [¹¹C] nomifensine uptake using positron emission tomography. *J. cerebral blood flow Metab.* **10**, 307–16.

Spokes, E. G. S., Bannister, R., and Oppenheimer, D. R. (1979). Multiple system atrophy with autonomic failure: clinical, histological, and neurochemical observations in four cases. *J. neurol. Sci.* **43**, 59–82.

Toghi, H., Tabuchi, M., Tomonaga, M., and Izumiyana, N. (1982). Selective loss of small myelinated and unmyelinated fibres in Shy–Drager syndrome. *Acta neuropathol., Berlin* **57**, 282–6.

Vanderhaeghen, J. J., Périer, O., and Sternon, J. E. (1970). Pathological findings in idiopathic orthostatic hypotension: its relationship with Parkinson's disease. *Arch. Neurol.* **22**, 207–14.

Ziegler, M. C., Lake, C. R., and Kopin, I. J. (1977). The sympathetic nervous system defect in primary orthostatic hypotension. *New Engl. J. Med.* **296**, 293–7.

30. The neuropathology and neurochemistry of multiple system atrophy

Susan E. Daniel

Introduction

Multiple system atrophy (MSA) is a primary degenerative disorder of the nervous system. The disease is characterized by asynchronous and progressive degeneration of 'at-risk' neurons which appear to be heterogeneous and are widely distributed in a selection of well-defined sites (Table 30.1). There is a considerable variety of pathology and for individual cases different selections of nuclear groups may be affected. In a large proportion of cases, when specifically looked for, nerve cell loss and gliosis occur at the following major sites: putamen, substantia nigra, basis pons, inferior olives, cerebellar folia and spinal cord intermediolateral column, and Onuf's nucleus. Neuronal degeneration without evidence of an inflammatory response is characteristic of the disease and there is no known association with any infectious, metabolic, or toxic agent.

Graham and Oppenheimer (1969) reported the clinicopathological findings of a patient with idiopathic hypotension and suggested use of the term MSA to encompass a group of presenile system degenerations which shared certain overlapping clinical and pathological features. In the original description of MSA, both familial and sporadic disease were included (Graham and Oppenheimer 1969). More recently, however, it has been recognized that familial examples are clinically distinct from the sporadic cases and only the latter are now included under the rubric of MSA. In a morphological classification the use of terms such as 'idiopathic orthostatic hypotension' and 'Shy–Drager syndrome' is best avoided.

Whether MSA represents variable expression of a single disease or several possibly related disease entities remains uncertain. The group as a whole is large and can be subclassified according to the predominant clinical signs of either parkinsonism—striatonigral degeneration (SND) type—or cerebellar involvement—olivopontocerebellar atrophy (OPCA) type. The relationship of such a classification to neuropathological findings remains to be fully elucidated. In my experience, patients with parkinsonism show a preponderance of pathology in the striatonigral system, while equal

Table 30.1.   Neuronal degeneration in MSA

Site	Severity	Reference*
Putamen	+ + +	
Caudate	+	
Pallidum	+	
Thalamus	±	Martin (1975); Borit *et al.* (1975)
Subthalamic nucleus	±	Andrews *et al.* (1970)
Hypothalamus	±	Shy and Drager (1960)
Cerebral cortex	±	Adams *et al.* (1969); Takei and Mirra (1973)
Substantia nigra	+ + +	
Edinger–Westphal nucleus	±	Shy and Drager (1960)
Pontine neurons	+ + +	
Locus ceruleus	+ +	
Vestibular nuclear complex	+	
Cerebellar cortex	+ + +	
Dentate nucleus	±	Berciano (1982); Mizutani *et al.* (1988)
Dorsal vagal nucleus	+ +	
Inferior olives	+ + +	
Arcuate nuclei	±	Takei and Mirra (1973); Berciano (1982)
Optic nerve/tract	±	Buonanno *et al.* (1975)
Intermediolateral cells	+ + +	
Onuf's nucleus	+ + +	
Anterior horn cells	+	
Clarke's nucleus	±	Sung *et al.* (1979)
Pyramidal tracts	+	
Sympathetic ganglia	±	Chapter 32
Sensory ganglia	±	Bannister and Oppenheimer (1972)
Peripheral nerves	±	Bannister and Oppenheimer (1972); Galassi *et al.* (1982)

±, loss in only some cases; +, commonly affected; + +, nearly always affected; + + +, always affected.
*Reference cited only where involvement is infrequently documented.

involvement of the striatonigral and olivopontocerebellar systems is more unusual. Patients with predominant cerebellar signs are less common; in these cases it appears that the principal pathology occurs in the olivopontocerebellar system with variable SND. In all varieties of MSA there is usually involvement of the autonomic nervous system which may precede any clinical signs of autonomic failure (Oppenheimer 1980). When pathology is confined to the autonomic nervous system the diagnosis of MSA cannot be made. However, many patients with MSA present with autonomic disturbance and it is conceivable that early in the course of the disease this might be the sole site of involvement.

The post-mortem in MSA

A complete general post-mortem and thorough neuropathological examination ensure that the best use can be made of available tissue. Knowledge of any coincidental disease together with the cause of death are essential and of particular importance for accurate interpretation of neurochemistry and *in situ* hybridization histochemistry. When there is a short post-mortem delay (usually less than 36 h) it is useful to freeze tissue; the brain is divided midsagittally and one-half frozen while the other half is formalin-fixed. Frozen tissue is required for biochemical investigations and is also preferable for many *in situ* hybridization studies. From a neuropathological viewpoint, the main limitation of such a procedure, as compared with using a fixed whole brain, is that it prevents the study of disease symmetry and of making a good clinico-anatomical correlation. Although the pathology of neurodegenerative diseases is generally symmetrical (Oppenheimer 1984) and this is often stated to be the case for MSA, it is worth noting that asymmetrical involvement of striatum and substantia nigra is occasionally reported (e.g. Adams *et al.* 1964; Fearnley and Lees 1990) and may have some relevance to clinical signs.

Once the tissue has been formalin-fixed and processed to paraffin wax, antigenicity is well preserved; thus archival material can be used for more recent histological techniques such as immunocytochemistry and *in situ* hybridization histochemistry.

Gross neuropathology of MSA

The external examination of the brain may be normal. However, when there is significant involvement of the olivopontocerebellar system the appearances are characteristic. The cerebellum is small with the hemispheres far from covering the occipital poles. The pons is reduced in size with a wedge-shaped appearance and there is atrophy of the middle cerebellar peduncles (Fig. 30.1). In the medulla the protuberances of the inferior olives may be reduced.

Brain weight is usually normal for age or only slightly reduced. The percentage weight of the detached brainstem and cerebellum to that of the whole brain is a useful indicator to the site of major pathology. In MSA

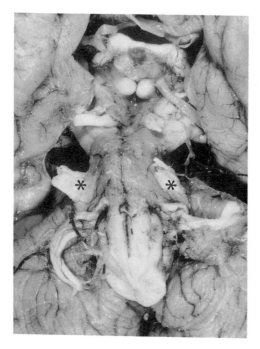

Fig. 30.1. Macroscopic appearance of the brainstem in MSA, from a 61 year-old female with disease lasting 10 years. The pons and middle cerebellar peduncles are atrophic and the trigeminal nerves (*) are prominent.

with predominant SND the proportion of brainstem and cerebellum to whole brain weight remains normal and comprises about 10 per cent; conversely with significant OPCA this percentage is considerably less.

Usually the diagnosis of MSA is evident when the brain is cut, although the extent of the disease cannot be fully appreciated before miscroscopic examination. In SND the putamina show orange-brown discoloration and are shrunken and, when pathology is severe, there may be a cribriform appearance resembling état lacunaire; atrophy and discoloration of the caudate nuclei and the pallida (Fig. 30.2) is less common. The substantia nigra invariably shows decreased pigmentation and the loci cerulei may also appear pale. In OPCA the basis pons and middle cerebellar peduncles are reduced (Fig. 30.3) while in the cerebellum white matter appears rather grey and the folia atrophic. Occasionally, macroscopic abnormality is confined to the brainstem pigmented nuclei and in these instances it is impossible to make a distinction from idiopathic Parkinson's disease (PD) on naked eye appearances alone.

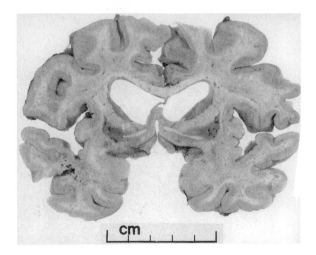

Fig. 30.2. Coronal slice of the brain at the level of anterior commissure, from a patient with MSA for 8 years. There is severe symmetrical atrophy of the caudate, putamen, and globus pallidus.

Microscopic neuropathology in MSA

Striatonigral degeneration (SND)

This condition was first described by Adams *et al.* (1961, 1964). The striatonigral system is the main site of pathology. However, it is important to emphasize that additional sites may also be involved (Oppenheimer 1984) although usually to a lesser degree.

The putamen shows a variable amount of nerve cell loss and astrocytic hyperplasia. In some cases the entire putamen may be affected (Figs 30.4(b) and 30.5), while in others gliosis is restricted to the lateral border and may be difficult to identify with certainty without the aid of immunostaining for glial fibrillary acidic protein (GFAP). Many reports suggest that the small neurons, which normally outnumber the large by about 170 to 1, are preferentially affected (e.g. Adams *et al.* 1964), while other workers describe equal depletion of both neuronal types (Fearnley and Lees 1990). When atrophy is severe the neuropil becomes rarefied with very few remaining nerve cells lying among hypertrophic astrocytes (Fig. 30.6); around blood vessels the perivascular spaces are widened (Fig. 30.5). Bundles of striopallidal fibres are narrowed and poorly stained for myelin (Fig. 30.4(b)). Much attention has been given to the nature of brown pigment granules (Fig. 30.6) which accumulate in astrocytes, macrophages, and around blood vessel walls; they have been identified as containing lipofuscin, neuromelanin, and acid

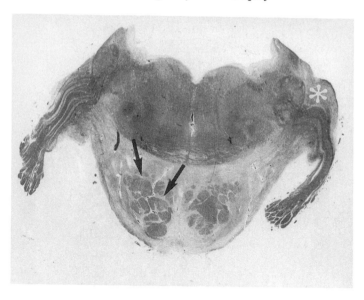

Fig. 30.3. Section of pons stained for myelin. The tegmentum is normal while the ventrodorsal diameter of basis pons is greatly reduced. Intact pyramidal tracts and trigeminal fibres stand out against more palely stained transverse fibres (arrows) and the middle cerebellar peduncle (*).

'haematin'. Borit *et al.* (1975) suggest that the neuromelanin may be derived from polymerization of dopamine in axon terminals of the nigrostriatal pathway, implying that the striatal lesion precedes nigral involvement. In my experience the amount of pigment may be quite variable but is usually greater than that associated with age and other neurodegenerative conditions, in particular, PD; furthermore, in these conditions pigment occurs predominantly in a perivascular distribution.

The putaminal lesion, like that of Huntington's disease (Richardson 1990), shows a distinct topographical distribution with a predilection for the posterior two-thirds and dorsolateral putamen (Adams *et al.* 1964; Takei and Mirra 1973). Fearnley and Lees (1990) have found that when atrophy is severe the ventral and anterolateral putamen are also involved. This characteristic pattern is seen in a large number of cases but exceptions do occur particularly with regard to the preponderance of dorsolateral over ventrolateral distribution.

In the caudate nucleus there is nerve cell loss and gliosis but rarely to the extent of that found in the putamen; alternatively, appearances may be normal. Fearnley and Lees (1990) report a regional distribution of atrophy in this nucleus with a predilection for the dorsal part of the body. The authors also report a positive correlation between nerve cell loss in the caudate and that occurring in the putamen.

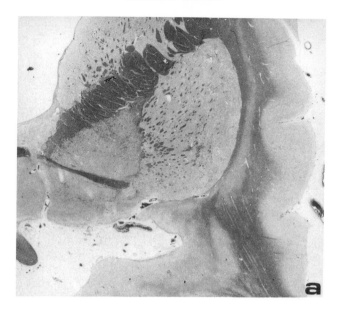

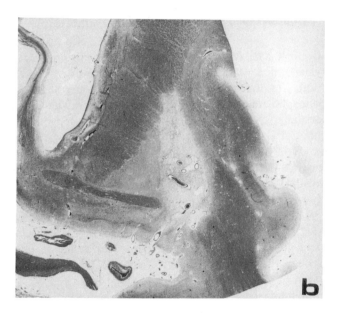

Fig. 30.4. Coronal section of striatum and globus pallidus stained for myelin. (a) Normal. Bundles of myelinated fibres are clearly identifiable in the caudate and putamen. (b) From a patient with MSA. Myelinated bundles of the striatum are unidentifiable and the pallidus is atrophic.

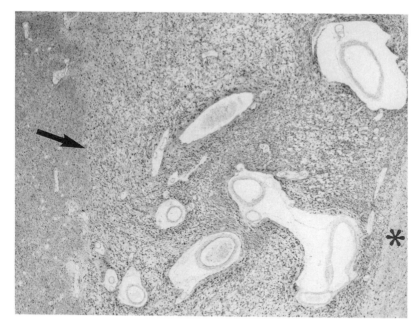

Fig. 30.5. Photomicrograph showing atrophy of putamen with ectatic perivascular spaces. Gliosis extends from the lateral border with external capsule (*) medially to the globus pallidus (arrow). Patient with MSA of 6 years' duration, responsive to levodopa. Immunocytochemistry for GFAP, 17 × .

The globus pallidus may appear uninvolved or show a reduction of myelinated fibres with gliosis and variable neuronal depletion, which is usually most severe in the external segment. The ansa lenticularis and lenticular fascicularis may appear narrowed. Pallidal atrophy is generally considered to be secondary to loss of putaminal efferent and afferent fibres; when there is also neuronal degeneration this may represent a transsynaptic effect or primary involvement.

The interpretation of subtle changes of gliosis and nerve cell loss in the basal ganglia is fraught with difficulty and requires careful comparison with control material; due allowance must be made for atrophy related to age or cerebrovascular disease. Oppenheimer (1984) has emphasized the value of myelin preparations when assessing the striatum and globus pallidus (Figs 30.4(a),(b)) and immunocytochemistry for GFAP is also very helpful (Fig. 30.5). Furthermore, in the absence of morphometry, nerve cell loss in these nuclei cannot be accurately predicted and may, as has recently been described for Huntington's disease (Richardson 1990), occur prior to gliosis. Unquestionably there is a need for a thorough quantitative morphological approach to investigation of the basal ganglia in MSA.

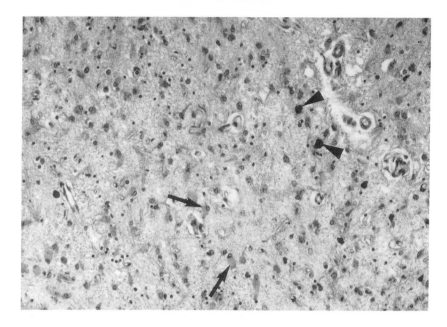

Fig. 30.6. Higher power view of putaminal atrophy with reactive astrocytes (some arrowed) and granules of pigment (arrowheads). No nerve cells remain in this field. Haematoxylin and eosin, 142 ×.

Degeneration of pigmented nerve cells occurs in the substantia nigra zone compacta. Non-pigmented cells of the pars reticulata are reported as normal; however, these cells are notoriously difficult to count and in MSA as well as in other nigral degenerations this observation requires clarification using unbiased stereological methods (Pakkenberg *et al.* 1991). The distribution of cell loss resembles that occurring in PD except that the dorsal tier is also involved (Fearnley 1991). The lateral region is most severely affected with neuronal depletion, astrocytic and microglial hyperplasia, and granules of neuromelanin lying free in the neuropil and within macrophages. The appearances are usually of a more active type of degeneration when compared with that of PD; the neuropil is often vacuolated and occasionally there are microglial nodules and evidence of neuronophagia in addition to a diffuse increase of microglia (Fig. 30.7).

Depletion of pigmented neurons also occurs in the locus ceruleus. Involvement of the dorsal vagal motor nucleus with cell loss has not, to my knowledge, been localized specifically to the pigmented cells. There remain many additional pigmented brainstem nuclear groups known to be affected in PD that are yet to be investigated in MSA.

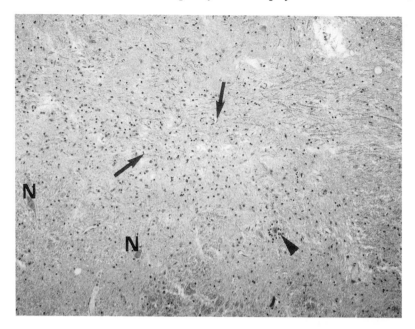

Fig. 30.7. The substantia nigra in MSA. There are only a few remaining non-pigmented neurons (N) and evidence of neuronophagia (arrowhead). The neuropil is rarefied and contains astrocytes and rod-shaped microglia (some arrowed). Haematoxylin and eosin, 92 × .

Olivopontocerebellar atrophy (OPCA)

The original description of the pathology of sporadic OPCA was made by Dejerine and Thomas in 1900. Although the familial OPCAs are excluded from discussion here, the majority show neuropathology which is indistinguishable from that of sporadic disease.

The basis pons is atrophic. Loss of pontine neurons and transverse pontocerebellar fibres occurs with replacement astrocytosis. In sections stained for myelin the intact descending corticospinal tracts stand out against the degenerate transverse fibres and middle cerebellar peduncles (Fig. 30.3). Many authors report a disproportionate depletion of fibres from the middle cerebellar peduncles compared with the loss of pontine neurons—an observation which has led to the suggestion of a 'dying-back' process (Oppenheimer 1984).

In MSA, cerebellar atrophy is often stated to be greatest in the neocerebellum whereas the palaeocerebellum is involved in primary cerebellar cortical degenerations. However, in several examples of MSA, pathology is most severe in the vermis (Takei and Mirra 1973) or, alternatively, vermis and hemispheres may be equally affected. There is loss of Purkinje nerve

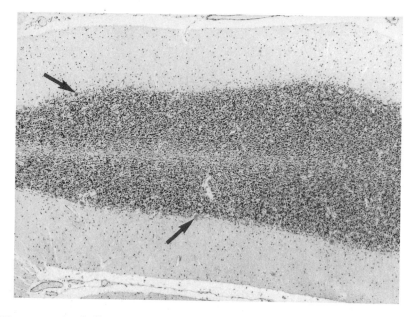

Fig. 30.8. Cerebellar cortex showing severe loss of Purkinje cells, some of those remaining are arrowed. The granule cell layer and folial white matter are atrophic. Haematoxylin and eosin, 38 × .

cells (Fig. 30.8) which is rarely complete and may be quite focal. The site of degenerate Purkinje cells is marked by the presence of empty basket formations (Fig. 30.9(a)); the persistence of these structures provides a useful distinguishing feature from cerebellar anoxic change where Purkinje and basket cells are both vulnerable. A Bergmann astrocytosis accompanies the Purkinje cell depletion and produces isomorphic gliosis in the molecular cell layer (Fig. 30.9(b)). In the granule cell layer it is usual to find some neuronal depletion together with axon torpedoes of degenerating Purkinje cells (Fig. 30.9(a)). Both the folial and central hemispheric white matter is reduced in amount while that around the dentate nucleus and within the hilus is well preserved. Due to the loss of Purkinje cell axon terminals, increased gliosis occurs in the dentate nucleus but there is usually no neuronal depletion at this site.

In the medulla there is loss of neurons in the inferior (Fig 30.10(a),(b)) and accessory olivary nuclei with increased gliosis. Either the whole olive is affected or there is a preponderance of neuronal depletion in the dorsal laminae (Takei and Mirra 1973). In several personal cases cell loss in the dorsal laminae (Fig. 30.10(b)) appeared to be related to severe involvement of the cerebellar vermis, presumably reflecting the neuroanatomical relationship between these nuclei. The olivary hilum is collapsed and there is pallor of myelin staining in olivocerebellar pathways.

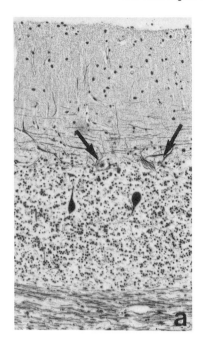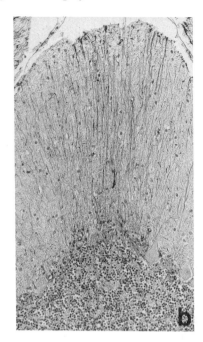

Fig. 30.9.   Cerebellar cortical degeneration in MSA. (a) In the granule cell layer there are torpedo-like swellings of Purkinje cell axons. Empty baskets (arrows) are present in the Purkinje cell layer. Modified Bielschowsky, 105 × . (b) A Bergmann astrocytosis has produced isomorphic gliosis in the molecular layer. Immunocytochemistry for GFAP, 105 × .

Autonomic failure

The separation of cases of primary autonomic failure into different groups was originally proposed by Graham and Oppenheimer (1969) and is now well established. Histologically, cases either show changes characteristic of PD or are typical of MSA. Each group, as well as being pathologically distinct, also presents different clinical features (Bannister and Oppenheimer 1972).

Orthostatic hypotension has been attributed to degeneration of sympathetic preganglionic neurons in the intermediolateral column of the thoracolumbar spinal cord. Oppenheimer (1980) has stressed the importance of a quantitative assessment before excluding involvement of this site in MSA; most of the cells lie within the lateral horn of grey matter where they are irregularly distributed and prone to shrink according to agonal state and post-mortem fixation. Several investigators have found, using quantification, a 50 per cent depletion of intermediolateral cells in cases which were previously thought to be normal. If one considers only those reports in which formal cell counts

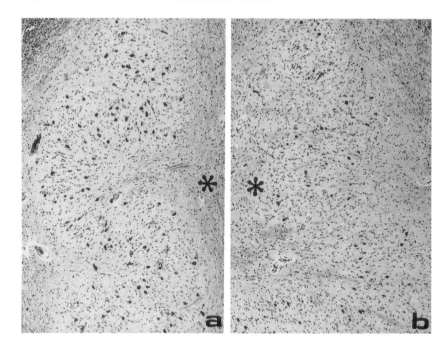

Fig. 30.10. Inferior olives in MSA. (a) Ventral lamina shows well-preserved neurons and adjacent white matter of the olivary hilum (*). (b) In the dorsal lamina, nerve cells are depleted and there is increased gliosis. The white matter (*) is also degenerate. Haematoxylin and eosin, 37 × .

have been made, with very few exceptions (e.g. Evans *et al.* 1972) all cases of MSA with predominant pathology in either the striatonigral or olivopontocerebellar system show loss of intermediolateral cells. Oppenheimer (1980) examined 21 cases of MSA and found lateral horn cell counts in patients with autonomic failure were on average 25 per cent of the controls, while in cases without autonomic failure there was about a 50 per cent depletion with some overlap occurring between the two groups.

Disordered bladder, rectal, and sexual function in SND and OPCA have been associated with cell loss in parasympathetic preganglionic nuclei of the sacral spinal cord (Sung *et al.* 1979; Konno *et al.* 1986). These neurons are localized rostrally in Onuf's nucleus between sacral segments S2 and S3 and more caudally in the inferior intermediolateral nucleus chiefly in the S3 to S4 segments (Konno *et al.* 1986). Although neurons of Onuf's nucleus morphologically resemble somatic motor neurons the sparing of this cell column in motor neuron disease and its involvement in MSA supports the view that it is part of the parasympathetic system (Sung *et al.* 1979) concerned with innervation of the anal and urethral sphincters.

In the majority of cases, a strong correlation exists between cell loss in preganglionic autonomic neurons and autonomic failure. However, exceptions do occur and undoubtedly there are additional contributory factors. Orthostatic hypotension in MSA has been reported in the absence of quantifiable cell change in the intermediolateral columns (Evans *et al.* 1972). Furthermore, Gray *et al.* (1988) describe 15 cases of MSA showing a greater than 50 per cent cell loss in the lateral horns but no relationship between severity of cell depletion and autonomic disturbance. These findings suggest that cells may be present but not functioning efficiently and that there may also be pathology at other autonomic sites.

The contribution of supraspinal lesions to autonomic failure is uncertain. Cell loss is commonly reported in the dorsal motor nucleus of the vagus (e.g. Sung *et al.* 1979). Shy and Drager (1960) found a reduction of Edinger–Westphal neurons but, subsequently, this site has rarely been commented upon. The same authors also describe mild cell loss in the posterior hypothalamus while Graham and Oppenheimer (1969) report this area as normal. Other central areas concerned with autonomic function are more difficult to identify and consequently have been less thoroughly investigated. Occasionally, nerve cell depletion and gliosis have been reported in the brainstem reticular formation (Adams and Salam-Adams 1986) but these changes are hard to quantify and no consistent abnormality has been documented.

In the peripheral component of the autonomic nervous system, Bannister and Oppenheimer (1972) have described atrophy of the glossopharyngeal and vagus nerves. No pathology has been reported in the visceral enteric plexuses or in the innervation of glands, blood vessels, or smooth muscles. The sympathetic and parasympathetic ganglia are discussed in Chapter 32.

Additional sites of pathology

A variety of other neuronal populations are noted to show cell depletion and gliosis with considerable differences in vulnerability from case to case. These sites are listed in Table 30.1 and only some of the reported lesions are discussed here. Martin (1975) describes thalamic degeneration occurring in 15 of 108 cases of 'multiple system atrophy' with the centrum medianum most frequently affected; unfortunately, the cases include a wide variety of system degenerations and the number of SND and OPCA is not detailed. The vestibular nuclear complex, notably the medial component, often shows neuronal depletion—what influence this may have on clinical signs is undetermined. Laryngeal stridor is a common feature of MSA particularly in later stages of the disease (Bannister *et al.* 1981). However, despite atrophy of the posterior cricoarytenoid muscles careful pathoanatomical evaluation has failed to reveal abnormality of motor neurons in the nucleus ambiguus (Bannister *et al.* 1981); the authors suggest a biochemical defect may be the basis of functional impairment. Similarly, the neuropathological background of abnormal eye movements in MSA is ill-defined although Mizutani *et al.* (1988) describe degeneration in the pathways concerned with the cerebellifugal control of ocular movement.

Degeneration of the anterior and lateral corticospinal tracts is commonly noted and may represent a 'dying-back' phenomenon as no consistent deficits of upper motor neurons, internal capsule, and upper brainstem corticospinal tracts are reported; occasionally the medullary pyramids are also involved. Anterior horn cells may show some depletion but not to the same extent as that occurring in motor neuron disease (Konno *et al.* 1986). Occasionally in MSA, degeneration of Clarke's column, spinocerebellar pathways, posterior columns, and gracile and cuneate nuclei are reported; Berciano (1982) has discussed the increased frequency of non-pyramidal spinal involvement in cases of familial OPCA.

Cytoplasmic inclusions in MSA

An argyrophilic cellular inclusion (Fig. 30.11) which appears to be characteristic for MSA has recently been described in oligodendrocytes of brain and spinal cord from patients with various combinations of SND, OPCA, and autonomic failure (Papp *et al.* 1989; Nakazato *et al.* 1990). Highest concentrations of inclusions occur in some but not all of the areas which are most frequently damaged, e.g. striatum, basis pons, and the white matter of cerebellum (Fig. 30.11). However, they are also found in large numbers in regions which appear morphologically spared, e.g. cerebral cortex, external capsule, and the medullary reticular formation. The electron microscope shows the inclusions to comprise a meshwork of 20 and 30 nm fibrils. They are immunostained by antibodies to ubiquitin and alpha and beta subunits of tubulin and tau protein and are interpreted as being related to altered microtubules. No such inclusions have been reported in a total of 329 brains so far examined from normal individuals or patients suffering from other neurodegenerative conditions including PD, Alzheimer's disease, and progressive supranuclear palsy. The study by Nakazato *et al.* (1990) included two cases of familial OPCA and in only one of these, in whom the clinical course was more typical of sporadic disease, were inclusions identified.

Kato and Nakamura (1990) have reported argyrophilic inclusion bodies in neurons of the basis pons of some patients with sporadic but not familial OPCA. It is clear from the data presented that the sporadic cases are examples of MSA although the authors have avoided use of the term. The inclusions appear to be distinct from those reported in oligodendrocytes and show a different antigen profile with positive immunostaining only with ubiquitin antisera. Ultrastructurally they are composed of granule-coated fibrils of diameter ranging from 24 to 40 nm.

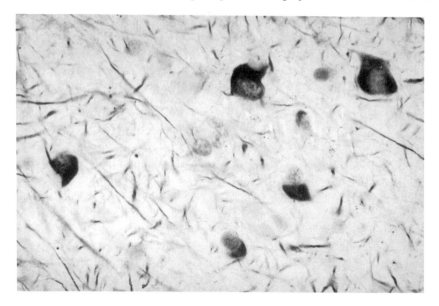

Fig. 30.11. Argyrophilic inclusions in oligodendrocyte-like cells of cerebellar hemispheric white matter. Patient had MSA for 5 years. Modified Bielschowsky, 850 × .

The specificity of both oligodendroglial and neuronal inclusions to MSA remains to be fully determined. However, it seems likely that they may represent a cell marker which could prove a useful adjunct to diagnosis as well as providing information concerning sites of involvement and pathogenesis.

The pathology of levodopa response

Often patients with early MSA show improvement with levodopa (Rajput *et al.* 1990) but sustained benefit is reported rarely (Chapter 34). At the Parkinson's Disease Society Brain Bank, London, of 22 cases with pathologically proven MSA, only 13 were diagnosed ante-mortem. Nineteen patients had a parkinsonian syndrome: 13 responded to levodopa treatment early in their disease and five remained at least partially levodopa-responsive at the time of death (Hughes, personal communication). Furthermore, in a series of 100 consecutive cases of clinically diagnosed PD (by definition responsive to levodopa), post-mortem examination found 5 per cent had MSA (Hughes *et al.* 1991*b*). Patients with MSA who respond to levodopa usually show relatively well-preserved putamina (Fearnley and Lees 1990) and a lack of response has previously been attributed to striatal damage and loss of postsynaptic dopamine receptors. However, exceptions do occur where, despite severe putaminal involvement (Fig. 30.5), there is a good levodopa response. Furthermore, striatal D2 receptor levels have recently been reported as comparable to those of patients with PD (Brooks *et al.* 1991). Rather than striatal damage being the sole determinant of levodopa responsiveness, it is likely that the functional connections of the whole basal ganglia are also involved.

Lewy bodies in MSA

Lewy bodies have been reported in the brainstem and intermediolateral cell columns of between 8 to 10 per cent of MSA cases in whom the predominant findings were either SND or OPCA; the frequency of Lewy bodies in MSA is similar to that in controls and suggests an incidental finding. There appear to be no distinguishing characteristics between the Lewy bodies of PD and those of MSA. In both conditions they are widely distributed in the brainstem and lack a disease-specific localization; using ubiquitin immunostaining it has been possible to identify Lewy bodies in the cerebral cortex of 100 per cent of PD cases (Hughes *et al.* 1991*b*) and cortical Lewy bodies also occur in MSA when brainstem Lewy bodies are present (personal observations). In some MSA cases the Lewy body may be attributable to coincidental PD which might be clinically concealed; we have recently had experience of a patient in whom the clinical history and neuropathological findings strongly supported PD with later development of MSA (Hughes *et al.* 1991*a*). Alternatively, and as has been suggested for the occurrence of Lewy bodies in neurologically normal cases, the Lewy body in MSA may represent a normal ageing phenomenon or be indicative of presymptomatic PD.

Neurochemistry of MSA

Immunocytochemical studies

Using immunocytochemistry, significant progress has been made in demonstrating regional neurotransmitter abnormalities and involvement of specific neuronal types. Recent evidence has shown that the striatum comprises a mosaic of neurochemically defined subdivisions termed matrix and striosomes. This arrangement is related to the different neurotransmitter interactions and to the striatal input and output systems. Immuno-cytochemical studies are in progress to investigate the pattern of striatal cell loss and its relationship to striatal organization and projection pathways. In SND the medium-sized spiny neurons, which are major projection neurons sending axons to the globus pallidus and substantia nigra, appear to be particularly severely affected. Areas of maximum putaminal damage show depletion of calcineurin immunoreactivity, one of the markers for medium-sized spiny neurons; results suggest a compartmental as well as a subregional distribution for the degenerative process, with calcineurin immunoreactive neurons of the matrix more severely affected than those of the striosomes (Goto and Hirano 1990). Loss of calcineurin immunoreactivity occurs to a much lesser extent in the caudate. As a consequence of degeneration of striatal efferent nerve terminals there is depletion of calcineurin, met-encephalin, and substance P immunoreactivity in the globus pallidus (Goto et al. 1989a).

In the substantia nigra, tyrosine hydroxylase-containing dopaminergic neurons are depleted particularly in the lateral portion; these neurons project primarily to the putamen. Furthermore, in the same area, loss of calcineurin immunoreactive striatonigral projection fibres occurs. Thus, the reciprocal relationship between substantia nigra and putamen, which forms part of the nigrostriatal loop, appears to be damaged. These findings contrast with those of PD where nigral dopaminergic neurons are depleted but the striatonigral projection fibres are preserved (Goto et al. 1989b).

Biochemical alterations in MSA

Due to the difficulties in obtaining suitable tissue there is a paucity of information concerning the biochemical alterations of MSA. Reduced dopamine (DA) and noradrenaline (NA) levels have been reported in striatum, substantia nigra, septal nuclei, nucleus accumbens, hypothalamus, and locus ceruleus (Spokes et al. 1979). Consistent with these findings there are low levels of homovallinic acid (the metabolite of DA) and NA in the cerebrospinal fluid (Williams 1981). Regional analyses of choline acetyltransferase (ChAT), an enzyme localized in cholinergic neurons, showed a variable degree of involvement; ChAT activity was consistently reduced in the red nucleus, dentate, pontine, and inferior olivary nuclei. In some but not all cases the enzyme was also reduced in the striatum and additional areas (Spokes et al. 1979). Gamma aminobutyric acid-containing neurons of the striatum and substantia nigra appear to be uninvolved, while levels of this enzyme in the dentate nucleus are reduced, reflecting the damage to Purkinje cells (Kwak 1985).

Over the past few years there has been considerable emphasis on glutamate dehydrogenase (GDH) levels in platelets and leucocytes; it now seems clear that reduced GDH activity does not distinguish between subtypes of MSA and is a non-specific finding which occurs in other neurodegenerative conditions including PD.

In MSA, depletion of DA in the striatum and substantia nigra is similar to that observed in PD (Spokes and Bannister 1981) and is consistent with the clinical state of parkinsonism. The contribution of other biochemical deficits to clinical symptomatology in MSA is less clear. It seems probable that reduced concentrations of NA in septal nuclei and hypothalamus may be an important factor resulting in autonomic failure. Depletion of NA could result from damage to the medullary reticular formation albeit in the absence of supportive morphological evidence.

Pathogenesis

The pathogenesis of MSA remains speculative. Involvement of different neuronal populations could represent a primary event. Alternatively, changes in some neurons occur either when fibres afferent to them are lost (anterograde or transsynaptic degeneration), or when the cells they project to malfunction (retrograde degeneration). Transneuronal degeneration is observed only at certain nervous system sites and is not an invariable neuronal response; furthermore, there are differences according to age and species. In the olivopontocerebellar system, degeneration of inferior olives, pontine neurons, and Purkinje cells occurs in MSA and a variety of other conditions. A 'linked' degeneration is postulated; however, neither the site of initial pathology nor the direction of degeneration is known. Whereas lesions of the striatonigral system in MSA show an anatomical correlation, there is no convincing evidence to suggest that this is due to transneuronal degeneration. In several conditions, for example, PD, postencephalitic parkinsonism, and progressive supranuclear palsy, nigral degeneration may occur without significant involvement of the striatum. In the autonomic nervous system, cell loss in the intermediolateral columns may be a primary event or could represent a transsynaptic consequence of degeneration in the upper sympathetic pathway; the problems of identifying these pathways and any pathology therein has been mentioned. Furthermore, functionally impaired nerve cells may appear morphologically normal; altered biochemical profiles and cell function may precede degeneration by an unknown period which could conceivably be several years. The finding of cytoplasmic inclusions in MSA suggests altered cytoskeletal structure and might represent an early change; in preliminary studies inclusions appear more numerous in cases where pathology is less severe and in addition they are found in areas previously considered uninvolved.

While the sites of pathology in MSA appear to be anatomically somewhat diverse, the nerve cells may well share certain physiological and/or biochemical properties which render them vulnerable to an aetiological agent. From both the clinical and pathological findings, it is unlikely that the different neuronal populations are involved simultaneously. Furthermore, if neurons are affected disparately the pattern of involvement may not be identical for each case. Several authors (for example, Borit *et al.* 1975) have suggested that the striatal lesion precedes nigral degeneration. However, there are cases where nigral damage is severe while lesions in the striatum are barely discernible. Rather than a single disease entity, MSA probably represents a group of conditions within which variation of individual expression is likely. *In situ* hybridization techniques are now being applied to MSA tissue and will provide more detailed information concerning the nature of cytoarchitectural disturbance. These results, together with molecular genetic studies, may identify the underlying biological deficit(s) and lead to a better understanding and classification of this disorder.

Acknowledgements

This work is supported by a grant from the Parkinson's Disease Society of the United Kingdom. I wish to thank Dr D. Oppenheimer for helpful discussion, Miss S. Blankson and Miss L. Kilford for technical assistance, Mrs S. Stoneham and Miss Kilford for photographic work, and Miss R. Nani for secretarial support.

References

Adams, R. D. and Salam-Adams, M. (1986). Striatonigral degeneration. In *Handbook of clinical neurology*, Vol. 5 (ed. P. J. Vinken, G. W. Bruyn, and H. L. Klawans), pp. 205–12. Elsevier Science, Amsterdam.

Adams, R. D., van Bogaert, L., and vander Eecken, H. (1961). Dégénérescences nigro-striées et cérébello-nigro-striées. *Psychiatria Neurologia*, **142**, 219–59.

Adams, R. D., van Bogaert, L., and vander Eecken, H. (1964). Striato-nigral degeneration. *J. Neuropathol. exp. Neurol.* **23**, 584–608.

Andrews, J. M., Terr, R. D., and Spataro, J. (1970). Striatonigral degeneration: clinical-pathological correlations in response to stereotaxic surgery. *Arch. Neurol., Chicago* **23**, 319–29.

Bannister, R. and Oppenheimer, D. R. (1972). Degenerative diseases of the nervous system associated with autonomic failure. *Brain* **95**, 57–74.

Bannister, R., Gibson, W., Michaels, L., and Oppenheimer, D. R. (1981). Laryngeal abductor paralysis in multiple system atrophy. A report on three necropsied cases with observations on the laryngeal muscles and the nuclei ambigui. *Brain* **104**, 351–68.

Berciano, J. (1982). Olivopontocerebellar atrophy. *J. neurol. Sci.* **53**, 253–72.

Borit, A., Rubinstein, L. J., and Urich, H. (1975). The striatonigral degenerations, putaminal pigments and nosology. *Brain* **98**, 101–12.

Brooks, D. J., Ibanez, V., Sawle, G. V., Playford, E. D., Quinn, N., Mathias, C. J., Lees, A. J., Marsden, C. D., Bannister, R., and Frackowiak, R. S. J. (1991). Striatal D_2 receptor status in Parkinson's disease, striatonigral degeneration, and progressive supranuclear palsy, measured with ^{11}C-Raclopride and PET. *Ann. Neurol.* (In press.)

Buonanno, F., Nardelli, E., Ounis, L., and Rizzuto, N. (1975). Striatonigral degeneration. Report of a case with an unusually short course and multiple system degenerations. *J. neurol. Sci.* **26**, 545–53.

Dejerine, J. and Thomas, A. (1900). L'atrophie olivo-ponto-cérébelleuse. *Nouv. Iconographie Salpêtrière* **13**, 330–70.

Evans, D., Lewis, P., Malhotra, O., and Pallis, C. (1972). Idiopathic orthostatic hypotension. Report of an autopsied case with histochemical and ultrastructural studies of the neuronal inclusions. *J. neurol. Sci.* **17**, 209–18.

Fearnley, J. M. (1991). Regional substantia nigra selectivity in the pathology of movement disorders. MD thesis, University of London.

Fearnley, J. M. and Lees, A. J. (1990). Striatonigral degeneration. A clinico-pathological study. *Brain* **113**, 1823–42.

Galassi, G., Nemni, R., Baraldi, A., Gibertoni, M., and Columbo, A. (1982). Peripheral neuropathy in multiple system atrophy with autonomic failure. *Neurology, NY* **33**, 1116–20.

Goto, S. and Hirano, A. (1990). Inhomogeneity of the putaminal lesion in striatonigral degeneration. *Acta neuropathol., Berlin* **80**, 204–7.

Goto, S., Hirano, A., and Rojas-Corona, R. R. (1989*a*). Calcineurin immunoreactivity in striatonigral degeneration. *Acta neuropathol., Berlin* **78(1)**, 65–71.

Goto, S., Hirano, A., and Matsumoto, S. (1989*b*). Subdivisional involvement of nigrostriatal loop in idiopathic Parkinson's disease and striatonigral degeneration. *Ann. Neurol.* **26**, 766–70.

Graham, J. G. and Oppenheimer, D. R. (1969). Orthostatic hypotension and nicotine sensitivity in a case of multiple system atrophy. *J. Neurol. Neurosurg. Psychiatr.* **32**, 28–34.

Gray, F., Vincent, D., and Hauw, J. J. (1988). Quantitative study of lateral horn cells in 15 cases of multiple system atrophy. *Acta neuropathol., Berlin* **75**, 513–18.

Hughes, A. J., Daniel, S. E., and Lees, A. J. (1991*a*). Idiopathic Parkinson's disease combined with multiple system atrophy: a clinicopathological report. *Movement Disorders* **6**, 342–6.

Hughes, A. J., Daniel, S. E., Kilford, L., and Lees, A. J. (1991*b*). The accuracy of clinical diagnosis of idiopathic Parkinson's disease: a clinicopathological study of 100 cases. *J. Neurol. Neurosurg. Psychiatr.* (In press.)

Kato, S. and Nakamura, H. (1990). Cytoplasmic argyrophilic inclusions in neurons of pontine nuclei in patients with olivopontocerebellar atrophy: immunohistochemical and ultrastructural studies. *Acta neuropathol., Berlin* **79**, 584–94.

Konno, H., Yamamoto, T., Iwasaki, Y., and Iizuka, H. (1986). Shy–Drager syndrome and amyotrophic lateral sclerosis: cytoarchitectonic and morphometric studies of sacral autonomic neurons. *J. neurol. Sci.* **73**, 193–204.

Kwak, S. (1985). Biochemical analysis of transmitters in the brains of multiple system atrophy. *No Shinkei* **37**, 691–4.

Martin, J. J. (1975). Thalamic degenerations. In *Handbook of clinical neurology*, Vol. 21 (ed. P. J. Vinken and G. W. Bruyn), pp. 587–605. Elsevier Science, Amsterdam.

Mizutani, T., Satoh, J., and Morimatsu, Y. (1988). Neuropathological background of oculomotor disturbances in olivopontocerebellar atrophy with special reference to slow saccade. *J. Neurol. Neurosurg. Psychiat.* **7**, 53–61.

Nakazato, Y., Yamazaki, H., Hirato, J., Ishida, Y., and Yamaguchi, H. (1990). Oligodendroglial microtubular tangles in olivopontocerebellar atrophy. *J. Neuropathol. Exp. Neurol.* **49**, 521–30.

Oppenheimer, D. (1980). Lateral horn cells in progressive autonomic failure. *J. neurol. Sci.* **46**, 393–404.

Oppenheimer, D. (1984). Diseases of the basal ganglia, cerebellum and motor neurons.

In *Greenfield's neuropathology* (4th edn), (ed. J. H. Adams, J. A. N. Corsellis, and L. W. Duchen), pp. 699–747. Wiley, New York.

Pakkenberg, A., Møller, Gundersen, H. J. G., Mouritzen Dam, A., and Pakkenberg, H. (1991). The absolute number of nerve cells in substantia nigra in normal subjects and in patients with Parkinson's disease estimated with an unbiased stereological method. *J. Neurol. Neurosurg. Psychiatr.* **54**, 30–3.

Papp, M. I., Kahn, J. E., and Lantos, P. L. (1989). Glial cytoplasmic inclusions in the CNS of patients with multiple system atrophy (striatonigral degeneration, olivopontocerebellar atrophy and Shy–Drager syndrome). *J. neurol. Sci.* **94**, 79–100.

Rajput, A. H., Rozdilsky, B., Rajput, A., and Ang, L. (1990). Levodopa efficacy and pathological basis of Parkinson syndrome. *Clin. Neuropharmacol.* **13**, 553–8.

Richardson, E. P. (1990). Huntington's disease: some recent neuropathological studies. *Neuropathol. appl. Neurobiol.* **16**, 451–60.

Shy, G. M. and Drager, G. A. (1960). A neurological syndrome associated with orthostatic hypotension. A clinicopathological study. *Arch. Neurol., Chicago* **2**, 511–27.

Spokes, E. G. S. and Bannister, R. (1981). Catecholamines and dopamine receptor binding in parkinsonism. In *Research progress in Parkinson's disease* (ed. F. C. Rose and R Capildeo), pp. 195–204. Pitman Medical, London.

Spokes, E. G. S., Bannister, R., and Oppenheimer, D. R. (1979). Multiple system atrophy with autonomic failure—clinical, histological and neurochemical observations on four cases. *J. neurol. Sci.* **43**, 59–82.

Sung, J. H., Mastri, A. R., and Segal, E. (1979). Pathology of Shy–Drager syndrome. *J. Neuropathol. exp. Neurol.* **38**, 353–68.

Takei, Y. and Mirra, S. (1973). Striatonigral degeneration: a form of multiple system atrophy with clinical parkinsonism. In *Progress in neuropathology*, Vol. 2 (ed. H. M. Zimmermann) pp. 217–51. Grune & Stratton, New York.

Williams, A. (1981). CSF biochemical studies on some extrapyramidal diseases. In *Research progress in Parkinson's disease* (ed. F. C. Rose and R. Capildeo), pp. 170–80. Pitman Medical, London.

31. Pathological studies of the sympathetic neuron

Phillip A. Low and R. D. Fealey

The normal preganglionic sympathetic neurone

The splanchnic mesenteric capacitance bed is of large volume, comprising approximately 25–30 per cent of total blood volume and is a low-resistance system of great importance in the maintenance of postural normotension (Rowell *et al.* 1972). The splanchnic veins are densely innervated and are markedly baroreflex responsive, responding to a reduction in pulse pressure by α-mediated venoconstriction (Thirlwell and Zsoter 1972). In humans, the splanchnic mesenteric bed appears to be more important than the muscle bed in raising total peripheral resistance in response to assuming the erect posture (Mancia *et al.* 1985). While muscle sympathetics are baroreflex responsive, the responses are not well sustained. The major sustained resistance changes occur in the splanchnic bed (Mancia *et al.* 1985).

The sympathetic nerve supply to the mesenteric bed is mainly the greater splanchnic nerve. This is a predominantly cholinergic preganglionic nerve with its cell body in the intermediolateral column (mainly T4 to T9) and synapses at the coeliac ganglion from whence postganglionic fibres go on to supply effector cells. There is much research and clinical evidence to support the importance of the sympathetic outflow in the maintenance of postural normotension (Low *et al.* 1975; Low 1984). Bilateral splanchnicectomy regularly results in orthostatic hypotension while neither bilateral lumbar sympathectomy (decentralizing the lower extremities) nor cardiac denervation cause orthostatic hypotension (Low *et al.* 1975). Orthostatic hypotension regularly occurs in spinal cord lesions above T4 (decentralizing the splanchnic outflow) but is absent in lesions below T9.

Because of the above considerations we studied the splanchnic outflow in fresh autopsy material of 12 persons aged 4.5 to 79 years who had died of disorders not affecting the splanchnic outflow (cardiac arrest, automobile accident, suicide, pulmonary embolus). Tissue was harvested within 4–6 h of death. The spinal cord was celloidin-embedded to avoid cellular shrinkage (as happens in paraffin-embedded tissues). The predominant cell type within the intermediolateral column had the staining characteristics of motor neurons with coarse and irregular Nissl substance.

The nucleus was large and often eccentric and neurons were oval, polygonal, spindle, or club-shaped. The mean preganglionic cell count in the intermediolateral column at T6, T7, and T8 spinal cord segments were 5002, 5004, and 4654 respectively (Low et al. 1977). There was no significant sex difference. Most cells ranged in diameter from 6 to 23 μm with the major peak at 12–13 μm. There was a progressive reduction of preganglionic neuron numbers with age. In adults, 370 preganglionic neurons (8 per cent) were lost per decade (Fig. 31.1). No significant differences in neuron numbers were found between segments.

Morphometric studies were also done on the corresponding ventral spinal root (Low and Dyck 1977) and autonomic rami (Low and Dyck 1978). There was good concordance between intermediolateral column neurons and ventral spinal root preganglionic axon numbers (0.81) and with autonomic rami (0.95). The preganglionic axon numbers in ventral spinal root and rami underwent attrition with age (8 and 5 per cent, respectively).

Morphometry of the splanchnic sympathetic outflow in multiple system atrophy (MSA) and pure autonomic failure (PAF)

The published reports on MSA are in good general agreement that there is a marked reduction in preganglionic sympathetic neurons qualitatively and quantitatively (Johnson et al. 1966; Bannister and Oppenheimer 1972; Low et al. 1978; Kennedy and Duchen 1985). In our study of two patients with

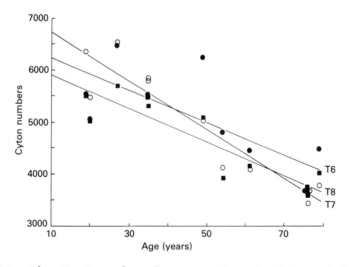

Fig. 31.1. Alteration in numbers of neurons with age for T6 (open circles), T7 (closed circles), and T8 (closed squares). (Taken with permission from Low et al. (1977).)

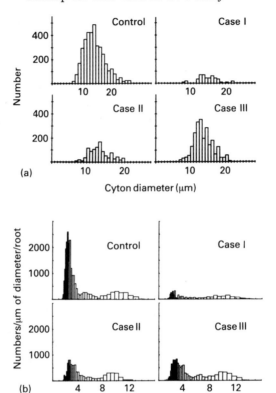

Fig. 31.2. Diameter histograms of (a) intermediolateral column neurons and (b) ventral spinal root myelinated fibres in a control, two patients with MSA (cases I and II) and a patient with PAF (case III). (Modified with permission from Low *et al.* (1978).)

MSA and one with PAF we measured preganglionic neuron sizes as well and related our neuron counts to axonal counts (Fig. 31.2). In the patients with MSA the T7 preganglionic neuron numbers were 10 and 24 per cent of age-matched controls. Their corresponding preganglionic axon numbers were 10 and 33 per cent of controls. Abnormalities in the preganglionic axons were milder in the patient with PAF. The preganglionic neurons and axons were 52 and 41 per cent of normal. The diameter distribution of neurons and axons was not different to that of controls.

Pathological changes in the postganglionic neuron in autonomic ganglia has been described in MSA (Thapedi *et al.* 1971) but is usually absent. We have reported morphometric studies on the splanchnic sympathetic outflow in MSA, PAF (Low *et al.* 1978), amyloid neuropathy and Tangier disease (Low *et al.* 1978), familial dysautonomia (Dyck *et al.* 1978), and diabetic autonomic neuropathy (Low *et al.* 1975; Low 1984). Based on the correlation between orthostatic hypotension and preganglionic neuron numbers with age and in disorders where the brunt of the pathology falls on the preganglionic system, we suggested that orthostatic hypotension does not occur until an attrition of at least 50 per cent of preganglionic neurons has occurred. This observation does not apply to disorders such as PAF and the peripheral autonomic neuropathies where there is an additional postganglionic lesion.

There is recent pharmacological evidence of postganglionic adrenergic failure in PAF leading to the suggestion that PAF is a postganglionic disorder and MSA a preganglionic disorder (Polinsky et al. 1981). Our morphometric study also suggested that the preganglionic neurons were more severely affected in MSA. To pursue this question we studied 97 consecutive patients with PAF or MSA (38 PAF: 59 MSA) seen at the Mayo Autonomic Reflex and Thermoregulatory Sweat laboratories over a 3.5-year period. These patients had severe generalized autonomic failure as indicated by the finding of orthostatic hypotension, widespread anhidrosis on the thermoregulatory sweat test (Fealey et al. 1985), and impairment of heart period responses to deep breathing and the Valsalva manoeuvre.

Postganglionic sudomotor and vasomotor functions were studied using the Quantitative Sudomotor Axon Reflex test (QSART; see Chapter 21) and supine plasma noradrenaline, respectively. Since axon reflex sudomotor function varies with sex (Low et al. 1983; Ahmed and Le Quesne 1986), the results were expressed as a sex-matched percentile of control values ($n = 100$). Postganglionic failure occurred at the forearm in 45 per cent and at the foot in 61 per cent of PAF patients providing clear evidence that sympathetic sudomotor fibres are also involved.

However, abnormalities were not confined to the postganglionic axon. The thermoregulatory sweat test and QSART have similar sensitivity so that it is possible to define the site of the sudomotor lesion (pre- or postganglionic) from the combined use of the two tests on the same patient. Postganglionic function was completely normal in some patients with anhidrosis on thermoregulatory sweat test indicating a preganglionic lesion in these patients. More commonly, there was combined pre- and postganglionic involvement in PAF (Cohen et al. 1987).

Plasma noreadreneline results from a spillover of noradrenaline from sympathetic postganglionic nerve terminals and the supine value is an index of net sympathetic activity (Polinsky et al. 1981). Supine plasma free noradrenaline values were significantly reduced in PAF ($p < 0.001$) but not in MSA. Plasma noradrenaline increment on standing was reduced in both PAF ($p < 0.001$) and MSA ($p < 0.001$) and the difference was not significant. We concluded that PAF is mainly a postganglionic disorder, although the preganglionic neuron may be affected to some degree (Cohen et al. 1987).

Apart from its association with involvement of other central nervous structures, especially striatonigral and olivopontocerebellar, MSA is usually but not invariably associated with a normal resting supine noradrenaline.

Compared with disorders with a similar degree of autonomic failure, such as acute panautonomic neuropathy (Low *et al.* 1983) or diabetic autonomic neuropathy, the reduction in supine noradrenaline is much less, suggesting a preganglionic site. The significantly reduced noradrenaline response to standing in MSA is thought to indicate a failure to activate central sympathetic pathways. These findings are consonant with published reports of a marked reduction in preganglionic sympathetic neurons, including morphometric studies. The splanchnic autonomic outflow is of crucial importance in the maintenance of orthostatic normotension and the attrition of 5–8 per cent of neurons per decade (Low *et al.* 1977; Low and Dyck 1977, 1978) may be responsible for the age-related orthostatic hypotension (Low 1984).

Autonomic preganglionic neuropathies with prominent orthostatic hypotension (OH) are associated with loss of intermediolateral column neurons (Low *et al.* 1978, 1981; Low 1984) and OH correlates with the attrition of approximately 50 per cent of intermediolateral column neurons (Low 1984). Although MSA patients appear to be a relatively homogeneous group with only a minor subset with postganglionic adrenergic failure, the latter has been well demonstrated pharmacologically and on catecholamine fluorescence and electron microscopy of peripheral arterioles (Bannister *et al.* 1981).

In contrast to adrenergic failure, where there is separation between PAF and MSA, postganglionic sudomotor failure occurred as frequently in MSA as it did in PAF occurring at the forearm in 42 per cent and at the foot in 64 per cent of MSA patients (Cohen *et al.* 1987). Our data lends some support to the hypothesis that the postganglionic sympathetic sudomotor failure in MSA is due to a transsynaptic effect. If the mechanism is transsynaptic the degree of postganglionic failure should vary with the severity of autonomic failure. There was a significant regression with severity of the percentage of anterior body-surface anhidrosis on thermoregulatory sweat test and with supine plasma noradrenaline in MSA supporting the hypothesis. The greater percentage of postganglionic failure in the foot than the forearm suggest a length-dependent transsynaptic mechanism. The insignificant regression with duration is not surprising since all cases are chronic.

Although there is good statistical separation between groups of patients with PAF and MSA using supine plasma noradrenaline, there is also considerable overlap, so that supine plasma noradrenaline cannot be relied on to always separate the individual patient with PAF from MSA (Fealey *et al.* 1985). Patients with PAF often have normal supine plasma noradrenaline. Moreover, some patients with MSA have reduced noradrenaline. The most reliable way to diagnose MSA is still the demontration of central nervous system involvement. Finally, the occasional patient will progress from apparent PAF to MSA.

In conclusion, generalized autonomic failure occurs in both MSA and PAF. However, while PAF is characterized by combined postganglionic sudomotor and adrenergic failure, postganglionic adrenergic denervation is less common in MSA while the preganglionic neuron is more severely affected. We speculate that the postganglionic sympathetic sudomotor failure in MSA may be due to a transsynaptic effect since the degree of postganglionic sudomotor failure increases with the severity of autonomic failure, the percentage of anhidrosis of anterior body surface on thermoregulatory sweat test, and the degree of reduction in supine plasma noradrenaline. Somatic neuropathy is more common in MSA and is usually mild or asymptomatic. The more frequent occurrence of somatic neuropathy seems to be in keeping with the more widespread involvement of neurological and autonomic systems in MSA than in PAF clinically and neuropathologically. These recent studies suggest that multiple system atrophy extends to involve the peripheral nervous system as well. Indeed the number of systems involved in MSA continue to grow as investigators evaluate more systems. From the clinical standpoint the neurological examination, seeking for multisystem involvement continues to be a more reliable discriminator of MSA from PAF than nuances of the degree or site of autonomic failure.

References

Ahmed, M. E. and Le Quesne, P. M. (1986). Quantitative sweat test in diabetics with neuropathic foot lesions. *J. Neurol. Neurosurg.* **49**, 1059–62.

Bannister, R. and Oppenheimer, D. R. (1972). Degenerative diseases of the nervous system associated with autonomic failure. *Brain* **95**: 457–74.

Bannister, R., Crowe, R., Eames, R., and Burnstock, G. (1981). Adrenergic innervation in autonomic failure. *Neurology* **31**, 150–6.

Cohen, J., Low., P. A., Fealey, R. D., Sheps, S., and Jiang, N-S. (1987). Somatic and autonomic function in progressive autonomic failure and multiple system atrophy. *Ann. Neurol.* **22**, 692–9.

Dyck, P. J., Kawamura, Y., Low, P. A., Shimono, M., and Solovy, J. S. (1978). The number and sizes of reconstructed peripheral autonomic, sensory and motor neurones in a case of dysautonomia. *J. Neuropathol. exp. Neurol.* **37**, 741–55.

Fealey, R. D., Schirger, A., and Thomas, J. E. (1985). Orthostatic hypotension. In *Clinical medicine*, Vol. 7 (ed. J. A. Spittell, Jr), pp. 1–12. Harper & Row, Philadelphia.

Johnson, R. H., Lee, G. de J., Oppenheimer, D. R., and Spalding, J. M. K. (1966). Autonomic failure with orthostatic hypotension due to intermediolateral column degeneration. A report of two cases with autopsies. *Quart. J. Med.* **35**, 276–292.

Kennedy, P. G. E. and Duchen, L. W. (1985). A quantitative study of intermediolateral column cells in motor neuron disease and the Shy–Drager syndrome. *J. Neurol. Neurosurg. Psychiat.* **48**, 1103–6.

Low, P. A. (1984). Quantitation of autonomic function. In *Peripheral neuropathy* (2nd edn) (ed. P. J. Dyck, P. K. Thomas, E. H. Lambert, and R. Bunge), pp. 1139–66. Saunders, Philadelphia.

Low, P. A. and Dyck, P. J. (1977). Splanchnic preganglionic neurons in man. II. Preganglionic ventral root fibers. *Acta neuropathol.* **40**, 219–26.

Low, P. A. and Dyck, P. J. (1978). Splanchnic preganglionic neurons in man. III. Morphometry of myelinated fibers of rami communicantes. *J. Neuropathol. exp. Neurol.* **37**, 734–40.

Low, P. A., Walsh, J. C., Huang, C. Y. and McLeod, J. G. (1975). The sympathetic nervous system in diabetic neuropathy. A clinical and pathological study. *Brain* **98**, 341–56.

Low, P. A., Okazaki, H., and Dyck, P. J. (1977). Splanchnic preganglionic neurons in man: I. Morphometry of preganglionic cytons. *Acta neuropathol.* **40**, 55–61.

Low, P. A., Thomas, J. E., and Dyck, P. J. (1978). The splanchnic autonomic outflow in Shy–Drager syndrome and idiopathic orthostatic hypotension. *Ann. Neurol.* **4**, 511–14.

Low, P. A., Dyck, P. J., Okazaki, H., Kyle, R., and Fealey, R. D. (1981). The splanchnic autonomic outflow in amyloid neuropathy and Tangier disease. *Neurology* **31**, 461–3.

Low, P. A., Dyck, P. J., Lambert, E. H., *et al.* (1983). Acute panautonomic neuropathy. *Ann. Neurol.* **13**, 412–17.

Mancia, G., Grassi, G., Ferrari, A., and Zanchetti, A. (1985). Reflex cardiovascular regulation in humans. *J. Cardiovasc. Pharmacol.* **7** (suppl. 3) 152–9.

Polinsky, R. J., Kopin, I. J., Ebert, M. H., and Weise, V. (1981). Pharmacologic distinction of different orthostatic hypotension syndromes. *Neurology* **31**, 1–7.

Rowell, L. B., Detry, J. M., Blackmore, J. R., and Wyss, C. (1972). Importance of the splanchnic bed in human blood pressure regulation. *J. appl. Physiol.* **32**, 213.

Thapedi, I. M., Ashenhurst, E. M., and Rozdilsky, B. (1971). Shy–Drager syndrome. *Neurology* **21**, 26–32.

Thirlwell, M. P. and Zsoter, T. T. (1972). The effect of propranolol and atropine on venomotor reflexes in man. *J. Med.* **3**, 65.

32. Autonomic ganglia in multiple system atrophy and pure autonomic failure

Margaret R. Matthews

Introduction

Since the first clear distinction was made, by Bannister and Oppenheimer in 1972, between two presentations of autonomic failure (AF), one occurring in multiple system atrophy (MSA) and the other found in association with Parkinson's disease (AF with PD), or occurring rarely as an apparently isolated phenomenon (pure autonomic failure, PAF), it has become increasingly evident that there are important differences between these two types, and that these differences may have causal significance. Thus, clinically the defect is in MSA mainly preganglionic and in PAF, ganglionic or postganglionic. None the less, the identity of the primary cause or causes of the autonomic failure in either group of cases still remains elusive.

Neuropathological studies of many cases of autonomic failure, notably by Oppenheimer (1980), who also reviewed earlier work, strongly support the possibility of a primary lesion at preganglionic level in MSA, by showing that there is, in almost all cases of MSA with AF, considerable loss of inter-mediolateral column (IML) neurons, amounting to 75 per cent or more of control numbers. Cases of PD with AF, however, also showed severe loss of IML neurons, and moderate loss was found in PD without AF. Oppenheimer's work has emphasized the importance of systematic counting of neurons in samples of adequate extent, with age-matched controls for comparison. More recent series have produced similar results (see, for example, Gray *et al.* 1988). It was already apparent that in the IML a loss of 50 per cent of neurons may be overlooked if no adequate counts are made, and it is now confirmed that 50 per cent or even more of IML neurons may be lost without overt AF.

Counts of preganglionic parasympathetic neurons at sacral spinal levels have likewise shown severe neuron loss in MSA (Konno *et al.* 1986). Loss of neurons has also been reported in the dorsal motor nucleus of the vagus, both in MSA and in PD with AF; and in PD this nucleus consistently shows Lewy bodies, typical of the disease, in common with other pigmented nuclei of the brainstem. (Similar Lewy bodies have sometimes been seen in the IML in PD.) Other parasympathetic central nuclei are less consistently examined, but in MSA there have been occasional reports of neuron loss in the Edinger–Westphal nucleus, and loss of facial and glossopharyngeal central parasympathetic neurons has also been suspected.

In view of the incomplete distinction between MSA and PAF, or AF with PD, in terms of central autonomic neuropathology it becomes crucial to consider the peripheral autonomic ganglia. Sympathetic ganglia have been examined in only about half of the reported pathological studies of AF, and seldom described quantitatively. Here, however, there begins to emerge a clearer distinction between the two types of AF.

In MSA with AF (Table 32.1) it has been typical to report either no obvious abnormality in sympathetic ganglia, or some foci of gliosis and possible loss of neurons, or sometimes neuronophagia, not quantified. Spokes *et al.* (1979) in silver preparations noted some depletion of nerve fibres, and argentophil debris. Gliosis could itself indicate loss of nerve fibres and terminals, and not exclusively loss of neurons: gliosis may be seen in the globus pallidus in MSA in conjunction with severe loss of neurons from the putamen. Any morphological changes reported in sympathetic ganglionic neurons in MSA have tended to be non-specific, falling within the normal range of appearances (Table 32.1), and published micrographs have indicated at least a moderate density, and sometimes quite a high density, of surviving neurons. Four cases of presumptive MSA, diagnosed retrospectively by Gray *et al.* (1988), are unusual in this respect.

In PAF, however, and in PD with AF, it has been characteristic to find Lewy bodies (and often numerous 'eosinophilic bodies' of bizarre form) in the sympathetic ganglia, with or without obvious neuronal loss, just as also in the pigmented neurons of the brainstem (Table 32.1). This suggests the possibility of a primary lesion affecting in common neurons of similar or related phenotype. Rajput and Rozdilsky (1976) found Lewy bodies in sympathetic ganglia in five of six PD cases, with 'axonal swellings' in the other and reported (without formal counting) slight-to-severe loss and atrophy of the ganglionic neurons, roughly correlated with the degree of orthostatic hypotension, in the three cases of PD who also showed AF. The subject with the most severe AF and greatest loss of sympathetic neurons showed only 'minimal reduction' of neurons in the IML, whereas a subject with MSA and AF was judged to have moderate loss of IML neurons and no more than slight neuron loss in the sympathetic stellate ganglion. More recently, Wakabayashi (1989) has confirmed the consistency of occurrence of Lewy bodies in sympathetic ganglia in 10 cases of PD (and also in five non-parkinsonian subjects with many Lewy bodies in the central nervous system) and has reported in such cases an increased incidence of Lewy bodies in enteric neurons and in cardiac and pelvic plexuses, in comparison with an extensive control series. Thus, there may be widespread involvement of peripheral autonomic neurons, sympathetic, parasympathetic, and enteric, in the pathological process which leads to the formation of Lewy bodies in PD and the presumptive pre-parkinsonian state.

Table 32.1. Neuropathological studies in autonomic failure in which sympathetic ganglia have been examined, and observations as reported. The findings are repeated in some cases verbatim, since they may be open to differences of interpretation. There has been a tendency among reviewers not primarily focusing on ganglia to equate all comments which are suggestive of pathological changes, regardless of degree and with little or no attempt at interpretation. It should be borne in mind that autonomic ganglionic neurons, like primary sensory neurons, could be subject to some degree of age-related cell death, which is likely to become manifest as a sporadic dropping-out of neurons leading to scattered nodules of Nageotte or clumps of satellite cells. Loss of nerve endings, as discussed in the text, or nerve sprouting, could also provoke focal or general increases of satellite cells. It should also be noted that in none of these ganglia were systemic neuron counts made.

Authors*	Case	Sex	Age at death (years)	Duration of OH (years)	Findings in sympathetic ganglia
Reports from cases accepted as MSA					
Shy & Drager (1960)	I	M	46	6+	Many neurons pale with decreased Nissl substance, scattered neurons hyperchromatic, a few vacuolated No mention of neuronal loss
Johnson et al. (1966)	II	M	54	5+	Appearance normal
Nick et al. (1967)		F	67	5+	Much lipofuscin in most neurons. Some loss of neurons (no counts); moderate proliferation of interstitial elements All changes very moderate
Schwarz (1967)	I	F	41	4+	'The usual deeply stained and pale neurons, some well-filled with lipofuscin and some with pigment. There were areas in which neurons may have been destroyed and phagocytized and replaced by increased numbers of capsular cells'
Schwarz (1967)	II	M	57	2+	No abnormalities detected
Martin et al. (1968)	IV	M	59	1–3	No abnormalities detected
Graham et al. (1969)		M	69	3+	No neuron loss, no morphological changes in ganglion cells. Some loss of nerve fibres

Table 32.1. *(continued)*

Authors*	Case	Sex	Age at death (years)	Duration of OH (years)	Findings in sympathetic ganglia
Hughes *et al.* (1970)	I	M	59	3 +	'Some loss of neurons with proliferation of satellite cells. All stages seen from cell shrinkage with slight excess of satellite cells to disappearance of neurons leaving nests of closely packed satellite nuclei. Endoneurial sheaths of both pre- and post-ganglionic fibre bundles abnormally thickened. Ganglia of normal appearance found in sections of bowel and bladder'
Bannister and Oppenheimer (1972)	I	M	47	4 +	Neurons appeared normal in form and numbers
	II	M	57	1 +	Ganglia appeared normal
Evans *et al.* (1972)		M	53	8 +	'Occasional fenestrated cells and extensive hydropic degeneration'. (Illustration shows perineuronal spaces, possibly shrinkage artefact; area well populated with neurons but showing one compact cluster of satellite cells)
Rohmer *et al.* (1973)		M	61	5 +	Sympathetic ganglia, intestinal and vascular plexuses, normal
Schober *et al.* (1975)	I	F	56	3 +	'A few atypical axonal swellings consisting of well-defined rounded structures with faintly eosinophilic fine and coarse granular content', examined ultrastructurally and authoritatively pronounced not to be Lewy bodies (authors include L. S. Forno). These they regarded as non-specific
De Lean and Deck (1975)		M	58	4 +	'A minimal loss of neurons. No Lewy bodies or hyaline eosinophilic bodies'
Rajput and Rozdilsky (1976)	VII	M	52	1 +	'Slight neuron loss' in stellate ganglion
Spokes *et al.* (1979)	I	M	70	1 +	No neuron loss. Some argyrophilic debris. Nil abnormal found in silver preparations of gut wall, bladder, coeliac

					Description
	II	M	49	1 +	No detectable neuron loss; some axon fragments
	III	M	51	4 +	No detectable neuron loss
	IV	F	53	4–5	No detectable neuron loss
Reports from cases accepted as PAF or PD with AF					
Fichefet et al. (1965)		F	72	1 +	Obvious neuron loss; Lewy bodies, numerous eosinophilic bodies of variable shape
Johnson et al. (1966)	I	M	66	4 +	No obvious neuron loss, relative poverty of nerve fibres; numerous sausage- or staghorn-shaped eosinophilic bodies
Vanderhaeghen et al. (1970)	II	M	74	1 +	Lewy bodies, elongated and spherical
Roessmann et al. (1971)	I	M	69	13 +	Nageotte nodules in many sections. A few small mononuclear infiltrates. A few Lewy bodies; many eosinophilic bodies of variable shape. Enteric ganglia, vagi, appeared normal
Schober et al. (1975)	II	M	73	3 +	Lewy bodies, a few in somata but much more numerous in processes
Rajput and Rozdilsky	I–VI			Various	Five cases showed neuron loss and Lewy bodies, roughly in proportion to degree of AF
An exceptional case combining features of MSA and PD					
Thapedi et al. (1971)		M	58	1/2	Moderate neuron loss; a few Nageotte nodules, some neurons chromatolytic. No Lewy bodies but several eosinophilic bodies

OH, orthostatic hypotension.

*All references relevant to this table are contained within Rohmer et al. (1973) or Spokes et al. (1979).

Since the autonomic ganglia appear to differ distinctively in these two forms of AF, it is clearly important to examine them carefully for any further evidence which may throw light on the pathological processes involved.

Why is it so difficult to be sure about the underlying changes? There are various reasons, some of which are common to all neuropathological studies while others are peculiar to the autonomic nervous system. First, the basic defect may be biochemical, metabolic, or regulatory and may not express itself in gross structural terms. Second, the condition may be well advanced before it presents clinically. This is perhaps particularly true of the autonomic nervous system, which, unlike the somatic motor system, shows no clearly defined functional demarcation between an upper (higher centres) and a lower motor neuron (IML) lesion. There are both divergence and convergence of preganglionic neurons on to ganglionic neurons, and the latter may receive multiple inputs which have the characteristic that they are subthreshold, requiring coincidence of several inputs to bring the neuron to the threshold for firing. The peripheral effectors are smooth or cardiac muscle and gland cells, neuroeffector contacts are typically not close, and electrotonic coupling in the effector organ is frequent or invariable. The interstitial dropping-out of peripheral sympathetic nerve endings may be initially compensated by diffusion of transmitter, since fewer nerve endings mean less high-affinity re-uptake; by increase in receptor density; and by electrotonic coupling, until the changes have become extreme. Moreover, collateral sprouting of preganglionic nerves in the ganglia (cf. Liestøl *et al.* 1986) and also of postganglionic nerves in the periphery is further able to compensate to a remarkable extent. A slowly progressive change may thus not become clinically evident until the underlying pathological changes are severe, as in the case of IML neuron loss in postural hypotension (Oppenheimer 1980).

By this time, secondary trophic and degenerative changes may well have occurred, involving not only neurons but also satellite or Schwann cells, supporting tissues, and vasculature. As far as the neurons are concerned, these secondary changes are likely to be transneuronal in character, but could be either anterograde or retrograde. Much knowledge has accrued latterly concerning retrograde trophic influences on neurons, and this has arisen largely from studies of autonomic and sensory ganglia, relating to nerve growth factor and, more recently, to brain-derived, ciliary and other tissue-derived neurotrophic factors, which govern the development and maintenance of peripheral ganglion cells (Thoenen 1991). A similar control may be expected to apply in the case of the preganglionic neurons. Survival and phenotypic specification may be governed by different factors, and a neuron may be induced to change its phenotype by target-derived factor(s) after it has reached and innervated the target, as in the case of the sympathetic sudomotor neuron, which is initially adrenergic but undergoes a cholinergic transformation after it has innervated the sweat glands. Anterograde influences may also be important, as is well exemplified by the striated muscle fibre: trophic maintenance is influenced by activation and, in its absence, shrinkage and a varying degree of dedifferentiation may occur. Whether in the long term denervation may lead to neuronal death is uncertain: it depends strongly on age, on the type of neuron, and the presence or absence of other inputs.

From the time of onset of AF a patient may survive for several or even many years. The availability of biopsy is strictly limited, e.g. to the peripheral autonomic terminals as seen in muscle or skin biopsies, since the removal of ganglia would be too destructive; and the possibility of early biopsy is virtually ruled out by the lateness of presentation. Post-mortem changes may preclude the finer aspects of the eventual analysis, and agonal changes, involving intense nervous discharges, may also have supervened, as the terminal event is often apparently asphyxial.

Desiderata for studying the ganglia post-mortem

These include early chilling of the body and early removal of tissues, to optimize tissue preservation; extensive sampling within the autonomic nervous system; the obtaining of adequate age-matched control material for comparison; and the use of appropriate fixation schedules—for example, buffered 4 per cent formaldehyde followed by paraffin-embedding for conventional histology, including neuron counting (Konigsmark 1970), or by cryostat or frozen sections for enzyme histochemistry and immunohisto-chemistry; buffered 3 per cent glutaraldehyde followed by resin-embedding for electron microscopy and for light microscopy of 1-μm sections; or alternatively, especially where little tissue may be obtainable, Bouin's fluid, or Zamboni's fixative (buffered 2 per cent formaldehyde with 15 per cent saturated picric acid), which is compatible with both immunohistochemistry and electron microscopy as well as conventional histology. In practice, for various reasons, it may only be possible to fulfil a limited number of these criteria.

Experimental results

The following account is based upon the examination of control material obtained through the courtesy of Drs David Oppenheimer and M. M. Esiri, and material from subjects dying with AF who had been in the care of Sir Roger Bannister. The material falls into three categories.

1. Various sympathetic ganglia from six subjects with MSA, confirmed at autopsy, aged 46–77 years, of whom two are represented only by paraffin-embedded specimens.

2. Superior cervical ganglia (SCGs), and in one case other ganglia, from two subjects with clinically pure AF, aged 58 and 70 years. One of the SCGs

was formaldehyde-fixed and cut serially for cell counting; the other was fixed for electron microscopy.

3. SCGs from three subjects dying of other causes, all female, aged 16, 64, and 98 years; causes of death were, respectively, road accident, cerebral vascular accident, and empyema. These were osmium- or glutaraldehyde-fixed and resin-embedded for electron microscopy.

4. Ganglia from three young male subjects dying from road accidents, aged 17, 19, and 27 years, and from four older male subjects dying of myocardial infarction, aged 57, 66, 68, and 85 years. These were fixed in formaldehyde or in Zamboni's fixative.

Light microscopy

No Lewy bodies were found in any ganglia from the control or MSA subjects. The ganglia of subjects with MSA were well populated with neurons which appeared within the range seen in the control ganglia in respect of size, general cytology, and packing density in the neuropil. Almost all neurons had conspicuous aggregates of lipofuscin granules. Nissl material was however relatively scanty. In silver-stained preparations many neurons were seen to have well preserved dendritic arborizations (Fig. 32.1). Some of these dendritic patterns were perhaps unusually complex and profuse, and some processes

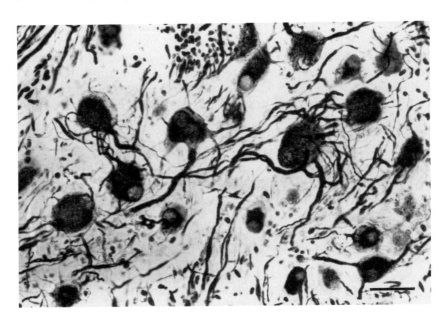

Fig. 32.1. Neurons of a thoracic sympathetic ganglion from a subject with MSA. Silver preparation (Glees and Marsland). Scale bar, 50 μm.

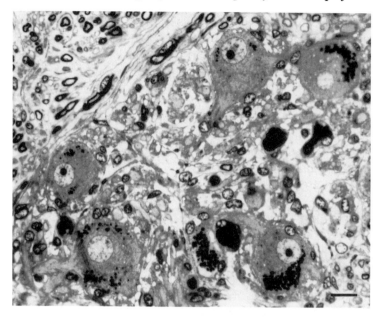

Fig. 32.2.   1-μm section of an Araldite-embedded thoracic ganglion of a subject with MSA, stained with methylene blue and Azur II. Most of the neurons have eccentric nuclei and contain arcs or masses of darkly stained lipofuscin bodies, but also contain some distinct Nissl material (intermediate grey clumps). Scale bar, 20 μm.

unusually stout, but no gross distortions were observed. Some of the smaller neurons showed no stainable arborizations; but failure to stain processes in this material cannot necessarily be taken to imply their absence.

The use of 1-μm resin-embedded sections from comparable mid-ganglion levels (Fig. 32.2) permitted semi-quantitative cytological comparisons. In SCGs of three control subjects, the mean packing density of neurons in areas of neuropil averaged 7.1 nucleated neuronal profiles in the area of a standard photoframe graticule at 325× magnification (range of means 5.6–8.3). In SCGs of three subjects with MSA the corresponding average was 8.9 nucleated neuronal profiles (range of means 6.8–10.4). This does not suggest severe neuronal loss, but might indicate compaction consequent on reduction of other elements such as preganglionic nerve fibres and extent of dendritic trees.

Nucleated neuronal profiles (NNP) in these 1-μm sections were assessed for various features (sample size 45–320, median 137). These included the presence of distinct Nissl granules, the incidence of lipofuscin bodies, the degree of nuclear eccentricity, and the size range of the neuron population. In the three control subjects, a mean of 91 per cent (range 84–95 per cent) showed distinct Nissl granules. In all three subjects with MSA, fewer neurons (37, 46, and 72 per cent of NNP) showed distinct Nissl granules. In the youngest control subject only 35 per cent of NNP showed heavy clumps or masses of lipofuscin bodies, but the incidences in the other two were 87 and 84 per cent. In the subjects with MSA, the mean incidence per NNP of massed lipofuscin bodies was 84 per cent (range 78–93 per cent). The proportion of NNP showing centrally situated, rather than eccentric, nuclei was similar in the two groups (control mean 15 per cent, range 11–24 per cent; MSA mean 13 per cent, range 8–18 per cent). The mean diameters of the five to eight largest and smallest neurons were compared, for two subjects from each group, and were not found to differ markedly (*smallest NNP*: control youngest 15.6 μm, oldest 22.3 μm; MSA 21.1 and 21.1 μm; *largest NNP*: control youngest 41.3, oldest 44.3 μm; MSA 45.3, 51.4 μm).

Thus, in the MSA group of subjects with AF, the principal observed difference from the controls lay in the reduced incidence of distinct Nissl granules in the neuronal cell bodies. No consistent abnormalities were noted in the vasculature or in adventitious cells in the ganglia; but in one of the MSA subjects there was some perivenular lymphocytic infiltration, part of a generalized distribution associated with a longstanding leukaemic condition (Waldenström macroglobulinaemia).

In sympathetic ganglia from the two subjects with PAF the packing densities of NNP in the neuropil were strikingly reduced, to means of 3.4 and 2.2 per standard graticule area, and there was similar heavy depopulation of neurons, with scattered evidence of neuronophagia, in all ganglia studied. Lewy bodies were seen in both subjects, with mean incidences of 1.1 and 1.25 per NNP; these were sometimes in neuronal somata and sometimes in enlarged neuronal processes. In the surviving neurons, however, the mean incidence of visible Nissl granules was high (92 and 93 per cent of NNP), and the proportions of NNP which showed massed lipofuscin bodies (82 per cent in each case) resembled those reported above for the MSA and control subjects. In these ganglia, therefore, the salient and distinctive features were the evidence of loss of neurons and the presence of Lewy bodies. In the younger PAF subject an entire SCG was available for neuron-counting in serial paraffin sections. Counts of all neuronal nuclei in every fiftieth section, of 10-μm thickness (cf. Ebbesson 1963), with application of correction factors according to the formula of Konigsmark (1970), yielded an estimate of 214 002 neurons in the entire ganglion. When compared with the mean figure of approximately 937 000 (range 760 370–1 041 652) obtained from four ganglia of young adults by Ebbesson (1963), this suggests a loss of over 75 per cent of neurons, which is much greater than might be expected to occur with age in normal subjects.

Histochemistry, immunohistochemistry, *in situ* hybridization

In frozen sections of a thoracic ganglion from the younger PAF subject, specific acetylcholinesterase activity was demonstrable, after prolonged incubation, with a normal distribution in the few surviving neuronal cell bodies and in parts of the surrounding neuropil, but not in nerve bundles.

Immunofluorescence histochemistry by the indirect method was performed on sections from ganglia of two subjects with MSA (males aged 56 and 77 years) and one with PAF (female, aged 58 years, from whom neuron counts were made in the SCG), in comparison with ganglia from the three young and four older male control subjects, with the following results.

Sensory nerve collaterals

In the control subjects prevertebral ganglia (coeliac–superior mesenteric) contained perineuronal networks of finely varicose nerve fibres immuno-reactive for substance P (SP), and likewise for calcitonin gene-related peptide (CGRP), which surrounded individual neurons or clusters of neurons. Both these peptides are found in certain primary sensory neurons, in many of which they coexist, and the intraganglionic networks are attributable to collateral terminal branches of sensory nerve fibres from the viscera which traverse the prevertebral ganglia en route to the dorsal root ganglia and spinal cord (Matthews and Cuello 1982). (It is not yet clear whether, as in the rat, some human preganglionic axons may also contain CGRP). In thoracic and lumbar paravertebral ganglia only occasional, solitary varicose trails were seen which were immunoreactive for SP or CGRP. No obvious differences were found between the younger and older control subjects. Similar networks in a prevertebral ganglion, resembling those in the controls both in distribution and in density, and occasional solitary fibres in paravertebral ganglia were found in one of the MSA subjects (Fig. 32.3 (b),(c)). (No prevertebral ganglion was available from the other MSA subject.) The coeliac ganglion of the subject with PAF showed localized 'baskets' of SP- and CGRP-immunoreactive varicosities surrounding some of the residual neurons, but not those with Lewy bodies or dystrophic neurites. These findings suggest that such trophic interactions as may be required for the maintenance of these sensory collateral networks are still present and operative, not only in older control subjects equally with younger subjects, but also in MSA, and in relation to some surviving neurons in PAF.

Encephalin-immunoreactive elements

In the control prevertebral ganglia, equally in younger and older subjects, short trails and perineuronal arcs of coarse encephalin-immunoreactive varicosities were scantily distributed from place to place. Similar encephalin-immunoreactive nerve elements, similarly distributed, were found in the prevertebral ganglion of the MSA subject (Fig. 32.3(a)) and occasionally, near to some of the surviving neurons, in the PAF subject.

In the paravertebral ganglia of all the control subjects profuse pericellular networks of finely varicose, slender, encephalin-immunoreactive nerve fibres were seen, surrounding clusters of neurons from place to place throughout the ganglia (Fig. 32.4(a)). In the two MSA subjects, although the post-mortem

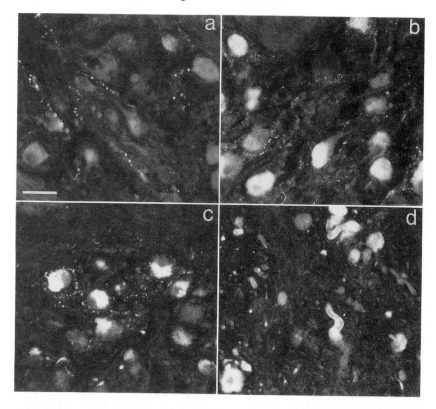

Fig. 32.3. Immunofluorescent staining for neuropeptides in the coeliac ganglion: (a) encephalin, (b) substance P, (c) CGRP, all from a case of MSA; (d) neuropeptide Y in dystrophic neurites from a case of pure autonomic failure. Scale bar, 50 μm. Some neurons in (b) and (c) show intensely autofluorescent lipofuscin masses.

intervals (10 h, 13 h) had been shorter for them than for any of the controls (21–48 h, mean 31 h), only slight and scanty encephalin-immunoreactive networks were found in thoracic and lumbar paravertebral ganglia (Fig. 32.4(b)). In a thoracic ganglion of the PAF subject, no encephalin-immunoreactive fibres or varicosities could be detected. This could have either of two causes: (1) ante-mortem loss, through degeneration; (2) post-mortem degradation of these very fine nerve fibres, since in this case the post-mortem interval was long (84 h), although cooling had been begun early. The question must remain open.

The fine encephalin-immunoreactive networks in the paravertebral ganglia are attributable to preganglionic nerve fibres. Clearly, these do not represent all the preganglionic nerve endings, since not all neurons are surrounded by them. In the rat, encephalin and choline acetyltransferase, the

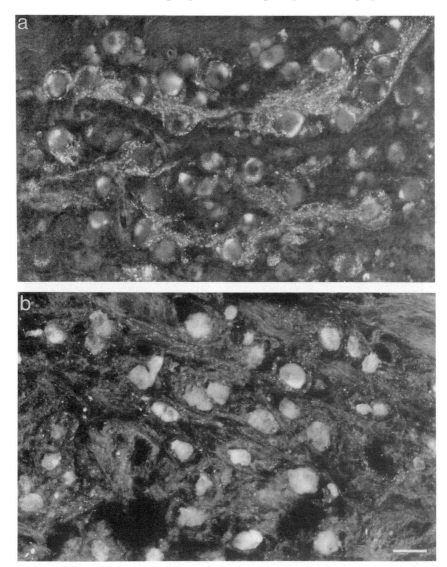

Fig. 32.4. Immunofluorescent staining for encephalin in thoracic paravertebral ganglia: (a) from a young control subject; (b) from a case of MSA. Very few trails of fine encephalin-immunoreactive fibres are present in (b). Most of the solitary bright points in this field represent lipofuscin autofluorescence. Scale bar, 50 μm.

acetylcholine-synthesizing enzyme, have been shown to coexist in some of the preganglionic sympathetic neurons (Kondo *et al.* 1985). The severe depletion of encephalin-immunoreactive networks in paravertebral ganglia in MSA suggests, first, that the corresponding IML neurons are heavily

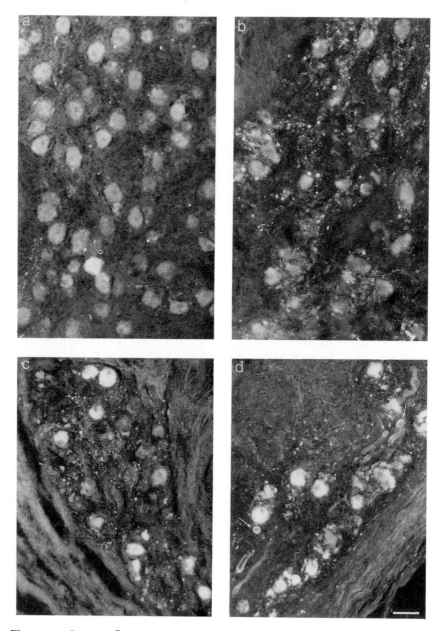

Fig. 32.5. Immunofluorescent staining for NPY in the coeliac ganglion: (a) From
a young control subject, aged 17 years; (b) from a case of MSA, subject aged
77 years; (c) from an old control subject, aged 85 years. NPY immunoreactivity
is visible in most of the neurons in (a) and (b), but in (c) is partly obscured by
lipofuscin masses. Irregular varicose trails and larger foci of bright
immunofluorescence are much more numerous in (c) than in (a) and are

depleted and, second, that this loss has not been fully compensated by whatever intraganglionic sprouting may have occurred from the nerve endings of surviving IML neurons. The same could well also apply to the other, non-encephalin-immunoreactive preganglionic neurons. In the PAF subject, absence of encephalin-immunoreactive networks could indicate loss of the preganglionic neurons from target deprivation, consequent upon the severe neuron depopulation of the ganglion. It is appropriate to consider whether death of preganglionic neurons from the target deprivation could also account for the loss of encephalin-immunoreactive nerve networks in the MSA subjects, since there is evidence for selective loss of sudomotor ganglionic neurons in this condition (see Chapter 31). Upon this point, however, the available evidence is conflicting, one study (Schmitt *et al.* 1988) suggesting that presumptive sudomotor neurons in human paravertebral sypathetic ganglia are not innervated by encephalin-immunoreactive nerve fibres and another (Järvi and Pelto-Huikko 1990) indicating the contrary.

Neuropeptide Y (NPY) immunoreactivity in ganglia

A proportion of sympathetic ganglionic neurons contains NPY-immuno-reactive material in addition to noradrenaline. These are vasoconstrictor neurons. In the young control subjects many ganglionic neurons showed moderate immunoreactivity for NPY, and a few short varicose trails and somewhat larger foci of more intense immunoreactivity were seen in the surrounding neuropil (Fig. 32.5(a)). In older subjects these additional foci of more intense immunoreactivity were more numerous and widespread, and the NPY immunoreactivity of the cell bodies also appeared more intense (Fig. 32.5 (c)). In the ganglia of MSA subjects this difference was at least as strongly marked, and possibly greater, placing them in sharp contrast with the ganglia of the younger subjects (Fig. 32.5(b)). The additional foci may represent NPY-rich short intracapsular dendrites or additional dendritic branches of the neurons, which increase with age, and might be particularly profusely developed, or strongly charged with NPY, in the MSA subjects, there perhaps reflecting low recruitment and engorgement with undischarged secretory materials, and perhaps the formation of local collateral sprouts and synapses (cf. Ramsay and Matthews 1985). In the PAF subject, many of the Lewy bodies and dystrophic neurites showed NPY immunoreactivity in their peripheral zone, marginal to the halo (Fig. 32.5(d)).

Fig. 32.5. (*continued*)   particularly conspicuous in (b). (d) is from the case of PAF illustrated also in Fig. 32.3(d), and shows the prevalence of Lewy bodies and dystrophic neurites, some with strong peripheral NPY immunoreactivity (arrows), in a region unusually well populated with surviving neurons. Scale bar, 50 µm.

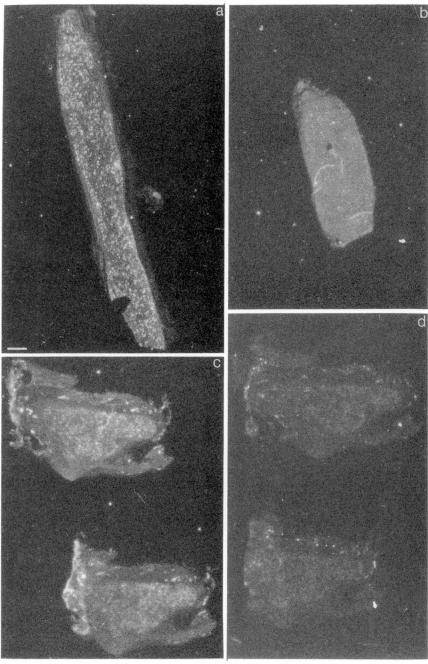

Fig. 32.6. *In situ* hybridization autoradiographs (reverse phase) from slide-mounted cryostat sections. (a) Paravertebral (lumbar) ganglion from a case of MSA, (b) coeliac ganglion from a case of PAF, (c) stellate ganglion from a control subject aged 66 years, all showing extent of binding of the antisense probe for tyrosine hydroxylase mRNA; (d) coeliac ganglion of the same control subject,

Tyrosine hydroxylase immunoreactivity

Tyrosine hydroxylase (TOH) is a cytoplasmic enzyme of the sympathetic neuron which is of interest as being the rate-limiting enzyme in catecholamine synthesis. It is also subject to up-regulation via incoming nerve impulses. A low cytoplasmic level of immunofluorescent signal for TOH, approximately $1.8 \times$ primary–antibody blank level, was demonstrable in neurons of a ganglion from a young control subject by image densitometry of film micrographs exposed for a standard interval. Similar measurements in the corresponding ganglion of an MSA subject gave a value of approximately $1.2 \times$ antibody blank level. These measurements were made with precautions to avoid deposits of lipofuscin in the neurons. They indicate that TOH-like material and a presumptive catecholamine productive capacity may persist in sympathetic ganglionic neurons in MSA despite a severe degree of decentralization, which harmonizes with the observation of normal supine plasma noradrenaline levels in this condition.

In situ hybridization for tyrosine hydroxylase mRNA

In a collaborative study with Dr O. J. F. Foster, working in the laboratory of Dr S. L. Lightman, cryostat sections of ganglia of the same two MSA subjects and the PAF subject and ganglia from the three younger and three older male control subjects, all from the above series and alternating with sections used in the immunohistochemical analysis, were examined by in situ hybridization for TOH mRNA. Sections from MSA subjects and both older and younger controls showed similar levels of binding of the 35S-labelled TOH mRNA antisense oligonucleotide probe used (Fig. 32.6(a), (c) and 32.7(a)). In contrast, sections from the PAF subject showed very low levels of probe binding over the few remaining neurons (Figs 32.6(b) and 32.7(b)); neurons containing Lewy bodies did not differ noticeably from those without such inclusions. All the sections studied showed low levels of hybridization to a TOH sense probe, employed to reflect non-specific binding (Fig. 32.6(d)). Binding of this probe was localized almost exclusively to collections of lipofuscin in the ganglionic neurons. This study indicates that TOH mRNA is detectable post-mortem in human sympathetic neurons by in situ hybridization. The finding that TOH probe binding was similar in MSA and in control ganglia suggests that TOH biosynthetic pathways may be functioning normally in the ganglionic neurons of MSA subjects, despite the deficiencies in preganglionic pathways. In the case of PAF studied, the low level of TOH anti-sense probe binding did not differ appreciably from the level of non-specific binding indicated by the sense probe. Any conclusion that

Fig. 32.6. (continued)   adjacent sections to those in (c), showing low level of non-specific binding of the sense probe. Scale bar, 1 mm.

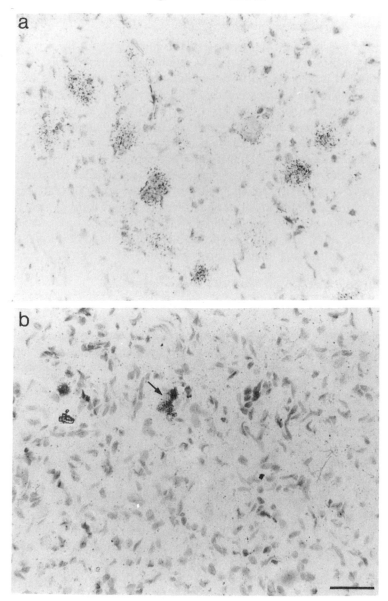

Fig. 32.7. *In situ* hybridization autoradiographs, lightly counterstained with toluidine blue, light micrography. Scale bar, 50 µm. (a) Lumbar ganglion of a 66-year-old control subject, showing heavy binding of antisense probe for tyrosine hydroxylase mRNA over ganglionic neurons; (b) coeliac ganglion of the PAF subject showing some binding of the same probe over a neuron containing a Lewy body (arrow) but little or no binding elsewhere; the binding in this specimen did not differ appreciably from the non-specific binding of the sense probe.

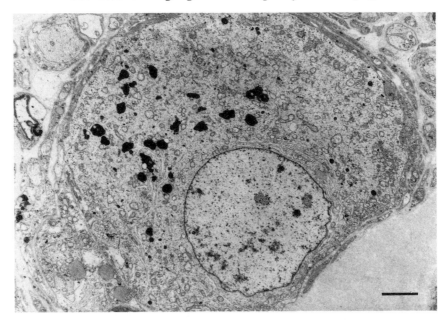

Fig. 32.8. Electron micrograph of a typical neuron from the SCG of a subject with MSA. The nucleus is markedly eccentric. The cytoplasm shows numerous lipofuscin bodies and little rough endoplasmic reticulum (Nissl material). At the lower right the satellite sheath of the neuron is very thin and in places deficient (cf. Fig. 32.12). Scale bar, 5 μm.

TOH biosynthesis was reduced in this case must, however, be tentative because of the long post-mortem delay of over 80 h already noted.

Electron microscopy

Not all the material was sufficiently well preserved to be informative. Questions which were addressed included general neuronal cytology (Fig. 32.8), the presence and type of synapses, the completeness of satellite cell cover of the neurons, and the state of the pre- and postganglionic nerve fibres.

In the youngest control subject, synapses were readily localizable with an incidence of approximately 6 to 10 per grid square of side 100 μm; they were of cholinergic preganglionic type (Fig. 32.9; Matthews 1983) and were mostly axodendritic. In the subjects with MSA similar synapses were present (Fig. 32.10), occurring in clusters in areas of dendritic neuropil, but were much less frequent, and tended to be greatly expanded and depleted of vesicles. This appearance was not necessarily just a post-mortem artefact, since it appeared equally in ganglia fixed within 8 h and over 36 h post-mortem: it recalled the appearance of nerve endings heavily overstimulated by black widow spider venom, and could possibly have reflected intense sympathetic

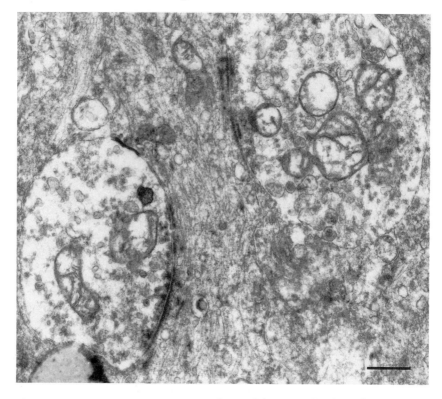

Fig. 32.9. Two synapses on opposite faces of the same dendrite, from the SCG
of a control subject aged 16. Scale bar, 0.5 μm.

discharges in surviving preganglionic endings in the ante-mortem period.
In addition, occasional synapses were seen containing tubular vesicles with
a relatively electron-dense content (Fig. 32.11); these resemble a type of
adrenergic nerve ending and could be intrinsic synapses, which can increase
appreciably in incidence in denervated (and presumably in partly denervated)
ganglia (Ramsay and Matthews 1985).

Neuro-neuronal attachment plaques were seen both in control and in MSA
ganglia (Fig. 32.11).

Neuron–satellite relations did not seem to differ markedly between control
and MSA ganglia. In both, neurons or their dendrites could show short,
sometimes multiple, regions of their surfaces devoid of satellite cell cover
(Fig. 32.12); these appeared to be at least at frequent in the MSA ganglia.
There was possibly some tendency for the enveloping satellite cell processes
to be thinner in the MSA ganglia, but further study, of material better
matched as to age and preservation, would be required to clarify this question.

In one MSA subject, the pre- and postganglionic nerve fibres were
sufficiently well preserved for ultrastructural study. Among the preganglionic

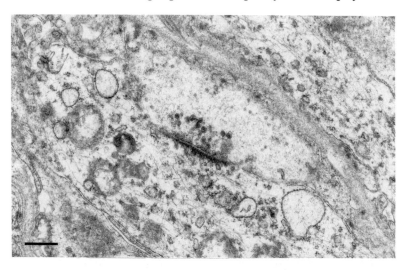

Fig. 32.10. Axodendritic synapse from the SCG of a subject with MSA. The presynaptic profile is heavily depleted of synaptic vesicles and shows evidence of numerous coated vesicles, suggesting recent extensive liberation of transmitter. Scale bar, 0.5 μm.

nerve fibres there was evidence of loss of axons, in the form of collagen-filled Schwann cell channels; myelinated fibres were few and other Schwann-axon units contained each only one or two unmyelinated axons (Fig. 32.13). The indications of fibre loss are consistent with the well-documented loss of IML neurons in MSA. Some of the unmyelinated axons were singly ensheathed and of relatively large diameter, up to 4 μm, which suggests possible demyelination, or hypertrophy without accompanying myelination. These axons were well populated with microtubules and neurofilaments, and did not appear to be pathologically swollen. Among the postganglionic fibres in the internal carotid trunk there was also some suggestion of fibre loss, in the form of collagen-filled channels in Schwann cells, and here also there was a wide range of diameters of unmyelinated axons, suggesting possible denervation atrophy of some neurons and hypertrophy of others. The number of fibres per Schwann unit was not unduly high, ranging mostly from two to six; thus, there was little evidence of axon sprouting at this level.

In the older subject with PAF, although preservation of the interneuronal neuropil was poor, information was obtained on the nature of the Lewy bodies in these sympathetic neurons (Fig. 32.14): a mass of densely fibrillar material with an amorphous denser core was surrounded by a rim of dense-cored vesicles, which were associated with the marginal filaments of the mass (cf. Forno and Norville 1976). Densely packed lysosomal bodies in addition to much lipofuscin were seen in some neurons, but, as was noted earlier, the surviving neurons, apart from those containing Lewy bodies, did not look grossly abnormal.

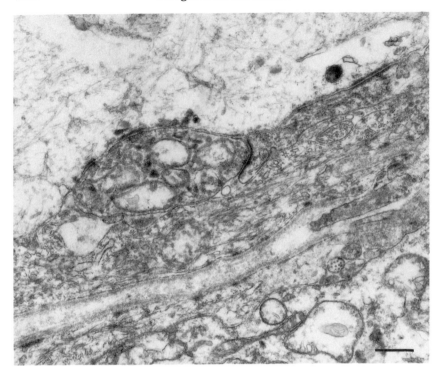

Fig. 32.11. Two synapses of possible adrenergic type from the same presynaptic profile, one axodendritic and the other probably axosomatic, from the SCG of a subject with MSA (same ganglion as Fig. 32.10). On the right the dendrite is linked with the presumptive soma by an attachment plaque. Scale bar, 0.5 μm.

Conclusions and comment

This ongoing study has indicated a clear difference in ganglionic pathology, and hence presumably in underlying cause of the AF, between MSA and PAF.

In MSA the neurons of sympathetic ganglia are not in general severely reduced in number and do not exhibit major abnormalities, except that considerably fewer may show distinguishable Nissl granules than in control subjects. This relative lack of Nissl material might indicate a denervation atrophy of long standing. There is confirmatory evidence of the loss of preganglionic nerve fibres, and there is evidence which suggests that, despite any regenerative sprouting from surviving fibres, by the time AF supervenes there is a severe deficiency of preganglionic nerve endings in the ganglia and possible overdriving of surviving endings. The loss of preganglionic nerve endings appears to be selective, since other demonstrable fibre systems, for example sensory collateral nerve networks, seem at least as profuse as in

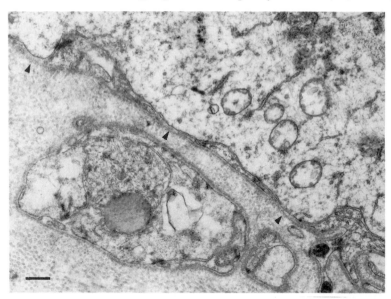

Fig. 32.12.   Arrowheads indicate short deficiencies in the satellite sheath of a neuron, from the SCG of a subject with MSA. Scale bar, 0.5 μm.

normal subjects. It has not so far proved feasible to determine whether they may actually be increased in MSA ganglia, by some mechanism of sprouting in response to the partial denervation. It is possible, however, that NPY immunoreactivity in neurons and their processes may be increased in these ganglia, by more than the increment with age which this study has revealed in control subjects. Tyrosine hydroxylase and its mRNA may still be demonstrable in these sympathetic neurons, in MSA with AF.

In PAF, on the other hand, the packing density of ganglionic neurons may be severely reduced, and counts in one complete SCG have indicated a loss of over 75 per cent of the neurons, which resembles the proportional loss of IML neurons at which autonomic failure occurs (Oppenheimer 1980). Some of the surviving ganglionic neurons show Lewy bodies, many display eosinophilic bodies in distorted, dystrophic neurites, and some show evidence of an intense lysosomal activity, but almost all of the remainder show well-defined Nissl granules and do not appear grossly abnormal for the age of the subject.

It therefore seems reasonable to assume, as a working hypothesis, that these two forms of AF result, respectively, from the loss of preganglionic and of ganglionic neurons. This might ultimately prove too simple a view. The initial causes of the loss of neurons remain obscure, though in the case of 'Lewy body disease' it might be the same metabolic dysfunction which causes the fibrillar accumulations that also leads to neuronal death. It remains to be

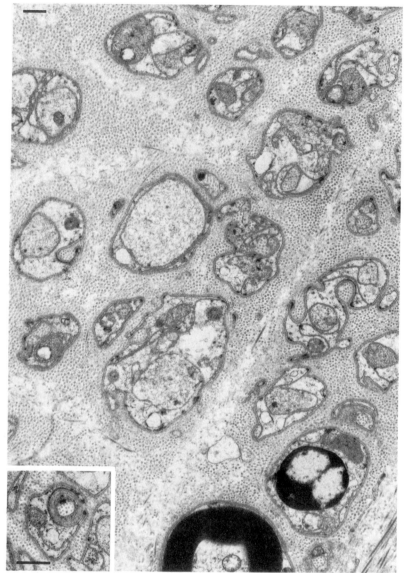

Fig. 32.13. Unmyelinated axons, and part of a myelinated axon, from the cervical sympathetic trunk of a subject with MSA, taken close to the SCG. Schwann-axon profiles are widely separated by dense endoneurial collagen. Most of the Schwann profiles contain only one or two axons, which are of 0.6 to 4 μm diameter; even large axons are unmyelinated in this field. The small numbers of axons per Schwann unit, and the occurrence of collagen-filled channels in the Schwann cells, sometimes lined by basal lamina, suggest appreciable loss of axons. Inset, Schwann unit containing one small axon and a collagen-filled channel, lined by reduplicated basal lamina. Scale bars, 1 μm.

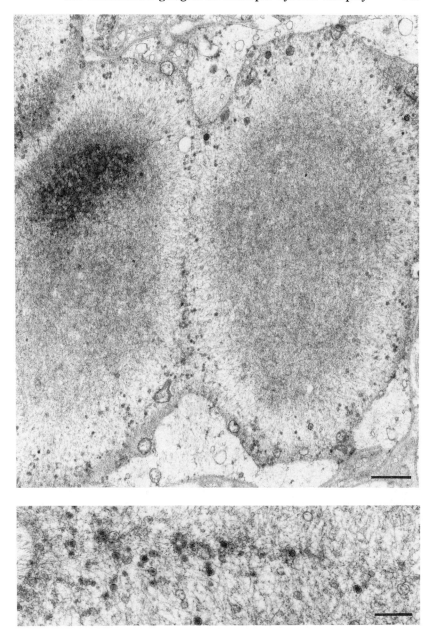

Fig. 32.14. Electron micrograph of two Lewy bodies filling adjacent parts of a neurite, possibly an axon, from the SCG of a subject with pure autonomic failure. Scale bar, 2 μm. Below is shown at higher magnification part of the periphery of the Lewy bodies, where dense-cored vesicles are associated with the margins of the fibrillary masses. Scale bar, 0.5 μm.

confirmed by counting whether there may be comparable loss of ganglionic neurons in the AF that can develop in PD, but it seems probable that PAF, PD, and AF with PD are different manifestations of the same disease process. The ramifications of the secondary consequences remain likewise to be unravelled. As Oppenheimer (1980) has clearly shown, loss of IML neurons in PAF, or in AF with PD, can be quite as severe as that found in MSA. This could be a retrograde neuronal death, consequent upon target deprivation and related to the profundity and duration of the latter. Indeed, the loss of IML neurons in MSA might itself be due to disruption of a retrograde trophic influence from the ganglionic neurons, which might arise, for example, from inadequate production or release of essential neurotrophic factor(s), without overt morphological changes in the ganglionic neurons. The demonstration of apparently normal prevertebral sensory collateral nerve networks in MSA suggests, however, that any deficiency of trophic substance could be highly specific for the preganglionic neurons.

Lewy bodies have recently been shown to be immunoreactive for neurofilament proteins (variably, in their haloes) and also for ubiquitin (both in their periphery and in the core) (Bancher *et al.* 1989). Ubiquitin is an 8.6 kDa cytoplasmic polypeptide of very widespread distribution which is involved in the adenosine triphosphate (ATP)-dependent hydrolysis of abnormal or short-lived proteins. Kuzuhara *et al.* (1988) describe 'decoration' of the filaments of the halo with ubiquitin immunoreactivity at ultrastructural level. Peptide or catecholamine neurotransmitters, or neurotransmitter-synthesizing enzymes, appropriate to the neuron type, have been detected immunohistochemically at the periphery of Lewy bodies (for example, Wakabayashi *et al.* 1990), as was also found for NPY in the present material. This mirrors the finding of many dense-cored vesicles at the periphery of the Lewy bodies in dystrophic neurites. Selective immunohistochemical studies indicate that the neurofilaments included within the Lewy body are chiefly phosphorylated, rather than non-phosphorylated (Bancher *et al.* 1989), thus resembling axonal rather than dendritic or intrasomatic neurofilaments. The conjoint presence of dense-cored vesicles and of phosphorylated neuro-filaments suggests that the dystrophic neurites are in fact axons or frustrated axonal forms.

The interpretation of these findings is at present unclear. It has been suggested that an abnormal level of phosphorylation may be preventing degradation of filamentous proteins; but this would not explain how, or why, the neurofilaments and other material should accumulate in this highly ordered manner. Moreover, we do not know the dynamics of the Lewy body: how long does it take to form? How long does it persist? Is the cell in which it is forming making a maximal productive effort, and of what? Will the cell survive? Can it recover? Possibly not: neuron numbers may be heavily depleted in nuclei such as the substantia nigra or locus ceruleus, or in sympathetic ganglia, in cases in which Lewy bodies are found. In the absence of an adequate animal model the answers to these and other relevant questions will perhaps not easily be determined.

Finally, the distribution of anhidrosis in AF is another topic illuminated by recent findings. Anhidrosis in AF, whether patchy or generalized, is often symmetrical. Not infrequently the limbs may be affected selectively, or the trunk and lower limbs. Of particular interest is the occasional sparing of the head, including the face and root of neck, with almost total anhidrosis elsewhere in the body (Bannister *et al.* 1967; Hughes *et al.* 1970). In both forms of AF, anhidrosis may be found on local testing of secretomotor function to be due to failure of ganglionic neurons, selectively so in the case of MSA; there is thus postganglionic denervation of the sweat glands. Recent immunohistochemical studies in experimental animals and suggestive evidence in man indicate that the cutaneous blood vessels in the head and neck receive a vasodilator innervation from cranial parasympathetic ganglia (Gibbins 1990), in addition to both vasoconstrictor and vasodilator sympathetic nerve fibres (Drummond and Finch 1989). It may therefore be proposed that the selective sparing of sweat secretion in the head and neck in some cases of AF could result from sprouting of, or diffusion of transmitter from, surviving parasympathetic vasodilator nerve fibres. This is the same territory (co-extensive with that of the superior cervical ganglion) as that within which gustatory sweating may also occur, following lesions of peripheral sympathetic pathways, and the latter is likely to have the same underlying mechanism. The distance from a sweat gland to the nearest parasympathetically innervated small artery or arteriole is unlikely to be excessive. The parasympathetic vasodilator fibres are cholinergic and show immunoreactivity for vasoactive intestinal polypeptide, and could therefore provide appropriate agonist stimulation for sweat gland activity. In physiological gustatory sweating, secretion is provoked by intense gustatory or painful oral stimulation, and the response is not susceptible to sympathetic blockade (Drummond and Lance 1987). The reflex which leads to the sweating is likely to be generated centrally, but to the extent that trigeminal afferents are involved it could be reinforced via 'axon reflex' release of transmitter from sensory nerve collaterals given in the cranial parasympathetic ganglia.

The observations reported here denote some advances to date but also present challenges for verification and raise various questions for exploration. The wider range of approaches and techniques now available offers renewed hope of progress, perhaps ideally by way of collaborative studies, in resolving the basic problems of causation in these devastatingly disabling conditions of autonomic failure.

Acknowledgements

This work was supported by a grant from the Medical Research Council. Thanks are due to Mr P. J. Belk and Mr M. Masih for technical assistance,

Mr B. Archer, Mr T. Barclay, and Mr C. Beesley for photographic work, and Miss J. Ballinger for secretarial assistance. Generous gifts of primary antibodies from Professors A. C. Cuello (SP, Enk, TOH) and J. M. Polak (CGRP, NPY) are gratefully acknowledged. The author thanks Drs D. R. Oppenheimer, M. M. Esiri, J. R. Ponsford, M. Rossi, N. D. Francis, and F. Scaravilli for obtaining ganglia, and Professor L. W. Duchen for access to paraffin-embedded material.

References

Bancher, C., Lassmann, H., Budka, H., Jellinger, K., Grundke-Iqbal, I., Iqbal, K., Wiche, G., Seitelberger, F., and Wisniewski, H. M. (1989). An antigenic profile of Lewy bodies: immunocytochemical indication for protein phosphorylation and ubiquitination. *J. Neuropathol. exp. Neurol.* **48**, 81–93.

Bannister, R. and Oppenheimer, D. R. (1972). Degenerative diseases of the nervous system associated with autonomic failure. *Brain* **95**, 457–74.

Bannister, R., Ardill, L., and Fentem, P. (1967). Defective autonomic control of blood vessels in idiopathic orthostatic hypotension. *Brain* **90**, 725–46.

Drummond, P. D. and Finch, P. M. (1989). Reflex control of facial flushing during body heating in man. *Brain* **112**, 1351–8.

Drummond, P. D. and Lance, J. W. (1987). Facial flushing and sweating mediated by the sympathetic nervous system. *Brain* **110**, 793–803.

Ebbesson, S. O. E. (1963). A quantitative study of human superior cervical sympathetic ganglia. *Anat. Rec.* **146**, 353–6.

Forno, L. S. and Norville, R. L. (1976). Ultrastructure of Lewy bodies in the stellate ganglion. *Acta neuropathol., Berlin* **34**, 183–97.

Gibbins, I. L. (1990). Target-related patterns of co-existence of neuropeptide Y, vasoactive intestinal peptide, enkephalin and substance P in cranial parasympathetic neurons innervating the facial skin and exocrine glands of guinea-pigs. *Neuroscience* **38**, 541–60.

Gray, F., Vincent, D., and Hauw, J. J. (1988). Quantitative study of lateral horn cells in 15 cases of multiple system atrophy. *Acta neuropathol., Berlin* **75**, 513–18.

Hughes, R. C., Cartlidge, N. E. F., and Millac, P. (1970). Primary neurogenic orthostatic hypotension. *J. Neurol. Neurosurg. Psychiat.* **33**, 363–71.

Järvi, R. and Pelto-Huikko, M. (1990). Localization of neuropeptide Y in human sympathetic ganglia: correlation with met-enkephalin, tyrosine hydroxylase and acetylcholinesterase. *Histochem. J.* **22**, 87–94.

Kondo, N., Kuramoto, H., Wainer, B. H., and Yanaihara, N. (1985). Evidence for the coexistence of acetylcholine and enkephalin in the sympathetic preganglion neurons of rats. *Brain Res.* **335**, 309–14.

Konigsmark, B. W. (1970). Methods for the counting of neurons. In *Contemporary research methods in neuroanatomy* (ed. W. J. H. Nauta and S. O. E. Ebbesson), pp. 315–40. Springer, Berlin.

Konno, H., Yamamoto, T., Iwasaki, Y., and Iizuka, H. (1986). Shy–Drager syndrome and amyotrophic lateral sclerosis: cytoarchitectonic and morphometric studies of sacral autonomic neurons. *J. neurol. Sci.* **73**, 193–204.

Kuzuhara, S., Mori, H., Izumiyama, N., Yoshimura, M., and Ihara, Y. (1988). Lewy bodies are ubiquitinated. A light and electron microscopic immunocytochemical study. *Acta neuropathol., Berlin* **75**, 345–53.

Liestøl, K., Maehlen, J., and Nja, A. (1986). Selective synaptic connections: significance of recognition and competition in mature sympathetic ganglia. *Trends Neurosci.* **9**, 21–4.

Matthews, M. R. (1983). The ultrastructure of junctions in sympathetic ganglia of mammals. In *Autonomic ganglia* (ed. L.-G. Elfvin), pp. 27–66. John Wiley, Chichester.

Matthews, M. R. and Cuello, A. C. (1982). Substance P-immunoreactive peripheral branches of sensory neurons innervate guinea pig sympathetic neurons. *Proc. natl. Acad. Sci., USA* **79**, 1668–72.

Oppenheimer, D. R. (1980). Lateral horn cells in progressive autonomic failure. *J. neurol. Sci.* **46**, 393–404.

Rajput, A. H. and Rozdilsky, B. (1976). Dysautonomia in Parkinsonism: a clinico-pathological study. *J. Neurol. Neurosurg. Psychiat.* **39**, 1092–100.

Ramsay, D. A. and Matthews, M. R. (1985). Denervation-induced formation of adrenergic synapses in the superior cervical sympathetic ganglion of the rat and the enhancement of this effect by postganglionic axotomy. *Neuroscience* **16**, 997–1026.

Rohmer, F., Warter, J.-M., Coquillat, G., Schupp, C., and Maitrot, D. (1973). "Maladie" de Shy et Drager. A propos d'une observation anatomoclinique. Revue de la littérature. *Ann. Méd. Interne* **124**, 665–75.

Schmitt, M., Kummer, W., and Heym, C. (1988). Calcitonin gene-related peptide (CGRP)-immunoreactive neurons in the human cervico-thoracic paravertebral ganglia. *J. Chem. Neuroanat.* **1**, 287–92.

Spokes, E. G. S., Bannister, R., and Oppenheimer, D. (1979). Multiple system atrophy with autonomic failure—clinical, histological and neurochemical observations on four cases. *J. neurol. Sci.* **43**, 59–82.

Thoenen, H. (1991). The changing scene of neurotrophic factors. *Trends Neurosci.* **14**, 165–70.

Wakabayashi, K. (1989). Parkinson's disease: the distribution of Lewy bodies in the peripheral autonomic nervous system. *No To Shinkei* **41**, 965–71. [English abstract.]

Wakabayashi, K., Takahashi, H., Ohama, E., and Ikuta, F. (1990). Parkinson's disease: an immunohistochemical study of Lewy body-containing neurons in the enteric nervous system. *Acta neuropathol.* **79**, 581–3.

33. Management of postural hypotension

Roger Bannister and Christopher J. Mathias

General principles

Treatment of postural hypotension due to autonomic failure is fraught with difficulties, many caused by inaccurate localization of the sites of the lesions. Treatment requires targeting; as Ehrlich commented on chemotherapy, 'we must learn to aim and aim in a chemical sense'. In autonomic failure, treatment has to be directed to overcoming precisely identified defects. This chapter focuses on the management of orthostatic hypotension due to primary autonomic failure but many of the principles outlined here are applicable to postural hypotension due to other causes.

In secondary autonomic failure (see Chapter 1) there may be special factors which are covered in other chapters. Some examples of these special factors may be listed:

(1) insulin affecting postural hypotension in diabetes (see Chapter 26);

(2) difficulties in managing postural hypotension in tetraplegics with drugs, as pressor drugs can lead to severe hypertension (see Chapter 43);

(3) The aggravating effects of hypoalbuminaemia due to protein loss in amyloid, making treatment with fludrocortisone very difficult.

Some principles of management are common to all patients.

Cerebral blood flow

First, it is important not to be overconcerned about a low standing blood pressure if the patient is without symptoms. Patients can sometimes tolerate a standing systolic blood pressure as low as 70 mm Hg without dizziness or syncope, probably because their cerebral blood flow is maintained at an adequate level because of the capacity of their cerebral circulation for autoregulation. There have been several studies attempting to clarify whether in autonomic failure there is a reduced fall of cerebral blood flow for a standard fall of mean arterial pressure. Thomas and Bannister (1980) studied five patients with autonomic failure (AF) and multiple system atrophy (MSA) and found that autoregulation was preserved down to a systolic blood pressure close to 60 mm Hg which is well below the 80 mm Hg at which autoregulation fails in normal subjects. The results in a further three patients with pure autonomic failure (PAF) showed a similar trend. A shift of autoregulation to the left in AF almost certainly occurs and the reason some have failed to record it is probably that, when cerebral blood flow was measured during tilt, the arterial pressure may have been transiently much lower than the recorded pressure. They found evidence of this in one patient with AF who developed symptoms of cerebral ischaemia when his systolic pressure fell transiently to 40 mm Hg and the clearance curve changed, implying a transient fall in flow (Fig. 33.1). The change in autoregulation may be the result of prolonged exposure to lower than normal arterial pressure, causing some changes in the response of normally innervated vessels, or be due to the fact that the cerebral vessels, like muscle vessels, are partially or completely sympathectomized in autonomic failure. It has been suggested that the major sympathetic innervation is to the extraparenchymal vessels, the intraparenchymal vessels being under myogenic and metabolic control. If this

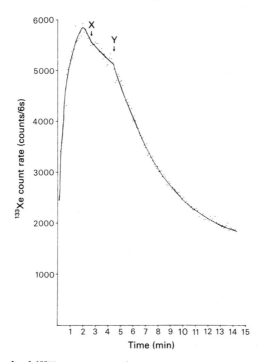

Fig. 33.1. Cerebral ^{133}Xe count rates/6 s in patient G. K. with pure autonomic failure tilted to 45°. At point X, the blood pressure fell suddenly to a systolic pressure of 40 mm Hg. The rate of ^{133}Xe clearance decreased and the patient developed symptoms of cerebral ischaemia. At point Y, the tilt table was lowered, blood pressure rose, and the rate of clearance increased. (Taken with permission from Thomas and Bannister (1980).)

is so, the sympathetic innervation at the lower level of autoregulation may normally reduce cerebral blood flow by constricting extraparenchymal vessels. Whatever the explanation, it is certain that patients with autonomic failure have a remarkable tolerance to low blood pressure without developing postural hypotensive symptoms.

Recumbent hypertension

A second principle that has to be considered in treatment is the tendency of patients to develop recumbent hypertension owing principally to defective baroreceptor reflexes, supersensitivity, and treatment with drugs such as fludrocortisone. Clearly, this may result in a reactive increase of cerebrovascular resistance leading to the likelihood of cerebral ischaemic symptoms when such patients stand suddenly. Some patients, if nursed lying flat, may develop severe hypertension and run the risk of developing complications such as papilloedema, other features of hypertensive retinopathy, and cerebral haemorrhage.

Control of blood volume

A third principle is that, although loss of baroreflexes determines the immediate response of blood pressure to standing, control of blood volume, determined by low-pressure receptors and the kidney, through antidiuretic hormone, possibly the atrial natriuretic factor, and the renin–angiotensin–aldosterone system, is the long-term and more important adjustment to postural hypotension in autonomic failure.

Limitations of treatment

All methods of treatment, directly or indirectly, aim either at reducing the vascular volume into which pooling occurs on standing or increasing the volume of blood available for pooling. A reduction of the volume into which the blood may pool by pressor drugs has its limitations. Unless the drugs increase the responsiveness of vessels to small amounts of noradrenaline that can still be liberated, they will aggravate the tendency to recumbent hypertension. An increase in blood volume runs the risk of overloading the circulation and leading to cardiac failure and peripheral oedema. Many patients with autonomic failure have defects of renal preservation of sodium when recumbent and are sensitive to sodium depletion which leads to a reduction of intravascular and extracellular fluid volume. Though we are aware that many patients continue to receive a variety of treatments in different medical centres, it is probable that any treatment with pressor drugs that temporarily enables a patient to become more mobile will improve the patient's other homeostatic responses to standing. Hence, an improvement, even if sustained, may be erroneously attributed to a particular form of treatment when it might, under controlled conditions, be possible to withdraw or replace it with a safer method.

Testing of drugs

There have been a series of reports of treatment with many different drugs, usually given empirically for a short uncontrolled trial, often in patients with an imprecise diagnosis of AF. It may reasonably be asked whether any pressor drug is effective when so many different treatments have been proposed. It is also reasonable to question whether the effect of drugs can be monitored when the lack of baroreceptor reflexes in autonomic failure leads to such marked fluctuations with changes of posture and other events such as food ingestion over the course of 24 h so that adequate maintenance of blood pressure is as difficult as targeting in a video space game. In any attempt to measure the benefit of a drug in AF, the standing and recumbent blood pressure must be taken under standard conditions, preferably four times a day by trained staff. As the blood pressure of these patients usually continues to fall when they stand, the duration of standing has to be recorded. We aim to record the blood pressure 2 min after the onset of standing because arterial recording has shown that any fall in blood pressure will then be clearly apparent. Prior to drug treatment it is advisable to have an equilibrium period of a week on a standard daily sodium diet of 150 mmol with monitoring of position and physical activity during the day and measurement of head-up tilt at night. It is also advisable to measure the haematocrit, plasma proteins, urea, creatinine, and electrolytes every 3 days, weigh the patient on accurate scales twice daily, measure day and night fluid balance and urinary sodium and potassium excretion, and measure blood pressure four times a day before meals.

Drug combinations

Since patients with autonomic failure have lesions at more than one site, it should always be considered whether a combination of drugs may be more effective than a single drug. For example, drugs with central, ganglionic, and postganglionic effects may have synergistic actions. At the sympathetic

Table 33.1. Approaches to treatment

Advice on factors which influence blood pressure

1. Straining during micturition and defecation
2. Diurnal changes in blood pressure
3. Exposure to a warm environment
4. The effects of food
5. Effects of drugs with vasoactive properties

Head-up tilt at night
External support
Cardiac pacing
Drugs (see Table 33.2)

---

terminals drugs which increase noradrenaline release may be combined with drugs which reduce re-uptake of the transmitter or increase the sensitivity of receptors. Similarly, drugs which influence plasma volume (such as desmopressin) or release of vasodilatatory hormones (such as octreotide) and factors influencing blood pressure may be of value in combination.

Approaches to treatment (Table 33.1)

Advice on factors which influence blood pressure

A number of factors have been now defined, which can considerably lower blood pressure and thus enhance the postural fall and therefore the symptoms accompanying postural hypotension. The pathophysiological mechanisms accounting for a number of these have been worked out and in a number of situations avoidance measures can be instituted. Patients should therefore be advised on these factors.

Straining during micturition and defecation

A number of patients suffer from either urinary bladder problems or from constipation. Straining might result in a Valsalva manoeuvre being performed. This can result in a substantial reduction in blood pressure without the recovery mechanisms which normally come into play. Episodes of hypotension in some situations may be particularly dangerous, as patients may lose consciousness while propped against a lavatory wall and may not fall to the ground and thus correct their blood pressure.

Diurnal changes in blood pressure

The supine blood pressure in patients with AF is lowest in the morning and rises gradually during the day. This has been confirmed by non-invasive measurements and also by using continuous ambulatory intraarterial blood pressure recording (see Fig. 33.2). The circadian changes in blood pressure are the reverse of those in normal subjects, in whom the blood pressure falls during sleep and rises prior to awakening. The low level of blood pressure in the morning appears to be the result of nocturnal polyuria and natriuresis, which can result in a substantial overnight weight loss, at times over 1 kg. The reduction in extracellular fluid volume is likely to contribute to the low blood pressure as it is improved by administration of desmopressin (see below). The low blood pressure aggravates the symptoms of postural hypotension in the morning, and some patients find it extremely difficult to conduct their normal activities for a few hours after waking. Methods of preventing morning postural hypotension are described below.

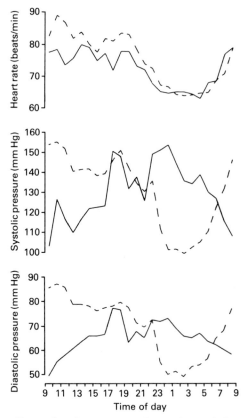

Fig. 33.2. Overall trend in heart rate and systolic and diastolic pressures of six subjects with autonomic failure (——) compared with those derived from a matched group of six subjects with normal or elevated blood pressure (-----). Lines join pooled hourly means. (Taken with permission from Mann *et al.* (1983).)

Exposure to a warm environment

Patients exposed to tropical or subtropical temperatures tend to have greater symptoms for a variety of reasons. They often lack the ability to sweat, and their core temperature can therefore rise. Uncompensated vasodilatation often ensues and the blood pressure can fall. Adequate precautions should therefore be taken by patients travelling to warm countries, who should be aware of the possible worsening of postural hypotension. Patients should be warned of the probability of a deterioration after a hot bath, especially if prolonged.

The effects of food

The majority of patients with AF have substantial postprandial hypotension. This occurs soon after food ingestion and may last for up to 3 h after a standard meal. The supine blood pressure can be lowered to levels of

80/50 mm Hg even in the supine position and therefore these patients often exhibit increased symptoms of postural hypotension. Carbohydrate appears to be the major component causing the hypotension, and this may be linked to the release of insulin and other gastrointestinal hormones which have vasodilatory properties. Vasodilatation in the gut, not compensated for by defective sympathetic reflexes, is the probable cause of the reduction in pressure. The pathophysiology and management of this important condition is described in Chapter 26. It is likely that alcoholic drinks, with their potential to cause vasodilatation, will lower blood pressure in these patients.

Effect of drugs with vasoactive properties

Both the patient and the physician should be aware that drugs with vasoactive properties, even if only a minor action of the agent, may result in substantial vascular changes because of supersensitivity. The responses to pressor agents, particularly sympathetic agents, have already been described. Vasopressor responses may occur to a variety of agents acting on receptors other than adrenoceptors, including drugs used via the intraocular or intranasal route. The list of drugs includes sympathomimetics which cause supine hypertension and β-adrenoceptor blockers which can cause bradycardia. The reverse, marked hypotension, may also occur with drugs which have vasodilatory properties. An example is provided by the agent glyceryl trinitrate, which is routinely used sublingually in patients with angina pectoris. This drug, even when given with patients in the supine position, can result in severe hypotension.

Head-up tilt at night

The first line of treatment in a patient with AF is to attempt to increase the patient's blood volume by the use of head-up tilt at night. Figure 33.3 (Bannister *et al.* 1969) shows the change in lying and standing blood pressure and body weight in a patient placed in the head-up position at night. The increase of 2.6 kg in body weight points to a progressive increase in extracellular fluid volume, which was reversed on the 1 night when the patient slept flat. The effect of this procedure was studied further in one patient in whom water and sodium balance were followed on a 90 mmol per day sodium diet. As shown in Fig. 33.4 (Sever and Bannister, unpublished) the patient was losing more sodium and water during the night than during the day for each of 5 days until head-up tilt at night was introduced, when the nocturnal loss of sodium and water was reversed over the subsequent 5 days. Head-up body tilt at night is likely to operate by reducing renal arterial pressure and promoting renin release with consequent angiotensin II formation, aldosterone stimulation, and thus increasing blood volume for patients with AF who can still release renin (Bannister *et al.* 1977). The excessive nocturnal polyuria was studied by Wilcox *et al.* (1977) and there

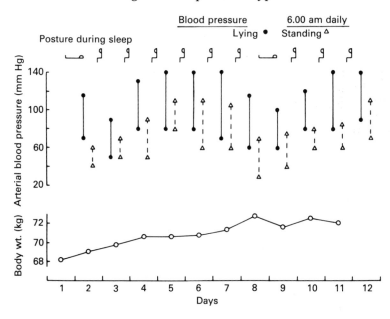

Fig. 33.3. The change in the early-morning blood pressure (lying and standing) in a patient (H) with autonomic failure and MSA studied when he slept in the sitting position for 10 days with one interruption. The changes in blood volume and body weight are also shown. (Taken with permission from Bannister *et al.* (1969).)

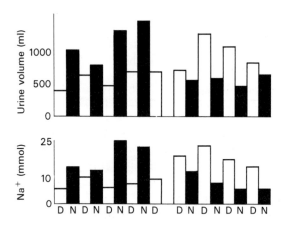

Fig. 33.4. Diurnal changes in water and sodium excretion in a patient with autonomic failure and multiple system atrophy during 5 days lying flat at night and 5 days of head-up tilt at night. D, day; N, night.

are more complex defects of renal sodium conservation in AF (see Chapter 10). Many patients with PAF, with incapacitating postural hypotension until the introduction of head-up tilt, have been maintained satisfactorily for years solely by this form of treatment.

Active support to raise blood pressure

There are a number of position changes which patients with severe postural hypotension find helpful. These include crossing the legs while standing, squatting, and stooping as if to tie shoe laces. They have been shown to raise blood pressure presumably by increasing vascular resistance or increasing venous return (van Lieshout *et al.* in press).

Passive external support to prevent pooling

The application of graduated pressure to the lower half of the body and legs reduces the amount of blood pooling in the legs on standing and so temporarily improves central blood volume and left ventricular filling. However, there must be concern that this treatment is in danger of reducing the intrinsic myogenic reaction of smooth muscle in response to stretch caused by increased intravascular pressure on standing, in addition to preventing other compensatory hormone and other responses to a low pressure. Thus the patient with orthostatic hypotension is even more vulnerable when not wearing the support garment. In practice it may be necessary temporarily in order to achieve mobility in a patient who has been recumbent as a result of severe postural hypotension for some time. Then, as the effect of head up-tilt and drugs such as fludrocortisone produce the benefit, a counter-pressure garment may be abandoned.

Originally antigravity suits were used which were certainly effective (see Fig. 33.5), but these were uncomfortable. More comfortable are the graded counterpressure support garments of the Jobst type (Sheps 1976).

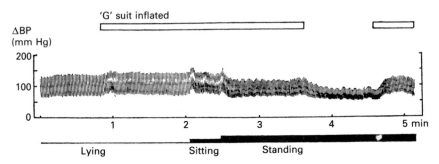

Fig. 33.5.   The effect of an antigravity suit on the changes of brachial arterial blood pressure (ΔBP) which occur on sitting and standing on a patient with pure autonomic failure. (Taken with permission from Bannister *et al.* (1969).)

Cardiac pacing

There have been reports of benefits obtained by implantation of a cardiac pace-maker and elevation of heart rate during postural change. The benefit noted by Moss *et al.* (1980) occurred in a patient who apparently had an incomplete autonomic lesion, and therefore had the potential to vasoconstrict at times. In patients with more severe lesions, with very low plasma noradrenaline levels at rest and in response to tilt, there appeared to be no benefit. Beneficial effects of tachypacing are unlikely in patients who have maximal arteriolar and venous dilatation, as cardiac output is dependent upon venous return which is often considerably reduced in such patients. Occasionally, cardiac pacing may be needed to prevent excessive bradycardia in response to elevation of blood pressure by drugs. We have described a patient in whom atrial demand pacing was needed to protect against vagal overactivity in the presence of a severe sympathetic autonomic neuropathy (Bannister *et al.* 1986). In this patient administration of drugs to raise the blood pressure resulted in severe bradycardia and consequent dysrhythmias (see Fig. 33.6). Assessment was initially made with atropine, which raised the heart rate but resulted in unacceptable side-effects. Atrial pacing was performed, initially with a temporary pace-maker which was clearly

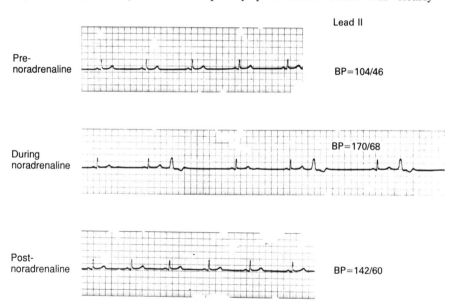

Fig. 33.6. ECG tracings before, during, and after intravenous infusion of noradrenaline. Sinus bradycardia and coupled beats occur when the blood pressure (BP) is elevated to 170/68 mm Hg. This is reversed when the BP returns to normal. (Taken with permission from Bannister *et al.* (1986).)

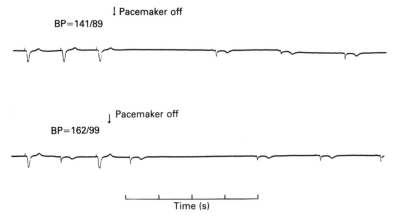

Fig. 33.7. ECG tracings, initially with the pace-maker on (upper trace). There are pace-maker triggered complexes followed by a pause and then sinus bradycardia. During noradrenaline infusion (lower trace) with the BP elevated, there are alternating pace-maker-induced and intrinsic complexes. Following exclusion of the pace-maker there is a longer pause before endogenous rhythm takes over. The elevation in BP appears to enhance sinus node suppression. (Taken with permission from Bannister *et al.* (1986).)

beneficial, and later with permanent implantation. This enabled effective use of pressor agents without the fear of development of either cardiac arrest or a serious dysrhythmia (see Fig. 33.7).

Noradrenaline infusion device

One potential future advance may be the utilization of devices which are closely linked to blood pressure control and postural change and which administer short-acting drugs such as noradrenaline when needed. One such device is that of Polinsky *et al.* (1983). They used an electromechanical device, utilizing the arterial transducer, to record blood pressure from one arm while controlling the rate of an intravenous infusion of noradrenaline into the opposite arm (see Fig. 33.8). Advances in this approach, using either implantable devices or mini-infusion pumps, linked to a non-invasive method of measuring blood pressure might be the way ahead in severely impaired patients in whom multiple drug therapy has failed.

Drugs in postural hypotension

A variety of agents has been used to raise supine blood pressure and so reduce postural hypotension. In Table 33.2 an attempt has been made to classify these agents on the basis of their main actions in helping postural hypotension. They are described below.

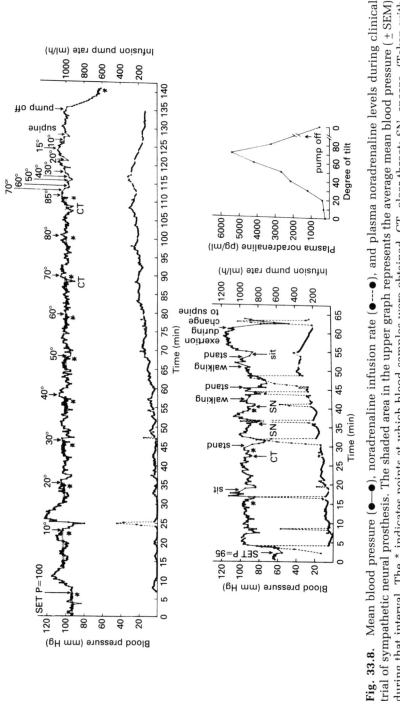

Fig. 33.8. Mean blood pressure (●—●), noradrenaline infusion rate (●--●), and plasma noradrenaline levels during clinical trial of sympathetic neural prosthesis. The shaded area in the upper graph represents the average mean blood pressure (± SEM) during that interval. The * indicates points at which blood samples were obtained. CT, clear throat; SN, sneeze. (Taken with permission from Polinsky *et al.* (1983).)

Table 33.2. Drugs used in the treatment of postural hypotension

Site of action	Drugs	Predominant action
Vessels: vasoconstriction (adrenoceptor-mediated)		
Resistance vessels	Ephedrine	Indirectly acting sympathomimetic
	Midodrine, phenyl-ephrine, methyl-phenidate	Directly acting sympathomimetics
	Tyramine	Release of noradrenaline
	Clonidine	Postsynaptic α_2-adreno-ceptor agonist
	Yohimbine	Presynaptic α_2-adreno-ceptor antagonist
	DL-DOPS and L-DOPS	Pro-drugs result in formation of noradrenaline
	Triglycyl-lysine-vasopressin (glypressin)	V_1-receptors on blood vessels
Capacitance vessels	Dihydroergotamine	Direct action on α-adrenoceptors
Vessels: prevention of vasodilatation	Propranolol	Blockade of β_2-adrenoceptors
	Indomethacin	Prevents prostaglandin synthesis
	Metoclopramide	Blockade of dopamine receptors
Vessels: prevention of postprandial hypo-tension	Caffeine	Blockade of adenosine receptors
	Octreotide	Inhibits release of vasodilator peptides
Heart: stimulation	Pindolol, xamoterol	Intrinsic sympathomimetic action (I.S.A.)
Plasma volume: expansion	Fludrocortisone	1. Mineralocorticoid effects 2. Increased plasma volume (large dose) 3. Sensitization of α-adreno-receptors to noradrenaline (small dose)
Kidney: reducing diuresis	Desmopressin	V_2-receptors on renal tubules

Plasma volume expansion and reducing natriuresis

Fludrocortisone

Fludrocortisone is the most commonly used drug treatment and has multiple pharmacological effects (Chobanian *et al.* 1979). In an initial dose of 0.1 mg at night, in some patients with AF, fludrocortisone approaches most closely to the ideal of a drug which increases effective vasoconstriction on standing, by augmenting the action of noradrenaline released by normal sympathetic efferent activity but without aggravating recumbent hypertension. In normal subjects fludrocortisone sensitizes vascular receptors to pressor amines (Schmidt *et al.* 1966). Studies by Tobian and Redleaf (1958) indicated that fludrocortisone may also increase the fluid content of vessel walls, so increasing their resistance to stretching.

In a study of four patients with AF and MSA, 0.1 mg of fludrocortisone daily did not increase body weight but caused a shift to the left of the noradrenaline infusion sensitivity curve and a significant rise in standing blood pressure (Davies *et al.* 1979). This effect may be less apparent in patients with pure autonomic failure (Chobanian *et al.* 1979). We speculated whether fludrocortisone might either increase the number of α-receptors or change their structure, or decrease the clearance rate by the uptake$_2$ mechanism by smooth muscle of blood vessels. Bannister *et al.* (1981) and Davies *et al.* (1982) have shown that there is an increase in the α-receptors of platelets and β-receptors of lymphocytes in autonomic failure and these changes are increased further after treatment with fludrocortisone. In AF there is also an increase in the pressor response to angiotensin II which is not affected by fludrocortisone, indicating a probable change in angiotensin vascular receptors as well as α-adrenoceptors (Davies *et al.* 1979).

In a higher dose fludrocortisone can, with careful supervision, expand the blood volume, improve cardiac output, and so reduce postural hypotension. Patients with AF have a normal or slightly low plasma volume when supine but this does not, as in normal subjects, fall on standing owing to the lack of vasoconstriction, probably because the lowered arterial pressure compensates for the raised hydrostatic pressure in the legs on standing. Patients with AF lose twice as much body weight as control subjects when on a low-sodium diet, with a corresponding increase in their postural hypotension. The resting plasma renin activity in AF is usually low, with a reduced rise on standing, though this is increased by sodium restriction or by dopamine infusion. This suggests that renin synthesis and storage are intact but release may be defective. Aldosterone secretion may be reduced in autonomic failure but the defect is likely to be the result of a chronic reduction of angiotensin stimulation of aldosterone secretion rather than an adrenal defect. The dose of fludrocortisone likely to increase the blood volume by replacing aldosterone levels without overloading the circulation requires delicate and continuous adjustment, in contrast to the situation in a patient with Addison's disease, probably because of the baroreflex defect. As with other forms of treatment, each patient shows variations in response which are the result of the different types of lesion present in each patient.

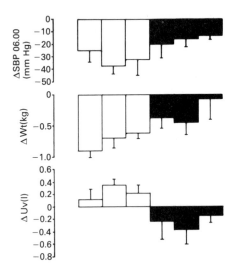

Fig. 33.9. Desmopressin (DDAVP) in the treatment of autonomic failure. From above, morning postural hypotension, difference between sitting and lying systolic pressure (ΔSBP), change in body weight overnight (ΔWt), and change in urine volume between night and day (ΔUv). The open rectangles show the changes during a 3-day control period and the closed rectangles the changes after 2 μg i.m. of DDAVP each evening for 3 days. The mean results in five patients with autonomic failure show after DDAVP a reduction in postural hypotension and a gain in extracellular and intravascular fluid volume as measured by the reduction in nocturnal weight loss and nocturnal urinary volume.

Desmopressin

Desmopressin (DDAVP) is a vasopressin-like agent which acts specifically upon the V_2-receptors on the renal tubules, which are responsible for the antidiuretic effects of vasopressin. It has virtually no activity on the V_1-receptor, which is responsible for the vasoconstriction induced by vasopressin. In patients with AF, nocturnal polyuria, overnight weight loss, and the subsequent reduction in extracellular fluid volume and intravascular volume account for the low morning blood pressures and for the increased severity of symptoms from postural hypotension. Intramuscular DDAVP prevents nocturnal polyuria and reduces overnight weight loss, and raises the supine blood pressure in the morning, thus improving symptoms resulting from postural change (Mathias *et al.* 1986; Fig. 33.9). Because of the lack of direct vascular effects of DDAVP an increased tendency to supine hypertension is not present. Studies with intranasal DDAVP indicate that it is equally effective in the short term and also in the long term: doses between 5 and 40 μg given at bedtime as a single dose are of benefit both in relation to preventing nocturia (which can also be a problem especially in those with bladder involvement) and also in morning postural hypotension.

DDAVP, however, has the potential to cause side-effects. Some patients, and in particular those with PAF, may be exquisitely sensitive to its action and hyponatraemia can readily ensue. This is best evaluated by determining the patient's responses to intramuscular DDAVP in a hospital environment and under close supervision. Small doses of intra-nasal DDAVP can then be administered in appropriate doses, again under careful supervision to ensure that hyponatraemia does not occur, before stabilization on an out-patient basis. In some patients natriuresis continues as before and occasionally is in excess and DDAVP needs to be combined with fludrocortisone and sodium supplements to ensure that the patient remains in sodium balance. We have treated patients with intra-nasal DDAVP for years with no long-term side-effects by monitoring of plasma osmolality or even plasma sodium levels on a 6-weekly or 2-monthly basis.

Drugs causing vasoconstriction

Drugs acting as vasoconstrictors can be broadly divided as follows.

1. *Directly acting agents.* A variety of agents have been used which act directly on α-adrenoceptors. These include agents such as phenylephrine, methylphenidate, and midodrine. These drugs are α-agonists which in some trials have been reported to be of benefit. A factor to be kept in mind is the potential of these agents to cause severe constriction in peripheral vessels. This might be a disadvantage especially in the elderly who are more likely to have peripheral vascular abnormalities.

2. *Indirectly acting agents.* Ephedrine acts by both releasing noradrenaline and also acting directly on adrenoceptors. This drug may have a role in patients with incomplete lesions, where a combination of its direct effects and the release of noradrenaline may be of benefit (Brooks *et al.* 1989). As with this and with other agents the potential to cause supine hypertension is always present. The value of the drug in patients with severe sympathetic lesions is probably minimal. With large doses of ephedrine (in excess of 45 mg t.d.s.) side-effects such as tachycardia or tremulousness may occur due to central stimulation.

Drugs releasing noradrenaline predominantly

Tyramine is an agent which raises blood pressure by the release of noradrenaline at the sympathetic nerve endings. In some patients with autonomic failure there may be sufficient sparing of nerve endings for this to be achieved, and the effects of tyramine can be potentiated by the concurrent administration of a monoamine oxidase inhibitor. A number of

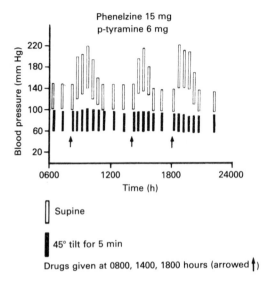

Fig. 33.10.   Blood pressure and heart rate before and after treatment of a patient with pure autonomic failure with phenelzine and *p*-tyramine. (Taken with permission from Davies *et al.* (1978).)

foods, such as cheese, contain *p*-tyramine and this may have been partially responsible for the erratic response, except that these were also obtained using chemically pure *p*-tyramine. Studies with the combination of *p*-tyramine and phenelzine in our unit resulted in marked fluctuation of blood pressure, with pronounced supine hypertension which was potentially hazardous (Fig. 33.10; Davies *et al.* 1978). It appeared that the improvement in postural hypotension caused by this combination was less effective than that caused by phenylephrine or ephedrine alone.

α_2-adrenoceptor agonists: clonidine

Clonidine is an α_2-adrenoceptor agonist, which is highly lipophilic and has actions both centrally and peripherally. Its central actions, which result in withdrawal of sympathetic tone, are responsible for the fall in supine blood pressure in both normal subjects and hypertensive patients. In tetraplegics, therefore, with a decentralized sympathetic nervous system clonidine does not lower resting blood pressure; however, it is capable of attenuating the pressor response to bladder stimulation, indicating that it may have effects either on spinal sympathetic neurons or on presynaptic α_2-receptors in the periphery (Mathias *et al.* 1979). When given intravenously to tetraplegics there is an initial pressor response (Mathias and Frankel, unpublished observations) which results from its normally transient peripheral postsynaptic effects causing vasoconstriction. These are probably a combination of both α_1- and α_2-receptor effects. These effects are probably the basis for the observations of the benefit of clonidine in some patients with AF. Our own experience with the use of clonidine in autonomic failure patients has not been favourable and it may be that the drug is only of benefit in those with complete lesions involving postganglionic fibres where there is extreme pressor sensitivity to α-adrenoceptor agents.

Presynaptic α_2-adrenoceptor antagonists: yohimbine

Yohimbine is an α_2-adrenoceptor antagonist which can act both centrally and peripherally. The blockade of presynaptic α_2-adrenoceptors may facilitate the release of noradrenaline at nerve terminals. The drug has been used in single doses with benefit in six patients with AF where it was likely that they had partial lesions, thus resulting in accentuation of noradrenaline release (Onrot et al. 1987). The drug may, therefore, have a role in certain patients with AF and incomplete lesions. It has not been evaluated in the long term and it may not have any advantages over ephedrine.

Increased endogenous production of noradrenaline

The pro-drugs, DL-DOPS or L-DOPS, can increase production of endogenous noradrenaline. This is described in detail in Chapter 38, along with its efficacy in different autonomic disorders, including DBH deficiency.

V_1-receptors in blood vessels

Stimulation of V_1-receptors in blood vessels results in constriction. The drug TGLVP (glypressin), an analogue of vasopressin with predominant V_1 effects, resulting in constriction of arteries mainly on the splanchnic and skin circulation, may be found to be helpful in reducing postural hypotension (Rittig et al. 1991).

Predominantly venoconstrictor agents with direct action on α-receptors: dihydroergotamine

Dihydroergotamine has a long history in treatment of postural hypotension since reports by Nordenfelt and Mellander (1972). It acts as a direct α-agonist, stimulating venous capacity vessels although resistance vessels may even show slight dilatation when normally innervated. It increases central blood volume by about 120 ml with only a slight rise in venous pressure. Nordenfelt and Mellander (1972) studied patients with intact sympathetic function but liable to syncope (so-called 'sympathotonic' orthostatic hypotension) and their results are not applicable to AF. When there is sympathetic denervation as in AF, dihydroergotamine almost certainly causes constriction of resistance vessels (Bevegard et al. 1974). It is highly effective after venous injection and abolishes postural hypotension almost completely for half an hour even in severe cases of AF, these benefits being obtained at the price of severe recumbent hypertension. The effectiveness of intravenous dihydroergotamine was confirmed by Jennings *et al.* (1979) in two patients with PAF and two with AF and MSA. They showed reduction of the excessive fall of central blood volume on standing. An oral dose of 30 mg daily was needed in three out of four patients to improve their postural hypotension and the addition of fludrocortisone resulted in further improvement.

The major disadvantage of dihydroergotamine is its poor bioavailability. One approach has been to combine it with oral glyceryl trinitrate, which was reported to increase its bioavailability and thus increase its efficacy. Studies in our unit, however, using such a combination in our patients with AF, did not provide any evidence of beneficial effect, when dihydroergotamine with placebo was compared with dihydroergotamine in combination with 0.5 mg of glyceryl trinitrate. In some patients there may even have been a fall in blood pressure, presumably because of the vasodilator effects of glyceryl trinitrate. Increasing the daily oral dose of dihydroergotamine may be of benefit in some patients, keeping in mind the potential complication of peripheral vasoconstriction. Dihydroergotamine can also be given parenterally, either subcutaneously or intramuscularly, as in the prevention of thromboembolic complications. It has been used with benefit intramuscularly in patients with AF resulting from alcoholism and diabetes. Other ergot derivatives have also been assessed in patients with autonomic failure. Ergotamine tartrate can be given orally, and has been used in doses of 2 to 5 mg daily with some benefit in patients with AF.

Prevention of vasodilatation

A variety of drugs have been used on the premise that blood pressure control can be improved by preventing vasodilatatory mechanisms.

β-adrenoceptor blockade: propranolol

Propranolol was introduced in the treatment of autonomic failure on the grounds, despite the obvious α-adrenoceptor defect, that β-agonist induced vasodilatation might also contribute to the orthostatic hypotension and should be reversed by the β-adrenoceptor blocking properties of propranolol. It may also act on presynaptic β-receptors and so reduce the release of noradrenaline. Chobanian *et al.* (1977) reported beneficial effects in four patients with a diagnosis of PAF on oral propranolol in doses of 40 to 240 mg daily but, as they were already taking 0.3 to 0.5 mg fludrocortisone daily and had an excessive salt intake, no clear conclusion can be drawn. Chobanian *et al.* later withdrew propranolol in one patient because it caused severe recumbent hypertension and they reported that in two patients episodes of 'syncope' still occurred in the early morning when orthostatic intolerance was most severe. In practice propranolol has not proved sufficiently encouraging for other trials to be reported, possibly because of its cardiac β-blocking effects.

Other forms of orthostatic hypotension have been treated with propranolol. Some patients, who have not been studied in detail physiologically or pharmacologically, appear to have no autonomic defect but have so-called orthostatic tachycardia or hyperadrenergic orthostatic response leading to postural hypotension due to a decreased output. The tachycardia is probably emotionally determined and is accompanied by a mounting sense of anxiety when standing, associated with overbreathing, and then sometimes, paradoxically, increasing bouts of vagally induced bradycardia, which may eventually lead to syncope. Propranolol reduces the initial tachycardia and may benefit such patients. Some patients with AF or diabetes and with sparing of cardiac sympathetic efferents but impaired sympathetic tone to the arterial bed have a compensatory tachycardia and deteriorate if this compensatory mechanism is blocked by propranolol.

Prostaglandin synthetase inhibitors: indomethacin and flurbiprofen

Indomethacin was first proposed on the theoretical basis that some prostaglandins are potent vasodilators and their effect may be inhibited by indomethacin, which also may have several other effects which modify pressor responses. Kochar and Itskovitz (1978) reported improvement in four patients with postural hypotension due to AF and MSA. However, the diagnosis was uncertain in one of them in that the standing blood pressure was within the normal range for her age and, in all, the diagnosis of AF and MSA was based on clinical features without the benefit of physiological tests. Davies *et al.* (1980) showed that oral indomethacin (50 mg t.d.s.) increased sensitivity to infused noradrenaline and angiotensin II in four patients with AF and MSA but the pressor effect was only significant on recumbent blood pressure, probably because the hydrostatic stresses on standing require compensatory constriction of different blood vessels in different vascular beds. Inhibition of prostaglandin synthesis may be a factor because urinary prostaglandin excretion was greater than in normal subjects and was decreased by indomethacin. The lack of improvement in the standing blood pressure might also have been due to a decrease in plasma renin activity due to indomethacin. Watt *et al.* (1981) have shown benefit from the combined effect of fludrocortisone and flurbiprofen in PAF. Since both prostaglandin inhibitors and fludrocortisone have pressor effects we have decided, in some cases failing to respond to fludrocortisone alone, to add indomethacin since both substances appear to increase smooth muscle sensitivity to noradrenaline and, in larger doses, may increase blood volume.

Dopamine antagonists: metoclopramide

Metoclopramide, a dopamine antagonist, has been used in the treatment of AF, on the basis that metoclopramide blocks the vasodilator effects of dopamine. In a single patient with postural hypotension after an extensive sympathectomy, Kuchel *et al.* (1980) reported an improvement in the postural hypotension. They postulated that this was the result of the drug inhibiting the vasodilator and natriuretic effects of the excess dopamine released. However, caution is necessary in patients with supersensitivity of central dopamine receptors who may be vulnerable to the extrapyramidal side-effects. Its effects in dopamine β-hydroxylase deficiency are described in Chapter 38.

Drugs preventing postprandial hypotension (see Chapter 26)

Dilatation within the splanchnic circulation following a meal is probably the cause of the marked postprandial fall in blood pressure in autonomic failure patients. Splanchnic vasodilatation may result from the release of vasodilatory neuropeptides. Drugs such as dihydroergotamine seem to have minimal effects in preventing postprandial hypotension. The use of other agents which have been used with benefit, caffeine and octreotide, is discussed in Chapter 26.

Drugs acting on the heart

Pindolol

Pindolol has additional partial β-agonist adrenoceptor activity (so-called intrinsic sympathomimetic activity) which should cause less reduction in resting heart rate than a pure β-blocker might be expected to cause. The initial encouraging report was by Frewin *et al.* (1980) on two patients with diabetic autonomic neuropathy who probably had supersensitivity to noradrenaline. It was followed by Man in't Veld and Schalekamp (1981), who showed benefits in three patients with AF, two of whom had amyloidosis and one following acute autonomic neuropathy. They argued that, when receptor occupancy is low as is assumed in the postganglionic lesion of AF, there was a strong possibility that even a partial β-agonist would act as a full agonist and its agonist effect would be enhanced by denervation hypersensitivity and lack of baroreflexes. They also raised the possibility that pindolol might have an effect on β-receptors in veins and, like dihydroergotamine, might increase venous tone. They showed that the improvement in postural hypotension was due to an improvement in cardiac output but vascular resistance was unchanged. Their patients had an increase in cardiac rate. However, this enthusiasm was premature. Davies *et al.* (1981) reported briefly on five patients studied under standard conditions after a control period. Pindolol was given in an adequate dose gauged by the heart rate response to intravenous isoprenaline but did not increase blood pressure or cause symptomatic benefit at any dose level. The trend was towards decrease in lying and standing pressure. Pindolol did not have a chronotropic action and there was instead a tendency for the pulse rate to decrease with increasing doses of pindolol. Two patients had raised jugular venous pressure after 3 days on 15 mg daily and frank cardiac failure after 45 mg daily for 3 days. Pindolol causes a rightward shift of the isoprenaline dose–response curve so that, although in theory pindolol acts more as a sympathetic agonist than competitive antagonist, its β-blocking action was still pronounced. In our patients there was evidence of increased receptor numbers and denervation supersensitivity to noradrenaline. The view put forward by Man in't Veld and Schalekamp (1981) that their patients responded because of the partial agonist effect of pindolol may therefore not be the only explanation.

Prenalterol and xamoterol

Two other β-blockers with β_1-adrenoceptor partial agonist effects have been assessed in AF. Prenalterol was found to be effective (Goovaerts et al. 1984). Xamoterol has also been shown in a number of patients to benefit postural hypotension (Mehlsen and Trap-Jensen 1985). These drugs, unlike pindolol which has the potential to cause cardiac failure, should be less likely to induce this complication.

Management of postural hypotension in dopamine β-hydroxylase deficiency

In the genetically determined defect of dopamine β-hydroxylase deficiency, dopamine is not converted to noradrenaline and profound postural hypotension results. Treatment is possible using the synthetic amino acid D or L-threo-dihydroxy-phenylserine (D or L DOPS) which is converted to noradrenaline by dopa decarboxylase, either intra- or extraneuronally. This results in marked improvement in the postural hypotension, as described in Chapter 38.

References

Bannister, R., Ardill, L., and Fentem, P. (1969). An assessment of various methods of treatment of idiopathic orthostatic hypotension. *Quart. J. Med.* **38**, 377–95.

Bannister, R., Sever, P., and Gross, M. (1977). Cardiovascular reflexes and biochemical responses in progressive autonomic failure. *Brain* **100**, 327–44.

Bannister, R., Boylston, A. W., Davies, I. B., Mathias, C. J., Sever, P. S., and Sudera, D. (1981). Beta-receptor numbers and thermodynamics in denervation supersensitivity. *J. Physiol., London* **319**, 369–77.

Bannister, R., Da Costa, D. F., Hendry, W. G, Jacobs, J., and Mathias, C. J. (1986). Atrial demand pacing to protect against vagal overactivity in sympathetic autonomic neuropathy. *Brain* **109**, 345–56.

Bevegard, S., Castenfors, J., and Lindblad, L.-E. (1974). Haemodynamic effects of dihydroergotamine in patients with postural hypotension. *Acta med. scand.* **196**, 473–7.

Brooks, D. J., Redmond, S., Mathias, C. J., Bannister, R., and Syman, L. (1989). The effects of orthostatic hypotension on cerebral blood flow and middle cerebral artery velocity in autonomic failure, with observations on the action of ephedrine. *J. Neurol. Neurosurg. Psychiatry* **52**, 962–6.

Chobanian, A. V., Volicer, L., Liang, C. S., Kershaw, G., and Tifft, C. (1977). Use of propranolol in the treatment of idiopathic orthostatic hypotension. *Trans. Ass. Am. Physcns* **90**, 324–34.

Chobanian, A. V., Volicer, L., Tifft, C., Gavras, H., Liang, C., and Faxon, D. (1979). Mineralocorticoid-induced hypotension in patients with orthostatic hypotension. *New Engl. J. Med.* **301**, 68–73.

Davies, B., Bannister, R., and Sever, P. (1978). Pressor amines and monoamine oxidase inhibitors for treatment of postural hypotension in progressive autonomic failure. Limitations and hazards. *Lancet* **i**, 172–5.

Davies, B., Bannister, R., Sever, P., and Wilcox, C. S. (1979). The pressor actions of noradrenaline, angiotensin II and saralasin in chronic autonomic failure treated with fludrocortisone. *Br. J. clin. Pharmacol.* **8**, 253–60.

Davies, B., Bannister, R., Hensby, C., and Sever, P. (1980). The pressor actions of noradrenaline, angiotensin II in chronic autonomic failure treated with indomethacin. *Br. J. clin. Pharmacol.* **10**, 223–9.

Davies, B., Bannister, R., Mathias, C., and Sever, P. (1981). Pindolol in postural hypotension; the case for caution. *Lancet* **i**, 982–3.

Davies, B., Sudera, D., Sagnella, E., Marchese-Saviotti, E., Mathias, C., Bannister, R., and Sever, P. (1982). Increased numbers of alpha-receptors in sympathetic denervation supersensitivity in man. *J. clin. Invest.* **69**, 779–84.

Frewin, D. B., Leonello, P. P., Pentall, R. K., Hughes, L., and Harding, P. E. (1980). Pindolol in orthostatic hypotension: possible therapy? *Med. J. Aust.* **1**, 128.

Goovaerts, J., Ver faillie, C., Fagard, R., and Knochaert, D. (1984). Effect of prenalterol on orthostatic hypotension in the Shy–Drager syndrome. *Br. med. J.* **288**, 817–18.

Jennings, G., Esler, M., and Holmes, R. (1979). Treatment of orthostatic hypotension with dihydroergotamine. *Br. med. J.* **ii**, 307–8.

Kochar, M. S. and Itskovitz, H. D. (1978). Treatment of idiopathic orthostatic hypotension (Shy–Drager syndrome) with indomethacin. *Lancet* **i**, 1011–14.

Kuchel, O., Buu, N. T., Gutkowska, J., and Genest, J. (1980). Treatment of severe orthostatic hypotension by metoclopramide. *Ann. intern. Med.* **93**, 841–3.

Man in't Veld, A. J. and Schalekamp, M. A. D. H. (1981). Pindolol acts as beta-adrenoceptor agonist in orthostatic hypotension: therapeutic implications. *Br. med. J.* **282**, 929–31.

Mann, S., Altman, D. G., Raftery, E. B., and Bannister, R. (1983). Circadian variation of blood pressure in autonomic failure. *Circulation* **68**, 477–83.

Mathias, C. J., Reid, J. L., Wing, L. M. H., Frankel, H. L., and Christensen, N. J. (1979). Antihypertensive effects of clonidine in tetraplegic subjects devoid of central sympathetic control. *Clin. Sci.* **57**, 425–6.

Mathias, C. J., Fosbraey, P., de Costa, D. F., Thorley, A., and Bannister, R. (1986). Desmopressin reduces nocturnal polyuria, reverses overnight weight loss and improves morning postural hypotension in autonomic failure. *Br. med. J.* **293**, 353–4.

Mehlsen, J. and Trap-Jensen, J. (1985). Use of xamoterol, a new selective beta-adrenoreceptor partial agonist, in the treatment of postural hypotension.

Proceedings of the International Symposium on Cardiovascular Pharmaco-therapy, Geneva, Abstract 73, ICI.

Moss, A. J., Glaser, W., and Topol, E. (1980). Atrial tachypacing in the treatment of a patient with primary orthostatic hypotension. *New Engl. J. Med.* **302**, 1456–7.

Nordenfelt, I. and Mellander, S. (1972). Central haemodynamic effects of dihydroergotamine in patients with orthostatic hypotension. *Acta med. scand.* **191**, 115–20.

Onrot, J., Goldberg, M. R., Biaggioni, I., Wiley, R. G., Hollister, A. S., and Robertson, D. (1987). Oral yohimbine in human autonomic failure. *Neurology* **37**, 215–20.

Polinsky, R. J., Samaras, G. M., and Kopin, I. J. (1983). Sympathetic neural prosthesis for managing orthostatic hypertension. *Lancet* **i**, 901–4.

Rittig, S., Arentsen, J., Sørensen, K., Matthiesen, T., and Dupont, E. (1991). The hemodynamic effects of triglycyl-lysine-vasopressin (glypressin) in patients with parkinsonism and orthostatic hypotension. *Movement Disorders* **6**, 21–8.

Schmidt, P. G., Eckstein, J. W., and Abboud, F. M. (1966). Effect of 9-alpha-fluorohydrocortisone on forearm vascular responses to norepinephrine. *Circulation* **34**, 620–6.

Sheps, S. G. (1976). The use of an elastic garment in the treatment of idiopathic orthostatic hypotension. *Cardiology* **62** (suppl. 1), 271–9.

Thomas, D. J. and Bannister, R. (1980). Preservation of autoregulation of cerebral blood flow in autonomic failure. *J. neurol. Sci.* **44**, 205–12.

Tobian, L. and Redleaf, P. D. (1958). Ionic composition of the aorta in renal and adrenal hypertension. *Am. J. Physiol.* **192**, 325–30.

van Lieshout, J. J., ten Harkel, A. D. J., and Wieling, W. (in press). Manoeuvres beneficial to patients with orthostatic hypotension. *Clin. Aut. Res.*

Watt, S. J., Tooke, J. E., Perkins, C. M., and Lee, M. (1981). The treatment of idiopathic orthostatic hypotension: a combined fludrocortisone-flurbiprofen regime. *Quart. J. Med.* **50**, 205–12.

Wilcox, C. S., Aminoff, M. J., and Slater, J. D. H. (1977). Sodium homeostasis in patients with autonomic failure. *Clin. Sci. mol. Med.* **53**, 321–8.

34. The treatment of multiple system atrophy

A. J. Lees

Introduction

It has become clear from recent clinicopathological studies in the United Kingdom Parkinson's Disease Brain Bank at the Institute of Neurology that multiple system atrophy (MSA) presenting as a parkinsonian syndrome is considerably underdiagnosed. Most of these patients confirmed at post-mortem as MSA have minimal or no cerebellar signs, but involutional changes of the cerebellar folia may be demonstrable on neuroimaging. Autonomic signs and symptoms, on the other hand, are more frequent and include urgency of micturition, impotence, and symptomatic orthostatic hypotension. In many cases they are indistinguishable from Parkinson's disease (PD) in life, although a more malignant clinical course, early gait disturbance with falls, early severe dysarthria, and absence of rest tremor are helpful clinical pointers. A minority have bilateral Babinski signs which, provided cervical spondylotic myelopathy has been excluded, is incompatible with a diagnosis of PD.

In the last 3 years 140 cases of the parkinsonian syndrome have been examined in the United Kingdom Parkinson's Disease Brain Bank at the Institute of Neurology. Twenty-four of these were found to have striatonigral degeneration (SND) at post-mortem and half had been diagnosed incorrectly in life. Of the first 100 cases prospectively diagnosed as having PD, seven were found to have SND (Hughes *et al.* 1991*b*). In another post-mortem study of 59 cases of the parkinsonian syndrome, 13 (22 per cent) had MSA but no information is given in this paper as to how many were correctly diagnosed in life (Rajput *et al.* 1990). A few patients have also been reported to have the pathological lesions of both PD and MSA (Gibb and Lees 1989). SND, therefore, probably constitutes between 5 and 10 per cent of all causes of the parkinsonian syndrome due to brainstem degeneration.

The pathological lesion in the striatonigral degeneration of multiple system atrophy

Severe loss of neuromelanin-containing neurons in the zona compacta of the substantia nigra occurs in SND. In the early stages the regional distribution of cell loss mirrors closely that seen in PD with a greater cell fall-out in the ventrolateral cell groups. In the fully established case, however, there appears to be rather more depletion of neurons in the dorsal tier than is seen in PD (Spokes *et al.* 1979; Goto *et al.* 1989). In contrast to PD there is additional marked nerve cell loss, gliosis, and pigmentation of the putamen, the caudate nucleus, and globus pallidus. In mild cases the involvement of the putamen is confined to its posterior two-thirds, dorsolaterally, and, with increasing severity, nerve cell loss extends in a dorsal to ventral and posterior to anterior direction. In addition there is damage to the pontine nuclei, inferior olives, and the cerebellar Purkinje cells (Adams *et al.* 1961; Fearnley and Lees 1990).

There have been relatively few neurochemical studies on MSA. Striatal dopamine, noradrenaline, choline acetyltransferase, and glutamate decarboxylase are all depressed (Spokes *et al.* 1979). The pattern of depression of striatal dopamine levels in MSA also seems to resemble that seen in PD with relative preservation of caudate levels (Spokes *et al.* 1979). In the only published study on dopamine receptor function in SND, Quik *et al.* (1979) found normal caudate D_2 densities in four patients, two of whom were receiving regular L-dopa therapy. *In vivo* imaging using positron emission tomography revealed heterogeneous results in MSA using ^{18}F-dopa uptake (see Chapter 28A). Some patients showed a similar pattern to PD with relative sparing of caudate uptake, whereas others had uniform striatal involvement with comparable reductions of caudate and putaminal dopamine. There was no clear difference in the pattern of clinical involvement between the patients with MSA who had mild and those who had more severe caudate involvement. The authors suggested that these findings might be a measure of the extent of individual nigral involvement in the patients studied (Brooks *et al.* 1990). *In vivo* imaging, using raclopride to investigate striatal dopamine receptor function in SND, has revealed a modest 13 per cent fall in D_2 binding activity in the putamen with preservation of caudate ^{11}C-raclopride binding, supporting the histological finding that the putamen is preferentially targeted in this condition (Brooks *et al.* 1991). The majority of striatal D_2 sites are postsynaptic on intrinsic striatal neurons and similar reductions in striatal D_2 function have been found in patients with L-dopa-treated PD and on–off disabilities, indicating that it is unlikely that the poor response in patients with MSA to L-dopa is due simply to loss of striatal D_2 receptors. In SND striatal and external pallidal degeneration is marked, lesions which in theory at least could counterbalance one another with respect to function. It may be, therefore, that the response to L-dopa in SND is crucially dependent on the degree and regional distribution of nigral cell loss (Fearnley and Lees 1990).

Acute challenges with oral L-dopa or subcutaneous apomorphine in multiple system atrophy

After withdrawal of oral dopaminergic drugs for 12 h a single dose of L-dopa/dopa decarboxylase inhibitor (250/25 mg) is given in the fasting state.

The motor response is assessed by timed tapping and walking tests at 15-min intervals and 4-point scales for tremor and dyskinesia. A Modified Webster Scale is also used at baseline and peak response to assess the amplitude of motor response. The peripheral dopamine receptor antagonist drug, domperidone is given in a dose of 30 mg three times a day for at least 24 h before the apomorphine test, which should also be given in the fasting state using serial challenges of 1.5, 3.0, 4.5, and 7.0 mg. The test is continued until either an unequivocal response occurs, intolerable side-effects are experienced, or the maximum dose is reached. One of four clinically definite MSA patients responded to both apomorphine and L-dopa and subsequently to sustained L-dopa therapy. The other three patients had negative responses to the acute challenges and failed to benefit from L-dopa therapy. A further eight patients with possible MSA were tested, five of whom had negative responses to the challenges and failed to respond to L-dopa therapy. One had positive responses to both apomorphine and the L-dopa test and responded well to chronic L-dopa, and a further two patients had equivocal responses to both apomorphine and L-dopa and subsequently responded to long-term L-dopa therapy (Hughes *et al.* 1990). In contrast, however, Oertel and colleagues (1989) found that none of five patients with clinically definite MSA responded positively to apomorphine. In a recent study evaluating the apomorphine and oral L-dopa tests in 45 previously untreated patients with PD, nine cases failed to respond either to challenge or to long-term L-dopa therapy and one of these developed pyramidal signs and autonomic nerve dysfunction in the 12 months of follow-up, suggesting a diagnosis of MSA. One of the other patients died after a rapidly progressive akinetic-rigid syndrome, a further two developed signs strongly suggestive of Steele–Richardson–Olszewski disease, while the other five patients had physical signs still consistent with PD (Hughes *et al.* 1991*a*). These challenge tests with L-dopa and apomorphine give supportive evidence that a parkinsonian patient may have MSA.

Clinical studies with L-dopa and dopaminergic agonists

The therapeutic results of L-dopa therapy in presumed cases of MSA are difficult to interpret because of the variablity. Aminoff and colleagues (1973) treated five cases of MSA with autonomic failure with doses of L-dopa between 1.25 and 3.5 g per day and four of the five got worse with respect to their parkinsonian disabilities, although two had some modest increase in the level of their standing blood pressure and three in their lying blood pressure. These were all patients with MSA and marked autonomic failure. Sharpe and colleagues (1973) treated a 58-year-old man with MSA with small doses of L-dopa and a non-selective monoamine oxidase inhibitor in an attempt to produce antiparkinsonian benefit and a controlled improvement in postural hypotension. Worthwhile benefit occurred with respect to tremor and rigidity, but only minimal improvement in bradykinesia. Goetz and colleagues (1984) reported that 16 or 19 patients with presumed MSA treated with L-dopa obtained definite improvement in rigidity and bradykinesia, and postural tremor was improved in two. The mean duration of disease in this study was long, averaging 10 years with a range of 5–20 years. Eleven of the patients presented with a parkinsonian syndrome, six with cerebellar signs, and the rest with a mixed picture. Fourteen had a definite or suspected family history of a similar condition, presenting with cerebellar symptoms alone, which raised the possibility that some patients may have had a familial cerebellar degeneration. Ten of the patients experienced drug-induced chorea and five had visual hallucinations. Lang and colleagues (1986) reported three patients diagnosed initially as having PD who derived sustained benefit from L-dopa preparations with the emergence of on–off oscillations. Limb ataxia and cerebellar dysarthria developed in two of the cases and a third was unable to stand or walk within 5 years of the onset of the disease. All three had marked involutional changes of the cerebellar folia on computerized axial tomography (CAT) scan. In a further study of 23 cases with possible SND (Staal *et al.* 1990), no response to L-dopa occurred in 15, four developed on–off effects, and four acute psychotic reactions. A prompt and sustained improvement to L-dopa is therefore a contra-indication to the diagnosis of MSA, but it does not exclude the diagnosis.

Results with the new synthetic ergolines, lisuride and pergolide, have been even more disappointing. Goetz and colleagues (1984), using doses of 10–80 mg daily of bromocriptine, reported benefit in five patients who had responded to L-dopa and one patient who had failed to respond to L-dopa. Williams and colleagues (1979) also reported temporary benefit in an occasional patient; others, however, have had more disappointing results. Gautier and Durand (1977), in a controlled trial with lisuride (mean dose 2.4 mg daily), found that only one of seven patients with MSA and autonomic failure derived improvement in parkinsonian features and another, who had been deriving considerable benefit from L-dopa before the study began, failed to respond at all to large doses of lisuride. Severe psychiatric side-effects occurred in six patients on lisuride, with nightmares, isolated visual hallucinations, and toxic confusional states (Lees and Bannister 1981).

Clinicopathological studies

If one reviews the therapeutic effects of L-dopa on histologically proven cases of SND, the results are generally disappointing (see Tables 34.1 and 34.2). Of the 33 patients in the literature only five derived sustained improvement (Feve *et al.* 1977; Fearnley and Lees 1990). Another 10, however, derived definite initial benefit lasting for periods up to several months, and one of

Table 34.1. The therapeutic effects of levodopa on histologically proven cases of striatonigral degeneration ($\pm$ autonomine failure); all patients had severe rigidity and bradykinesia

Reference	Sex	Age at onset (years)	Duration of disease (years)	Tremor	Dysarthria	Pyramidal signs	Cerebellar signs	Postural hypotension	Sphincter dysfunction	Duration at onset	Max. dosage (mg/day)	Results	Adverse effects
Izumi et al. 1971	M	51	2	+		+				1	6 400	No effect	None
Greer et al. 1971	F	53	3							2	2 600	No effect	None
	F	73	4	+						3	12 000	Marked benefit for 6 months	None
Bannister and Oppenheimer 1972	F	48	6		+	+		+		3	3 000	No effect	Severe postural hypotension
Raiput et al. 1972	F	56	7	7	+	+			+	7	5 000	No effect	None
	F	63	7		+	+	+			7	5 000	No effect	Severe postural hypotension
Trotter 1973	F	66	8	+		+				4	8 000	Modest benefit for 3 months	Orofacial dyskinesia
Sharpe et al. 1973	F	41	6	+	+	+				5	6 000	Modest benefit for 2 months	Nausea
Takei and Mirra 1973	F	66	2		+					1	3 000	No effect	None
Schober et al. 1975	F	53	3	+	+	+		+	+	1	2 000*	Modest benefit for 6 months	Rise in erect pressure
											3 000	No effect	
Michel et al. 1976	M	61	3		+	+			+	2	3 000	No effect	None
	F	61	2		+	+			+	1	600*	No effect	None
											3 000	No effect	None

Reference	Sex	Age	Dur.	1	2	3	4	5	Dose (mg)	No.	Effect	Side-effects
Boudin et al. 1976	F	59	7	+				+	600* 5 000 800*	3	No effect	None
	F	56	4	+			+	+	4 000	2	Modest benefit for 6 months	Orofacial and limb dyskinesia
DeLean and Deck 1976	M	54	6	+	+		+	+	1 000	4	Modest benefit for 3 months	Rise in erect blood pressure
Rajput and Rozdilsky 1976	M	46	5	+	+		+	+	750*	4	No effect	Severe postural hypotension
Feve et al. 1977	F	61	4	+	+				3 000		Marked benefit for 3 years	Dyskinesias
Spokes et al. 1979	M	70	9	+			+	+			No effect	None
	M	49	9	+		+	+	+			No effect	None
	M	51	4	+	+		+	+			No effect	None
	F	53	5	+	+		+	+			No effect	None
Van Leuwen and Perquin 1989	M	68	4				+	+	N/S	2	Modest benefit for 3 months; bromocriptine 45 mg: good response for 10 months	Severe postural hypotension

*In combination with a peripheral dopa decarboxylase inhibitor.
N/S = not stated.

Table 34.2. The therapeutic effects of L-dopa on histologically proven cases of striatonigral degeneration (± autonomic failure) from the UK–PDS Brain Bank (Fearnley and Lees 1990)

			Clinical features							Levodopa treatment		
Sex	Age at onset (years)	Duration of disease (years)	Tremor	Dysarthria	Pyramidal signs	Cerebellar signs	Postural hypotension	Sphincter dysfunction	Duration at onset (years)	Max. dosage (mg/day)	Results	Adverse effects
F	64	3	+	+			+	+	1	800*	Modest benefit for 3 years	Increased postural hypotension
M	47	4			+	+		+	2	500*	Modest benefit for 2 years	On–off effects and dyskinesia
M	70	8		+				+	2	600*	Modest benefit for 5 years	Dyskinesias
F	67	5	+				+	+	2	400*	Modest benefit for 3 years	Dyskinesias
F	51	5					+		1	300*	Mild benefit for 3 months	—
F	49	10					+		2	400	Modest benefit for 6 months	Severe postural hypotension, orofacial chorea
F	51	10	+	+	+		+		2	1 200	Modest benefit for 5 years	Hypotension, visual hallucinations dyskinesia
F	64	8	+					+	3	300	No response	None
M	62	6		+				+	2	N/K	No response	None
M	68	2		+			+		1	300	No response	None

*In combination with a peripheral dopa decarboxylase inhibitor.

these patients who could not tolerate L-dopa subsequently improved in a sustained fashion on high doses of bromocriptine (Van Leuwen and Perquin 1989). Taken alone, the results recently reported by Fearnley and Lees (Table 34.2) are somewhat better, suggesting that as many as 60 per cent of patients might derive worthwhile initial benefit. Half of these patients were misdiagnosed in life as having PD and in the responders autonomic dysfunction was not severe. Coexisting severe autonomic dysfunction greatly reduces the chances of a worthwhile therapeutic response to L-dopa in MSA as intolerable orthostatic hypotension may occur on initial challenge with the drug.

Conclusion

Patients with MSA presenting with a parkinsonian syndrome without severe autonomic dysfunction may respond to therapeutic doses of L-dopa, but the progression of the illness will be more rapid than that seen in PD. Although a negative response to acute challenges with oral L-dopa and subcutaneous apomorphine favour SND over PD, these challenges are not useful as a diagnostic test for PD. Attempts to improve the motor disabilities of MSA by modification of other neurotransmitter systems have so far proved disappointing, but greater understanding of the complexity and interrelationships of the neuronal circuits within the basal ganglia may in time lead to new, useful therapeutic approaches. In the meantime much of course can be done to make more tolerable the life of a patient with MSA by means of physiotherapy, the judicious use of aids to daily living, and speech therapy.

References

Adams, R. D., van Bogoert, L., and van der Eecken, H. (1961) Dégénerescences nigro-striées et cérébello-nigro-striées. *Psychiatria et Neurologia* **142**, 219–59.

Aminoff, M. J., Wilcox, C. S., Woakes, M. M., and Kremer, M. (1973). Levodopa therapy for parkinsonism in the Shy–Drager syndrome. *J. Neurol. Neurosurg. Psychiatr.* **36**, 350–3.

Bannister, R. and Oppenheimer, D. R. (1972). Degenerative diseases of the nervous system associated with autonomic failure. *Brain* **95**, 457–74.

Boudin, G., Guillard, A., Mikol, J., and Galle, P. (1976). Dégénérescence striato-nigrique—à propos de l'étude clinique, thérapeutique et anatomique de 2 cas. *Rev. Neurol. Paris* **132**, 137–56.

Brooks, D. J., Ibanez, V., Sawle, G. V., Quinn, N., Lees, A. J., Mathias, C. J., Bannister, R., Marsden, C. D., and Frackowiak, R. S. J. (1990). Differing patterns of striatal 18F-dopa uptake in Parkinson's disease, multiple system atrophy and progressive supranuclear palsy. *Ann. Neurol.* **28**, 547–55.

Brooks, D. J., Ibanez, V., Sawle, G. V., Playford, E. D., Quinn, N., Mathias, C. J., Lees, A. J., Marsden, C. D., Bannister, R., and Frackowiak, R. S. J. (1991). Striatal D2 receptor status in Parkinson's disease, striatonigral degeneration and progressive supranuclear palsy measured with ^{11}C-raclopride and PET. *Ann. Neurol.* (In press.)

DeLean, J. and Deck, J. H. (1976). Shy–Drager syndrome—neuropathological correlation and response to levodopa therapy. *Can. J. neurol. Sci.* **3**, 167–77.

Fearnley, J. M. and Lees, A. J. (1990). Striatonigral degeneration—a clinicopathological study. *Brain* **113**, 1823–42.

Feve, J., Mussini, J. M., Cler, J-L, and Nombalais, M-F. (1977). Dégénérescence striato-nigrique—étude clinique et anatomique d'un cas ayant réagi très favorablement à la L-dopa. *Rev. Neurol., Paris* **133**, 271–8.

Gautier, J-C. and Durand, J. P. (1977). Traitement des syndromes parkinsoniens par la bromocriptine. *Nouv. Presse Méd.* **6**(3), 171–4.

Gibb, W. R. G. and Lees, A. J. (1989). The significance of the Lewy body in the diagnosis of idiopathic Parkinson's disease. *Neuropathol. appl. Neurobiol.* **15**, 27–44.

Goetz, C. G., Tanner, C. M., and Klawans, H. L. (1984). The pharmacology of olivopontocerebellar atrophy. *Adv. Neurol.* **41**, 143–8.

Goto, S., Hirano, A., and Matsumoto, S. (1989). Subdivisional involvement of nigrostriatal loop in idiopathic Parkinson's disease and striatonigral degeneration. *Ann. Neurol.* **26**, 766–70.

Greer, M., Collins, G. H., and Anton, A. H. (1971). Cerebral catecholamines after levodopa therapy. *Arch. Neurol.* **25**, 461–7.

Hughes, A. J., Lees, A. J., and Stern, G. M. (1990). Apomorphine test to predict dopaminergic responsiveness in Parkinsonian syndrome. *Lancet* **335**, 32–4.

Hughes, A. J., Lees, A. J., and Stern, G. M. (1991*a*). Challenge tests to predict the dopaminergic response in untreated Parkinson's disease. *Neurology* **41**, 1723–5.

Hughes, A. J., Daniel, S. E., Kilford, L., and Lees, A. J. (1991*b*). The accuracy of clinical diagnosis of idiopathic Parkinson's disease: a clinicopathological study of 100 cases. *J. Neurol. Neurosurg. Psychiat.* (In press.)

Izumi, K., Inoue, N., Shirabe, T., Miyazaki, T., and Kuroiwa, Y. (1971). Failed levodopa therapy in striato-nigral degeneration. *Lancet* **i**, 1355.

Lang, A. E., Birnbaum, A., Blair, R. D. G., and Kierans, C. (1986). Levodopa dose-related fluctuations in presumed olivopontocerebellar atrophy. *Movement Disorders* **1**, 93–102.

Lees, A. J. and Bannister, R. (1981). The use of lisuride in the treatment of multiple system atrophy with autonomic failure (Shy–Drager syndrome). *J. Neurol. Neurosurg. Psychiat.* **44**, 347–51.

Michel, D., Tommasi, M., Laurent, B., Trillet, M. and Schott, B. (1976). Dégénérescence straito-nigrique—à propos de 2 observations anatomocliniques. *Rev. Neurol., Paris* **132**, 3–22.

Oertel, W., Gasser, T., Ippisch, R., Trenkwalder, C., and Poewe, W. H. (1989). Apomorphine test for dopaminergic responsiveness. *Lancet* **ii**, 1261–2.

Quik, M., Spokes, E., Mackay, A., and Bannister, R. (1979). Alterations in 3H-spiperone binding in human caudate nucleus, substantia nigra and frontal cortex in the Shy–Drager syndrome and Parkinson's disease. *J. neurol. Sci.* **43**, 429–37.

Rajput, A., Kazi, K. A., and Rozdilsky, B. (1972). Striatonigral degeneration—response to levodopa therapy. *J. neurol. Sci.* **16**, 331–41.

Rajput, A. H. and Rozdilsky, B. (1976). Dysautonomia in Parkinsonism—a clinicopathological study. *J. Neurol. Neurosurg. Psychiat.* **39**, 1092–100.

Rajput, A. H., Rozdilsky, B., Rajput, A., and Ang, L. (1990). Levodopa efficacy and pathological basis of Parkinson's syndrome. *Clin. Neuropharmacol.* **13**, 553–8.

Schober, R., Langston, J. W., and Forno, L. S. (1975). Idiopathic orthostatic hypotension. Biochemical and pathologic observations in 2 cases. *Eur. Neurol.* **13**, 177–88.

Sharpe, J. A., Rewcastle, N. B., Lloyd, K. G., Hornykiewicz, O., Hill, M., and Tasker, R. (1973). Striato-nigral degeneration response to levodopa therapy with pathological and neurochemical correlation. *J. neurol. Sci.* **19**, 275–86.

Spokes, E. G. S., Bannister, R., and Oppenheimer, D. R. (1979). Multiple system atrophy with autonomic failure. Clinical, histological and neurochemical observations in 4 cases. *J. neurol. Sci.* **43**, 59–82.

Staal, A., Van der Meerwaldt, J. D., Van Dongen, K. J., Mulder, P. G. H., and Busch, H. F. M. (1990). Non-familial degenerative disease and atrophy of brain stem and cerebellum. *J. neurol. Sci.* **95**, 259–69.

Takei, Y. and Mirra, S. A. (1973). A form of multiple system atrophy with clinical Parkinsonism. In *Progress in neuropathology*, Vol. 2 (ed. H. M. Zimmerman), pp. 217–51. Grune & Stratton, New York.

Trotter, J. (1973). Striato-nigral degeneration. Alzheimer's disease and inflammatory changes. *Neurology* **23**, 1211–16.

Van Leeuwen, R. B. and Perquin, W. V. M. (1988). Bromocriptine therapy in striatonigral degeneration. *J. Neurol. Neurosurg. Psychiat.* **51**, 592.

Williams, A. C., Nutt, J., Lake, C. R., Pfeiffer, R., Teychenne, P. E., Ebert, M. and Calne, D. B. (1979). Actions of bromicriptine in the Shy–Drager and Steele–Olszewski syndromes. In *Dopaminergic ergots and motor control* (ed. K. Fuxe and D. B. Calne), pp. 271–83. Pergamon Press, Oxford.

PART V

Peripheral autonomic neuropathies

35. Autonomic dysfunction in peripheral nerve disease

J. G. McLeod

Introduction

The autonomic nervous system is affected to some extent in many peripheral neuropathies, although the clinical manifestations may be mild. When small-diameter myelinated and unmyelinated fibres in afferent and efferent nerves are pathologically involved by the disease process (e.g. diabetes, amyloid) or when segmental demyelination affects myelinated autonomic fibres in the vagus or sympathetic pathways (e.g. Guillain-Barré syndrome, diabetes) autonomic disturbances will be present. The clinical features of this autonomic dysfunction may range from the frequent mild impairment of sweating on the extremities to the more serious postural hypotension. The mechanisms and manifestations of autonomic dysfunction in peripheral nerve diseases are summarized in this chapter.

Histology of the autonomic nervous system

Sympathetic nervous system

The sympathetic chain, white rami, and splanchnic nerve in man consist of myelinated and unmyelinated fibres. The fibre diameter distribution of myelinated fibres is similar in all three nerves (McLeod 1980). Most of the fibres are in the range 2–6 μm but there is another distinct group of larger fibres with a peak at about 12 μm; the larger myelinated fibres and some of the smaller myelinated fibres are afferent. Internodal lengths in the sympathetic chain and in the white rami are shorter in relation to fibre diameter than those in the peripheral nervous system (Fig. 35.1). Morphometric analysis of the preganglionic neurons in the spinal cord of man and of the sympathetic preganglionic fibres in the ventral roots has shown that the preganglionic fibres range in diameter from 1.5 to 4.7 μm with a peak at 2.5 μm. There is progressive reduction of numbers of both cells and fibres with age.

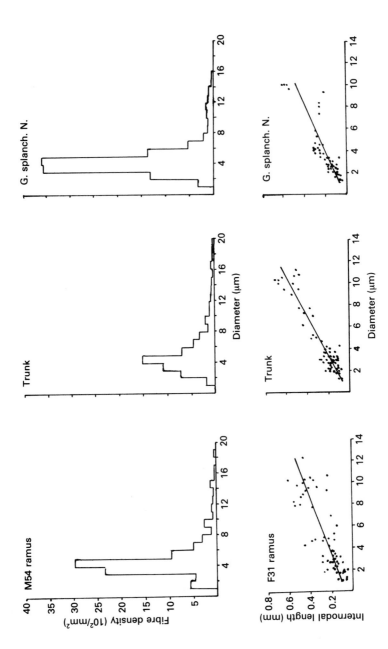

Fig. 35.1. Control subjects. (Above) diameter distribution of myelinated fibres in white ramus, sympathetic trunk, and greater splanchnic nerve. (Below) relationship between internodal length and diameter of myelinated fibres in white ramus, trunk, and greater splanchnic nerve. (From McLeod (1980).)

Parasympathetic nervous system

The histological structure of the vagus nerve has been studied in man. Only a small proportion (about 20 per cent) of the afferent and efferent fibres in the cervical vagus are myelinated and most of these are 3 μm or less in diameter.

The carotid sinus nerve has been studied in different animal species including man and contains myelinated fibres which range in diameter from 2 to 14 μm, most of these being in the 2–5μm diameter range; it also contains many unmyelinated fibres (Tamura *et al.* 1988). Afferent fibres from the aortic arch receptors are both myelinated and unmyelinated; the myelinated fibres in the cat range from 2 to 10 μm, although most are in the 2–6μm range.

Manifestations of autonomic dysfunction in peripheral nerve diseases

Impaired sweating of the extremities is common and probably results from degeneration of cholinergic postganglionic sympathetic unmyelinated fibres that travel with the peripheral nerves to innervate sweat glands, or to degeneration or demyelination of preganglionic sympathetic efferent fibres. Hyperhidrosis may be seen in partial nerve injuries that cause causalgia or when there is pressure on the nerve roots such as occurs in malignancy and in some toxic neuropathies. When sweating is impaired in the extremities, excessive compensatory sweating may occur on trunk and face.

Orthostatic postural hypotension results from damage to the small-diameter myelinated and unmyelinated fibres in afferent and efferent nerves in the baroreflex pathways and in the splanchnic outflow. Postural hypotension, therefore, most commonly occurs in diseases such as diabetes and amyloidosis in which the small fibres degenerate and in the Guillain–Barré syndrome in which segmental demyelination affects the myelinated autonomic fibres in the vagus and sympathetic pathways. It is more likely to occur when fibres in the splanchnic vascular bed are pathologically involved since the latter plays an important part in human blood pressure regulation (Low *et al.* 1975; McLeod 1980). Orthostatic hypotension is uncommon in dying-back neuropathies which initially affect predominantly the large-diameter fibres of the longest nerves. Impaired heart rate control results from vagal impairment in patients with autonomic neuropathy, particularly diabetes. Bladder dysfunction, impotence, and pupillary abnormalities are other clinical manifestations of autonomic dysfunction in peripheral nerve disease.

Investigation of autonomic function
in peripheral nerve diseases

The physiological and pharmacological tests of autonomic function in peripheral nerve disease are described in Part III of this volume. Biopsy techniques are not widely used in the investigation of autonomic function but have provided useful information in some conditions. In peripheral autonomic failure, such as that due to diabetes, amyloidosis, chronic alcoholism, and the inflammatory neuropathies, the findings on sural nerve biopsy generally reflect the changes in the autonomic nervous system. In some cases biopsy of the vagus or sympathetic nerves at abdominal operations has shown characteristic degenerative changes and has increased the understanding of the pathophysiology of some autonomic neuropathies. Rectal biopsy may demonstrate degenerative changes in the myenteric plexus but is rarely diagnostic. Skin biopsy may demonstrate reduction in the number of sweat glands. Muscle biopsy studied with histochemical techniques may demonstrate absence of catecholamine fluorescence in perivascular nerves in pure autonomic failure (Bannister *et al.* 1981). In general, biopsy techniques have little place in the investigation of peripheral autonomic failure but in selected cases have been helpful research tools.

Autonomic disorders with
no associated peripheral neuropathy

Acute and subacute autonomic neuropathy

Three types of acute and subacute autonomic neuropathy are recognized: pure pandysautonomia; pure cholinergic dysautonomia; and acute autonomic and sensory neuropathy. Young and his colleagues (1969) were the first to describe a definite clinical entity of pure pandysautonomia involving both sympathetic and parasympathetic nervous systems with a subacute onset followed by recovery. There had been some earlier reports of the condition in the literature although it was not clearly defined. The disorder differs from other neurological causes of autonomic dysfunction in that normal function of the central and peripheral somatic nervous systems is preserved. Since these first reports, a number of other patients with acute and subacute pandysautonomia have been described as well as some cases of pure cholinergic dysautonomia. Some cases of dysautonomia with associated sensory disturbances have also been reported, in some but not all of which there is electrophysiological and pathological evidence of loss of small-diameter myelinated and unmyelinated fibres (Kanda *et al.* 1990).

Acute and subacute pandysautonomia affects both sexes and all ages. There are no known familial or hereditary factors. The onset may be rapid, over a period of days, or more gradual over weeks or months. There may be a prodromal febrile or viral illness. The initial symptoms may be non-specific autonomic symptoms of postural hypotension, blurred vision, abdominal pain and constipation (sometimes preceded by diarrhoea), loss of sweating (which may be preceded by excessive sweating), urinary retention and incontinence, impotence, and dry mouth and eyes. On examination the pupils may be fixed or poorly reactive, the skin is dry, lacrimation is impaired, and the abdomen and bladder may be distended. Tests of autonomic function reveal impairment of both sympathetic and parasympathetic systems. Recovery occurs over a variable period ranging from months to years. The cerebrospinal fluid protein may be elevated. Electromyography and nerve conduction studies are normal in the pure form.

A number of the cases of pure cholinergic dysautonomia have been in children. Symptoms consist of blurred vision, impaired lacrimation, dry mouth, constipation, urinary retention and incontinence, and absence of sweating, but there is no postural hypotension. In the initial stages of the illness excessive salivation and sweat secretion have been reported. Cerebrospinal fluid findings have been normal in these patients. The illness tends to be more chronic and recovery less complete than is usual with pure pandysautonomia. In none of the cases of acute pandysautonomia or cholinergic dysautonomia has there been any abnormality of mental function, muscle strength, sensation, reflexes, or ocular movements.

The cause of these conditions remains uncertain but they are possibly a form of acute idiopathic polyneuritis restricted to autonomic nerves. Some cases have been associated with viral illnesses. The differential diagnosis includes botulism and acute autonomic neuropathy associated with the Guillain–Barré syndrome, porphyria, diabetes, toxic causes, systemic lupus erythematosus, and other connective tissue diseases.

Sympathomimetic drugs and 9-α-fluorohydrocortisone have been of value in treating postural hypotension in cases of pandysautonomia. In the cases of cholinergic dysfunction, carbachol may be helpful in the management of urinary retention and impaired gastrointestinal motility.

Botulism

Botulism is characterized by muscle paralysis, acute autonomic dysfunction, and gastrointestinal symptoms caused by absorption from the alimentary tract of toxins produced by strains of *Clostridium botulinum*. The toxin impairs the release of acetylcholine from nerve terminals; electrophysiological features are similar to those seen in the Eaton–Lambert syndrome. Acute autonomic dysfunction may be present without associated muscular weakness; in this circumstance the condition may be difficult to distinguish clinically from acute autonomic neuropathy.

Autonomic neuropathy associated with peripheral sensorimotor neuropathy (Table 35.1)

The autonomic nervous system is affected in many peripheral neuropathies, although the clinical manifestations may be mild (McLeod and Tuck 1987). Autonomic dysfunction is clinically important in the neuropathies associated with diabetes, amyloid disease, porphyria, and in the Guillain–Barré syndrome and some cases of hereditary sensory and autonomic neuropathy, particularly the Riley–Day syndrome. In most of the other conditions described below it is usually of only minor clinical importance.

Hereditary neuropathies

Charcot–Marie–Tooth disease (hereditary motor and sensory neuropathies (HMSN) types I and II)

Autonomic function has been investigated in Charcot–Marie–Tooth disease by a number of workers with conflicting results. There is general agreement that pupillary reflexes may be abnormal and that there is impairment of sweating distally. A recent study found no abnormality of cardiovascular reflexes in patients with HMSN types I and II when compared with control subjects (Ingall and McLeod 1991a). The impairment of sweating is most probably caused by distal degeneration of postganglionic sympathetic fibres and is consistent with the hypothesis that HMSN results from neuronal atrophy, the extremities of the nerve cell being affected first and most severely.

Friedreich's ataxia

Autonomic function studies, including sweat tests, are normal with no evidence of postural hypotension or impairment of baroreflex function (Ingall and McLeod 1991b). Since there is a reduction in the number of large-diameter myelinated fibres but small myelinated and unmyelinated fibres remain relatively intact in the peripheral nerves of patients with Friedreich's ataxia, the findings of normal autonomic function support the hypothesis that it is necessary for small fibres in the peripheral nerve to be affected to cause autonomic disturbances.

Hereditary sensory and autonomic neuropathy (HSAN)

The autonomic nervous system may be affected in hereditary sensory and autonomic neuropathies (HSAN), particularly familial dysautonomia (Riley–Day syndrome, HSAN type III), HSAN type IV, originally described by Swanson, in which there is a marked loss of small myelinated and unmyelinated fibres, and HSAN type V in which there is a marked reduction of small-diameter myelinated fibres but normal unmyelinated fibres.

Table 35.1.   Causes of peripheral autonomic dysfunction

Disorders with no associated peripheral neuropathy

Acute and subacute autonomic neuropathy
  Pandysautonomia
  Cholinergic dysautonomia

Botulism

Disorders associated with peripheral neuropathy

Autonomic dysfunction clinically important

  Diabetes
  Primary amyloidosis and familial amyloid neuropathy type I (Portuguese)
  Acute inflammatory neuropathy
  Acute intermittent and variegate porphyria
  Hereditary sensory and autonomic neuropathy (HSAN):
    HSAN type III (Riley–Day syndrome, familial dysautonomia); HSAN
    type IV (Swanson); HSAN type V

Autonomic dysfunction usually clinically unimportant
  Hereditary neuropathies
    Hereditary motor and sensory neuropathies
    Fabry's disease
    Hereditary sensory and autonomic neuropathy (HSAN types I & II)
    Amyloid disease (some familial amyloid polyneuropathies, secondary
      amyloidosis)

  Chronic inflammatory demyelinating polyradiculoneuropathy

  Metabolic disorders
    Chronic renal failure
    Chronic liver disease
    Vitamin B_{12} deficiency

  Alcoholism and nutritional disorders

  Malignancy

  Toxic causes (vincristine, acrylamide, heavy metals, perhexiline maleate,
    organic solvents)

  Connective tissue diseases
    Rheumatoid arthritis
    Systemic lupus erythematosus
    Mixed connective tissue diseases

  Infection
    Leprosy
    Human immunodeficiency virus (HIV)
    Chagas' disease

Amyloidosis

Amyloidosis is the collective name for a heterogeneous group of diseases characterized by the deposition in the body tissues of amyloid, a proteinaceous material consisting of polypeptide fibrils arranged in β-pleated sheets. The disease has been classified in various ways according to clinical and biochemical criteria. Several major types are recognized (Hersch and McLeod 1987).

1. Immunocyte dyscrasia with amyloidosis, including primary amyloidosis, multiple myeloma, and Waldenström's macroglobulinaemia.

2. Heredofamilial amyloidosis. This was originally classified on clinical and genetic criteria into four major types. The amyloid fibrils contain prealbumin (transthyretin) and a number of mutations of the prealbumin gene on chromosome 18 have now been identified by techniques of molecular biology, accounting for the different familial types (Mendell *et al.* 1990).

3. Secondary amyloidosis.

4. Organ-limited amyloidosis.

5. Senile amyloidosis.

The types most frequently complicated by autonomic dysfunction are primary amyloidosis and the Portuguese type of familial amyloid polyneuropathy (FAP type I).

Peripheral neuropathy is present in about 15–20 per cent of patients with primary amyloidosis and all the cases of FAP type I. Symptoms of autonomic dysfunction, which are often disabling, frequently accompany and may precede the other manifestations of peripheral neuropathy. Symptoms of postural hypotension are common; other manifestations of autonomic dysfunction include genitourinary disturbances (impotence, loss of bladder sensation, incomplete bladder emptying, and incontinence), gastrointestinal disturbances (dysphagia due to abnormal oesophageal motility, diarrhoea, and constipation), and irregular pupils reacting poorly to light and accommodation. Tests of autonomic function (sweat tests, Valsalva response, tests for postural hypotension, baroreflex sensitivity, heart-rate response to change in posture and breathing, vasomotor responses to cold and inspiratory gasp) are abnormal. The clinical course is one of steady progression and treatment is symptomatic.

Autonomic dysfunction is attributable to predominant loss of unmyelinated and small myelinated fibres in the peripheral autonomic nerves and reduction in the number of cells in the intermediolateral columns. Widespread deposition of amyloid in the autonomic nerves and ganglia has been frequently seen (Fig. 35.2).

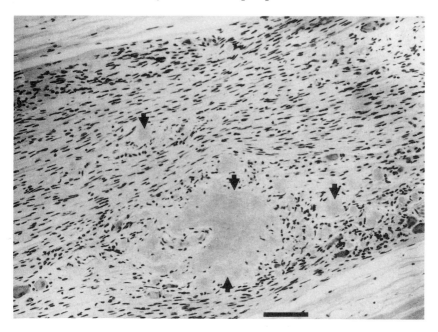

Fig. 35.2.   Amyloid deposits (arrows) in thoracic sympathetic trunk of a patient with primary amyloidosis. Bar, 100 μm.

Inflammatory neuropathies

Acute inflammatory neuropathy (Guillain–Barré syndrome)

Disturbances of autonomic function are well recognized in the Guillain–Barré syndrome. Tachycardia, which may remain fixed and unresponsive to postural change, has been reported by a number of workers (Tuck and McLeod 1982). Elevated or fluctuating arterial blood pressure has been documented as well as postural hypotension (Tuck and McLeod 1982; Fagius and Wallin 1983).

Abnormalities of the heart rate and of the blood pressure response to Valsalva manoeuvre have been described. The heart rate response to elevated arterial blood pressure induced by intravenous injection of phenylephrine may be impaired (Fig. 35.3) and the sweat test is commonly abnormal (Fig. 35.4). The nature of the abnormalities of autonomic function is variable and depends upon the site of the demyelinating lesions, which may be present in the afferent fibres in the vagus and glossopharyngeal nerves, in the arterial baroreceptors, in the efferent parasympathetic fibres in the vagus nerves, and in the sympathetic nerves that innervate the heart and control sweating and vasomotor tone. Pathological studies have demonstrated demyelinating lesions in the glossopharyngeal and vagus nerves and in the sympathetic chains and white rami. The severity of the involvement of the autonomic nervous

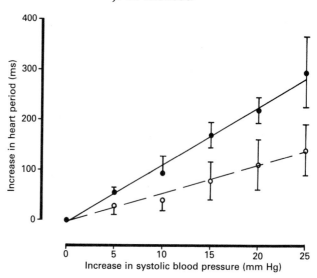

Fig. 35.3. Relationship of increase in heart period to increase in systolic blood pressure in control subjects (closed circles) and in patients with Guillain–Barré syndrome (open circles) following intravenous phenylephrine. Vertical bars represent ± 1SE. (From Tuck and McLeod (1982).)

system does not appear to be related to the degree of motor or sensory disturbance. In most patients the consequences of involvement of the autonomic nervous system are not serious but on some occasions they can be life-threatening. Postural hypotension may lead to syncope and irreversible brain damage in a paralysed patient who is inadvertently left in a sitting position or who requires an anaesthetic; sudden death due to cardiac arrhythmias or to asystole may also occur.

Chronic inflammatory neuropathy

In chronic inflammatory demyelinating polyradiculoneuropathy, postural hypotension and other symptoms of autonomic nervous system dysfunction are very uncommon (Ingall *et al.* 1990). These findings are in contrast to those in acute inflammatory neuropathy in which the more severe disturbances of autonomic function are presumed to be related to acute conduction block and possibly more extensive involvement of unmyelinated fibres in the acute stages.

Metabolic disorders

Diabetes

Autonomic neuropathy is commonly associated with diabetic peripheral neuropathy in which degenerative change can be demonstrated in the

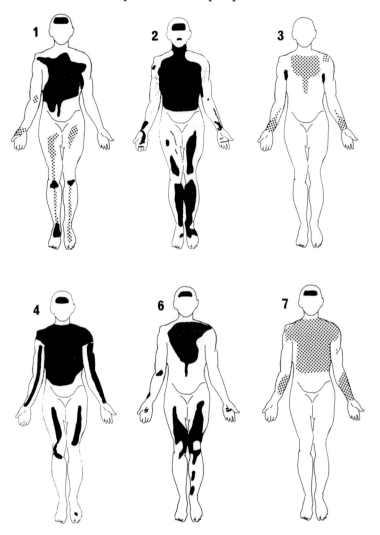

Fig. 35.4. Patterns of sweating in Guillain–Barré syndrome. Black areas indicate regions of normal sweat production; spotted areas are those in which sweating was patchy. (From Tuck and McLeod (1982).)

peripheral autonomic nerves (Fig. 35.5). It is considered in detail in Chapters 36 and 37.

Porphyria

Postural hypotension may occur in acute intermittent and variegate porphyria, although hypertension is more common and may precede the manifestation of peripheral neuropathy. Persistent tachycardia may be an early feature of

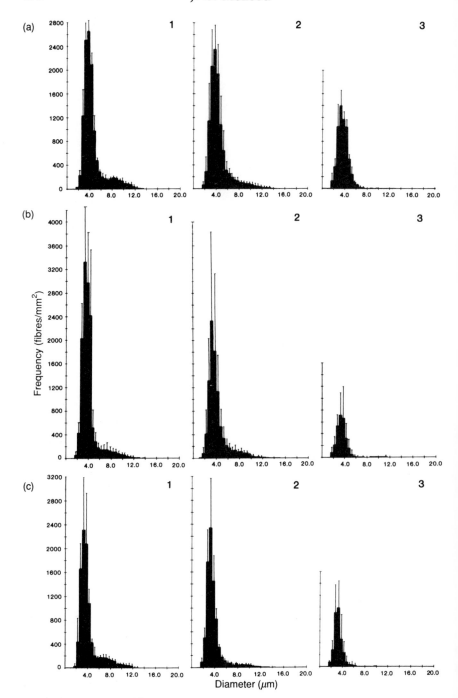

Fig. 35.5.

an attack and may also precede the onset of neuropathy. Other clinical features of autonomic neuropathy include abdominal pain, nausea and vomiting, constipation, diarrhoea, bladder distension, and disorders of sweating. Autonomic function studies have demonstrated abnormalities of sympathetic and parasympathetic function (Yeung Laiwah *et al.* 1985). There is pathological evidence of involvement of brainstem and spinal cord cells and vagus and sympathetic nerves.

Chronic renal failure

Impairment of autonomic function is common in patients with terminal uraemia and disturbances of sympathetic and parasympathetic function have been demonstrated by many authors. Improvement follows renal transplantation. Persistent hypotension in patients on chronic haemodialysis can be an important clinical problem and has been investigated by several groups of workers to determine whether it is due to autonomic failure or to other factors such as plasma volume depletion, cardiomyopathy, and coronary artery disease. Sympathetic efferent function is normal, as are most other tests of autonomic function except for baroreceptor sensitivity. It may be concluded that autonomic dysfunction alone is not a sufficient explanation for the haemodialysis hypotension, although damage to baroreceptors or their afferent fibres or central nervous system connections may play a part (Nies *et al.* 1979; Naik *et al.* 1981).

Chronic liver disease

Autonomic dysfunction, predominantly affecting the parasympathetic system, is present in about 40–50 per cent of patients with both alcoholic and non-alcoholic chronic liver disease, the latter including primary biliary cirrhosis and chronic active hepatitis. Disordered autonomic function is present in some patients without evidence of peripheral neuropathy. The mechanism of autonomic neuropathy in chronic liver disease remains uncertain but is most likely to be due to damage to the peripheral autonomic nervous system resulting from nutritional and metabolic disorders consequent upon hepatic failure or, alternatively, to immunoglobulin or immune complex deposition (Thuluvath and Triger 1989).

Vitamin B_{12} deficiency

Orthostatic hypotension may be the initial manifestation of pernicious anaemia. It usually responds well to replacement therapy. The pathological

---

Fig. 35.5. (*opposite*)   Mean myelinated fibre density distribution of vagus nerves from: (a) controls; (b) diabetics; and (c) alcoholics at (1) midcervical; (2) lung hilum; and (3) diaphragm levels. Bars indicate one standard deviation from mean. (From Guo *et al.* (1987).)

findings in the peripheral neuropathy of vitamin B_{12} deficiency are those of axonal degeneration but this alone is unlikely to cause postural hypotension which may possibly be due to some central mechanism (McCombe and McLeod 1984).

Alcoholism and nutritional disorders

Postural hypotension is common in patients with Wernicke's encephalopathy and is probably the result of impaired sympathetic outflow at central or peripheral levels. Clinical manifestations of autonomic dysfunction are unusual in uncomplicated alcoholic peripheral neuropathy (Low et al. 1975; Duncan et al. 1980), although postural hypotension may occur in patients who are severely affected (Novak and Victor 1974). These findings indicate that peripheral sympathetic vasomotor control is relatively well preserved in alcoholics until the peripheral neuropathy reaches an advanced stage, even though abnormal sweat tests indicate that there is early involvement of sympathetic efferent fibres (Low et al. 1975). Duncan et al. (1980) have provided definite evidence of vagal damage in chronic alcoholics by demonstrating impaired heart rate responses to Valsalva manoeuvre, deep breathing, change in posture, neck suction, and atropine. Novak and Victor (1974) reported hoarseness and weakness of the voice and dysphagia as clinical manifestations of vagal neuropathy in patients with severe alcoholic neuropathy. Other possible manifestations of disordered parasympathetic function in alcoholics include impaired oesophageal motility, abnormal pupillary reflexes, and impotence. Alcoholics with vagal neuropathy have an increased mortality rate (Johnson and Robinson 1988). Morphometric studies have demonstrated a significant reduction in the density of myelinated fibres in the distal parts of the vagus (Fig. 35.5) and carotid sinus nerves in chronic alcoholics (Guo et al. 1987; Tamura et al. 1988), but the splanchnic nerves are relatively spared (Low et al. 1975).

Alcoholic neuropathy is a dying-back neuropathy identical to that of beriberi (Novak and Victor 1974). The most distal parts of the longest fibres in the vagus nerve are affected earliest and the shorter and more proximal myelinated fibres of the sympathetic system are not affected until later in the illness when the peripheral neuropathy is severe. The absence of postural hypotension and the relatively normal baroreflex function are consistent with a lack of pathology in the splanchnic nerves since postural hypotension is more likely to occur if the splanchnic outflow is involved.

Malignancy

Impairment of sweating occurs in association with the peripheral neuropathy of remote malignancies. Pandysautonomia was reported in a patient with small cell carcinoma of the bronchus in whom there was no clinical or electrophysiological evidence of peripheral neuropathy; in addition to severe orthostatic hypotension there was an abnormal Valsalva response, impaired oesophageal and gastrointestinal motility, abnormal sweat and Schirmer tests, denervation supersensitivity to noradrenaline, and a flat cystometrogram (Chiappa and Young 1973). Other patients with postural hypotension and other manifestations of autonomic dysfunction have been reported with carcinoma of the lung and pancreas and with lymphoma. Local hyperhydrosis and piloerection may result from direct irritation of nerves or roots.

Autonomic dysfunction is well documented in the Lambert–Eaton myasthenic syndrome, manifestations including dry mouth, impaired lacrimation and sweating, impotence, constipation, and orthostatic hypotension (Khurana *et al.* 1988). Abnormalities of cholinergic function predominate but abnormalities of sympathetic function have also been reported. The Lambert–Eaton syndrome is an autoimmune disorder in which antibodies to voltage-gated calcium channels of peripheral cholinergic nerve terminals impair the release of acetylcholine. It seems likely that autoimmune mechanisms affecting the autonomic nervous system are responsible for many of the paraneoplastic causes of autonomic dysfunction.

Toxic causes

Vincristine

The vinca alkaloids are cytotoxic drugs used in the treatment of lymphoma, leukaemia, and some other malignancies. Vincristine, and occasionally vinblastine, cause peripheral neuropathy, the predominant pathological change in the peripheral nerve being axonal degeneration. Postural hypotension has been reported as a neurotoxic side-effect of vincristine and constipation, abdominal pain, paralytic ileus, urinary retention, and other bladder disturbances are well recognized complications. Published accounts of autonomic function studies in patients with vincristine-induced autonomic neuropathy are limited but have demonstrated abnormalities of postganglionic sympathetic efferent function and abnormal Valsalva responses in patients with postural hypotension (Hancock and Naysmith 1975). The sympathetic nerves and ganglia were normal in two cases in whom autopsy material was examined pathologically.

Autonomic dysfunction may develop within days of commencement of vincristine therapy. The mechanism of action is not clear, although there is some evidence in man and other animals that the primary site of damage is the unmyelinated noradrenergic fibres of the sympathetic nervous system. However, the symptoms in man of constipation, paralytic ileus, and bladder disturbances indicate that parasympathetic fibres are also affected. Ultra-structurally, vinca alkaloids disrupt microtubules and cause an increase in the neurofilaments and the appearance of paracrystalline structures in axons. Unmyelinated fibres are more susceptible to the neurotoxin than myelinated fibres.

Heavy metal poisoning

There have been very few cases of heavy metal poisoning in which autonomic function has been adequately studied. In thallium poisoning, tachycardia and hypertension have been reported in association with peripheral neuropathy. In arsenical poisoning excessive sweating and impairment of sweating on the extremities have been described. Subacute or chronic inorganic mercury poisoning is the cause of acrodynia, which occurs mainly in children and includes amongst its manifestations tachycardia, hypertension, and profuse sweating.

Organic solvents

Autonomic function has been shown to be disturbed in some workers who had experienced prolonged chronic occupational exposure to a variety of organic solvents containing mainly aliphatic, aromatic, and other hydrocarbons, alcohols, ketones, esters, and ethers, as well as to carbon disulphide and toluene. They had significant impairment of heart rate variation with respiration and Valsalva ratio compared to controls. The most severely affected patients were those exposed to carbon disulphide. Some of the patients had clinical and electrophysiological evidence of peripheral neuropathy (Matikainen and Juntunen 1985).

Inhalation of *n*-hexane and methyl-*n*-butyl-ketone may result in a rapidly progressive polyneuropathy associated with autonomic features of excessive or impaired sweating on the extremities, postural hypotension, and impotence.

Acrylamide

Acrylamide is neurotoxic in its soluble monomeric form, in which it is manufactured and distributed. After transformation to a polymer it is used in industry as a flocculator for separating solids from aqueous solutions. It is also used in the preparation of grouts for the sealing of pipes and subterranean tunnels. The major toxic effect in man is a predominantly sensory polyneuropathy, often preceded by blueness and excessive sweating of the extremities due to a disturbance of sympathetic function. Other autonomic disturbances in man are rarely seen although they have been studied extensively in experimental animals.

Perhexiline maleate

Perhexiline maleate, used in the treatment of angina pectoris, may cause a peripheral neuropathy. Fraser *et al.* (1977) described three patients who developed autonomic neuropathy manifested by postural hypotension and an abnormal Valsalva ratio related to perhexiline maleate-induced neuropathy.

Connective tissue diseases

Rheumatoid arthritis

Impairment of sweating on the extremities is relatively common in rheumatoid arthritis and is probably related in most cases to damage of postganglionic sympathetic efferent fibres in the peripheral nerves. In addition, there may be vagus nerve involvement since the heart rate response to standing, to the Valsalva manoeuvre, and to respiration may be impaired particularly in patients with peripheral neuropathy. Rarely, autonomic neuropathy may be secondary to amyloidosis.

Systemic lupus erythematosus and mixed connective tissue diseases

Autonomic neuropathy has been reported as a complication of systemic lupus erythematosus (Gledhill and Dessein 1988) and mixed connective tissue diseases (Gudesblatt *et al.* 1985).

Infections

Leprosy

Leprosy, one of the most common causes of peripheral neuropathy, may be associated with autonomic disturbances. Loss of sweating over the skin supplied by the diseased nerves is the usual finding but, in addition, cardiac denervation, postural hypotension, decreased sweating, and impaired response to the cold pressor test, even in the absence of other features of peripheral neuropathy, have been described.

Human immunodeficiency virus (HIV) infection

Autonomic dysfunction affecting both sympathetic and parasympathetic divisions may be associated with HIV infections. Abnormalities of autonomic function tests may be demonstrated in asymptomatic patients or there may be specific symptoms of postural hypotension, disorders of sweating, diarrhoea, impotence, and disturbed bladder function. Autonomic dysfunction is more frequent and of greater severity in patients with AIDS but may be present in the early stages of HIV infection and appears to progress during the illness (Freeman *et al.* 1990). The mechanism of the disordered autonomic function is not clear; it is not necessarily related to the presence of peripheral neuropathy (Cohen and Laudenslager 1989).

Chagas' disease

Chagas' disease is very common in South America. It is caused by the protozoal parasite, *Trypanasoma cruzi*, and in its chronic form it is manifested clinically by cardiac failure, arrhythmias, disturbances of gastrointestinal motility including mega-oesophagus and megacolon, and other autonomic disturbances including postural hypotension. Tests of autonomic function including blood pressure and heart rate response to tilting, and the Valsalva manoeuvre, baroreceptor sensitivity, and plasma noradrenaline levels are abnormal (Iosa *et al.* 1990). In the heart, there are pathological changes in the myocardium and conducting system as well as in autonomic ganglia and postganglionic nerves; in the gastrointestinal system there is destruction of autonomic ganglia and the myenteric plexus. Multifocal inflammatory lesions associated with demyelination are present in the peripheral nervous system in humans and in the murine experimental model (Said *et al.* 1985). There is evidence that the destruction of the peripheral and sympathetic nervous systems has an autoimmune basis, T lymphocytes and possibly humoral factors being responsible for an attack on neural elements. Antigenic determinants may be shared by the parasite and host. A recent placebo-controlled clinical trial of mixed gangliosides has demonstrated improved blood pressure control with treatment possibly due to an indirect neurotrophic effect (Iosa *et al.* 1991).

Experimental autonomic neuropathy

Autonomic neuropathy has been induced in experimental animals in order to study its pathophysiology in greater detail than is possible in man. A number of different methods have been employed for inducing experimental autonomic neuropathy, including sympathectomy with 6-hydroxydopamine, nerve growth factor antiserum, and guanethidine; experimental allergic neuritis; injection of extracts of sympathetic chain; acrylamide; and diabetes.

6-hydroxydopamine sympathectomy

6-hydroxydopamine (6-OHDA) causes selective destruction of peripheral adrenergic nerve terminals. Its effect on mesenteric vascular control was studied in cats (McLeod 1980). There was no clinical or electrophysiological evidence of peripheral neuropathy in the animals but studies of mesenteric blood flow demonstrated that neural control of the mesenteric vascular bed was abnormal. There was denervation supersensitivity to noradrenaline and phenylephrine, there was no response to intravenous tyramine, and there was a markedly impaired vasoconstrictor response to electrical stimulation of the splanchnic nerve. No morphological changes were demonstrated in the posterior tibial or splanchnic nerves. 6-OHDA therefore produces a chemical sympathectomy in animals resulting in impaired vasomotor control, but there does not appear to be any precise counterpart in man of the sympathetic failure seen in these animals.

Nerve growth factor antiserum

Nerve growth factor antiserum induces immunosympathectomy by causing degeneration of sympathetic ganglion cells and other postganglionic fibres.

It results in impaired vasoconstriction and blood pressure control (Brody 1964). There is no precise counterpart in man of this experimental autonomic neuropathy.

Guanethidine-induced sympathectomy

Guanethidine causes degeneration of postganglionic sympathetic nerves. Rats treated with guanethidine have low arterial blood pressure, ptosis, loss of neurons in the cervical sympathetic ganglia, and a decreased C fibre action potential in the cervical sympathetic trunk, while normal function is preserved in somatic and vagus nerves (Zochodne *et al.* 1988).

Autoimmune preganglionic sympathectomy

Injection of monoclonal antibodies to neural acetylcholinesterase in adult rats causes destruction of presynaptic fibres in sympathetic ganglia and the adrenal medulla. The animals develop ptosis, hypotension, bradycardia, and postural syncope. There is failure of ganglionic transmission when preganglionic fibres are stimulated, but there is a normal response on direct ganglionic stimulation. The preganglionic terminals are inactivated but postganglionic neurons remain intact. Parasympathetic function and motor function are normal. Morphological and histochemical studies demonstrate depleted presynaptic acetylcholinesterase and loss of presynaptic terminals with preservation of the ganglion cells. This example of preganglionic immunosympathectomy in rats may be a useful model for studying some forms of autonomic failure in man (Brimijoin and Lennon 1990).

Experimental immune autonomic neuropathy

Appenzeller and colleagues (1965) sensitized rabbits with antigen extracted from human sympathetic nerves and ganglia. Although the animals were not clinically ill, they had impaired reflex vasodilatation of the ear vessels. The defect in reflex vasomotor function was attributed to involvement of efferent sympathetic cholinergic fibres. Basophils were abundant in the perivascular spaces of the ear vessels in the immunized animals but there were no abnormalities detected histologically in the sympathetic nervous system although morphometric studies suggested regeneration of unmyelinated fibres.

Experimental allergic neuritis

Autonomic function has been studied in animals with experimental allergic neuritis (EAN) (Tuck *et al.* 1981). Slowed conduction and dispersion of the compound action potential were demonstrated in the splanchnic and vagus nerves and light and electron microscopy confirmed the presence of demyelination. In some animals unmyelinated fibres were also damaged. Since the clinical, histopathological, and electrophysiological features of EAN and the Guillain–Barré syndrome are similar, the findings are relevant to the pathogenesis of autonomic dysfunction in the Guillain–Barré syndrome.

Acrylamide neuropathy

Acrylamide causes a distal symmetrical axonopathy in man and animals. The autonomic nervous system has been studied in animals with acrylamide neuropathy in order to help understand the pathophysiology of autonomic dysfunction in the common peripheral neuropathies in which axonal degeneration is the underlying pathological abnormality (e.g. alcoholic, nutritional, and toxic neuropathies). Comparison of the histological changes in the peripheral, somatic, and autonomic nerves of cats demonstrated that the longest fibres were the most profoundly damaged: the peripheral somatic nerves were more severely affected than the autonomic nerves and the vagus nerves showed greater degrees of fibre loss than the shorter splanchnic nerves. Vasomotor control of the mesenteric vascular bed was impaired in the more severely affected animals. The findings are consistent with the clinical observations in alcoholic and other dying-back neuropathies that the earliest autonomic abnormalities are those of vagal function and that postural hypotension occurs only in the more severe peripheral neuropathies when the splanchnic nerves are likely to be involved (McLeod 1980).

Studies of baroreflexes in animals with acrylamide neuropathy have shown that aortic arch baroreceptors, innervated by the vagus nerve, are more greatly affected than the carotid sinus baroreceptors which are innervated by the shorter carotid sinus nerves (Satchell 1990). It is likely that blood pressure control in man would remain relatively normal in dying-back neuropathies until the carotid sinus and splanchnic nerves became pathologically involved.

Dogs with acrylamide neuropathy develop mega-oesophagus which has been shown to be caused by damage to the vagally innervated oesophageal mechanoreceptors (Satchell and McLeod 1984). Pulmonary stretch receptors are affected in relatively mild acrylamide neuropathy in dogs, resulting in abnormalities of respiratory reflexes. The cough reflex is also impaired (Hersch *et al.* 1989). These experimental findings suggest that damage to vagal afferent fibres may contribute to respiratory complications in humans with peripheral nerve disease.

Experimental diabetic autonomic neuropathy

Autonomic neuropathy has been studied in rats with streptozocin-induced diabetes and diabetic BB Wistar rats (Sima *et al.* 1987). The diabetic Wistar rat has clinical, pathological, and physiological evidence of sympathetic and parasympathetic dysfunction. Dystrophic axonal changes are widely distributed throughout the sympathetic nervous system, but not the parasympathetic nervous system which is characterized by progressive axonal degeneration.

Summary and conclusions

Disturbances of autonomic function are frequently present in patients with peripheral neuropathy, but may be mild and asymptomatic. Severe autonomic dysfunction is most likely to result from conditions such as amyloidosis and diabetes that affect the small myelinated and unmyelinated fibres in the baroreceptor afferents, the vagal innervation of the heart, and the sympathetic efferent fibres in the mesenteric vascular bed, or from the Guillain–Barré syndrome in which there is acute segmental demyelination in the sympathetic and parasympathetic nerves.

References

Appenzeller, O., Arnason, B. G., and Adams, R. D. (1965). Experimental autonomic neuropathy: an immunologically induced disorder of reflex vasomotor function. *J. Neurol. Neurosurg. Psychiat.* **28**, 510–15.

Bannister, R., Crowe, R., Eames, R., and Burnstock, G. (1981). Adrenergic innervation in autonomic failure. *Neurology* **31**, 1501–6.

Brimijoin, S. and Lennon, V. A. (1990). Autoimmune preganglionic sympathectomy induced by acetylcholinesterase antibodies. *Proc. nat. Acad. Sci. USA* **87**, 9630–4.

Brody, M. J. (1964). Cardiovascular responses following immunological sympathectomy. *Circulation Res.* **15**, 161–7.

Chiappa, K. H. and Young, R. R. (1973). A case of paracarcinomatous pandysautonomia. *Neurology* **23**, 423.

Cohen, J. A. and Laudenslager, M. (1989). Autonomic nervous system involvement in patients with human immunodeficiency virus infection. *Neurology* **39**, 1111–12.

Duncan, G., Johnson, R. H., Lambie, D. G., and Whiteside, E. A. (1980). Evidence of vagal neuropathy in chronic alcoholics. *Lancet* **ii**, 1053–6.

Fagius, J. and Wallin, G. (1983). Microneurographic evidence of excessive sympathetic outflow in the Guillain–Barré syndrome. *Brain* **106**, 589–600.

Fraser, D. M., Campbell, I. W., and Miller, H. C. (1977). Peripheral and autonomic neuropathy after treatment with perhexiline maleate. *Br. med. J.* **iii**, 675–6.

Freeman, R., Roberts, M. S., Friedman, L. S., and Broadbridge, C. (1990). Autonomic function and human immunodeficiency virus infection. *Neurology* **40**, 575–80.

Gledhill, R. F. and Dessein, P. H. M. C. (1988). Autonomic neuropathy in systemic lupus erythematosus. *J. Neurol. Neurosurg. Psychiat.* **51**, 1238–40.

Gudesblatt, M., Goodman, A. D., Rubenstein, A. E., Bender, A. N., and Choi, H-SH. (1985). Autonomic neuropathy associated with autoimmune disease. *Neurology, New York* **35**, 261–4.

Guo, Y-P., McLeod, J. G., and Baverstock, J. (1987). Pathological changes in the vagus nerve in diabetics and chronic alcoholics. *J. Neurol. Neurosurg. Psychiat.* **50**, 1449–53.

Hancock, B. W. and Naysmith, A. (1975). Vincristine-induced autonomic neuropathy. *Br. med. J.* **3**, 207.

Hersch, M. I. and McLeod, J. G. (1987). Peripheral neuropathy associated with amyloidosis. In *Handbook of clinical neurology*, Vol. 7 (51). *Neuropathies* (ed. P. J. Vinken, G. W. Bruyn, and H. L. Klawans), pp. 413–28. Elsevier, Amsterdam.

Hersch, M. I., McLeod, J. G., and Sullivan, C. E. (1989). Abnormal cough reflex in canine acrylamide neuropathy. *Ann. Neurol.* **26**, 738–45.

Ingall, T. J. and McLeod, J. G. (1991*a*). Autonomic function in hereditary motor and sensory neuropathy (Charcot–Marie–Tooth disease). *Muscle Nerve* **14**, 1080–3.

Ingall, T. J. and McLeod, J. G. (1991*b*). Autonomic function in Friedreich's ataxia. *J. Neurol. Neurosurg. Psychiat.* **64**, 162–4.

Ingall, T. J., McLeod, J. G., and Tamura, N. (1990). Autonomic function and unmyelinated fibres in chronic inflammatory demyelinating polyradiculoneuropathy. *Muscle Nerve* **13**, 70–6.

Iosa, D., Dequattro, V., Lee, D. De-P., Elkayam, U., Caeiro, T., and Palmero, H. (1990). Pathogenesis of cardiac neuro-myopathy in Chagas' disease and the role of the autonomic nervous system. *J. autonom. nerv. Syst.* **30**, 583–8.

Iosa, D., Massari, D. C., and Dorsey, F. C. (1991). Chagas' cardioneuromyopathy: effect of ganglioside treatment in chronic dysautonomic patients—a randomised, double-blind, parallel placebo controlled study. *Am. Heart J.* **122**, 775–85.

Johnson, R. H. and Robinson, B. J. (1988). Mortality in alcoholics with autonomic neuropathy. *J. Neurol. Neurosurg. Psychiat.* **51**, 476–80.

Kanda, F., Uchida, T., Jinnai, K., Tada, K., Shiozawa, S., Fujita, T., and Ohnishi, A. (1990). Acute autonomic and sensory neuropathy: a case report. *J. Neurol.* **237**, 42–4.

Khurana, R. K., Koski, C. L., and Mayer, F. (1988). Autonomic dysfunction in Lambert–Eaton myasthenic syndrome. *J. neurol. Sci.* **85**, 77–86.

Low, P. A., Walsh, J. C., Huang, C.-Y., and McLeod, J. G. (1975). The sympathetic nervous system in alcoholic neuropathy. A clinical and pathological study. *Brain* **98**, 357–64.

Matikainen, E. and Juntunen, J. (1985). Autonomic nervous system dysfunction in workers exposed to organic solvents. *J. Neurol. Neurosurg. Psychiat.* **48**, 1021–4.

McCombe, P. A. and McLeod, J. G. (1984). The peripheral neuropathy of vitamin B12 deficiency. *J. neurol. Sci.* **66**, 117–26.

McLeod, J. G. (1980). Autonomic nervous system. In *The physiology of peripheral nerve disease* (ed. A. J. Sumner), pp. 432–83. Saunders, Philadelphia.

McLeod, J. G. and Tuck, R. R. (1987). Disorders of the autonomic nervous system. *Ann. Neurol.* **21**, 419–31, 519–30.

Mendell, J. R., Jiang, X-S., Warmolts, J. R., Nichols, W. C., and Benson, M. D. (1990). Diagnosis of Maryland/German familial amyloidotic polyneuropathy using allele-specific enzymatically amplified, genomic DNA. *Ann. Neurol.* **27**, 553–7.

Naik, R. B., Mathias, C. J., Wilson, C. A., Reid, J. L., and Warren, D. J. (1981). Cardiovascular and autonomic reflexes in haemodialysis patients. *Clin. Sci.* **60**, 165–70.

Nies, A. S., Robertson, D., and Stone, W. J. (1979). Hemodialysis hypotension is not the result of uremic peripheral autonomic neuropathy. *J. lab. clin. Med.* **94**, 395–402.

Novak, D. J. and Victor, M. (1974). The vagus and sympathetic nerves in alcoholic neuropathy. *Arch. Neurol., Chicago* **30**, 273–84.

Said, G., Joskowicz, M., Barreira, A. A., and Eisea, H. (1985). Neuropathy associated with experimental Chagas' disease. *Ann. Neurol.* **18**, 676–83.

Satchell, P. M. (1990). Baroreceptor dysfunction in acrylamide axonal neuropathy. *Brain* **113**, 167–76.

Satchell, P. M. and McLeod, J. G. (1984). Abnormalities of oesophageal mechanoreceptors in canine acrylamide neuropathy. *J. Neurol. Neurosurg. Psychiat.* **47**, 692–8.

Sima, A. A. F., Brismar, T., and Yagihashi, S. (1987). Neuropathies encountered in the spontaneously diabetic BB Wistar rat. In *Diabetic neuropathy* (ed. P. J. Dyck, P. K. Thomas, A. K. Asbury, A. L. Winegrad, and D. Porte), pp. 253–9. Saunders, Philadelphia.

Tamura, N., Baverstock, J., and McLeod, J. G. (1988). A morphometric study of the carotid sinus nerve in patients with diabetes mellitus and chronic alcoholism. *J. autonom. nerv. Syst.* **23**, 9–15.

Thuluvath, P. J. and Triger, D. R. (1989). Autonomic neuropathy in chronic liver disease. *Quart. J. Med.* **72**, 737–47.

Tuck, R. R. and McLeod, J. G. (1982). Autonomic dysfunction in Guillain–Barré syndrome. *J. Neurol. Neurosurg. Psychiat.* **44**, 983–90.

Tuck, R. R., Pollard, J. D., and McLeod, J. G. (1981). Autonomic neuropathy in experimental allergic neuritis: an electrophysiological and histological study. *Brain* **104**, 187–208.

Yeung Laiwah, A. C., Macphee, G. J. A., Boye, P., Moore, M. R., and Goldberg, A. (1985). Autonomic neuropathy in acute intermittent porphyria. *J. Neurol. Neurosurg. Psychiat.* **48**, 1025–30.

Young, R. R., Asbury, A. K., Adams, R. D., and Corbett, J. L. (1969). Pure pandysautonomia with recovery. *Trans. Am. neurol. Ass.* **94**, 355–7.

Zochodne, D. W., Ward, K. K., and Low, P. A. (1988). Guanethidine adrenergic neuropathy: an animal model of selective autonomic neuropathy. *Brain Res.* **461**, 10–16.

36. The epidemiology of diabetic autonomic neuropathy

H. A. W. Neil

Introduction

Diabetes mellitus is the most common cause of autonomic neuropathy, and the development of simple non-invasive cardiovascular reflex tests has allowed autonomic function to be extensively studied in diabetic patients. However, the epidemiology and natural history of diabetic autonomic neuropathy remain poorly documented, although rather more is known about its prevalence than about its aetiology or incidence.

Epidemiology can be defined as the study of the distribution and determinants of disease frequency in specified populations. By definition, epidemiological studies have numerators, denominators, and rates. Descriptive studies involve the measurement of prevalence and incidence. Analytical studies are concerned with measurement of individual characteristics, including genetic host factors and possible environmental determinants, to try to identify aetiological associations. Experimental studies examine the effects of manipulating a particular study factor and can be subdivided into natural experiments and randomized clinical trials. Because so few epidemiological studies of diabetic autonomic neuropathy have been conducted, most of our knowledge of its epidemiology has to be inferred from clinical studies.

Definition of diabetic autonomic neuropathy

There is no standardized definition of cardiovascular autonomic neuropathy, which complicates comparison between studies. The American Diabetes Association and American Academy of Neurology (ADA 1988) have recommended three non-invasive tests for routine assessment of autonomic function: (1) heart rate response to Valsalva manoeuvre, deep breathing, and standing; (2) the response of blood pressure to standing or tilting and sustained handgrip; and (3) the sweat response to heat or chemicals such as acetylcholine or pilocarpine. Tests of heart rate variability (HRV) and the blood pressure response to sustained handgrip are simple and accurate enough for use in epidemiological studies, although the intraindividual coefficient of variation is wide, for instance, 15.4 per cent for the Valsalva ratio and 8.9 per cent for the expiratory:inspiratory (E:I) ratio (Smith 1982, 1984). Some other studies have reported smaller coefficients, and the intraindividual variation is reduced in patients with autonomic neuropathy. Since HRV depends on age, age-related normal ranges should be used to classify results of cardiovascular reflex tests. Using the ADA definition, abnormalities of cardiovascular reflex tests alone would not constitute autonomic neuropathy but might more properly be termed cardiovascular autonomic dysfunction. In practice, these terms are usually used interchangeably.

Descriptive studies

The prevalence of diabetic autonomic neuropathy

Clinical case-series and clinic surveys have reported abnormalities of cardiovascular autonomic function in between 17 and 70 per cent of Caucasian populations, although most estimates were no higher than 40 per cent (Ewing 1984). In Chinese and black South African populations higher estimates have been reported. The results of most studies are difficult to interpret because the denominator populations were unrepresentative due to referral or selection bias. The sex ratios observed may be unreliable, and no significance can be attached to geographical or ethnic differences. Apparent differences in prevalence may also partly be explained by differences in the definition of autonomic neuropathy and by differences in the inclusion criteria since some studies were restricted to younger age groups or to insulin-dependent patients and others made no distinction between patients with insulin-dependent (IDDM) and non-insulin-dependent diabetes (NIDDM). Most studies had relatively small sample sizes resulting in wide confidence intervals for the prevalence estimates.

A small number of studies have used protocols that are consistent in most respects with the ADA recommendations. The largest case series from Edinburgh studied 774 patients over a 10-year period (Ewing et al. 1985). For 543 patients complete cardiovascular autonomic function test results were available for HRV (Valsalva manoeuvre, deep breathing, and standing) and blood pressure response to standing and sustained handgrip. Predetermined lower normal limits, rather than age-related normal ranges, were used to classify the results and 40 per cent showed definite or severe impairment, but this figure does not provide a reliable estimate of the prevalence of cardiovascular autonomic neuropathy because the patients were a selected rather than representative sample. A clinic survey, however, randomly recruited 506 IDDM patients from four diabetic clinics to ascertain the prevalence of impaired HRV in IDDM (O'Brien et al. 1986). A computerized technique was used to measure HRV at rest and in response to a single deep breath, a Valsalva manoeuvre, and standing. The results were classified using age-related normal ranges. Heart rate responses below the 2.5 centiles were found for 9 to 16 per cent of the four tests, and the prevalence of one or more abnormal result was 26 per cent. Allowance must, however, be made for the proportion of abnormal results that would be expected in a control population—using four tests, up to 10 per cent might be expected to be abnormal. After adjusting for this, the prevalence of cardiovascular autonomic neuropathy in IDDM would be 16 per cent (95 per cent confidence intervals (CI) 13 to 19 per cent).

Referral and selection bias can be avoided by studying a geographically defined population. A population-based survey conducted in the UK identified 43 insulin-dependent and 202 non-insulin-dependent patients aged 20 years or more (Neil et al. 1988), and measured HRV by a computerized technique at rest and in response to both a single deep breath and a Valsalva manoeuvre. The prevalence of one or more abnormal test result was 17 per cent. After adjustment to allow for the 7.5 per cent of expected abnormal test results, the prevalence of impaired HRV overall was 10 per cent, in NIDDM was 8 per cent (95 per cent CI 5 to 12 per cent), and in IDDM was 14 per cent. Neither this, nor the study by O'Brien et al. (1986), were large enough to provide statistically reliable age- and sex-specific prevalence rates for IDDM or NIDDM.

The use of a geographically defined population reduces bias, but estimating the prevalence of autonomic neuropathy in an unselected population is complicated, particularly in the elderly, both by drugs and other pathology which may interfere with the measurement and interpretation of HRV. Severe arrhythmias obviously invalidate tests of HRV and are more common in the elderly. Limited expiratory reserve may preclude a Valsalva manoeuvre, some adrenergic blocking drugs enhance sinus arrhythmia, and ischaemic heart disease may impair HRV. The use of blood pressure response to standing may be unreliable since postural hypotension has been variously estimated to affect between 5 and 30 per cent of people over the age of 65 and may indicate vascular pathology rather than sympathetic dysfunction. Testing autonomic function in a different organ system may be useful in these patients.

Little is known about the epidemiology of autonomic dysfunction in any system other than the cardiovascular system despite the availability of simple, non-invasive, accurate, and reproducible tests of the sudomotor and ocular systems. A large case series of IDDM patients compared cardiorespiratory reflexes with quantative sweat testing (Kennedy et al. 1989) by determining the number of sweat glands on the dorsum of the foot secreting after iontophoresis of pilocarpine. Of 292 patients, 244 (84 per cent) were abnormal, 139 (48 per cent) were abnormal for both HRV and sweat gland count, 81 (28 per cent) were abnormal for HRV, and 24 (8 per cent) for sweat gland count alone. A significant correlation was found between HRV and the number of sweat glands activated ($r = 0.47$ for deep breathing; $r = 0.51$ for Valsalva ratio). Some data are also available for the ocular system. Polaroid photography can be used to assess pupillary innervation by measuring darkness pupil size in relation to age-related normal ranges. In a sequential series of 147 patients tested as part of a population-based study of impaired HRV described earlier, the prevalence of pupillometric abnormalities was 14 per cent (Neil, unpublished observation). A significant correlation between darkness pupil diameter and tests of HRV has been demonstrated, but the predictive value of the pupil test in identifying patients with abnormal HRV was only 55 per cent (Neil and Smith 1989). From these and other data, it seems likely that there are diffuse neurological changes to the autonomic nervous system with different degrees of damage to different parts of the nervous system either resulting from a generalized metabolic abnormality or possibly from a diffuse multifocal process.

The prevalence of symptomatic and asymptomatic diabetic autonomic neuropathy

Evaluating and quantifying the prevalence of symptomatic autonomic neuropathy is difficult because most symptoms are non-specific: impotence may be of vascular, neuropathic, or mixed aetiology; postural hypotension may be due to vascular pathology; and there is some dispute whether diarrhoea is a true manifestation of autonomic dysfunction. In a clinic study of 51 NIDDM patients diagnosed between the ages of 40 and 55 years, 23 patients (43 per cent) complained of symptoms but only 11 had any evidence of autonomic dysfunction (Bergstrom et al. 1990). In a cross-sectional study of a representative cohort of 168 IDDM patients aged 25 to 34 years, with a mean duration of diabetes of 20 years, the prevalence of most symptoms was less than 5 per cent and the only statistically significant association of impaired HRV was with decreased urinary frequency (Maser et al. 1990). Other studies have also demonstrated a poor correlation between symptoms and objective evidence of autonomic dysfunction.

Few published studies have systemically assessed the frequency of symptomatic autonomic neuropathy. A clinic-based review of the complications of NIDDM concluded that symptomatic autonomic neuropathy was rare (Watkins et al. 1987), and the population-based survey described earlier (Neil et al. 1988) found a prevalence of only 0.5 per cent in NIDDM, but a significantly higher prevalence of 12 per cent in IDDM (these estimates would be higher if impotence—a non-specific symptom present in 53 per cent of men—had been included in the diagnostic criteria). In summary, the available evidence suggests that symptoms of autonomic neuropathy are present in only a small proportion of all patients with measurable autonomic defects.

The natural history and prognosis
of diabetic autonomic neuropathy

Cross-sectional studies and follow-up of clinic case series have clarified the pattern and sequence of abnormal tests of cardiovascular autonomic function. Ewing *et al.* (1985) showed by repeated tests more than 5 years apart that worsening of cardiovascular tests followed a fairly uniform sequence with first heart rate and later blood pressure tests becoming abnormal. These authors also demonstrated a pattern of abnormal tests of HRV, which, in order of frequency, were an abnormal heart rate response to deep breathing, lying to standing, and a Valsalva manoeuvre. This is consistent with heart rate responses being mediated primarily via cardiac parasympathetic pathways with additional sympathetic influences altering the responses particularly to Valsalva manoeuvre. It suggests that the heart rate response to deep breathing is the most sensitive test. Some other studies, however, do not show the same frequency distribution of abnormal test results. In representative populations of IDDM and NIDDM patients (O'Brien *et al.* 1986; Neil *et al.* 1988) there was no significant difference between the prevalence of abnormal Valsalva and E:I ratios. This discrepancy may be explained by differences in the technique used or by use of age-related normal ranges in these latter studies.

The incidence of cardiovascular autonomic neuropathy is unknown, and its determination requires prospective follow-up of a representative inception cohort. Cross-sectional studies have reported impaired autonomic function in newly diagnosed diabetes which would be expected in NIDDM since unrecognized hyperglycaemia may precede the diagnosis by years. A study of 19 NIDDM patients with a duration of diabetes 12 months or less, and 14 IDDM patients with a duration of 24 months or less (Pfeifer *et al.* 1984), found that the mean R–R interval variation after β-adrenergic blockade was significantly less than in a control group. The dark-adapted pupil size after topical parasympathetic block was also significantly smaller, but most of the results for individual patients were within the age-related normal range. Although the incidence of autonomic neuropathy remains unknown, it is clear that abnormal cardiovascular and pupillary reflexes can be detected early in the clinical course of diabetes.

Asymptomatic autonomic neuropathy can be shown to precede symptomatic neuropathy, but it is unclear precisely what proportion of patients progress to become symptomatic. Using data from cross-sectional studies, Ewing and Clarke (1986) have proposed a sequence of autonomic damage that begins with loss of sweating in the feet, impotence, and bladder dysfunction, and progresses through abnormalities in the cardiovascular reflexes to a final stage of symptomatic postural hypotension, sweat disturbances of the upper body, gastroparesis, diarrhoea, and bladder atony. A recent review (Bilous 1990) emphasized that this sequence cannot be inevitable because the prevalence of cardiovascular autonomic dysfunction is about 8 per cent in NIDDM and 16 per cent in IDDM, but symptomatic patients are rare. This has been confirmed by a prospective study of IDDM patients aged less than 50 years which showed that the development of autonomic symptoms in asymptomatic patients with abnormal HRV was uncommon over a 10-year period (Sampson *et al.* 1990). In patients with symptoms of autonomic neuropathy, the main symptoms—diarrhoea, postural hypotension, and gustatory sweating—were very persistent but did not necessarily deteriorate. It is evident that most asymptomatic patients do not progress to symptomatic autonomic neuropathy, and that, when symptoms are present, deterioration is not inevitable.

Diabetic autonomic neuropathy and mortality

Few studies have attempted to assess the mortality associated with cardio-vascular autonomic neuropathy. Unfortunately, interpreting mortality data can be difficult unless a prospective cohort design is used, and a large, representative, and well-characterized population is studied by standardized methods with near complete follow-up. Not surprisingly, available data are derived from studies which do not meet these criteria in full and most are restricted to IDDM.

An important study by Ewing *et al.* (1980) has shown a high cumulative mortality in a heterogeneous cohort of patients with symptomatic autonomic neuropathy. It consisted of 62 men and 11 women with a mean age of 46 years (range 24–69), a mean duration of diabetes of 17 years (range 2–37), and a mean duration of symptoms of 3 years (range 1–18). Eight patients were treated with oral hypoglycaemic agents and the remaining 65 (89 per cent) were insulin-treated, but it is not clear what proportion had IDDM. Cardiovascular autonomic function was assessed using a Valsalva manoeuvre, the postural fall in blood pressure, and the blood pressure response to sustained handgrip. Forty patients (55 per cent) had abnormal autonomic function tests and significantly more of these patients had evidence of proteinuria, retinopathy, and peripheral neuropathy in comparison with a group of patients with normal autonomic function. There were 26 deaths over a 10-year period, 21 of the deaths occurred in patients with abnormal autonomic function tests, and the 10-year cumulative mortality in this group was 56 per cent. Patients with normal autonomic function had a cumulative mortality similar to an age- and sex-matched population of Edinburgh diabetic patients, and a somewhat lower mortality than the general popu-lation of Scotland (Fig. 36.1). Diabetic nephropathy accounted for half the deaths of patients with symptomatic autonomic neuropathy while sudden unexpected deaths accounted for about a quarter. The high morta-lity of patients with symptomatic autonomic neuropathy may partly be explained by a 50 per cent prevalence of proteinuria at entry to this cohort.

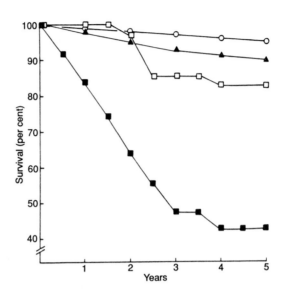

Fig. 36.1. Five-year survival curves for: (open circles) age- and sex-matched general population; (filled triangles) age and sex-matched diabetic population; (open squares) 37 diabetics with normal and (filled squares) 40 diabetics with abnormal autonomic function tests. (From Ewing *et al.* (1980).)

A recent study (Sampson *et al.* 1990) suggests that the prognosis of patients with symptomatic autonomic neuropathy may be less grave than reported by Ewing *et al.* (1980). This study was restricted to a younger population of 73 IDDM patients consisting of three groups: the first group were 49 patients with early symptomatic autonomic neuropathy; the second group, 24 patients with abnormal HRV alone; and the third group, 38 asymptomatic patients with normal HRV. HRV was initially assessed on deep respiration at 6 cycles/min. The 10-year cumulative mortality in the group with symptomatic autonomic neuropathy was about 27 per cent and was 10 per cent in the other two groups (Fig. 36.2). The results demonstrated that asymptomatic autonomic dysfunction did not appear to be associated with any excess mortality. There were 18 deaths in the group of patients with symptomatic autonomic neuropathy, 4 of which were due to renal failure, 3 to myocardial infarction, and 3 were sudden and unexpected. The rather less grave prognosis for symptomatic autonomic neuropathy demonstrated in this study may be explained by the shorter duration of symptoms, younger age of patients, and the lower prevalence of nephropathy at the beginning of the study.

A further study has investigated the 5-year mortality of IDDM patients with autonomic neuropathy. A detailed clinical and biochemical assessment was performed (O'Brien *et al.* 1991), and unlike other studies, the mortality

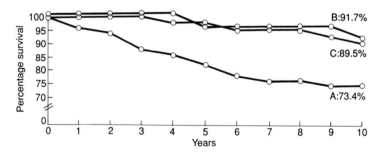

Fig. 36.2. Calculated 10-year survival (per cent) in groups A (symptomatic autonomic neuropathy; $n = 49$), B (abnormal HRV; $n = 24$), and C (asymptomatic normal HRV; $n = 38$). (From Sampson *et al.* (1990).)

was assessed in an unselected group of patients. Twenty two of the 506 patients were lost to follow-up and 44 (9 per cent) of the remaining 484 patients died. The cumulative 5-year mortality was 27 per cent in patients with cardiovascular autonomic neuropathy compared to 5 per cent in those with normal autonomic function. Autonomic neuropathy was associated with an increased mortality from renal failure but not from any other cause. It is not clear whether the higher mortality was confined to patients with symptomatic autonomic neuropathy. Survival analysis using a multivariate proportional hazard model to assess the contribution of autonomic dysfunction to mortality after adjusting for the effect of other variables was not used, but the relative importance of various factors associated with mortality was examined by discriminate analysis of survivors and non-survivors which showed that autonomic neuropathy was the best predictor of death.

Causes of mortality

Each of the three studies reviewed has shown that deaths in patients with autonomic neuropathy were due mainly to renal failure. This might simply indicate that autonomic neuropathy and nephropathy share, at least in part, a common complex aetiology, which may include microangiopathic damage, and that they develop in parallel. Some limited evidence, however, suggests that autonomic neuropathy may independently affect renal function and may be a contributory causal factor for the development of nephropathy. Autonomic dysfunction has been shown to be associated with increased urinary albumin excretion and renal blood flow, and changes in renal haemodynamics have been implicated in the development of diabetic nephropathy.

Sudden unexpected cardiorespiratory arrests in patients with symptomatic autonomic neuropathy were the second most frequent cause of death in two of the above studies. Various case reports have also described deaths from sudden cardiopulmonary arrest, particularly in association with anaesthesia. The evidence for the proposed mechanisms that could result in either respiratory arrests or fatal arrhythmias is conflicting. The evidence implicating sleep apnoea, impaired hypoxic ventilatory drive, or diminished bronchial response to cold air is limited. Cardiac arrhythmias may contribute to these deaths and a number of studies have demonstrated that QT interval prolongation is associated with autonomic dysfunction, at least in IDDM. This may increase the risk of ventricular arrhythmia, particularly in the presence of impaired vagal function, but there are no prospective data to confirm this. Indeed, ambulatory 24-hour electrocardiograms in diabetic patients fail to show any increased prevalence of arrhythmias, and the cause of these sudden unexpected deaths remains uncertain.

Analytical studies

A small number of epidemiological and clinical studies have examined cross-sectionally the characteristics of patients with and without autonomic neuropathy to identify features that may relate to its cause and prognosis. In the absence of prospective data for NIDDM, analytical studies are useful in trying to assess the clinical significance of asymptomatic autonomic neuropathy and in interpreting the limited prospective data available for IDDM.

Age and duration of diabetes

HRV declines with age in normal subjects (Smith 1982, 1984), and in diabetic patients declines at about three times the normal rate over a decade (Sampson *et al.* 1990). The combined effect of age and duration of diabetes on HRV during deep breathing was examined in a cross-sectional study of 143 control subjects, 102 IDDM patients, and 116 NIDDM patients (Masaoka *et al.* 1985). In IDDM both age and duration were significantly inversely related to HRV on multiple linear regression analysis. In NIDDM age was inversely related to HRV but there was no relationship with the duration of diabetes, which is consistent with the results of other studies. For IDDM the combined effect of age and duration could explain only 36 per cent of the observed difference in HRV from the control group, and only 8 per cent of the difference for NIDDM.

Peripheral and autonomic neuropathy

The association between peripheral and autonomic neuropathy has been assessed in a number of studies, but more detailed data are available for

IDDM than NIDDM. In the study described above (Masaoka *et al.* 1985), impaired HRV (below the 2.5 percentile) was present in 61 (64 per cent) of 96 patients with evidence of peripheral neuropathy (no distinction was made between IDDM and NIDDM). A larger study of 417 IDDM patients with a mean age of 34 years (range 13–80) and a mean duration of diabetes of 19 years (range 1–52) showed a significant correlation between HRV assessed by the response to breathing (6 cycles/min) and motor nerve conduction velocity, amplitude of compound muscle potential, distal latency, and amplitude of sensory nerve action potential (Kennedy *et al.* 1989). About 40 per cent of the patients found to have normal motor and sensory nerve function had abnormalities of HRV, whereas 85 per cent with any abnormality in nerve conduction also had abnormalities of HRV. It seems, therefore, that in most patients there is parallel involvement of the somatic and autonomic nervous systems.

The prevalence of both peripheral and autonomic neuropathy was examined in a survey of 506 randomly selected IDDM patients discussed earlier (O'Brien and Corrall 1988). Peripheral neuropathy was defined as the absence or impairment of ankle reflexes and a vibration perception threshold greater than the 95th percentile, for age-matched controls without diabetes, measured using biothesiometry. The overall prevalence of peripheral neuropathy was 24 per cent and of autonomic neuropathy was 16 per cent. Interestingly, a marked difference was found in the prevalence of both types of neuropathy with age: the prevalence of peripheral neuropathy increased

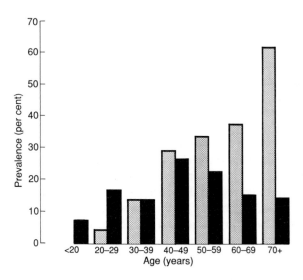

Fig. 36.3. The prevalence of peripheral neuropathy (hatched bars) and autonomic neuropathy (solid bars) in patients with insulin-dependent diabetes according to age. (From O'Brien and Corrall (1988).)

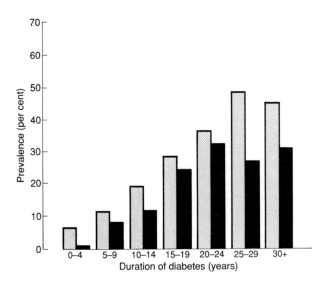

Fig. 36.4. The prevalence of peripheral neuropathy (hatched bars) and autonomic neuropathy (solid bars) in patients with insulin-dependent diabetes according to duration. (From O'Brien and Corrall (1988).)

progressively whereas that of autonomic neuropathy peaked in the fifth decade and then declined (Fig. 36.3). Both were related to the duration of diabetes (Fig. 36.4), but the prevalence of autonomic neuropathy apparently declined after 25 years duration.

It is unclear why the prevalence of peripheral and autonomic neuropathy should diverge in later life. Interpretation of these data is complicated because they are prevalence rather than incidence rates. There are a number of alternative explanations (Krolewski 1988). First, if the rate of selective removal due to mortality was small, adjustment for it would have increased only slightly the prevalence of autonomic neuropathy after 25 years, and would suggest that the risk of autonomic neuropathy increases during the first two decades of IDDM and declines thereafter. The second possibility is that the removal due to mortality was large and, after adjustment for it, the prevalence of autonomic neuropathy increased proportionately with the duration of diabetes, which would suggest that the risk of this complication is independent of the duration of diabetes. The third possibility is that selective removal due to mortality was very large, and the adjusted prevalence of autonomic neuropathy increased exponentially with the duration of diabetes. As Krolewski emphasizes, these three different hypothetical patterns of occurrence suggest different causes. The first implies that only a subset of patients are susceptible because of some genetic or environmental factor. The second implies a process that could be the result of multiple interactive factors, exclusive of duration. The third pattern implies that a cumulative process is responsible for the development of autonomic neuropathy and that all persons are at risk. Knowledge of the true pattern would provide an important insight into the cause of autonomic neuropathy.

Autonomic neuropathy and risk factors for coronary heart disease

The association between known risk factors for coronary heart disease and autonomic function has been studied in IDDM. A cross-sectional study, discussed earlier, of a representative cohort of 168 IDDM patients aged 25 to 34 years (Maser *et al.* 1990) used multiple logistic regression analysis to examine the relationship between the heart rate response to deep breathing and a number of independent variables. Retinopathy was significantly associated with HRV, and its severity has previously been demonstrated to correlate with the degree of autonomic dysfunction which suggests that they develop in parallel (Smith *et al.* 1981). After modelling potential correlates retinopathy, hypertension, low-density lipoprotein cholesterol, high-density lipoprotein cholesterol, and female gender were shown to be independently associated with impaired HRV. This association between autonomic dysfunction and cardiovascular risk factors may help explain the increased mortality observed in patients with autonomic neuropathy but prospective follow-up of this cohort is needed to confirm these findings.

The relationship in NIDDM between autonomic neuropathy, diabetic complications, and risk factors for coronary heart disease has been assessed in a small number of studies. A population-based survey of 202 NIDDM patients examined the relationship between HRV and other complications of diabetes (Neil *et al.* 1988). On univariate analysis, patients with impaired HRV were shown to have a significantly higher body mass index (BMI), systolic blood pressure, urinary albumin, and fasting insulin concentrations than patients with normal HRV, but there were no significant differences in age, duration of diabetes, glycosylated haemoglobin, or in the prevalence of retinopathy or impaired vibration perception. These findings are consistent with the results of a study of 51 NIDDM patients aged 41 to 59 years (Bergstrom *et al.* 1990), which found no significant association between autonomic dysfunction and duration of diabetes, peripheral neuropathy or retinopathy, and also demonstrated that patients with autonomic neuropathy had a significantly higher BMI than patients with normal autonomic function (BMI 31.0 ± 0.9 versus $27.5 \pm 0.8 \text{ kg/m}^2$). The aggregation of known risk factors for coronary heart disease with cardiovascular autonomic dysfunction suggests that mortality could be increased in NIDDM patients with asymptomatic autonomic neuropathy. It also suggests that the importance of asymptomatic autonomic neuropathy may lie in its association with other complications, although in a small proportion of patients it will precede symptomatic autonomic neuropathy.

Autonomic function and obesity

The association between autonomic dysfunction and a higher mean BMI indicates that obesity may be a possible link between autonomic neuropathy and NIDDM. Studies in non-diabetic individuals have shown statistically significant but weak associations between autonomic function and obesity. In 56 obese non-diabetic men (Peterson *et al.* 1988), the percentage of body fat correlated with the variation in R–R interval after β-adrenergic blockade, and with plasma noradrenaline and adrenaline concentrations, which suggests that alterations in autonomic function with obesity are not confined to a single system. A further study has also demonstrated an association between obesity and cardiac autonomic function in markedly obese men and women (Rossi *et al.* 1989). The authors suggested that autonomic dysfunction may account for the increased risk of sudden death in obese patients since changes in autonomic function have been implicated as a mechanism of sudden death. In NIDDM, however, autonomic dysfunction appears to be associated with overweight or mild obesity rather than morbid obesity.

The mechanisms which may relate autonomic dysfunction to obesity are speculative, and the prognostic implications are not clear. It has been proposed that a disordered homeostatic mechanism may promote an excessive storage of energy by decreasing sympathetic activity, while providing protection against weight gain by decreasing parasympathetic activity. With additional stress placed on an already stressed autonomic nervous system, further compensation may not be possible (Peterson *et al.* 1988). A simpler link between autonomic neuropathy and obesity would be mechanical. Obese individuals may have difficulty in lung expansion during deep breathing resulting in attenuation of respiratory reflexes. However, alterations in autonomic function are evident in only modestly overweight NIDDM patients who are unlikely to experience any difficulty with pulmonary inflation. Nevertheless, the possibility that the association may be mediated by mechanical factors is interesting. It would imply that abnormal test results may have different prognostic implications for obese NIDDM and non-obese IDDM patients. Although a high mortality has been reported among IDDM patients with symptomatic autonomic neuropathy, abnormal cardiovascular test results may not necessarily be associated with an equivalent additional mortality risk amongst overweight or obese patients with NIDDM. Longitudinal studies are needed to examine this possibility.

Experimental studies

The pathogenetic mechanisms responsible for the initiation and later progression of diabetic autonomic neuropathy are poorly understood, but it seems likely that both metabolic and vascular factors are involved. The metabolic factors may include chronic hyperglycaemia, glucose-induced disturbances of sorbitol and myo-inositol, and increased non-enzymatic glycosylation of nerve proteins. Small vessel angiopathy has also been implicated. There is no evidence as yet to support a genetically determined basis for autonomic damage and little evidence for an immunological basis. Unfortunately, knowledge of the epidemiology of diabetic autonomic neuropathy is too limited to have generated any convincing aetiological hypotheses.

Clinical studies have examined whether intensified glycaemic control or treatment with aldose reductase inhibitors can favourably influence autonomic function. Trials of aldose reductase inhibitors have been disappointing and have not significantly improved autonomic function. Pancreatic transplantation, however, appears to prevent further deterioration in autonomic function (Kennedy *et al.* 1990), but other studies of intensified glycaemic control using various insulin regimens show conflicting results. Arguably this may be because the deterioration in function was too advanced, a longer intervention period was required, or studies failed to achieve near-normoglycaemia. However, the explanation may be that any real effect is small and therefore can only be demonstrated by a large randomized controlled trial with adequate statistical power, such as the Diabetes Control and Complications Trial (DCCT Research Group 1986), which is studying over 1400 IDDM patients randomized to receive standard therapy or intensified insulin therapy designed to maintain near normoglycaemia for a period of up to 10 years. As part of the trial, the effect of treatment on autonomic function is being assessed which should help to clarify the relationship between cardiac autonomic damage and metabolic control.

Summary

Diabetes is a common cause of secondary autonomic neuropathy, and the overall prevalence of cardiac autonomic dysfunction is about 10 per cent but appears to be higher in IDDM than NIDDM. The incidence remains unknown. Most patients with evidence of autonomic damage are asymptomatic, and few progress to symptomatic autonomic neuropathy which is associated with a high mortality mainly from renal failure. The natural history of asymptomatic autonomic dysfunction is poorly documented, but the apparent association with cardiovascular risk factors implies that there may be an increased risk of coronary heart disease. However, prospective cohort studies are needed to confirm this. Obesity may be a link between autonomic dysfunction and NIDDM which would suggest that abnormal cardiac test results are not necessarily associated with an equivalent mortality risk for obese NIDDM and non-obese IDDM patients. Again, longitudinal studies are needed to examine this possibility. Unfortunately, knowledge of the epidemiology of diabetic autonomic neuropathy is too restricted to have generated any convincing aetiological hypotheses, and clinical studies have yet to demonstrate that improved metabolic control can favourably influence autonomic function.

References

ADA (American Diabetes Association and American Academy of Neurology) (1988). Report and recommendations of the San Antonio conference on diabetic neuropathy. *Diabetes Care* **11**, 592–7.

Bergstrom, B., Lilja, B., Osterlin, S., and Sundqvist, G. (1990). Autonomic neuropathy in non-insulin dependent (type II) diabetes mellitus. Possible influence of obesity. *J. intern. Med.* **227**, 57–63.

Bilous, R. W. (1990). Diabetic autonomic neuropathy. *Br. med. J.* **301**, 565–6.

DCCT Research Group. (1986). The Diabetes Control and Complications Trial (DCCT): design and methodologic considerations for the feasibility phase. *Diabetes* **35**, 530–45.

Ewing, D. J. (1984). Cardiac autonomic neuropathy. In *Diabetes and heart disease* (ed. R. J. Jarrett), pp. 99–132. Elsevier, Amsterdam.

Ewing, D. J. and Clarke, B. F. (1986). Diabetic autonomic neuropathy: present insights and future prospects. *Diabetes Care* **9**, 648–65.

Ewing, D. J., Campbell, I. W., and Clarke, B. F. (1980). The natural history of diabetic autonomic neuropathy. *Quart. J. Med.* **193**, 95–108.

Ewing, D. J., Martyn, C. N., Young, R. J., and Clarke, B. F. (1985). The value of cardiovascular autonomic function tests: 10 years experience in diabetes. *Diabetes Care* **198**, 491–8.

Kennedy, W. R., Navarro, X., Sakuta, M., Mandell, H., Knox, C. K., and Sutherland, D. E. R. (1989). Physiological and clinical correlates of cardiorespiratory reflexes in diabetes mellitus. *Diabetes Care* **12**, 399–408.

Kennedy, W. R., Navarro, X., Goetz, F. C., Sutherland, D. E. R., and Najarian, J. S. (1990). Effects of pancreatic transplantation on diabetic neuropathy. *New Engl. J. Med.* **322**, 1031–7.

Krolewski, A. S. (1988). Epidemiology of diabetes and its complications. *New Engl. J. Med.* **318**, 1620.

Masaoka, S., Lev-Ran, A., Hill, L. R., Vakil, G., and Non, E. H. G. (1985). Heart rate variability in diabetes: relationship to age and duration of the disease. *Diabetes Care* **8**, 64–8.

Maser, R. E., Pfeifer, M. A., Dorman, J. S., Kuller, L. K., Becker, J. D., and Orchard, T. J. (1990). Diabetic autonomic neuropathy and cardiovascular risk. *Arch. intern. Med.* **150**, 1218–22.

Neil, H. A. W. and Smith, S. A. (1989). A simple test of pupillary autonomic function. *Neuro-ophthalmology* **9**, 237–42.

Neil, H. A. W., Thompson, A. V., John, S., McCarthy, S. T., and Mann, J. I. (1988). Diabetic autonomic neuropathy: the prevalence of impaired heart rate variability in a geographically defined population. *Diabetic Med.* **6**, 20–4.

O'Brien, I. A. D. and Corrall, R. J. M. (1988). Epidemiology of diabetes and its complications. *New Engl. J. Med.* **318**, 1619–20.

O'Brien, I. A. D., O'Hare, J. P., Lewin, I. G., and Corrall, R. J. M. (1986). The prevalence of autonomic neuropathy in insulin-dependent diabetes mellitus: a controlled study based on heart rate variability. *Quart. J. Med.* **234**, 957–67.

O'Brien, I. A. D., McFadden, J. P., and Corrall, R. J. M. (1991). The influence of autonomic neuropathy on mortality in insulin-dependent diabetes. *Quar. J. Med.* **290**, 495–502.

Peterson, H. R., Rothschild, M., Weinberg, C. R., Fell, R. D., McLeish, K. R., and Pfeifer, M. A. (1988). Body fat and the activity of the autonomic nervous system. *New Engl. J. Med.* **318**, 1077–83.

Pfeifer, M. A., Weinberg, C. R., Cook, D. L., Reenan, A., Halter, J. B., Ensinck, J. W., and Porte, D. (1984). Autonomic neural dysfunction in recently diagnosed diabetic subjects. *Diabetes Care* **7**, 447–53.

Rossi, M., Marti, G., Ricordi, L., Gornasari, G., Finardi, G., Fratino, P., and Bernardi, L. (1989). Cardiac autonomic dysfunction in obese subjects. *Clin. Sci.* **76**, 567–72.

Sampson, M. J., Wilson, S., Karagiannis, P., Edmonds, M., and Watkins, P. J. (1990). Progression of diabetic autonomic neuropathy over a decade in insulin-dependent diabetics. *Quart. J. Med.* **278**, 635–46.

Smith, S. A. (1982). Reduced sinus arrhythmia in diabetic autonomic neuropathy: diagnostic value of an age-related range. *Br. med. J.* **285**, 1599–601.

Smith, S. A. (1984). Diagnostic value of the valsalva ratio reduction in diabetic autonomic neuropathy: use of an age-related normal range. *Diabetes Med.* **1**, 295–7.

Smith, S. E., Smith, S. A., and Brown, P. M. (1981). Cardiac autonomic dysfunction in patients with diabetic retinopathy. *Diabetologia* **21**, 525–8.

Watkins, P. J., Grenfell, A., and Edmonds, M. (1987). Diabetic complications of non-insulin-dependent diabetes. *Diabetic Med.* **4**, 293–6.

37. Clinical presentations of diabetic autonomic failure

M. E. Edmonds and P. J. Watkins

Introduction

Diabetic neuropathy is a common condition with highly characteristic features due to the early and extensive involvement of small nerve fibres. It is the most common cause of autonomic neuropathy causing functional defects and symptoms in a wide variety of systems. The gastrointestinal tract, the genitourinary system, the heart, and blood vessels are all affected; there are abnormalities of sweating, pupillary defects, and a wide variety of metabolic disorders. Early small-fibre damage is manifested by impairment of vagally controlled heart-rate variability, while diminished peripheral sympathetic tone leads to increased blood flow, which is detectable before there is clinical evidence of neuropathy, and thermal sensation (a small-fibre modality) is lost before vibration sensation (a large-fibre modality). Indeed, reduced thermal sensation is probably a very early marker of this and other neuropathies. Pain sensation has not been extensively assessed, but is abnormal in most diabetics with neuropathic ulcers and Charcot arthropathy.

Causes of diabetic autonomic neuropathy

The mechanisms which underlie the development of diabetic autonomic neuropathy are still poorly understood (Greene *et al.* 1988; Vinik and Mitchell 1988). Diabetes control and the resulting metabolic abnormalities are probably important, although it is disappointing that most studies of strict blood glucose control show little or no benefit on autonomic function; even 3½ years after successful pancreatic transplantation, autonomic function differs minimally from that of controls although motor and sensory function benefit seem to improve (Kennedy *et al.* 1990). Evidence for hypoxia resulting from reduced blood supply to diabetic nerves is widely discussed and still under investigation. More recently, possible immunological mechanisms have been considered.

Abnormal autonomic function tests in diabetes are common, and heart rate variation is diminished in about one-fifth of all diabetic patients (O'Brien *et al.* 1986). In contrast, symptomatic autonomic neuropathy is uncommon: we suggest that immunological mechanisms may play some role in causing sympathetic autonomic neuropathy. Thus, we have observed an association of severe symptomatic autonomic neuropathy with iritis (Guy *et al.* 1984); Rothova *et al.* (1988) have made similar observations in Holland. Immune complexes (Gilbey *et al.* 1986) and activated T cells (Gilbey *et al.* 1988) are increased in these cases. The discovery that sympathetic ganglion antibodies and antivagus nerve antibodies are present in a considerable number of diabetic patients lends further weight to the hypothesis (Sundqvist *et al.* 1991) although the role of these antibodies has not been determined. While their presence has been linked with orthostatic hypotension (Rabinowe *et al.* 1989), Sundqvist found no association with abnormal autonomic function tests. Finally, the demonstration at post-mortem of cellular infiltrations of lymphocytes, macrophages, and some plasma cells in relation to autonomic nerve bundles and ganglia, in or around bundles of unmyelinated nerve fibres, and in the superior cervical sympathetic ganglion also suggests the possibility of immunological mechanisms.

Nerve growth factor (NGF) regulates autonomic nerve development and is required to maintain their neurotransmitter levels in animals (Logan 1990). Antibodies to NGF can both damage autonomic nerves and cause pronounced atrophy of sympathetic ganglion cells in adult rats and mice (Ruit *et al.* 1990). The iris contains large amounts of NGF and even more when denervated. Thus NGF antibodies might both mediate iritis and cause damage to the autonomic nervous system. Bennett (1984) suggested that insulin antibodies might be responsible by cross-reacting with NGF, and there are some structural similarities between NGF and insulin.

Blood flow in the neuropathic foot

Peripheral neuropathy in the foot leads to both somatic and autonomic damage. Small-fibre loss may predominate leading to loss of pain and thermal sensation before light touch and vibration sense are blunted. A peripheral sympathetic nerve fibre defect has been demonstrated by direct measurement of sympathetic activity in postganglionic C fibres in the diabetic neuropathic limb (Fagius 1982). These studies show that damage to sympathetic nerves in diabetic polyneuropathy gives rise to loss of signal conduction in successively more fibres resulting in weak and eventually undetectable activity, whereas the fibre conducts with normal velocity as long as conduction capacity is retained. Autonomic denervation may be responsible for abnormalities in blood flow. Venous occlusion plethysmography, which measures total arterial inflow, has demonstrated increased peripheral blood flow (Archer *et al.* 1984). Spontaneous variations in resting flow, which are secondary to sympathetic activity, are considerably reduced in the neuropathic diabetic foot.

Increase in blood flow is associated with arteriovenous shunting in the neuropathic limb resulting in prominent turgid veins over the dorsum of the foot and lower part of the calf in the recumbent position. Furthermore, evidence from Doppler sonography, microsphere partitioning, and foot venous blood sampling supports the concept of arteriovenous shunting and this has recently been confirmed by laser flowmetry (Flynn *et al.* 1988). The presence of substantial arteriovenous shunting might, in theory, jeopardize capillary nutritional flow. However, television microscopy of the great toe-nail fold has shown that the nutritional capillary blood flow is increased in diabetics with neuropathy although it may be relatively insufficient to meet the increased metabolic requirements of the warmer skin of the neuropathic foot (see below).

All these observations were made in the supine patient, but high blood flows and overperfusion have also been demonstrated in the dependent foot. In normal subjects, standing causes precapillary vasoconstriction in the foot, limiting the increment in capillary pressure and reducing blood flow. This veniarteriolar response is dependent upon a sympathetic axon reflex. Laser Doppler flowmetry has shown that in the neuropathic foot the percentage fall in skin blood flow on dependency is less than normal. This suggests that postural control of blood flow is disturbed in patients with diabetic neuropathy and this abnormality is compatible with loss of sympathetic vascular tone.

However, in the neuropathic limb the major arterial walls are stiff, probably as a result of medial wall calcification, and sympathetic neuropathy may be an important aetiological factor (Fig. 37.1).

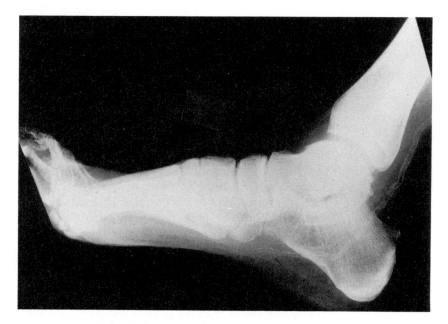

Fig. 37.1.   Medial calcification in the arteries of a young, severely neuropathic, insulin-dependent diabetic.

Deterioration of arterial smooth muscle cells has been demonstrated following sympathetic denervation in rabbits. Calcification has also been reported in familial amyloidosis with polyneuropathy and also in the ipsilateral leg following lumbar sympathectomy. Eleven out of 13 patients who underwent unilateral sympathectomy developed Monckeberg's sclerosis on the operated side, having had normal radiographs before the procedure. Bilateral sympathectomy was carried out in seven patients, all of whom showed calcification on both sides later (Goebel and Fuesse 1983). Autonomic neuropathy may be responsible for two other abnormalities in the foot, namely, disorders of thermal regulation and disturbances of sweating (see below). Increased blood flow leads to raised skin temperature in the resting neuropathic limb. However, local heating to the great toe causes a paradoxical fall in blood flow through arteriovenous anastomoses (Fig. 37.2; Stevens *et al.* 1991*a*). This is probably due to abnormal neurogenic control of a local axon reflex and not due to diabetic microangiopathy. This

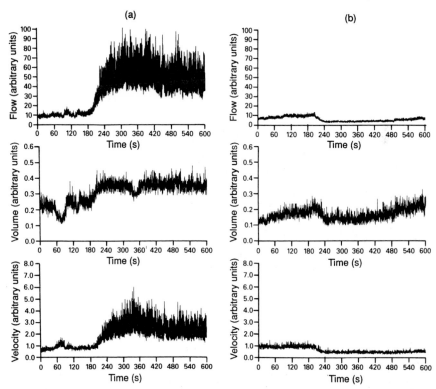

Fig. 37.2. Two typical skin blood flow recordings of (a) a normal subject and (b) a diabetic patient with neuropathy during local heating of the great toe. Local heating was started at 180 s after measuring basal flow for 3 min. Total skin blood flow is shown in the uppermost trace and the changes in microvascular volume and velocity are shown by the middle and lower traces, respectively.

is supported by the observation that there is a paradoxical vasoconstriction to heating in the ipsilateral limb of non-diabetic patients with a unilateral traumatic neuropathy compared with the physiological vasodilatation in the contralateral normal limb (Stevens *et al.* 1991*b*).

Abnormalities in blood flow thermoregulation and sweating that follow from autonomic neuropathy may be responsible for the complications of the neuropathic foot. Several studies have shown that there is greater autonomic impairment in diabetics with neuropathic ulceration compared to that in those with neuropathy but no ulceration (Edmonds *et al.* 1986). Rigid dilated arteries and shunting lead to a rapid increase of flow with raised venular pressure and venous distension. Indeed, in one animal study, arteriovenous shunting was a necessary requirement for neuropathic ulceration. Autonomic neuropathy also predisposes to ulceration by other mechanisms. Abnormal responses to temperature changes, in particular, vasoconstriction on exposure to heat, could be harmful. Loss of sweating leads to dry skin with thick plaques of hard callus which readily crack. This can lead to fissuring of the skin and eventually ulceration. The acetylcholine sweat spot test, a measure of peripheral autonomic denervation, was absent in all cases of diabetic neuropathic foot ulceration (Ryder *et al.* 1990).

Although less frequent, the Charcot joint can be a devastating complication of the neuropathic foot. Circulatory changes can lead to abnormalities in bone-structure (Fig 37.3). In the experimental animal increased blood flow leads to rarefaction and demineralization of bone and in the human there is a reduction in bony cortical thickness rendering the foot susceptible to even minor trauma. Thus there may be a primary vascular defect (secondary to autonomic neuropathy) which will encourage bone resorption and this theory is supported by a report of three cases, all of whom developed Charcot changes several months after successsful vascular surgery had increased blood flow to their feet (Edelman *et al.* 1987). Nevertheless, somatic neuropathy is also a prerequisite; patients with Charcot arthropathy have absent flare responses after axon-reflex stimutionindicatingdegeneration ofunmyelinated nociceptivefibres.The combination of somatic and autonomic neuropathy permits abnormal mechanical stress to occur, resulting in fracture and, finally, bone and joint disorganization.

Peripheral oedema, sometimes of considerable severity and resistance to treatment, is a rare feature of some cases of diabetic neuropathy. It may be related to overperfusion, especially in the dependent position, together with arteriovenous shunting, raised venous pressure, and venous distension. The use of sympathomimetic agents by stimulating vasoconstriction may be expected to reduce this form of oedema. We have shown that ephedrine is of value in treating neuropathic oedema. It results in a rapid decrease in weight, a reduction in peripheral diastolic flow, and an increase in sodium excretion, all associated with diminution of oedema. The effect of ephedrine is, however, complex and, as well as its peripheral effects, it may have central effects on the control of sodium and water homeostasis.

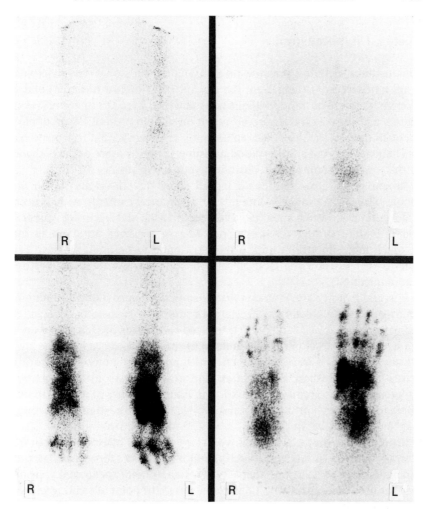

Fig. 37.3.   Isotope uptake in the feet of a normal subject (top pair) and a patient
with severe diabetic neuropathy (bottom pair) indicating the greatly increased bone
blood flow which occurs in diabetic neuropathy.

High peripheral blood flow and increased warmth have been observed in
the acutely painful neuropathic limb. Reduction of this blood flow, either
by sympathetic stimuli or by inflation by a sphygmomanometer cuff, was
associated with a reduction in pain. This finding could explain the observation
that this pain could be diminished by cooling the feet, and therapeutic
reduction of blood flow may be possible treatment for painful diabetic
neuropathy.

These abnormalities of blood flow secondary to autonomic neuropathy
may thus predispose to the complications of the diabetic neuropathic foot.

Postural hypotension

Maintenance of blood pressure on standing depends on afferent impulses from baroreceptors (namely in the carotid sinus and aortic arch) and on efferent sympathetic impulses to the heart and blood vessels. In normal people there is a 20 per cent fall in cardiac output on standing; about 700 ml of blood accumulates in the legs and splanchnic circulation, but compensatory mechanisms prevent a fall in blood pressure. If one or more of the pathways in this system are impaired, postural hypotension results.

Recent blood flow studies do indeed show that the reduction in foot blood flow on standing is diminished in diabetic patients with postural hypotension, although significant vasoconstriction still occurs (Flynn et al. 1988). Failure of the splanchnic bed to vasoconstrict on standing may be much more important and, using ultrasound techniques, we have been able to demonstrate the lack of this phenomenon (M. Stevens, personal communication).

Postural hypotension is an established complication of diabetic autonomic neuropathy and is chiefly due to efferent sympathetic vasomotor denervation. Failure of cardiac acceleration and reduced cardiac output (exhibited under the stress of exercise) both contribute to the problems. Noradrenaline levels are also generally reduced in diabetics with postural hypotension, although occasionally an excess of noradrenaline is found in some patients with hypotension due to reduced intravascular volume. Failure of renin responses on standing, though probably not responsible for acute postural hypotension, may or may not be abnormal.

Insulin is known to have cardiovascular effects. It causes a reduction in plasma volume, an increase of peripheral blood flow from vasodilatation, and an increase of heart rate. In patients with autonomic neuropathy, insulin may cause or exacerbate postural hypotension to the point of fainting whether it is given intravenously or subcutaneously (Fig. 37.4). It has a similar effect in sympathectomized patients. These cardiovascular effects of insulin are likely to be due to the insulin itself, and not to changes in blood glucose concentration.

Postprandial hypotension in various non-diabetic patients with autonomic neuropathy is well described in Chapter 26. The raised insulin level following the meal was thought to be responsible but observations on insulin-dependent diabetics show the same phenomenon. This suggests that other factors may be important since postprandial insulinaemias would not occur in such patients. The effectiveness of octreotide (somatostatin analogue) in preventing the meal-induced hypotension described in other autonomic neuropathic patients (Raimbach et al. 1989) might also be useful in diabetes although it has not been fully evaluated.

Postural hypotension (a fall of systolic pressure of more than 30 mm Hg)

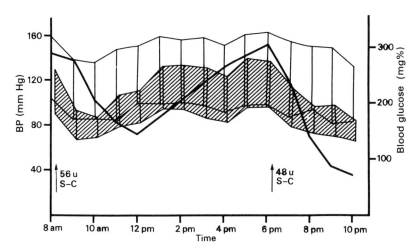

Fig. 37.4. Diurnal variation of lying and standing blood pressures in a 48-year-old man with severe autonomic neuropathy. Insulin was given subcutaneously (S–C) at times shown by the vertical arrows. The unhatched area shows supine blood pressure, the hatched area the standing blood pressure, and the continuous line the blood glucose

occurs in diabetics with advanced neuropathy although symptoms are infrequent and were noted in only 23 of 73 autonomic neuropathy patients described by Ewing and Clarke (1986) and eight of 125 neuropathy patients examined by Rundles (1945). Disabling hypotension, when systolic pressure falls below 70 mm Hg, is rare. Both hypotension and its symptoms fluctuate spontaneously to a remarkable degree, but may persist for many years without necessarily deteriorating (Sampson *et al.* 1990). The explanation for the variability is unclear, although insulin itself may be partly responsible by exacerbating the condition, and fluid retention (for example, from cardiac failure) may ameliorate it.

Treatment of postural hypotension

Few diabetics develop symptoms sufficiently severe to need treatment. When they do, it is first essential to stop any drugs which exacerbate hypotension, notably diuretics, tranquillizers, and antidepressants. Simple treatments should always be tried and include raising the head of the bed and wearing full-length elastic stockings, but the benefits are slight. Anti-g suits are not very helpful and are too cumbersome to be acceptable. Measures which increase plasma volume are the most effective, although oedema is a troublesome side-effect which often renders treatment unacceptable. A high salt intake or fludrocortisone sometimes in high doses (up to 0.4 mm daily) can, however, be effective. The use of an orally active adrenergic agonist, midodrine, can help; it has an exclusively peripheral pressor effect on arterial and venous capacitance vessels. We found that it improved both standing blood pressure and symptoms in two of three patients severely affected by postural hypotension.

Many other treatments have been suggested: their effectiveness is inconsistent, some regimes are hazardous, and supine hypertension is a common sequel. These treatments include β-blockers with partial agonist activity, such as pindolol, and the use of ergotamine, vasopressin, caffeine, non-steroidal inflammatory drugs, clonidine, and metoclopramide (Chapter 33). The value of the somatostatin analogue octreotide in these patients needs to be studied.

Sweating abnormalities

Defective sweating in diabetic neuropathy was described many years ago. The sweat gland is an important structure with a complex peptidergic as well as cholinergic innervation. Neuropeptide immunoreactivity, especially that of vasoactive intestinal polypeptide (VIP), is low in diabetic sudomotor nerves (Levy *et al.* 1989). There is a renewed interest in this field brought about by development of new techniques. Measurement of sweating in the periphery is one of the few quantitative methods for assessing cholinergic nerve function.

There are various methods for studying sweat responses. The thermo-regulatory sweat test adapted by Fealey *et al.* (1989) involves whole body heating and sweating is detected by the application of alizarin red powder: this method assesses peripheral sympathetic function (pre- plus postganglionic). The quantitative sudomotor axon reflex test (Q-SART) stimulates sweating by iontophoresis of acetylcholine and assesses postganglionic sympathetic function by the axon reflex. Direct stimulation of sweat glands either by iontophoresis of pilocarpine and counting sweat droplets on a silastic imprint or by acetylcholine injection and counting iodine starch sweat spots assesses postganglionic sweat gland denervation. Finally, the dermal sweat glands are normally activated by a sympathetic discharge and this provides the galvanic skin response. This is a biphasic charge of electrical potential that can be recorded from the skin using electrocardiogram electrodes. A recent technique can measure basal and stimulated sweating using a direct reading computerized sudorometer and this technique has shown that transepidermal water loss is reduced in diabetics with neuropathy and is consistent with the lack of spontaneous sympathetic activity measured on microneurography (Levy *et al.* 1991).

The most common sweating deficit is in the feet in the classical stocking distribution. There is close correlation with other autonomic defects, especially with postural hypotension, but also with cardiac vagal denervation, although the cardivascular function tests tend to be abnormal before there is evidence of peripheral sweating loss. Abnormal responses may be found in cases of painful neuropathy and patients with truncal mononeuropathies may have patchy sweaty defects. These tests all confirm the widespread small nerve damage which occurs in diabetic neuropathy.

Gustatory sweating is a highly characteristic and not uncommon symptom of diabetic autonomic neuropathy (Fig. 37.5). Sweating begins soon after starting to chew tasty food especially cheese. It starts on the forehead, and spreads to involve the face, scalp, and neck, and sometimes the shoulders and upper part of the chest, compelling patients to keep a towel at the dinner table. Distribution of the sweating is in the territory of the superior cervical ganglion. It may be of sudden onset; its cause is unknown, although aberrant nerve regeneration has been suggested. It is occasionally sufficiently severe to need treatment: anticholinergic drugs are highly effective though side-effects may limit their use. Poldine methylsupate (Nacton) is the best agent, and propantheline bromide (Pro-banthine) can also be used. They are given half an hour before meals, but may also be effective if given before single meals at social occasions.

Diabetic diarrhoea

Diarrhoea is a very disagreeable symptom of autonomic neuropthy. Borborygmi and discomfort precede attacks of water diarrhoea, without pain or bleeding, and usually without malabsorption. Faecal incontinence is common, especially at night, when exacerbations seem to be worse. Symptoms last from a few hours to a few days and then remit, with normal bowel action or even constipation (sometimes induced by treatment) in between attacks. Constipation is not otherwise, in our view, a particular problem experienced by neuropathic diabetics.

The cause of diabetic diarrhoea is not known, and there have been few recent advances. Abnormalities of gut motility, decreased gut transit time, bacterial overgrowth, and bile salt malabsorption have all been described (Chapter 27).

The diagnosis of diabetic diarrhoea must be established by confirming the presence of autonomic neuropathy and excluding other causes of diarrhoea.

Tetracycline offers effective treatment in approximately half the patients, and is given in one or two doses of 250 mg at the onset of an attack which is abruptly aborted. If this fails, a range of the antidiarrhoea remedies could be tried, notably codeine phosphate, lomotil, or loperamide (Imodium). The use of clonidine has also been described.

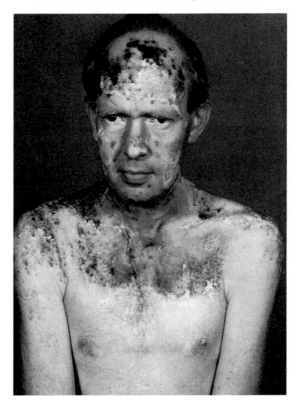

Fig. 37.5.   Severe facial and shoulder sweating (gustatory sweating) seen a few minutes after eating cheese. The area of sweating is clearly delineated by the application of quinazarin powder which turns blue when moist.

Gastroparesis

Vomiting from gastroparesis is a rare complication of autonomic neuropathy. It is usually intermittent, and only rarely so persistent that surgical measures may be needed. Gastroparesis is characterized by a gastric splash and, radiologically, by large food residues, absent peristalsis, a failure to empty the stomach, and a patulous pylorus. Failure to advance a jejunal biopsy capsule beyond the pylorus is also a feature.

Gastroparesis is most probably due to vagal degeneration. Several post-mortem studies have demonstrated loss of myelinated fibres in the vagus nerve but, only recently, loss of unmyelinated fibres has been shown in a vagus nerve removed at laparotomy from a patient with intractable vomiting from gastroparesis. Subtotal smooth-muscle cell atrophy in the muscularis propria of the stomach has been described in these patients, associated with transformed, smooth muscle cells undergoing a form of necrobiosis appearing as highly distinctive, homogeneous, round, eosinophilic bodies.

Gastric motility and emptying studies are generally difficult to perform and yield variable results. Liquids, solids, and indigestible solids are emptied by the stomach at different rates, and by different mechanisms. Radioisotope studies in diabetics with autonomic neuropathy have variously shown normal solid emptying, impairment of the usual differentiation between solid and liquid emptying, abnormal solid but normal liquid emptying, and abnormal solid and liquid emptying. Abnormal liquid emptying probably represents advanced disease; it can be assessed with relative simplicity by measuring epigastric impedance (Gilbey and Watkins 1987; Fig. 37.6). This technique seems to be a reliable diagnostic tool, and distinguishes those with vomiting from gastroparesis from the many patients with severe autonomic neuropathy who have normal gastric liquid emptying.

Dopamine antagonists (metoclopramide and domperidone) enhance gastric tone and emptying. They may accelerate gastric emptying in diabetic autonomic neuropathy with some effect. The motility stimulant cisapride can also be tried. These drugs form the mainstay of treatment during vomiting bouts. The use of erythromycin has been described recently (Janssens *et al.* 1990): this binds to motilin receptors and acts as a motilin agonist. Intravenous erythromycin causes a substantial acceleration of gastric emptying; oral administration is less effective and alleviation of symptoms still needs more investigation. The approach is promising.

Persistent and intractable vomiting from gastroparesis is very rare. Alleviation by surgical drainage using a Roux-en-Y gastrectomy has been described but may not succeed. This procedure has probably been superseded by the application of gastrostomy or jejunostomy: the tubes are inserted

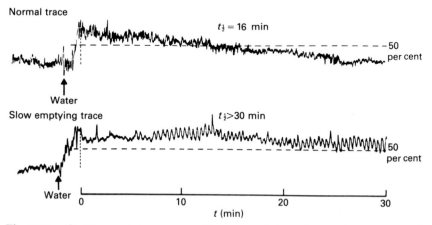

Fig. 37.6. Gastric emptying measured by epigastric impedance, showing normal emptying (above) and grossly delayed emptying in gastroparesis (below). $t\frac{1}{2}$ is the time taken for impedance to return to 50 per cent of maximum deflection.

endoscopically and may remain *in situ* for long periods. They can be removed or re-inserted with ease. Successful application of this technique has been reported in two cases and we have ourselves found it very effective in one patient. The long-term outlook after this treatment has still to be determined.

Oesophagus

Abnormal oesophageal motility has been described in diabetic autonomic neuropathy, although it is often asymptomatic. Studies by Maddern *et al.* (1985) describe relief of heartburn and dysphagia by domperidone, a peripherally acting dopamine antagonist; however, no improvement in solid emptying was noted.

Gall bladder

Enlargement of the gall bladder, probably due to poor contraction, may be a feature of diabetes related to autonomic neuropathy. Studies by ultrasonography have not confirmed the enlargement of the gall bladder, but do suggest impaired muscular contraction. There are no known clinical effects from this.

Neurogenic bladder (see Chapter 24)

Autonomic neuropathy affecting the sacral nerves causes bladder dysfunction. Bladder function tests are commonly abnormal in neuropathic diabetics but symptoms from neurogenic bladder in diabetes are relatively rare, usually occurring in diabetics who already have advanced complications. Most patients with neurogenic bladder are also impotent.

Impairment of bladder function is chiefly the result of neurogenic detrusor muscle abnormality, while pudendal innervation of perineal and periurethral striated muscle is usually unaffected in diabetic neuropathy. Afferent damage results in impaired sensation of bladder filling, and leads to detrusor areflexia: thus, the bladder pressure during cystometrography fails to increase as the bladder is filled. In advanced cases bladder emptying is reduced because of impaired detrusor activity and possibly failure of the internal sphincter to open adequately. Measurements of urine flow show that the peak flow rate is reduced and that duration of flow is increased.

There are no symptoms in the early stages, but later patients experience hesitancy during micturition, develop the need to strain, a feeble stream, and a tendency to dribble. Micturition is sometimes in short interrupted spurts which result from straining. Patients may be aware of lengthening intervals between micturition and also experience a sensation of inadequate bladder emptying. Gradually, residual urine volume increases and, in severe cases, gross bladder retention occurs with abdominal swelling and sometimes overflow incontinence as well. Bladder capacity may exceed 1 litre.

Diagnosis of neurogenic bladder is usually possible especially in those patients with clinical evidence of severe neuropathy. It is, however, important to exclude bladder-neck obstruction and, especially, prostatic obstruction in men. Ultrasound examination before and after emptying should be performed, and cystoscopy is usually needed: rarely, diabetic neurogenic bladder causes hydroureter and hydronephrosis. Occasionally, more sophisticated bladder function tests are needed. These include cystograms, cystometrography, and urine flow-rate measurements (see Chapter 24).

The principles of treatment are to compensate for deficient bladder sensation and thus prevent the development of a high residual urine volume. For those diabetics who have few symptoms of cystopathy, education is important and may suffice. In particular, the patient should be told to void every 3 hours during the daytime. Straining may be required, and the Crede manoeuvre (manual suprapubic pressure) can increase the efficiency of bladder emptying. With more severe symptoms, more active measures are needed. Cholinergic drugs such as bethanecol are used to increase intravesical pressure and maintain a small bladder capacity, although side-effects of sweating, salivation, and tachycardia can be a nuisance. Administration of prazosin, an α_1-adrenoceptor blocker may help by reducing urethral resistance. If it is ineffective alone, catheterization with regular clamping and release can help to overcome the problem. Surgery is sometimes needed. Careful bladder neck resection, even in women, provides very effective relief in the more severe cases by lowering the propulsive force needed to empty the bladder. In the most disabled patients, long-term catheterization is the only solution to the problem.

The most serious consequence of urinary retention is the development of urinary tract infections which are severe or even fatal. Diabetic cystopathy sometimes occurs in the presence of advanced nephropathy, and then infections may accelerate the decline of renal function. If the residual bladder volume is very large, renal transplantation may not succeed because postoperative sepsis is almost inevitable.

Impotence

Autonomic neuropathy is still considered to be the main aetiological factor in diabetic impotence (Chapter 24). It is due to erectile failure resulting from damage to both parasympathetic and sympathetic innervation of the corpora cavernosa. VIPergic nerves are also important in the vasodilatation of erection and the concentration of VIP is low in the penile corpora in diabetics with autonomic neuropathy. Failure to achieve erection may also be the result of a concomitant sensory deficit in the dorsal nerve of the penis. The onset of neuropathic impotence is usually gradual, progressing slowly over months, but complete erectile failure is usually present within 2 years of the onset symptoms. This history contrasts with psychogenic impotence which begins suddenly and in which nocturnal erections are present.

Impotence may also be due to vascular occlusion of the branches of the internal pudendal artery. Furthermore, in rare cases, erectile failure may be caused by the Leriche syndrome.

The diagnosis of neuropathic impotence in diabetes is difficult. The use of an intracavernosal injection of papaverine is to some extent useful in distinguishing neurogenic from vasculogenic impotence —it causes an erection in the former and fails to do so in the latter. This is helpful both in terms of diagnosis and giving guidance in the choice of treatment. For centres with particular interest, other techniques are available. Thus, it is possible to record nocturnal penile tumescence and rigidity during sleep: the absence of tumescence and rigidity over three successive nights is a strong indication for an organic cause of impotence. Vasculogenic impotence can be confirmed by a measurement of penile blood pressure and by comparing it with a brachial systolic pressure, thereby achieving a penile brachial index. When the ratio of penile-to-brachial pressure is 0.75 or less, a diagnosis of penile vascular disease can be considered. Autonomic function tests give some guidance as to the presence of autonomic neuropathy, but they do not establish conclusively in an individual whether it is the cause of the impotence. A neuropathic cause can be more exactly defined by electrophysiological testing of reflex sexual pathways. Conduction velocity is reduced in the dorsal nerve of the penis in diabetic impotent patients, and the latency of the bulbocavernosus reflex is prolonged.

The rational treatment of diabetic impotence depends on a careful history, in particular to evaluate any psychological component. If this factor is present, then the patient and his partner may be helped by appropriate discussion and advice. For the younger patients rigid penile implants are often successful, especially since ejaculation is often retained. Inflatable prostheses can also be inserted, but are more prone to failure. The intracavernous injection of the muscle relaxant, papaverine, causes an erection in patients not suffering from severe vascular disease, and offers a treatment which some men find satisfactory: potential problems exist from infection and penile fibrosis. The use of a vacuum pump applied to a condom is less invasive, and is a technique which some patients find satisfactory, especially if they are properly instructed. In vasculogenic impotence, arterial disease is often distal and arterial reconstruction is only likely to be useful in those patients with major arterial occlusions.

Respiratory responses and arrests

Sudden cardiorespiratory arrests have been well described in diabetes with autonomic neuropathy. In most of these episodes, there was some interference with respiration either by anaesthesia, drugs, or bronchopneumonia. These observations have led to further investigation of the respiratory system of diabetics with autonomic neuropathy: (1) the control of ventilation in response to hypoxia and hypercapnoea; (2) the pattern of respiration during sleep; and (3) the bronchial reactivity to chemical and physical agents.

The integrity of the ventilatory responses in autonomic neuropathy has been studied by measuring response to hypoxia and hypercapnoea in diabetics with and without neuropathy. The results of these investigations are conflicting. Normal increased ventilatory responses to transient hypoxia during exercise and to progressive hypoxia have been reported, implying that peripheral chemoreceptors and their afferent nerves are intact in diabetic autonomic neuropathy. However, other studies have found a defective response to hypoxia in autonomic neuropathy. The results regarding responses to hypercapnoea have also been conflicting; both normal ventilatory and reduced responses have been detected (Ewing and Clarke 1986). Thus the true importance of abnormal ventilatory responses as a cause of respiratory arrest has yet to be established.

In 1981, Guilleminault *et al.* reported four insulin-dependent diabetics with apnoeic episodes during sleep. These apnoeic episodes occurred not only during rapid eye movement sleep when they are a normal event, but also during non-rapid eye movement when they are definitely pathological. In the same year Rees *et al.* (1981) reported three further diabetics with autonomic neuropathy who also had sleep apnoea. However, two of these patients were older than any of the control group, and the incidence of sleep apnoea in normal subjects is known to rise with increasing age.

In recent studies of unselected diabetic patients, five of 12 insulin-dependent diabetic patients had abnormal breathing patterns, and four of these had evidence of autonomic neuropathy. Interestingly, the heart rate adaption to the apnoeic episodes was also abnormal in these patients. However, when well-matched groups of diabetics with and without autonomic neuropathy were studied, the number of apnoeic episodes per night was not significantly different in the two groups. It was concluded that diabetic patients with severe autonomic neuropathy have normal breathing patterns and oxygenation during sleep and that it is unlikely that sleep apnoea is a cause of respiratory arrest and sudden death in patients with autonomic neuropathy (Catterall *et al.* 1984).

The third area of study has assessed the integrity of respiratory reflexes which affect bronchomotor tone. Airways tone is mainly under vagal control and is reduced in diabetics with autonomic neuropathy. Administration of

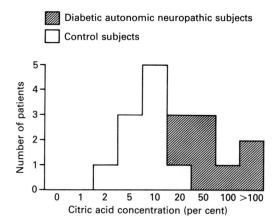

Fig. 37.7. Cough responses to inhaled citric acid in normal subjects and diabetics with severe autonomic neuropathy. The response may be impaired or even absent in autonomic neuropathy.

ipratropium, an anticholinergic bronchodilator, to normal subjects blocks efferent vagal tone in the airways, causing bronchial dilatation. This response is, however, reduced in diabetics with autonomic neuropathy, indicating that the patient has reduced airways tone. Furthermore, these patients also have an impaired cough reflex as demonstrated by a high cough threshold to inhalation of citric acid (Fig. 37.7). Diabetics with autonomic neuropathy have a diminished bronchial reactivity to cold air. To determine whether this defect was due to a neurodeficit or an abnormality of bronchial smooth muscle, reactivity to inhaled histamine, which has a direct effect on bronchial smooth muscle, was studied in diabetics with and without autonomic neuropathy. In one study there was no difference in reactivity, implying that the failure of patients with autonomic neuropathy to respond to cold-air inhalation is due to vagal impairment. In a further study, increased bronchial reactivity to histamine was observed in diabetics with autonomic neuropathy. Differential damage to the respiratory parasympathetic pathways could be a reason but an alternative explanation may be denervation hypersensitivity (Rhind *et al.* 1987).

The perception of respiratory sensations in diabetics was measured as they breathed through a tube manifold apparatus with resistance to air flow that was randomly varied. Diminished perception of respiratory resistance loads occurred in diabetics with neuropathy and this may render the patient prone to subclinical episodes of respiratory illness (O'Donnell *et al.* 1987).

Respiratory arrests in diabetics with autonomic neuropathy continue to be reported as do sudden deaths. Control of ventilation may contribute to these events although it is unlikely that sleep apnoea causes unexpected deaths in diabetics with autonomic deficit. Respiratory protective reflexes, including the cough reflex, are definitely impaired.

Hypoglycaemia

Hypoglycaemia is a powerful stimulus of autonomic function and the symptoms include sweating, tremor, and palpitations. Loss or blunting of autonomic symptoms of hypoglycaemia, 'hypoglycaemic unawareness', occurs in many insulin-treated diabetic patients. It probably occurs in as many as one in 10 insulin-treated diabetics within a year and may affect patients of almost any age or duration with or without diabetic complications. However, it is unlikely that autonomic neuropathy alone is responsible. In a study of 302 insulin-treated patients, loss of hypoglycaemic awareness was not invariably associated with abnormal cardiovascular function tests (Hepburn *et al.* 1990).

Autonomic neuropathy diminishes the secretion of adrenaline during insulin-induced hypoglycaemia and this may be the cause of loss of awareness. Tetraplegic subjects that are sympathectomized by cord transection lose both their awareness of hypoglycaemia and their adrenaline responses to it (Frier 1986; Chapter 43). However, in some diabetic patients who have described hypoglycaemic unawareness, the secretion of adrenaline following hypoglycaemia is normal, and it is possible that, in some diabetic patients with autonomic neuropathy, the reduction in intensity of autonomic symptoms is associated primarily with impairment of autonomic neural activity rather than a decreased rise in plasma adrenaline. Perception of hypoglycaemia can be reduced by non-selective β-adrenergic blocking drugs and a reduction in sensitivity of peripheral β-adrenoceptors may reduce symptoms of hypoglycaemia.

Loss of warning of hypoglycaemia may be caused by mechanisms other than peripheral autonomic dysfunction. Failure in activation of central autonomic centres during acute hypoglycaemia has been suggested as a possible reduced autonomic activity by Frier (1986) who described various deficits of hypothalamic (β-endorphins) and pituitary secretions (corticotrophin (ACTH), growth hormone, and prolactin).

Hypoglycaemia reliably stimulates the release of pancreatic polypeptide; this is blocked by atropine indicating that it is mediated by parasympathetic nerves. This response is defective or absent in diabetics with established autonomic neuropathy and this response is now considered to be a useful test for the integrity of the autonomic innervation of the pancreatic islets. Indeed, Kennedy *et al.* (1988) found that subnormal pancreatic polypeptide responses to insulin-induced hypoglycaemia predicted the development 2 to 3 years later of evidence of autonomic neuropathy.

Hypoglycaemia is also a powerful stimulus of glucagon release. There is indeed a defect of hypoglycaemia-induced glucagon release in long-term diabetics which is independent of autonomic neuropathy (Fig. 37.8).

The threshold for release of adrenaline can be affected by recent levels of blood glucose. Heller *et al.* (1987) showed that adrenergic responsiveness and awareness of hypoglycaemia may be diminished during mild hypoglycaemic clamping in some diabetic patients without autonomic neuropathy and Amiel *et al.* (1987) showed an appreciably lower threshold for triggering the release in diabetic patients with a mean haemoglobin A1 concentration of 7.6 per cent compared with those with a mean concentration of 11.5 per cent. Thus improved levels of blood glucose result in a lowering of the threshold for adrenaline release.

Recently, some patients have complained of loss of warning symptoms of hypoglycaemia since starting human insulin. However, a definite link between hypoglycaemic unawareness and human insulin has not yet been established.

In conclusion, unawareness of hypoglycaemia is a common problem in insulin-treated diabetics; autonomic neuropathy is, however, unlikely to be responsible for this phenomenon.

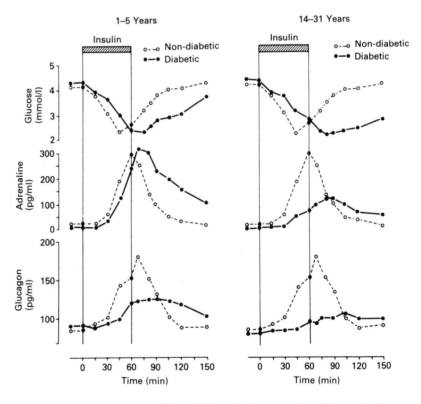

Fig. 37.8. Mean responses of blood glucose, plasma adrenaline, and glucagon in groups of non-diabetic and insulin-dependent diabetic subjects (duration shown above each graph) following intravenous infusion of insulin to induce hypoglycaemia. (Reproduced by kind permission of Frier (1986) and the editor of *Diabetic Medicine*.)

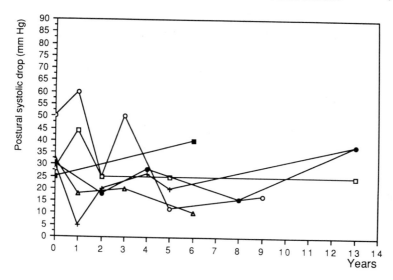

Fig. 37.9. Serial measurements of postural drop in systolic pressure in six patients with autonomic neuropathy who presented with a postural drop of more than 30 mm Hg.

Blood pressure changes

Insulin administration and hypoglycaemia cause major changes of blood pressure, which differ from normal in neuropathic patients and those on β-blockers. Insulin administration to sympathectomized or severe neuropathy patients causes a decrease of blood pressure and even severe hypotension when upright. This hypotensive effect of insulin may account for occasional black-outs in neuropathic patients erroneously attributed to hypoglycaemia. In normal subjects taking β-blocking drugs, hypertension occurs during hypoglycaemia (increase of systolic and diastolic pressures) in contrast to the normal response, which is an increase of systolic but a decrease of diastolic pressure. It is unlikely that the hypertensive effect of hypoglycaemia in diabetics on β-blocking drugs has serious consequences.

Prognosis

Autonomic function declines with age, but in diabetes it deteriorates, on average, faster than in normal subjects. Thus heart rate variation which normally decreases at approximately 1 beat/min/3 years declines about three times faster in the diabetic patient although there is substantial variation (Sampson *et al.* 1990). Most patients who develop abnormal autonomic function do not become symptomatic and the mortality of those with asymptomatic abnormalities is no different from that of patients with normal function: 90 per cent of our patients (all under 50 years old at the beginning of the study) were alive 10 years later. In contrast, the outcome for those with symptomatic autonomic neuropathy is not as good, although even in this group 73 per cent were still alive after a decade. Ewing *et al.* (1980) described a poorer prognosis, although patient selection was different and the patients were older. Most deaths are from renal failure or cardiac disease, and there are a few sudden unexplained deaths which may be from respiratory arrests or possibly arrythmias related to the prolonged QT interval associated with autonomic neuropathy (Chambers *et al.* 1990); neither cause has been proved, though we believe respiratory arrests to be the more likely. Patients with postural hypotension have the highest mortality.

Established symptoms of autonomic neuropathy run a very protracted, yet intermittent course; they rarely remit completely nor, on the whole, do they become disabling (Sampson *et al.* 1990). This is true for diabetic diarrhoea, vomiting from gastroparesis, and gustatory sweating in which disabling symptoms are rare indeed, even after 10 to 15 years. Postural hypotension fluctuates substantially with corresponding variation in the intensity of symptoms (Fig. 37.9). We have observed six patients for up to 13 years: in all of these cases postural hypotension persisted, but there was no overall deterioration and none of them became disabled. The explanation for this absence of progression is obscure, especially when the devastating hypotension in other autonomic neuropathies is observed.

References

Amiel, S. A., Tamborlane, W. V., Simpson, D. C., and Sherwin, R. S. (1987). Defective glucose counterregulation after strict glycaemia control of insulin-dependent mellitus. *New Engl. J. Med.* **316** 1376–83.

Archer, A. G., Roberts, V. C., and Watkins, P. J. (1984). Blood flow patterns in painful diabetic neuropathy. *Diabetologia* **27**, 563–7.

Bennett, T. (1984). Diabetic autonomic neuropathy and iritis. *Br. med. J.* **289**,123.

Catterall, J. R., Claverly, P. M. A., Ewing, D. J., Shapiro, C. M., Clarke, B. F., and Douglas, N. J. (1984). Breathing, sleep and diabetic autonomic neuropathy. *Diabetes* **33**, 1025–7.

Chambers, J. B., Sampson, M. J., Sprigings, D. C., and Jackson, G. (1990). QT prolongations in diabetic autonomic neuropathy. *Diabetic Med.* **7**, 105–10.

Edelman, S. V., Kosofsky, E. M., Paul, R. A., and Kozak, G. P. (1987). Neuroosteoarthropathy (Charcot's joints) in diabetes mellitus following revascularization surgery: three case reports and a review of the literature. *Arch. intern. Med.* **147**, 1504–8.

Edmonds, M. E., Nicolaides, K. H., and Watkins, P. J. (1986). Autonomic neuropathy in diabetic foot ulceration. *Diabetic Med.* **3**, 56–9.

Ewing, D. J., and Clarke, B. F. (1986). Autonomic neuropathy: its diagnosis and prognosis. In *Clinics in endocrinology and metabolism* (ed. P. J. Watkins), pp. 855–88. Saunders, London.

Ewing, D. J., Campbell, D., and Clarke, B. F. (1980). The natural History of diabetic autonomic neuropathy. *Quart. J. Med.* **193**, 95–100.

Fagius, J. (1982). Microneurographic findings in diabetic polyneuropathy with special reference to sympathetic nerve activity. *Diabetologia* **23**, 415–20.

Fealey, R. D., Low, P. A., and Thomas, J. E. (1989). Thermoregulatory sweating abnormalities in diabetes mellitus. *Mayo Clinic Proc.* **64**, 617–28.

Flynn, M. E., Edmonds, M. E., Tooke, J. E., and Watkins, P. J. (1988). Direct measurement of capillary blood flow in the diabetic neuropathic foot. *Diabetologia* **31**, 652–6.

Frier, B. M. (1986). Hypoglycaemia and diabetes. *Diabetic Med.* **3**, 513–25.

Gilbey, S. G., and Watkins, P. J. (1987). Measurement by epigastric impedance of gastric emptying in diabetic autonomic neuropathy. *Diabetic Med.* **4**, 122–6.

Gilbey, S. G., Guy, R. J. C., Jones, H., Vergani, D., and Watkins, P. J. (1986). Diabetes and autonomic neuropathy: an immunological association? *Diabetic Med.* **3**, 241–5.

Gilbey, S. G., Hussain, M. J., Watkins, P. J., and Vergani, D. (1988). Cell-mediated immunity and symptomatic autonomic neuropathy. *Diabetic Med.* **12**, 1–6.

Goebel, F. D., and Fusse, H. S. (1983). Monckeberg's sclerosis after sympathetic denervation in diabetic and non-diabetic subjects. *Diabetologia.* **24**, 347–50.

Greene, A. D., Lattimer, S. A., and Sima, A. A. F. (1988). Pathogenesis and prevention of diabetic neuropathy. *Diabetes/Metab. Rev.* **4**, 201–21.

Guilleminault, C., Briskin, J. G., Greenfield, M. S., and Silvestri, R. (1981). The impact of autonomic nervous system dysfunction on breathing during sleep. *Sleep* **4**, 263–78.

Guy, R. J. C., Richards, F., Edmonds, M. E., and Watkins, P. J. (1984). Diabetic autonomic neuropathy and ititis: an association suggesting an immunological cause. *Br. med. J.* **189**, 343–5.

Heller, S. R., MacDonald, I. A., Herbert, M., and Tattersall, R. D. (1987). Influence of sympathetic nervous system on hypoglycaemic warning symptoms. *Lancet* **ii**, 359–63.

Hepburn, D. A., Patrick, A. W., Eadington, D. W., Ewing, D. J., and Frier, B. M. (1990). Unawareness of hypoglycaemia in insulin-treated diabetic patients: prevalence and relationship to autonomic neuropathy. *Diabetic Med.* **7**, 711–17.

Janssens, J., Peeters, P. L., Vanprappen, G., *et al.* (1990). Improvement of gastric emptying in diabetic gastroparesis by erythromycin: preliminary studies. *New Engl. J. Med.* **322**, 1028–31.

Kennedy, F. P., Go, V. L. W., Cryer, P. E., Bolli, G. B., and Gerich, J. E. (1988). Subnormal pancreatic polypeptide and epinephrine responses to insulin induced hypoglycaemia identify patients with insulin dependent diabetes mellitus predisposed to develop overt autonomic neuropathy. *Ann. intern, Med.* **108**, 54–8.

Kennedy, W. R., Navarro, X., Goetz, F. C., Sutherland, D. E. R., and Najarian, J. S. (1990). The effects of pancreas transplantation on diabetic neuropathy. *New Engl. J. Med.* **322**, 1031–7.

Levy, D. M., Karanth, S. S., Springall, D. R., and Polak, J. M. (1989). Depletion of cutaneous nerves and neuropeptides in diabetes mellitus: an immuno-cytochemical study. *Diabetologia* **32**, 427–33.

Levy, D. M., Reid, G., Abraham, R. R., and Rowley, D. A. (1991). *Diabetic Med.* **8**,S78–81.

720   M. E. Edmonds and P. J Watkins

Logon, A. (1990). CNS growth factors. *Br. J. hosp. Med.* **43**, 428–37.
Maddern, G. J., Horowitz, M., and Jamieson, G. G. (1985). The effect of domperidone on oesophageal emptying in diabetic autonomic neuropathy. *Br. J. clin. Pharmacol.* **19**, 441–4.
O'Brien, I. A. D., O'Hare, J. P., Lewin, I. G., and Corral, R. J. M. (1986). The prevalence of autonomic neuropathy in insulin dependent diabetes mellitus: a controlled study based on heart rate variability. *Quart. J. Med.* **61**, 957–67.
O'Donnell, C. R., Friedman, L. S., Russomanno, J. H., and Rose, R. M. (1988). Diminished perception of inspiratory-resistive loads in insulin dependent diabetics. *New Engl. J. Med.* **319**, 1369–73.
Rabinowe, S. L., Brown, F. M., Watts, M., Kadrofske, M. M., and Vinik, A. I. (1989). Anti sympathetic ganglia antibodies and postural pressure in IDDM subjects of varying duration and patients at high risk of developing IDDM. *Diabetes Care* **12**, 1–5.
Raimbach, S. J., Cortelli, P., Kooner, J. S., Bannister R., Bloom, S. R., and Mathias, C. J. (1989). Prevention of glucose induced hypotension by the somatostatin analogue SMS 210-995 in chronic autonomic failure: haemodynamic and hormonal changes. *Clin. Sci.* **77**, 623–8.
Rees., P. J., Prior, J. C., Cochrane, G. M., and Clarke, T. J. H, (1981). Sleep apnoea in diabetic patients with autonomic neuropathy. *J. roy. Soc. Med.* **74**,192–5.
Rhind, G. B., Gould, G. A., Ewing, D. J., Clarke, B. F., and Douglas, N. J. (1987). Increased bronchial reactivity to histamine in diabetic autonomic neuropathy. *Clin. Sci.* **73**, 401–5.
Rothova, A., Meenken, C., Michels, R. P. J., And Kijlstra, A. (1988). Uveitis and diabetes mellitus. *Am. J. Ophthalmol.* **106**, 17–20.
Ruit, K. G., Osborne, P. A., Schmidt, R. E., Johnson, E. M., and Snider, W. D. (1990). Nerve growth factor regulates sympathetic ganglion cell morphology and survival in the adult mouse. *J. Neurosci.* **10**, 2412–19.
Rundles, R. W. (1945). Diabetic neuropathy: a general review with a report of 125 cases. *Medicine, Baltimore* **24**, 111–60.
Ryder, R. E. J., Kennedy, R. L., Newrick, P. G., Wilson, R. M., Ward, J. D., and Hardisty, C. A. (1990). Autonomic denervation may be a prerequisite of diabetic neuropathic foot ulceration. *Diabetic Med.* **7**, 726–30.
Sampson, M. J., Wilson, S., Karagiannis, P., Edmonds, M. E., and Watkins, P. J. (1990). Progression of diabetic autonomic neuropathy over a decade in insulin dependent diabetics. *Quart. J. Med.* **75**, 635–46.
Stevens, M. J., Edmonds, M. E., Douglas, S. L. E., and Watkins, P. J. (1991*a*). Influence of neuropathy on the microvascular response to local heating in the human diabetic foot. *Clin. Sci.* **80**, 249–56.
Stevens, M. J., Edmonds, M. E., and Watkins, P. J. (1991*b*). Abnormal vascular responses in the diabetic foot are a result of neuropathy and not microangiopathy. *Proc. Physiol. Soc.* **438**, 94.
Sundqvist, G., Lind, P., Bergstrom, B., Lilja, B., and Rabinowe, S. L. (1991). Autonomic nerve antibodies and autonomic nerve function in Type I & Type II diabetic patients. *J. Int. Med.* **229**, 505–10.
Vinik, A. and Braxton, M. (1988). Clinical aspects of diabetic neuropathies. *Diabetes/Metab. Rev.* **4**, 223–53.

38. Dopamine β-hydroxylase deficiency and other genetically determined causes of autonomic failure

A. Clinical features, investigation, and management

Christopher J. Mathias and Roger Bannister

Introduction

Dopamine β-hydroxylase (DBH) is the enzyme which converts dopamine into noradrenaline (Fig. 38.1). It is present within vesicles in sympathetic nerve endings and within the adrenal medulla and is released stoichiometrically with noradrenaline during sympathetic stimulation. It can be readily measured in plasma, and studies in both animals and man indicate that the major contribution to circulating levels is from sympathetic nerve endings. It was once thought that it might serve as a better indicator of sympathetic nervous activity than noradrenaline. Further studies, however, have indicated that there are marked differences within normal subjects and that plasma levels are largely genetically predetermined. Its half-life is probably in the region of about 30 min and is considerably longer than that of noradrenaline. This can be a disadvantage with short-lived sympathetic stimuli. Furthermore, it has a much larger molecular weight (290 kDa as compared to 169 Da for noradrenaline) and it reaches the circulation predominantly by lymphatic channels rather than through diffusion. Studies from a variety of sources indicate that, in man, it is not as sensitive an indicator of short- or long-term changes in sympathetic activity as is noradrenaline (Mathias *et al.* 1976; Weinshilboum 1979*a*).

Interest in DBH in autonomic disorders was stimulated by the lower plasma levels observed in familial dysautonomia (Weinshilboum and Axelrod 1971) and later in familial amyloid polyneuropathy (Suzuki *et al.* 1980). In the latter group further evidence of a functional DBH deficit was provided by successful treatment of their hypotension with the agent DL-dihydroxyphenylserine (DOPS) which bypassed the deficient enzymatic component (Fig. 38.2). There was a resurgence of interest in the late 1980s with the description of two patients with a congenital deficiency of DBH resulting in severe postural

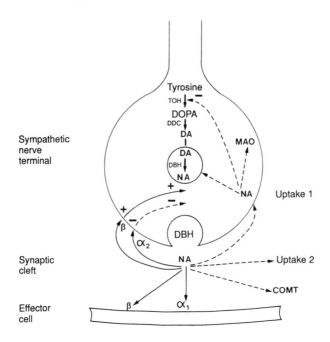

Fig. 38.1. Schema of some pathways in the formation, release, and metabolism of noradrenaline from sympathetic nerve terminals. Tyrosine is converted into dihydroxyphenylalanine (DOPA) by tyrosine hydroxylase (TOH). DOPA is converted into dopamine (DA) by dopa-decarboxylase (DDC). In the vesicles, DA is converted into noradrenaline (NA) by dopamine β-hydroxylase (DBH). Nerve impulses release both DBH and NA into the synaptic cleft by exocytosis. NA acts predominantly on α_1-adrenoceptors but has actions on β-adrenoceptors on the effector cell of target organs. It also has presynaptic adrenoceptor effects. Those on α_2-adrenoceptors inhibit NA release while those on β-adrenoceptors stimulate NA release. NA may be taken up by a neuronal (uptake 1) process into the cytosol, where it may inhibit further formation of DOPA through the rate-limiting enzyme TOH. NA may be taken into vesicles or metabolized by monoamine oxidase (MAO) in the mitochondria. NA may be taken up by a higher-capacity but lower-affinity extraneuronal process (uptake 2) into peripheral tissues such as vascular and cardiac muscle, and certain glands. NA is also metabolized by catechol-o-methyl transferase (COMT). NA measured in plasma is thus the overspill which is not affected by these numerous processes. (From Mathias (1991).)

hypotension due to sympathetic adrenergic failure (Robertson *et al.* 1986; Man in't Veld *et al.* 1987a). Since then four further cases have been described, two of whom are siblings (see Table 38.1).

The clinical features, autonomic deficits, results of routine, and specialized investigations, together with the management of DBH deficiency are described.

Table 38.1. Details of six patients with DBH deficiency

	USA		The Netherlands		UK	
	Patient 1	Patient 2	Patient 3	Patient 4	Patient 5*	Patient 6*
Reference	Robertson et al. (1986)	Biaggioni et al. (1990)	Man in't Veld et al. (1987a)	Man in't Veld et al. (1988)	Mathias et al. (1990)	Mathias et al. (1990)
Sex	F	M	F	F	M	F
Origin	Scotch–Irish	Dutch, Scotch–Irish, Cherokee	Dutch†	Dutch†	English	English
Consanguinity	—	—	None	—	None	None
Siblings	1 brother	—	1 brother, 1 sister	—	1 sister	1 brother
Family affected	No	No	No	—	Yes (sister)	Yes (brother)
Age when postural hypotension recognized (years)	25	33	21	20	29	21

*Patients 5 and 6 are siblings.
†Presumed, as no details provided.
—No details provided.

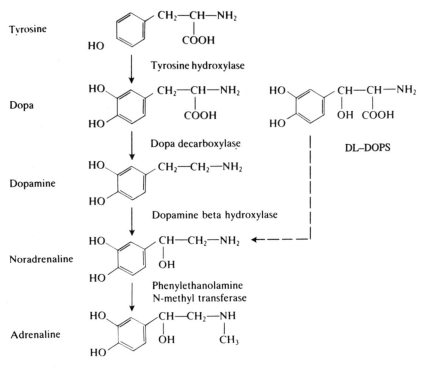

Fig. 38.2. Biosynthetic pathway in the formation of noradrenaline and adrenaline. The structure of DL-DOPS is indicated on the right. It is converted directly to noradrenaline by dopa-decarboxylase, thus bypassing the necessity of dopamine beta-hydroxylase.

There will also be a short discourse on the differential diagnosis and on genetic studies in such patients.

Clinical features

Presentation

Of the six patients, four are female (Table 38.1). All were diagnosed after the age of 20, although their history was suggestive of autonomic failure from birth or early childhood. In patients 2 and 3 there were other complicating features (hypoglycaemia, epilepsy probably incorrectly diagnosed), and both were unsuccessfully treated for what was thought to be recurrent epileptic seizures. The reason for investigation and subsequent diagnosis was directly related to symptoms and signs of postural hypotension. This was recognized only in their teens or later.

Family history

In none of the cases was there a history of a similar problem in previous generations. There was no evidence of consanguinity. The patients were of white Caucasian stock; of Scottish, Irish, Dutch, and northern English descent except for patient 2 who also had Cherokee Indian lineage. There was a history of miscarriages in some of their parents. The brother and sister in the UK (patients 5 and 6) were the only siblings in the family.

Pre-adult manifestations

All, except for patient 5, were unwell from early childhood. There was a strong association between their symptoms, syncope, and exercise, which was avoided in some, and especially in patients 3 and 6. As a child, patient 6 had difficulty in walking, which her mother attributed to her not trying. Epilepsy was considered in patients 2 and 3 who were unsuccessfully tried on anti-epileptic medication. At birth patient 3 had episodes of hypoglycaemia and hypothermia. Physical growth in all appeared to be normal, and sexual maturation was not delayed. Symptoms, however, became more apparent in their teens; in patient 5, however, this only emerged at 13 years. Whether the clinical manifestations were associated with greater activity, worsening of their condition, or sharpening of their ability to associate symptoms with specific events is not clear.

Clinical manifestations at diagnosis

Autonomic function

Symptoms pointed to postural hypotension, with blurring of vision, dizziness, and at times syncope (Table 38.2). This was often worse in the morning, during exercise, and during hot weather. Postural symptoms were not worse after food ingestion except in patient 2. Patient 5 occasionally had aching in the back of the neck and shoulders after meals. In patient 6 food often reduced postural symptoms but there was no evidence of hypoglycaemia. In patients 5 and 6 precordial pain occasionally occurred during exertion, which was reproduced during exercise testing with electrocardiography (ECG), but without concomitant evidence of ischaemia on the ECG. They both also had weakness and paraesthesiae in the legs during exertion, suggestive of ischaemia to the spinal cord. On formal testing immediately post-exercise, no objective evidence of a neurological or vascular deficit in the periphery was obtained.

Patients 1–4 had bilateral partial ptosis, presumably related to the lack of sympathetic tone to Muller's muscle in the upper lid. Patient 1 had nasal stuffiness probably due to vasodilatation secondary to lack of sympathetic

Table 38.2. Clinical symptoms and signs in six patients* with DBH deficiency

Symptoms and signs	USA		The Netherlands		UK	
	Patient 1	Patient 2	Patient 3	Patient 4	Patient 5	Patient 6
Autonomic						
Postural symptoms	+	+	+	+	+	+
Postural hypotension	+	+	+	+	+	+
Postural rise in heart rate	+	+	+	+	+	+
Sweating	+	+	+	+	+	+
Bowels	ID	ID	N	N	N	N
Urinary bladder	N	N	N	N	N	N
Sexual						
Maturation/ Menarche	N	N	N	N	N	N
Erection		Impaired			N	
Ejaculation		Retro- grade			Delayed or absent	
Partial ptosis	+	+	+	+	–	–
Neurological	N	Reduced deep tendon reflexes	Hypotonia, facial weakness, sluggish deep tendon reflexes		N	N
Higher function	N	N	N	N	N	N
Miscellaneous		Hyper- extensible joints	Brachydactyly, high palate			

N, normal; +, symptom or sign present; –, symptom or sign absent; ID, intermittent diarrhoea
*Patient details in Table 38.1.

vasoconstriction, as seen in acute tetraplegia (Guttmann's sign) and after α-adrenoceptor blockers such as phenoxybenzamine. It is recorded that patients 2, 5, and 6 were aware of their ability to sweat. There were no abnormalities in relation to lacrimation or salivation. There was normal gut and large bowel function, except for intermittent diarrhoea in patients 1 and 2.

Urinary bladder function was normal in all. Patient 6 had nocturia. In patient 5 erection was preserved but ejaculation took a prolonged time to achieve or was absent. Patient 2 was originally described as impotent (Biaggioni and Robertson 1987) but was later reported to have difficulty in maintaining an erection and to have retrograde ejaculation (Biaggioni *et al.* 1990).

Neurological and mental function

There were no major neurological abnormalities. Mild ptosis was present in patients 1–4. Patient 2 had reduced deep tendon reflexes. Muscle hypotonia, weakness of the facial musculature, and sluggish deep tendon reflexes were reported in patients 3 and 4. No neurological deficits were recorded in patients 5 and 6. There was no evidence of impairment of mental function and detailed psychometric examinations in patients 5 and 6 were normal.

Miscellaneous

Patients 2 and 6 had renal impairment with an elevated creatinine level (220 and 150 μmol/l, respectively). In patient 6 this was due to an episode of glomerulonephritis which had been treated successfully with steroids when she was 21, but which left her with an elevated but stable creatinine level; she had remained mildly anaemic (Hb 10 g/dl). Patients 3 and 4 had brachydactyly and a high palate. Patient 2 had atrial fibrillation and patient 3 had negative or flat T waves in the precordial leads of the ECG.

Autonomic investigations

Physiological

Cardiovascular

The investigations indicated sympathetic adrenergic failure (Table 38.3). All patients had severe postural hypotension, with an abnormal Valsalva manoeuvre, but with an adequate rise in heart rate when the blood pressure fell, showing preserved baroreceptor afferent and vagal efferent pathways. In patients 1, 5, and 6 there was a small rise in blood pressure and heart rate during some of the pressor tests. This suggested, in the absence of noradrenaline, the presence of alternative although less effective mechanisms which raise blood pressure. These include vagal withdrawal, which can raise heart rate and cardiac output, and pressor effects exerted through dopamine, neuropeptides (such as neuropeptide Y), or purines (such as adenosine triphosphate) released from otherwise intact sympathetic nerve terminals.

Heart rate responses to deep breathing and hyperventilation were present indicating functional cardiac vagus nerves.

The responses to food ingestion were tested in patients 5 and 6. In neither was there a fall in supine blood pressure or an accentuation of postural

Table 38.3. Summary of physiological autonomic investigations in six patients*
with DBH deficiency

Physiological investigations	USA		The Netherlands		UK	
	Patient 1	Patient 2	Patient 3	Patient 4	Patient 5	Patient 6
Sympathetic adrenergic						
Head-up postural change-BP	↓	↓	↓	↓	↓	↓
Valsalva manoeuvre						
-BP	A	A	A	A	A	A
-Phase IV-HR	A	A	A	A	A	A
Pressor tests	A	A	A	A	A	A
Sympathetic cholinergic						
Sweating	N	N	N	N	P	P
Parasympathetic						
Sinus arrhythmia	+	+	+	+	+	+
Hyperventilation-HR	↑	↑	↑	↑	↑	↑
Head-up postural change-HR	↑	↑	↑	↑	↑	↑
Valsalva manoeuvre Phase II-HR	↑	↑	↑	↑	↑	↑
Schirmer's test					N	N
Miscellaneous						
Food on BP					↔	↔
Nocturnal polyuria					+	+
Nocturnal natriuresis					+	+

BP, blood pressure; HR, heart rate; A, abnormal; N, normal; P, preserved but patchy;
↓, fall; ↑, rise; ↔, no change; +, symptom present; no symbol, not described.
*Patient details in Table 38.1.

hypotension, which differs from observations in patients with primary
autonomic failure (Fig. 38.3). The possible mechanisms for this difference
are discussed in Chapter 26.

Sweating

Sweating was preserved in all patients. Thermoregulatory sweating response
was tested in patients 3–6 and was present, although in patients 5 and 6 this
was patchy when compared with normals. Patient 3 sweated profusely when
hypoglycaemia was induced by insulin.

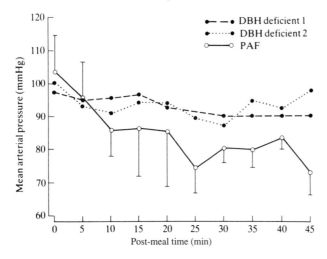

Fig. 38.3. Blood pressure before and after ingestion of a balanced liquid meal with measurements in the supine position, in five patients with pure autonomic failure (PAF) and in patients 5 and 6 (1 and 2, respectively, in figure). (From Mathias *et al.* (1990).)

Lacrimation and salivation

Schirmer's test was normal in patients 5 and 6 and there were no symptoms to suggest xerostomia.

Nocturnal polyuria and natriuresis

This was recorded in patients 5 and 6. Both excreted large amounts of urine and sodium at night (Fig. 38.4). In patient 3, sodium output was reported as high but details were not provided.

Electrophysiological studies

Sympathetic microneurography was performed in patient 2 (Rea *et al.* 1990). This demonstrated a rise in muscle sympathetic nerve activity with pressor stimuli (despite no change in blood pressure) and a fall in nerve discharge with phenylephrine, both consistent with functional preservation of sympathetic nerve activity (Fig. 38.5(a),(b)).

Biochemical investigations

Plasma catecholamines

The key findings were the virtual absence of circulating levels of noradrenaline and adrenaline, with abnormally elevated levels of dopamine (Fig. 38.6(a)). Patient 1 was reported to have detectable plasma adrenaline levels but this

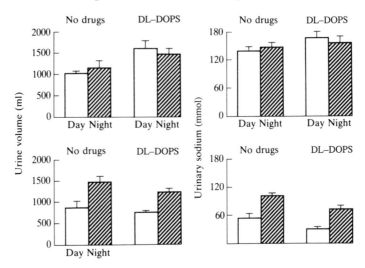

Fig. 38.4. Day (open histograms) and night (hatched histograms) urine volumes (left panels) and urinary sodium excretion (right panels) in patient 5 (upper panels) and patient 6 (lower panels) with DBH deficiency, before and after drug therapy with DL-DOPS. (From Mathias *et al.* (1990).)

was later retracted (Biaggioni *et al.* 1990) on the basis that the levels observed were probably due to cross-reactivity with high levels of dopamine. The evidence of an inability to convert dopamine to noradrenaline suggested a lack of DBH activity which was confirmed (Fig. 38.6(b)). In patients 2–4 the precursor substance to dopamine, dihydroxyphenylalanine, was also elevated in plasma. The high levels of dopamine suggested lack of inhibition of tyrosine hydroxylase, the rate-limiting enzyme, which is normally inhibited by intraneuronal noradrenaline. Despite these high basal levels, definite elevations in plasma dopamine levels were associated with physiological and/or pharmacological stimulation in all patients (Fig. 38.7). Neither intravenous tyramine (patients 1–4) nor insulin-induced hypoglycaemia (patients 3 and 4) caused an elevation in noradrenaline or adrenaline levels (respectively) as they normally do.

Cerebrospinal fluid catecholamines

In patients 2 and 3, noradrenaline and adrenaline were not detectable in cerebrospinal fluid, while dopamine and its metabolites were elevated (Fig. 38.8).

Urinary catecholamine measurements

The urinary metabolites of dopamine (homovanillic acid and 3-methoxytyramine) were normal or elevated while those of noradrenaline (normetanephrine)

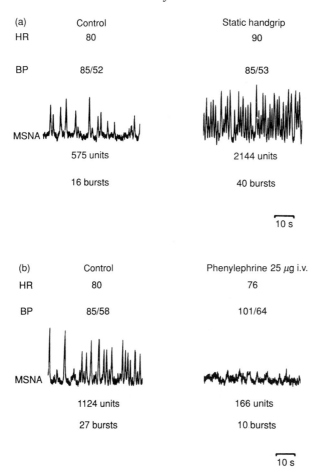

Fig. 38.5. Heart rate (HR), blood pressure (BP), and muscle sympathetic nerve activity (MSNA) recorded from the peroneal nerve in a patient with DBH deficiency (patient 2): (a) before and during isometric exercise (static handgrip); and (b) during injection of phenylephrine. Isometric exercise increases MSNA and phenylephrine decreases MSNA indicating that baroreflex pathways are intact. (From Rea *et al.* (1990).)

and adrenaline (metanephrine) were either extremely low or undetectable (Fig. 38.9). This was consistent with the plasma observations.

Tissue studies

Electron microscopy was performed on axillary and gluteal skin in patients 5 and 6 and did not show any structural abnormalities of sympathetic nerve terminals. In these patients, immunohistochemical staining indicated the

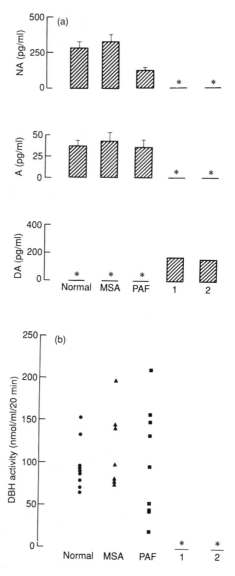

Fig. 38.6. (a) Mean levels (± SEM) of plasma noradrenaline (NA), adrenaline (A), and dopamine (DA) in 10 normal subjects, 12 patients with multiple system atrophy (MSA), and 8 patients with pure autonomic failure (PAF). Individual values on the first occasion in patients 5 and 6 (1 and 2, respectively, in figure) with DBH deficiency are indicated. The asterisk indicates undetectable levels, which were below 5 pg/ml for NA and A and 20 pg/ml for DA. (b) Scattergram showing DBH activity in 10 normal subjects, 7 MSA, and 9 PAF patients. In patients 5 and 6 (1 and 2, respectively, in figure) activity was undetectable. (From Mathias *et al.* (1990).)

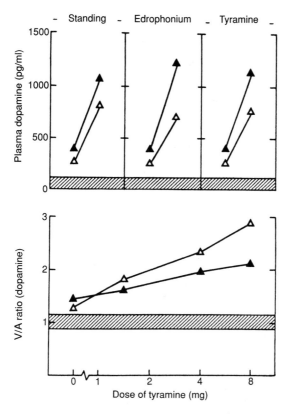

Fig. 38.7. Effect of standing, edrophonium, tyramine, and plasma dopamine and the venous/arterial (V/A) ratio for dopamine in two patients (3 and 4) with congenital DBH deficiency. (Filled triangles) patient 3; (open triangles) patient 4; (hatched area) 95 per cent confidence intervals in normals. (From Man in't Veld *et al.* (1988).)

presence of tyrosine hydroxylase but not DBH. In patient 3 immunohisto-chemistry of skin biopsy material was negative for DBH and noradrenaline and positive for dopamine, but no details of methodology were provided. Immunofluorescence to vasoactive intestinal polypeptide, neuropeptide Y, substance P, and calcitonin-gene related peptide was present in patients 5 and 6, similar to that in normal subjects.

Pharmacological

A series of investigations performed further emphasized the enzymatic deficiency and the associated autonomic abnormalities (Table 38.4). There was pressor supersensitivity to both noradrenaline and to clonidine, emphasizing α-adrenoceptor up-regulation (Figs 38.10(a) and 38.11). There

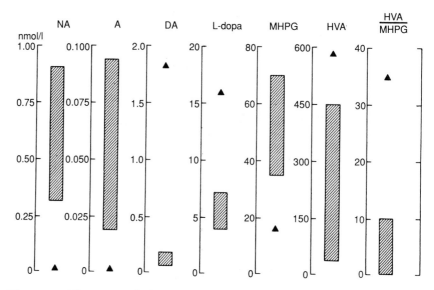

Fig. 38.8. Plasma catecholamine concentrations, 3-methoxy-4-hydroxyphenyl-ethylene glycol (MHPG) and homovanillic acid (HVA) in cerebrospinal fluid (CSF) of patient 3 with DBH deficiency. NA, noradrenaline; A, adrenaline, DA, dopamine, L-dopa = L-dihydroxyphenylalanine. (From Man in't Veld *et al.* (1987*a*).)

Table 38.4. Summary of pharmacological investigations in six patients* with DBH deficiency. Responses relate to blood pressure unless otherwise stated

Pharmacological investigations	USA		The Netherlands		UK	
	Patient 1	Patient 2	Patient 3	Patient 4	Patient 5	Patient 6
Noradrenaline	↑ + +	↑ + +	↑ + +	↑ + +	↑ + +	↑ + +
Isoprenaline (BP)	↓ + +	↓ + +	↓ + +	↓ + +	↓ + +	↓ + +
HR response	↑ + +	↑ + +	↑ + +	↑ + +	↑ + +	↑ + +
Tyramine	↔†	↔†	↔†	↔†		
Clonidine	↑ + +	↑ + +	↑ + +	↑ + +	↑ + +	↑ + +
Edrophonium			↔†	↔†		
Atropine (HR)	N	N	N	N	N	N
Metoclopramide	↔	↔	↑	↑	↓	↓
DL-DOPS	↑	↑	↑	↑	↑	↑
L-DOPS					↑	↑
L-DOPS + carbidopa					↔	↔

BP, blood pressure; HR, heart rate; N, normal; ↑, rise; ↓, fall; ↔, no response; + +, excessive response; no symbol, not described.
*Patient details in Table 38.1.
†Includes plasma noradrenaline response.

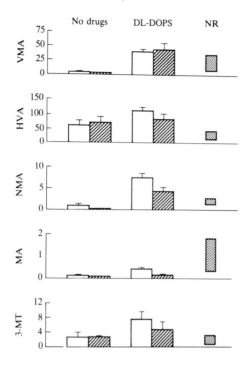

Fig. 38.9. Twenty-four hour urinary secretion of catecholamine metabolites in patient 5 (open histograms) and patient 6 (filled histograms) with DBH deficiency, before and after treatment with DL-DOPS. Bars indicate ± SEM and relate to collections over 3 consecutive days. VMA, vanillylmandelic acid; HVA, homovanillic acid; 3-MT, 3-methoxy-tyramine; MA, metadrenaline; NMA, normetadrenaline. Normal range (NR) indicated by stippled histogram on right. HVA and 3-MT are metabolites of dopamine. (From Mathias *et al.* (1990).)

was a depressor response to isoprenaline with an exaggerated heart rate response, probably due to a combination of β_1-adrenoceptor supersensitivity and also vagal withdrawal in response to the fall in blood pressure (Fig. 38.10(b),(c)). Tyramine did not raise levels of plasma noradrenaline in patients 1–4 (Fig. 38.12); edrophonium administration in patients 3 and 4 had no effect, but raised levels of plasma dopamine. The functional role of high circulating levels of dopamine varied: in patients 1 and 2 there was no response to oral metoclopramide, in patients 3 and 4 intravenous metoclopramide raised blood pressure, while an identical dose in patients 5 and 6 lowered blood pressure (Fig. 38.13). The reasons for these differences are not known.

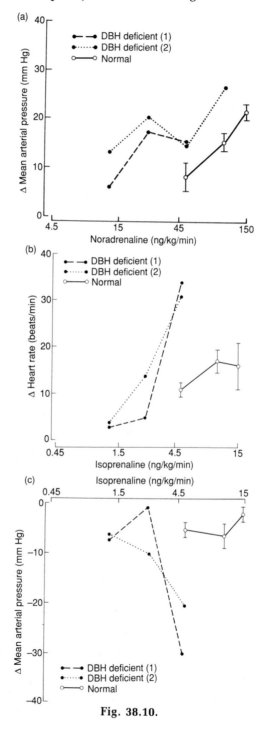

Fig. 38.10.

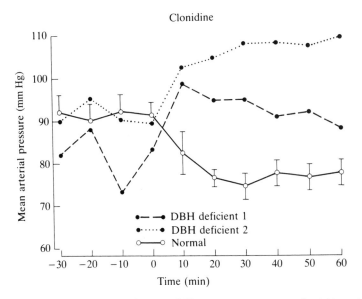

Fig. 38.11. Blood pressure changes following intravenous clonidine given at time 0 (2 μg/kg infused over 10 min) in six normal subjects and in patients 5 and 6 (1 and 2, respectively, in figure) with DBH deficiency. In the normal subjects there is a substantial and significant fall in blood pressure after clonidine. (From Mathias *et al.* (1990).)

Other familial and hereditary disorders with autonomic dysfunction and postural hypotension

The presence of the disorder at birth and the recognition of siblings with DBH deficiency places this condition among other familial and hereditary autonomic disorders, some of which are briefly described below. In the majority of these disorders there are associated neurological deficits which immediately separate them from congenital DBH deficiency.

Familial dysautonomia (Riley–Day syndrome)

This is an autosomal recessive disorder with autonomic abnormalities often present from birth (Axelrod and Pearson 1987). There is usually a strong

Fig. 38.10. (*opposite*)   (a) Change in mean blood pressure in normal subjects and in patients 5 and 6 (1 and 2, respectively, in figure) with DBH deficiency after incremental intravenous infusion of noradrenaline. In patient 5 the pulse rate fell to 40 beats/min after the third dose infusion and no further doses were administered. (b) and (c) Rise in heart rate (b) and fall in mean blood pressure (c) in normal subjects and in patients 5 and 6 (1 and 2, respectively, in figure) after incremental intravenous infusion of isoprenaline. (From Mathias *et al.* (1990).)

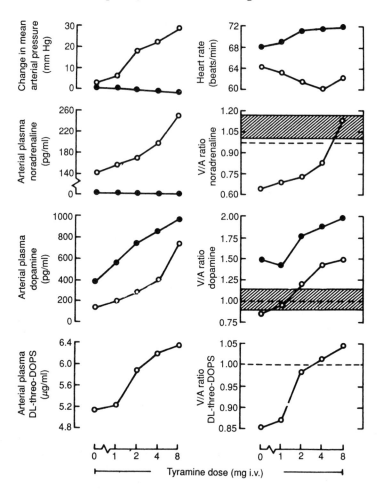

Fig. 38.12. Effects of tyramine before (●———●) and after (○———○) treatment with DOPS in patient 3. V/A, venous/arterial. Hatched areas indicate 95 per cent confidence interval of V/A ratios for noradrenaline and dopamine in 30 untreated patients with borderline hypertension under basal conditions. Prior to treatment with DL-DOPS, tyramine has no effects on blood pressure and plasma noradrenaline levels. This is changed after treatment with DOPS. (From Man in't Veld *et al.* (1987*b*).)

history of consanguinity. The parents are usually normal. There is a possibility that more than one child in the family may be affected. It mainly occurs in Ashkenazi Jews.

The clinical manifestations are disparate and not fully understood but mainly relate to autonomic and sensory abnormalities. Postural hypotension

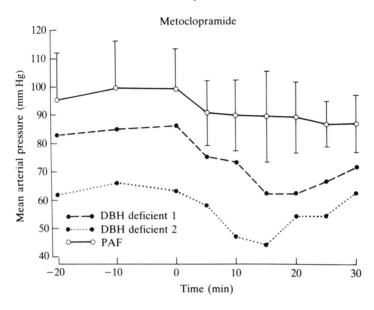

Fig. 38.13.   Blood pressure changes before and after the dopamine antagonist metoclopramide (10 mg given as 2.5 mg i.v. every 2.5 minutes from time 0) in four patients with pure autonomic failure (PAF) and patients 5 and 6 (1 and 2 in figure, respectively) with DBH deficiency. (From Mathias *et al.* (1990).)

is often observed, with impaired responses to pressor stimuli. Hypertension has also been reported together with episodes of sweating and blotchy erythema which may occur at meal times or when patients are excited. Excretion of both homovanillic acid (a metabolite of dopamine) and vanillylmandelic acid (a metabolite of noradrenaline and adrenaline) is reduced, unlike in DBH deficiency. Plasma DBH levels may be low. There are usually parasympathetic abnormalities. Periodic vomiting may occur, along with constipation and diarrhoea. These may be present at birth, with respiratory abnormalities, hypothermia, and hypotonic muscles. Urinary bladder control is often impaired. The eyes are usually affected with decreased tear secretion and hypersensitivity of the pupil to cholinomimetics such as dilute methacholine. Corneal hypoaesthesia may occur with complications such as ulceration and scarring. This is consistent with impairment of sensory systems which is also thought to account for the abnormal taste sensation and lack of fungiform papillae which results in a pale and smooth tongue. These are prominent features in helping make a clinical diagnosis. The intradermal histamine test is abnormal with an initial local area of erythema, not followed by pain or a flare, consistent with deficient sensory neuropeptides. Sexual maturation is often delayed in both sexes. Scoliosis is prominent, especially in girls. There is a wide variety of neurological disturbances which affect gait, reduce tendon reflexes, and impair sensation to heat and pain. There is a range of psychometric abnormalities. The prognosis varies with some dying early in life while an increasing number now reach adulthood. The cause of death may be sudden and related to dysrhythmias due to abnormal cardiac autonomic activity. Pulmonary causes and, in some adults, renal failure are contributory.

There is no specific therapy available. The possible involvement of nerve growth factor (NGF), which is in keeping with both the sensory and autonomic involvement, continues to be pursued.

Familial 'Shy–Drager' like syndrome

There have been two reports of a familial syndrome with postural hypotension, sphincter involvement, and multiple neurological deficits. The age of onset however was the late thirties or early forties in the first family (Lewis 1964) and even later in the second (Ilson *et al.* 1982). Details of the autonomic disorder in these patients are limited.

Familial amyloidosis (familial amyloid polyneuropathy, FAP)

This condition is characterized by abnormal deposition of fibrillar amyloid protein predominantly into peripheral and autonomic nerves. The amyloid is derived from abnormal transthyretin (prealbumin) which has a methionine valine substitution at position 30. This can be readily detected and serves as a genetic marker of the disease. It is an autosomal dominant condition, with an equal sex ratio and clinical manifestations usually between 20 and 40 years, involving both sensory and motor nerves often in the lower limbs, along with a range of autonomic disturbances. The latter include postural hypotension, urinary bladder dysfunction, constipation or diarrhoea, impotence, pupillary abnormalities, and anhidrosis. The condition is progressive, with death occurring in 10 to 20 years. Plasma DBH levels are low and the postural hypotension responds favourably to therapy with L-DOPS (Suzuki *et al.* 1980).

Fabry–Anderson disease

This is an X-linked glycolipid lysosomal storage disease. It results from mutation of the α-galactosidase genes situated on the X chromosome and there are a number of variants. The enzymatic deficiency results in accumulation of its main natural substrate, ceramide trihexoside being deposited in connective tissues. Globoside, a tetrahexoside which is its major precursor, is also found in red blood cells, blood vessels, and the kidney. A characteristic of the disease is skin deposits resulting in angiokeratoma, hence the alternative name angiokeratoma corporis diffusum. In addition, the peripheral and autonomic nervous systems, the kidney, the gastrointestinal tract, and the blood vessels themselves are affected. Vascular dilatation and constriction may be impaired directly or through autonomic involvement. In a detailed study of 10 males (Cable *et al.* 1982) impaired sweating was found in all. Lacrimal and salivary secretion and abnormal pupillary responses to pilocarpine were found in half the cases. The responses to postural change and the plasma noradrenaline levels were normal in all.

Other hereditary peripheral neuropathies

A range has been described (Chapter 35). These include porphyria (the acute intermittent, variegate, and coproporphyria forms) where the inheritance is autosomal dominant. Widespread autonomic involvement may occur including tachycardia and hypertension, which is thought to be related to baroreceptor denervation, in addition to other factors. There are a number of hereditary sensory and autonomic neuropathies (Thomas 1989) where the key feature is the sensory neuropathy. The autonomic abnormalities often include the urinary bladder or sweat glands.

Familial hyperbradykininism

These patients have symptoms suggestive of postural hypotension (Streeten *et al.* 1972). During head-up postural change the systolic blood pressure (but not necessarily the diastolic) usually falls and there is a marked rise in heart rate. Associated signs include cutaneous dilatation in the face and the lower limbs, which may turn purple. There are no neurological deficits. The findings have been attributed to excessive bradykinin levels. The postural hypotension is not therefore due to autonomic failure. These patients appear to benefit from propranolol, fludrocortisone, and the serotonin antagonist, cyproheptadine.

Adrenoleucodystrophy

This is an X-linked disorder which is related to the deposition of long-chain fatty acids (such as hexocosanoate C26:0) in cerebral white matter and in the adrenal cortex. This is thought to be due to an enzymatic defect in degradation of long-chain fatty acids.

   There are three forms which result in adrenocortical failure (Addison's disease) and may therefore cause a low supine blood pressure and postural hypotension (O'Neill 1987). In the childhood form, with presentation between the ages of 4 and 8 years, there may be deafness, dementia, cortical blindness, and tetraparesis. In the adult form the presentation is usually between 20 and 30 years with a longer life expectancy. In this form spastic paraparesis and polyneuropathy are common. A mixed form has been described. The symptomatic hetrozygote form, which may occur in females, does not appear to involve the adrenal cortex.

Like hyperbradykininism, there is no evidence of autonomic failure accounting for the postural hypotension, and deficiency of cortisol and aldosterone is responsible.

Tyrosine hydroxylase, DBH, and sensory neuropeptide deficiency

A patient with sympathetic adrenergic failure, and with sparing of sweating and parasympathetic function, similar to DBH deficiency, has been recently described (Anand *et al.* 1991). In addition she had undetectable plasma dopamine levels, along with immunohistochemical evidence of absent neuronal tyrosine hydroxylase, DBH, and the sensory neuropeptides, substance P and calcitonin gene-related peptide. Dopa decarboxylase activity was present and she could convert oral L-dopa into dopamine and L-DOPS to noradrenaline. There was an impaired histamine response on skin testing. Nerve growth factor (NGF) levels in skin were subnormal. The combined autonomic and sensory neuropeptide deficit appears related to a reduction in NGF. There are therefore marked differences from the patients with isolated DBH deficiency.

Aromatic L-amino acid decarboxylase deficiency (AADC)

Three children (including monozygotic twins) with AADC deficiency have recently been described (Clayton *et al.* 1991). The twins (1 year old) had reduced plasma dopamine, noradrenaline, and adrenaline levels, along with absent DBH in plasma. Whole blood serotonin levels were low. Cerebrospinal fluid levels of dopamine and serotonin metabolites were reduced. AADC was not present in liver tissue and was reduced in plasma. The previous sibling had died soon after birth and limited information indicated that this was very likely the reason. The autonomic abnormalities included temperature and blood pressure instability, excessive sweating, miosis, and ptosis. Heart rate variation was preserved. Neurological features were consistent with a cerebral deficiency of dopamine (oculogyric crises and abnormal movements) and responded to dopamine agonists (bromocriptine) and monoamine oxidase inhibitors. The parents appear normal, but have plasma AADC levels which are <20 per cent of controls. They are first cousins. The inheritance of the disorder appears to be autosomal recessive.

Menkes' kinky hair disease (trichopoliodystrophy)

This is a focal degenerative disorder of grey matter in which there is a maldistribution of body copper with low serum copper and caeruloplasmin levels (Menkes 1987). It is an X-linked trait. There is reduced activity of DBH, which is dependent on copper as a co-factor. This results in impaired conversion of dopamine to noradrenaline. It presents in infancy with vomiting, hypothermia, and neurological abnormalities such as hypotonia and poor head control. An important pointer to the diagnosis is the appearance of the hair which is colourless and friable. Most infants have delayed growth and development and the mean age at death is 19 months.

Fatal familial insomnia

This is an autosomal dominant condition characterized by selective degeneration of the anterior and dorsomedial thalamic nuclei. It presents in the third or fourth decade with progressive insomnia, ataxia, dysarthria, and myoclonus along with hypertension, tachycardia, and sweating. The autonomic investigations suggest preserved parasympathetic but higher background and stimulated sympathetic activity (Cortelli *et al.* 1991).

Management of DBH deficiency

The main problem in these patients is postural hypotension which responds unsatisfactorily to conventional approaches and drugs. In patients 1–4 details of drug combinations used were not provided. Patient 5 improved on fludrocortisone alone but, despite having nocturnal polyuria, did not benefit from desmopressin at night; patient 6 needed a combination of fludro-cortisone, dihydroergotamine, and desmopressin at night, which helped partially.

Metyrosine is a drug which inhibits the rate-limiting enzyme tyrosine hydroxylase and is used in patients with malignant phaeochromocytoma to prevent the formation of noradrenaline. In patient 1 it was used successfully to raise supine blood pressure and improve postural hypotension. This was thought to be due to reducing the formation of dopamine (Fig. 38.14; Biaggioni *et al.* 1987). However, in this same patient metoclopramide, the dopamine antagonist, had no effect on blood pressure. The reasons for this difference are not clear.

The drug that has been particularly beneficial in all six patients is dihydroxyphenylserine (DOPS). It is available either as the racaemic mixture (DL-DOPS) or in the laevo form (L-DOPS). The L form is thought to be the active form, based on both animal studies and on observations in patients with familial amyloidosis, where it was effective in half the dosage of the DL form. It is similar in structure to noradrenaline (Fig. 38.2), except that it has a carboxyl group as in DOPA (Fig. 38.2). It is therefore acted upon by dopa-decarboxylase, which is present both intraneurally and in a number of extraneuronal tissues including the kidney and liver, and is converted directly into noradrenaline, thus bypassing the DBH enzymatic step. The drug

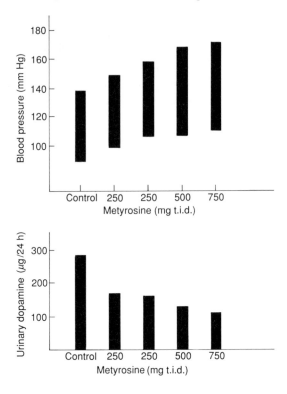

Fig. 38.14. Effects of increasing doses of metyrosine on supine blood pressure (upper panel) and on urinary dopamine levels (lower panel) in patient 2 with DBH deficiency. (From Biaggioni *et al.* (1987).)

crosses the blood–brain barrier, as has been demonstrated in animal studies (Kato *et al.* 1987).

In each of the patients, DL-DOPS had remarkable effects. There were definite improvements, with an elevation of supine blood pressure and, more importantly, a reduction in postural hypotension (Figs. 38.15 and 38.16(a), (b)). There were no mood changes in patients 1 and 2. In patients 3, 5, and 6 the description indicated that use of the drug effectively changed their lives. Patient 3 could cycle, climb stairs, and sit in the sun without feeling faint, which she could not do previously. Patients 5 and 6 were less tired and fatigued, especially in the morning. In patient 5 the symptoms of postural hypotension were virtually eliminated, and in patient 6 they were considerably improved. They both became far more active physically and noted perspiration to a greater extent on exertion, especially around the axillae and groins. Both noted cutis anserina (goose pimples) over the forearms and thighs, which they had not seen previously. The change in patient 6 improved a strained marital relationship. She was at times slightly more aggressive than previously

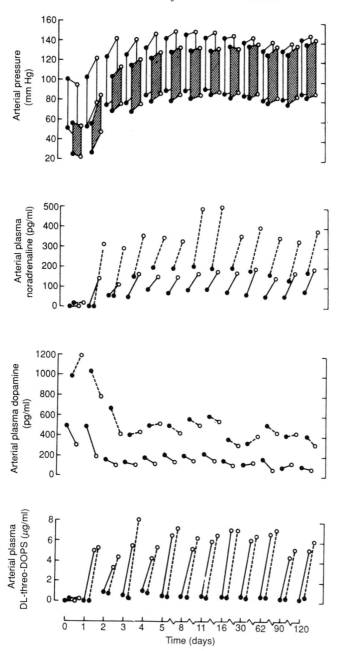

Fig. 38.15. Effects of DL-DOPS in patient 3 with DBH deficiency. Open columns and solid lines indicate values with the patient supine, hatched columns and broken lines with the patient standing. (Filled circle) 12 h after dosing; (open circle) 2 h after dosing. (From Man in't Veld *et al.* (1987*b*).)

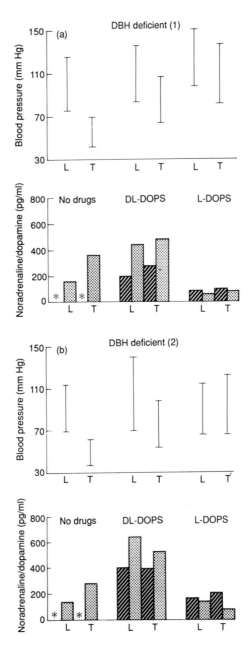

Fig. 38.16. Blood pressure (systolic and diastolic) while lying (L) and during head-up tilt (T) in (a) patient 5 and (b) patient 6 (b) with DBH deficiency (1 and 2, respectively, in figures), before and during treatment with DL-DOPS and L-DOPS. Plasma noradrenaline (hatched histogram) and dopamine (stippled

and even challenged her mother-in-law for the first time, having previously wished to do so but having been too timid. Neither patient 5 or 6 had difficulty in sleeping which is consistent with observations in patients 3 and 4 (Tulen *et al.* 1990). After DOPS, patient 5 may have had an increase in the number of nightmares, which she had suffered from for many years. There was little doubt, however, that on DL-DOPS and later with L-DOPS, patients 5 and 6 were symptomatically far better than when their blood pressure was raised to an equivalent degree on the conventional therapy described above (i.e. fludrocortisone in patient 5 and fludrocortisone, dihydroergotamine, and desmopressin in patient 6). The treatment with DL-DOPS had no effect on nocturia in patient 6, and in both patients the nocturnal diuresis and natriuresis continued (Fig. 38.4). Whether the overall improvement was related to the effects of the drug (including central effects) or non-specifically to the rise in blood pressure and reduction in postural hypotension was not entirely clear.

An additional advantage of DL- and L-DOPS in patient 5 was the improvement in sexual function, as he was able to achieve ejaculation, which had been difficult or impossible previously. The effect of DOPS on sexual function in patient 2 was not described.

Levels of plasma noradrenaline rose in each of the patients to whom DL-DOPS was administered; there was also a rise in patients 5 and 6 who were also given L-DOPS. In patients 1–3 there was a further increase in plasma noradrenaline levels with postural challenge (Fig. 38.15). This was not consistently observed in patients 5 and 6 (Fig. 38.16(a), (b)) when given either DL-DOPS or L-DOPS. In patients 5 and 6 this may imply inadequate intraneuronal replacement. In patient 3 the ability of tyramine to release noradrenaline after DL-DOPS was provided as evidence of intraneuronal replacement. However, noradrenaline formed extraneuronally (dopa decarboxylase is extensively distributed, especially in liver and kidneys) would have been incorporated by uptake$_1$ mechanisms into the cytosol and this could have been released by tyramine, not necessarily indicating intraneuronal conversion of DL-DOPS to noradrenaline and release of noradrenaline by neuronal impulses. The data in patients 5 and 6 suggest that extraneuronal formation of noradrenaline appeared to have played a more important role in them.

In patients 5 and 6, adrenaline remained undetectable in plasma and the metabolite of adrenaline in urine (metadrenaline) did not change (Fig. 38.9) until after 3 months of therapy. This raised the question of abnormalities in the conversion of noradrenaline to adrenaline, either because of an atrophic adrenal medulla or because of the absence of the enzyme phenylethanolamine

---

Fig. 38.16. (*continued*)   histogram) levels are indicated before and during tilt. Plasma noradrenaline was undetectable (∗ = < 5pg/ml) in both while off drugs. (From Mathias *et al.* (1990).)

Table 38.5. Summary of studies using DL-DOPS (or L-DOPS where stated) for the treatment of postural hypotension in different disorders

Disorder	No. of patients	Effect on postural hypotension	Reference
Familial amyloidosis	4	+	Suzuki *et al.* (1980)
	7	+	Suzuki *et al.* (1982)
L-DOPS	7	+	Suzuki *et al.* (1982)
Parkinson's disease	20	+	Birkmayer *et al.* (1983)
Pure autonomic failure	2	–	Hoeldtke *et al.* (1984)
Diabetic autonomic failure	4	–	Hoeldtke *et al.* (1984)
Shy–Drager syndrome	1	+	Sakoda *et al.* (1985)
L-DOPS	4	+	Senda *et al.* (1987)
	1	+	Kachi *et al.* (1988)
DBH deficiency	2	+	Biaggioni and Robertson (1987)
	1	+	Man in't Veld *et al.* (1987*b*)
	2	+	Mathias *et al.* (1990)
(L-DOPS)	2	+	Mathias *et al.* (1990)

+, Beneficial response; –, no benefit.

N-methyl transferase (PNMT). Further evidence of the inability to form adrenaline was obtained in patients 5 and 6 in whom insulin hypoglycaemia was induced while they were on treatment with L-DOPS. During hypoglycaemia, there was no rise in plasma adrenaline levels, and a small rise in plasma noradrenaline levels. The absence of a rise of metadrenaline excretion in urine was also noticed in patients with familial amyloidosis who were given L-DOPS (Suzuki *et al.* 1982).

In patients 5 and 6, the question of whether DOPS had direct pressor effects was tested by pre-treating them with the dopa-decarboxylase inhibitor carbidopa, in a dose sufficient to prevent peripheral decarboxylation. L-DOPS was then administered and, unlike in previous studies, it had no beneficial effect either on blood pressure or on their ability to stand (Table 38.5). This was consistent with a lack of its conversion to noradrenaline, which could not be detected in plasma. Clearly L-DOPS alone, even in patients with known adrenoceptor supersensitivity, has no direct pressor effects.

Another point of interest is the question of central effects of DOPS. This has been partially discussed in relation to behavioural and mood changes and may also be relevant to the blood pressure responses. Animal studies indicate that DL- and L-DOPS enter the brain (Kato *et al.* 1987). In patients 5 and 6, L-DOPS in the same dose as DL-DOPS was equally effective;

theoretically it should have been doubly effective. One possibility is greater formation of noradrenaline within the central nervous system which, as is clearly demonstrated in animal studies, reduces centrally induced sympathetic discharge and would thus have negated the peripheral effects of the drug (Araki *et al.* 1981). This would be consistent with the lower levels of plasma dopamine observed after L-DOPS, as compared with levels after L-DOPS (Fig. 38.16(a), (b)). There may also have been other effects including a central reduction of dopamine levels. Both patients 5 and 6 felt that DL-DOPS was 'better' than L-DOPS, though this has not been quantified. In repeat studies in patients 5 and 6 after 2 years of treatment with L-DOPS there was no evidence of any neurological or behavioural impairment and they continue to benefit considerably from the drug.

B. The molecular genetics of dopamine β-hydroxylase

Ian Craig, Christopher Porter, and Sally Craig

Introduction

There has been continuing interest in the possible existence of genetically determined variation in the activity levels of enzymes involved in the metabolism of neurotransmitters, with the hope that the characterization of such variation may provide insights into a range of behavioural and physiological disorders. Although complete deficiencies of some of the major enzymes involved in the synthesis and degradation of the catecholamine transmitters, e.g. phenylalanine hydroxylase and monoamine oxidase, have been shown to result from primary defects at the DNA level, much less profound, but nevertheless still genetically determined, alterations in levels may exist for many neurotransmitter enzymes. These may not result in clearly distinguishable phenotypes, but contribute as one of several factors to the aetiology of multifactorial disorders including autonomic failure, migraine, schizophrenia, and depression. In this context, dopamine β-hydroxylase (DBH) is remarkable in that simple Mendelian genetic variation, with high- and low-activity alleles segregating in the population, has been described: in addition, individuals with profound deficiencies in circulating enzyme are available for investigation. DBH therefore represents a paradigm for the investigation of genetic factors in complex disorders such as those discussed above.

Variation in DBH activity—genetic basis and possible relationship to clinical disorders

The existence of wide variation in activity levels of serum DBH in human populations has been established for a considerable time. Early studies showed greater than 20-fold variation in serum levels in normal individuals and noted very significant reductions of activity in some members of pedigrees with familial dysautonomia. Abnormal levels were also observed in patients with neuroblastoma, torsion dystonia, and Down's syndrome. The variation in activity correlated with amounts of DBH detected immunologically, suggesting that alterations in the total amount of enzyme protein rather than alterations to its specific activity were responsible (see Weinshilboum 1979*b*).

A strong familial element in determining activity levels was suggested by extensive sibling pair correlation studies; however, because of the extensive influence of environmental factors, such as stress, the genetic basis underlying the distribution of enzyme levels was not established until family and twin studies were undertaken. These, later, were to show that low levels of activity could apparently be determined by homozygosity for a recessive allele; however, perhaps the most appropriate description is that a single locus with codominantly inherited high- and low-activity alleles is responsible for the segregation of activity in the families studied (Goldin *et al.* 1982). The gene frequencies for high- and low-activity alleles indicated by such investigations were about 0.8 and 0.2, respectively, with 3–4 per cent of the population having substantially lower DBH activity than the normal range.

Convincing evidence has subsequently accumulated for a locus determining activity levels of serum DBH, which is linked to the ABO blood group gene on chromosome 9. No recombination was detected between ABO and the putative locus in a small number of informative families (Goldin *et al.* 1982). Other studies by Asamoah *et al.* (1987) also provided evidence for close linkage to the ABO locus in a detailed study of a single large pedigree. More recent studies (Wilson *et al.* 1988) have independently confirmed and extended this important observation and determined a very high probability of close linkage between ABO and the DBH activity gene.

Two questions remained unanswered concerning the nature of the genetic factors involved.

1. Is the model proposed sufficient to explain the major inherited contribution to enzyme activity?

2. Is the locus detected by segregation analysis the structural gene for the enzyme or an independent regulatory gene?

As regards the first question, Goldin (1985) reported that both a single locus and other contributing genetic factors were necessary to explain adequately the familial transmission of activity variants. Some evidence for the involvement of a second significant gene has also been provided by biochemical studies (Dunnette and Weinshilboum 1982) based on activity and thermostability determinations. Wilson *et al.* (1990) have examined the possible existence of a second locus by employing an approach which is based on identifying and removing from consideration the influence of the ABO-linked locus and testing for the segregation of additional genetic components. By this procedure, they were able to predict that about 90 per cent of the variance in activity is accounted for by the ABO-linked locus and the remaining 10 per cent by a putative, second locus which may be linked to the complement factor C3 gene on chromosome 19.

Although several investigations have compared the levels of DBH in patients with depression or schizophrenia with controls, it is surprising, given the clear inheritance pattern of DBH activity, that an examination of the predisposition of family members with genetically determined low enzyme activity to various disorders in which abnormalities in DBH levels may be a contributing factor (including autonomic failure) has not, as yet, been carried out systematically.

The possibility of exploring the molecular basis underlying the genetic variation and of addressing the second question raised above, was provided through the cloning of a cDNA (copy of the messenger RNA) for DBH by Lamouroux *et al.* (1987). Sequence analysis of the cDNA allowed the exclusion of any significant relationship of DBH to other enzymes of the catecholamine synthetic pathway, in particular to phenylethanolamine *N*-methyltransferase and tyrosine hydroxylase which had been predicted previously on the basis of apparent structural and immunological similarity (Joh *et al.* 1984). Furthermore, gene localization for DBH by *in situ* hybridization to chromosome preparations with labelled coding sequence was now possible, and Craig *et al.* (1988) showed a single peak of hybridization to 9q34—a position very close to that assigned for the ABO-linked locus determining levels of circulating enzyme (see Fig. 38.17). It is probable, therefore, that the activity variation results from the existence of alternative forms of the structural gene itself, or of its immediately adjacent regulatory sequences. This provides a way forward to investigate the molecular basis of variation at this locus and to examine the genetic factors responsible.

Activity levels themselves are not always the clearest indicator of genotype with respect to DBH status. Markers at the DNA level would provide more direct tools for linkage analysis within families, both to map disorders which have been localized to the same region of chromosome 9—including torsion dystonia and tuberous sclerosis—and to evaluate the possible involvement of the DBH locus in their aetiology. Simple variants in the DNA sequence can be revealed by analysis of fragments released by digestion of genomic DNA with restriction enzymes (restriction fragment length polymorphisms—RFLPs).

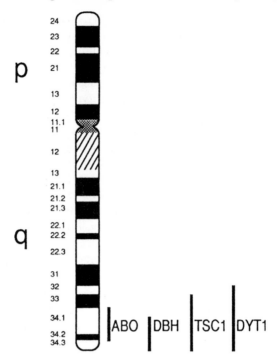

Fig. 38.17.   Localization on chromosome 9 of DBH gene and other significant loci in its vicinity. Vertical bars represent the limits on the cytogenetic ideogram within which the locus has been assigned. ABO, blood group; DBH, dopamine β-hydroxylase; TSC1, tuberous sclerosis 1; DYT1, torsion dystonia 1.

A variety of such genetic markers flanking or within the DBH gene can be detected with enzymes such as, *Xba*I, *Taq*I, *BamH*I, and *FnuD*II. It is hoped that their availability will lead both to an improved genetic map for the region and allow more precise ascertainment of the involvement of specific genetic variants at the DBH locus to the levels of circulating enzyme.

Studies are in progress to clone and sequence the structural gene and the adjacent regulatory regions from individuals expressing the high- or low-activity phenotype with a view to establishing the nature of the mutation responsible.

Genetic basis of individuals with profound deficiency in serum DBH

As discussed in part A of the chapter, there have been several reports of individuals with extremely low levels of serum DBH, which are presumed to result from a condition other than that associated with homozygosity for the ABO-linked, low-activity allele. During the last few years, at least six individuals have been identified and investigated in an attempt to determine the primary biological role of dopamine β-hydroxylase in man. Of particular interest is the report of Mathias *et al.* (1990) which concerns two affected siblings, suggesting a familial, rather than sporadic, aetiology. In examining the possible molecular lesions in such individuals, it is necessary to consider the various stages at which such defects might arise between the structural gene and the manifestation of DBH in serum. One important aspect is the relationship between the soluble and the membrane-associated forms of the enzyme.

During development of the peripheral nervous system, DBH appears initially in sympathoblasts which differentiate into sympathetic ganglia and adrenal medulla. DBH activity may be enhanced during development by nerve growth factor and other agents stimulating protein synthesis. Association with secretory granules is well established and it appears that the intragranular enzyme is present in soluble and membrane-bound forms in approximately equal amounts. There has been considerable debate concerning the structural basis for attachment of DBH to membranes; two major forms differing in size (75 and 72 kDa) have been discerned and the heavier of the two is thought to represent the membrane-associated form. There is evidence that the larger form may be posttranslationally modified to produce the smaller, soluble enzyme. This would be consistent with the tentatively identified, N-terminal, hydrophobic peptide capable of anchoring the protein to membranes and which is cleaved on its conversion into the soluble form (Talkjanidisz *et al.* 1989). Other studies have failed to distinguish between the N-terminal sequence of the two forms of the enzyme and reconstitution studies have suggested that, in contrast to a hydrophobic protein tail, the binding of phosphatidyl serine moieties are responsible for anchoring membranous DBH (Taylor *et al.* 1989).

Studies on gene organization and of the RNA transcripts show that the complete gene comprises 12 coding segments (exons) and that two alternative transcripts can be produced differing in length by 300 base pairs. The type A transcript, 2.7 kb, and the type B transcript, 2.4 kb, are produced by alternative selection between sites responsible for the initiation of the addition of poly A tails to the message (Kobayashi *et al.* 1989). Both forms carry the potential to produce a full length protein product and differ only in the untranslated region in the terminal segment; however, the functional significance of the alternative forms is not understood.

It is clear that the lack of serum DBH could reflect a defect in the coding sequence necessary for enzyme function or at one of the subsequent stages required for the correct modification, localization, or passage of the enzyme into the circulation. Patients presenting with complete lack of serum DBH provide an important opportunity to examine the possible critical steps involved and recent studies on some of these have provided relevant biochemical and genetical information. There is evidence that the lack of enzyme is not confined to the serum. Enzyme assays on cerebrospinal fluid (Man in't Veld *et al.* 1987*a*) and immunological studies on peripheral nerves in tissue sections (Mathias *et al.* 1990) suggest that the defect is also apparent at stages preceding its appearance in the circulation. Primary defects at the DNA level may be caused by alteration to one or a few bases and are difficult to detect other than by direct sequencing of the region containing

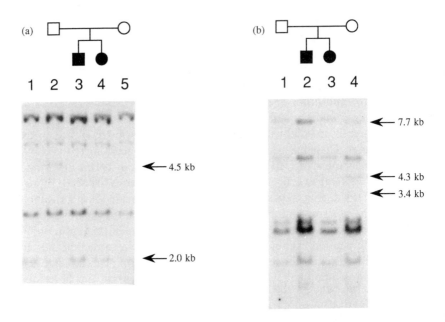

Fig. 38.18.   Segregation of a DBH restriction fragment length polymorphism in the family with two siblings with enzyme deficiency. (a) Illustration of a polymorphism for the restriction fragments produced by digestion with *Bam*HI and detected by electrophoresis and Southern blotting, followed by hybridization with the cDNA for DBH. Tracks 2–5 are digests from the father, the two affected siblings, and the mother, respectively. The father is heterozygous for alleles resulting in restriction fragments of 4.5 and 2.0-kb. The mother is homozygous for the 2.0-kb allele. Both siblings have received the 2.0-kb allele from the father. (b) Illustration of a polymorphism for the restriction fragments produced by digestion with *Taq*1 and detected by electrophoresis and Southern blotting, followed by hybridization with the cDNA for DBH. Tracks 1–4 are digests from the father, the two affected siblings, and the mother, respectively. The polymorphism is revealed by the presence/absence of an additional *Taq*I site in the large (7.7 kb) fragment detected, giving two additional bands of 4.3 and 3.4 kb. Whereas the father is homozygous for the 7-kb allele, the mother is heterozygous, having both the 7.0-kb allele and the 4.3 + 3.4-kb allele. Both siblings are homozygous for the 7.0-kb and must have inherited the same 7.0 allele from their mother. They can therefore be assumed to be genetically identical for the DBH region. (Other fragments are observed at 5.1, 2.8, 2.6, 2.4, and 1.6-kb).

the mutation. In other cases (usually involving more substantial alterations), genetic defects can be detected through observed alterations to the restriction enzyme fragment patterns discerned following hybridization with labelled cDNA. Investigations on the family with affected siblings (Mathias *et al.* 1990) have failed to detect any major alterations to the DBH gene; however, use of restriction fragment length polymorphisms in the family have clearly demonstrated that both affected individuals have inherited the same combination of alleles from their parents—consistent with the possibility that they both carry two defective versions of the DBH gene (see Fig. 38.18).

Further investigations are currently being undertaken, employing the polymerase chain reaction (PCR) to amplify the coding regions of the DBH gene and those regions involved in its regulation and transcriptional processing from the affected individuals. A sequence comparison with the equivalent regions in other family members and controls will allow the evaluation of the nature of the genetic defects involved. Furthermore, extension of these molecular studies should enable both the synthesis of new constructs involving genes from affected individuals which can be tested for possible functional defects following their introduction into test cell systems and, eventually, the development of mouse models with defective DBH genes to examine the significance of such a deficiency at various developmental stages.

References

Anand, P., Rudge, P., Mathias, C. J., Springall, D. R., Ghatei, M. A., Naher-Noe, M., Sharief, M., Misra, V. P., Polak, J. M., Bloom, S. R., and Thomas, P. K. (1991). New autonomic and sensory neuropathy with loss of adrenergic sympathetic functions and sensory neuropeptides. *Lancet* **337**, 1253–4.

Araki, H., Tanaka, C., Fujiwara, H., Nakamura, M., and Ohmura, I. (1981). Pressor effect of L-threo-3, 4-dihydroxyphenylserine in rats. *J. Pharm. Pharmacol.* **33**, 772–7.

Asamoah, A., Wilson, A. F., Elston, R. C., Dalferes, E. Jr, and Berenson, G. S. (1987). Segregation and linkage analysis of dopamine-β-hydroxylase activity in a six generation pedigree. *Am J. med. Genet.* **27**, 613–21.

Axelrod, F. B. and Pearson, J. (1987). Familial dysautonomia. In *Neurocutaneous diseases* (ed. M. R. Gomez), pp. 200–8. Butterworth, Stoneham, Massachusetts.

Biaggioni, I. and Robertson, D. (1987). Endogenous restoration of noradrenaline by precursor therapy in dopamine beta-hydroxylase deficiency. *Lancet* **ii**, 1170–2.

Biaggioni, I., Hollister, A. S., and Robertson, D. (1987). Dopamine in dopamine beta-hydroxylase deficiency. *New Engl. J. Med.* **317**, 1415–16.

Biaggioni, I., Goldstein, D. S., Atkinson, T., and Robertson, D. (1990). Dopamine beta-hydroxylase deficiency in humans. *Neurology* **40**, 370–3.

Birkmayer, W., Birkmayer, G., Lechner, H., and Riederer, P. (1983). DL-3, 4-threo-DOPS in Parkinson's disease: effects on orthostatic hypotension and dizziness. *J. neural Transmission* **58**, 305–13.

Cable, W. J. L., Kolodny, E. H., and Adams, R. D. (1982). Fabry disease: impaired autonomic function. *Neurology, NY* **32**, 498–502.

Clayton, P., Hyland, K., and Surtes, R. (1991). Autonomic effects of aromatic L-amino acid decarboxylase deficiency. *Clin. autonom. Res.* **1**, 83–4.

Cortelli, P., Parchi, P., Contin, M., Pierangeli, G., Avoni, P., Tinuper, P., Montagna, P., Barruzzi, A., Gambetti, P. L., and Lugaresi, E. (1991). Cardiovascular dysautonomia in fatal familial insomnia. *Clin. autonom. Res.* **1**, 15–22.

Craig, S. P., Buckle, V. J., Lamouroux, A., Mallet, J., and Craig, I. W. (1988). Localization of the human dopamine beta hydroxylase (DBH) gene to chromosome 9q34. *Cytogenet. Cell Genet.* **48**, 48–50.

Dunnette, J. and Weinshilboum, R. (1982). Family studies of plasma dopamine-β-hydroxylase thermal stability. *Am. J. human Genet.* **34**, 84–99.

Goldin, L. R. (1985). Segregation analysis of dopamine beta hydroxylase (DBH) and catechol-O-methyltransferase (COMT): identification of a major locus and polygenic components. *Genet. Epidmiol.* **2**, 317–25.

Goldin, L. R., Gershon, E. S., Lake, C. R., Murphy, D. L., McGinnis, M., and Sparkes, R. S. (1982). Segregation and linkage studies of plasma dopamine beta hydroxylase (DBH), erythrocyte catechol-O-methyltransferase (COMT) and platelet monoamine oxidase (MAO): possible linkage between the ABO locus and a gene controlling DBH activity. *Am. J. human Genet.* **34**, 250–62.

Hoeldtke, R. D., Cilmi, K. M., and Mattis-Graves, K. (1984). DL-Threo-3,4-dihydroxyphenylserine does not exert a pressor effect in orthostatic hypotension. *Clin. Pharmacol. Ther.* **36**, 302–6.

Ilson, J., Parrish, M., Fahn, S., and Cote, L. J. (1982). Familial Shy–Drager syndrome: clinical, biochemical and pathological findings. *Neurology* **32**, A160.

Joh, T. H., Baetge, E. E., Ross, M. E., and Reis, D. J. (1984). Biochemistry and biology of catecholamine neurons: a single gene or gene family hypothesis. *Clin. exp. Hypertension* **6A**, 11–21.

Kachi, T., Iwase, S., Mano, T., Saito, M., Kunimoto, M., and Sobue, I. (1988). Effect of L-threo-3,4-dihydroxyphenylserine on muscle sympathetic nerve activities in Shy–Drager syndrome. *Neurology* **38**, 1091–4.

Kato, T., Karai, N., Katsuyama, M., Nakamura, M., and Katsube, J. (1987). Studies on the activity of L-threo-3,4-dihydroxyphenylserine (L-DOPS) as a catecholamine precursor in the brain: Comparison with that of L-DOPA. *Biochem. Pharmacol.* **36**, 3051–7.

Kobayashi, K., Kurosawa, Y., Fujita, K., and Nagatsu, T. (1989). Human dopamine β-hydroxylase gene: two mRNA types having different 3'-terminal regions are produced through alternative polyadenylation. *Nucleic Acids Res.* **17**, 1089–102.

Lamouroux, A., Vigny, A., Faucon Biguet, N., Darmon, M. C., Franck, R., Henry, J.-P., and Mallet, J. (1987). The primary structure of human dopamine-β-hydroxylase: insights into the relationship between the soluble and the membrane-bound forms of the enzyme. *EMBO J* **6**, 3931–7.

Lewis, P. (1964). Familial orthostatic hypotension. *Brain* **87**, 719–28.

Man in't Veld, A. J., Boomsma, F., Moleman, P., and Schalekamp, M. A. D. H. (1987*a*). Congenital dopamine beta-hydroxylase deficiency. A novel orthostatic syndrome. *Lancet* **i**, 183–7.

Man in't Veld, A. J., Van den Meiracker, A. H., Boomsma, F., and Schalekamp, M. A. D. H. (1987*b*). Effect of unnatural noradrenaline precursor on sympathetic control and orthostatic hypotension in dopamine beta-hydroxylase deficiency. *Lancet* **ii**, 1172–5.

Man in't Veld, A. J., Boomsma, F., Lenders, J., Meiracker, A., Julien, C., Tulen, J., Moleman, P., Thien, T., Lamberts, S., and Schalekamp, M. A. D. H. (1988). Patients with congenital dopamine beta-hydroxylase deficiency. A lesson in catecholamine physiology. *Am. J. Hypertension* **1**, 231–8.

Mathias, C. J. (1991). Disorders of the autonomic nervous system. In *Neurology in clinical practice* (ed. W. G. Bradley, R. B. Daroff, G. M. Fenichel, and C. D. Marsden), pp. 1661–85. Butterworth, Stoneham, Massachusetts.

Mathias, C. J., Smith, A. D., Frankel, H. L., and Spalding, J. K. M. (1976). Dopamine beta-hydroxylase release during hypertension from sympathetic nervous overactivity in man. *Cardiovasc. Res.* **10**, 176–81.

Mathias, C. J., Bannister, R., Cortelli, P., Heslop, K., Polak, J. M., Raimbach, S., Springall, D. R., and Watson, L. (1990). Clinical, autonomic and therapeutic observations in two siblings with postural hypotension and sympathetic failure due to an inability to synthesize noradrenaline from dopamine because of a deficiency of dopamine beta-hydroxylase. *Quart. J. Med.* **75**, 617–33.

Menkes, J. H. (1987). Kinky hair disease. In *Neurocutaneous diseases* (ed. M. R. Gomez), pp. 284–93. Butterworth, Massachusetts.

O'Neill, B. P. (1987). Adrenoleukodystrophy. In *Neurocutaneous diseases* (ed. M. R. Gomez), pp. 273–83. Butterworths, Massachusetts.

Rea, R., Biaggioni, I., Robertson, R. M., Haile, V., and Robertson, D. (1990). Reflex control of sympathetic nerve activity in dopamine beta-hydroxylase deficiency. *Hypertension* **1**, 107–12.

Robertson, D., Goldberg, M. R., Onrot, J., Hollister, A. S., Wiley, R., Thompson, J. G., and Robertson, R. M. (1986). Isolated failure of autonomic noradrenergic neurotransmission. Evidence for impaired beta-hydroxylation of dopamine. *New Engl. J. Med.* **314**, 1494–7.

Sakoda, S., Suzuki, T., Higa, S., Ueji, M., Kishimoto, S., Matsumoto, M., and Yoneda, S. (1985). Treatment of orthostatic hypotension in Shy–Drager syndrome with DL-threo-3,4-dihydroxyphenylserine: a case report. *Eur. Neurol.* **24**, 330–4.

Senda, Y., Muto, T., Matsuoka, Y., Takahashi, A., and Sobue, I. (1987). Clinical effects of oral L-threo-3,4-dihydroxyphenylserine on orthostatic hypotension in patients with Shy–Drager syndrome. *Clin. Neurol.* **27**, 300–4.

Suzuki, S., Higa, S., Tsuga, I., Sakoda, S., Hayashi, A., Yamamura, Y., Takaba, Y., and Nakajima, A. (1980). Effects of infused L-threo-3,4-dihydroxyphenylserine in patients with familial amyloid polyneuropathy. *Eur. J. clin. Pharmacol.* **17**, 429–35.

Suzuki, T., Higa, S., Sakoda, S., Ueji, M., Hayashi, A., Takaba, Y., and Nakajima, A. (1982). Pharmacokinetic studies of oral L-threo-3,4-dihydroxy-phenylserine in normal subjects and patients with familial amyloid polyneuropathy. *Eur. J. clin. Pharmacol.* **23**, 463–8.

Taljanidisz, J., Stewart, L., Smith, A. J., and Klinman, J. P. (1989). Structure of bovine adrenal dopamine-β-monooxygenase, as deduced from cDNA and protein sequencing: evidence that the membrane form of the enzyme is anchored by an uncleaved signal peptide. *Biochemistry* **28**, 10054–61.

Taylor, C. S., Kent, U. M., and Fleming, P. J. (1989). The membrane-binding segment of dopamine-β-hydroxylase is not an uncleaved signal sequence. *J. Biol. Chem.* **264**, 14–16.

Thomas, P. K. (1989). Inherited autonomic neuropathies. In *New issues in neurosciences. Basic and clinical approaches.* Autonomic neuropathies, Vol. 1 (ed. P. K. Thomas), pp. 425–30 AIREN, Geneva.

Tulen, J. H. M., Man in't Veld, A. J., Mechelse, K., and Boomsma, F. (1990). Sleep patterns in congenital dopamine beta-hydroxylase deficiency. *J. Neurol.* **237**, 98–102.

Weinshilboum, R. M. (1979*a*). Serum dopamine beta-hydroxylase. *Pharmacol. Rev.* **30**, 133–66.

Weinshilboum, R. M. (1979*b*). Catecholamine biochemical genetics in human populations. In *Neurogenetics* (ed. X. O. Breakefield), pp. 257–82. Elsevier, New York.

Weishilboum, R. M. and Axelrod, J. (1971). Reduced plasma dopamine beta-hydroxylase in familial dysautonomia. *New Engl. J. Med.* **285**, 938.

Wilson, A. F., Elston, R. C., Siervogel, R. M., and Tran, L. D. (1988). Linkage of a gene regulating dopamine-β-hydroxylase activity and the ABO blood group locus. *Am. J. human Genet.* **42**, 160–6.

Wilson, A. F., Elston, R. C., Sellers, T. A., Bailey-Wilson, J. E., Gersting, J. M., Deen, D. K., Sorant, L. D., Tran, A. J. M., Amos, C. I., and Siervogel, R. M. (1990). Stepwise oligogenic segregation and linkage analysis illustrated with dopamine-β-hydroxylase activity. *Am. J. med. Genet.* **35**, 425–32.

PART VI

Other disorders affecting autonomic function

39. Syncope and fainting

Roger Hainsworth

Introduction

Syncope or fainting refers to a transient loss of consciousness resulting from inadequate cerebral blood flow. A syncopal attack is frequently preceded by sweating, pallor, blurring of vision, dizziness, and nausea. It is much less common in supine subjects and usually when subjects become supine during syncope they rapidly recover consciousness.

There is a wide variation in the susceptibility of individuals to syncope. The fainting of pregnant women or soldiers standing motionless on hot parade grounds is well known. On the other hand, patients in heart failure rarely, if ever, faint. Syncope does not usually point to organic disease, although it is clearly important to exclude diseases such as epilepsy, autonomic nervous disease, cerebrovascular disease, heart disease, particularly that involving the aortic valve, and various endocrine disorders. Most healthy individuals can precipitate at least presyncopal symptoms if, particularly in a warm environment (resulting in skin vasodilatation), they hyperventilate (to constrict cerebral blood vessels), and suddenly stand after having been in a crouching position (to allow abdominal blood vessels to fill with blood and to increase the height to which blood must be pumped to the brain). This is a well known 'mess trick'.

The actual onset of syncope can be quite abrupt. Usually preceding the faint there is an increased activity of the sympathetic nervous system leading to a maintained or sometimes increased blood pressure accompanied by increases in heart rate and vascular resistance. Then, quite suddenly, there is a profound fall in arterial blood pressure, inadequate cerebral perfusion, and loss of consciousness. Often the syncopal attack is accompanied by vasodilatation and bradycardia. This is the vasovagal attack, a term introduced in 1932 by Sir Thomas Lewis.

In this chapter, I first categorize the main causes of syncope. Then I discuss the control of cerebral blood flow since it is inadequacy of this that causes loss of consciousness. I also discuss the factors leading to vasodilatation and to bradycardia and the consequences of these responses for the maintenance of blood pressure. The vasovagal syncope is described and I suggest a number of physiological mechanisms which may trigger this response.

Causes of syncope

Syncope is due to cerebral hypoperfusion and this may result from either increased cerebral vascular resistance, as occurs when the carbon dioxide level is decreased by hyperventilation, or an inadequate cerebral perfusion pressure. Cerebral hypotension results from one or more of three possible deficiencies: deficient return of blood to the heart; deficient vasoconstriction; and deficient cardiac pumping.

Deficient venous return

It is axiomatic that the heart can pump no more than the quantity of blood returning from the veins. Venous return is impaired in the following.

1. *Postural hypotension.* In the upright position, more blood remains in dependent veins leading to a fall in cardiac output. Also, cerebral perfusion pressure decreases due to the altered position of the brain relative to the heart.

2. *Hypovolaemia.* Low blood volume, for example, following haemorrhage or treatment with diuretics, predisposes to postural fainting.

3. *Valsalva.* Deliberate Valsalva manoeuvres or increased straining in upright position, as in obstructed micturition or paroxysmal coughing, increases intrathoracic and intra-abdominal pressures and impedes return of blood to the heart.

4. *Capacitance vessel dilatation.* Accumulation of an excessive volume of blood in capacitance vessels (mainly veins), particularly those in the splanchnic vascular bed, may occur in response to some reflex stimuli and during vasodilator therapy.

Deficient vasoconstriction

Although cerebral blood flow shows autoregulation (see below) a minimum level of blood pressure is still required for adequate perfusion, particularly in the upright position, and blood pressure is directly related to the total systemic vascular resistance. Therefore, an inadequate vascular tone is a common cause of syncope. The following conditions are associated with failure of adequate vasoconstriction.

1. *Vagovagal syncope.* This is described in detail later in this chapter. The usual dominant feature is the sudden onset of vasodilatation immediately preceding syncope.

2. *Thermal stress.* Excessive cutaneous vasodilatation may lead to syncope.

3. *Reflex causes.* Changes in the level of stimulation of several reflexogenic areas may lead to vasodilatation. These include some visceral pain receptors, baroreceptors (e.g. 'carotid sinus syndrome'), decreased stimulation of visceral stretch receptors (e.g. voiding distended bladder resulting in micturition syncope).

4. *Drugs.* Particularly vasodilators.

5. *Peripheral neuropathy.* Autonomic impairment due to various diseases.

Cardiac causes

Failure of the heart to pump an adequate amount of blood may be the result of several conditions.

1. *Vascular stenosis or incompetence.* Aortic valve disease particularly is associated with syncope. In this condition, in addition to the obstruction to flow there may also be reflex vasodilatation due to stimulation of cardiac afferent nerves.

2. *Vasovagal syncope.* Although vasodilatation is the main cause of syncope, bradycardia occasionally may be so severe as to make a significant contribution.

3. *'Carotid sinus syndrome'.* Baroreceptor stimulation may lead to an exaggerated bradycardia, although the principal site of the abnormality along the reflex arc is uncertain.

4. *Bradyarrhythmias and tachyarrhythmias.* As explained below, abnormal increases as well as abnormal decreases in the heart rate substantially decrease cardiac output.

Cerebral blood flow

The blood flow to the human brain normally remains relatively constant. Unlike tissues such as muscle or glands, in which changes in metabolic activity result in large changes in blood flow, changes in cerebral activity result in changes in flow which are usually too localized and, overall, too small to be apparent in estimates of total flow. Typical values of cerebral blood flow are 50–60 ml/min per 100 g brain tissue, about 15 per cent of the resting cardiac output.

The brain cannot withstand more than a few seconds of total interruption of flow without loss of consciousness; interruption for prolonged periods results in irreversible damage.

Regulation of cerebral blood flow

Cerebral blood flow shows marked autoregulation. That is, over a wide range
of cerebral perfusion pressures, blood flow remains almost constant. There
are two mechanisms postulated for maintaining a constant flow to a region
when perfusion pressure decreases: a decrease in the degree of contraction
of arteriolar smooth muscle in response to decreased stretch (the myogenic
theory), and an increase in local concentrations of vasodilator metabolites
following a transient decrease in flow (the metabolic theory). In the brain
it seems likely that metabolic factors predominate although there may be a
myogenic component.

The innervation of cerebral blood vessels is relatively sparse and flow is
little affected by changes in activity in vasomotor nerves. Of much greater
importance is its control by vasodilator metabolic products. Changes in the
level of carbon dioxide in the arterial blood are particularly effective in causing
changes in cerebral blood flow. At normal levels of arterial pressure, an
increase in P_{CO_2} from 5.3 to 7 kPa approximately doubles cerebral flow
whereas a decrease to 4 kPa halves it. The level of CO_2 in the perfusing
blood also influences the autoregulation of cerebral blood flow. Autoregulation

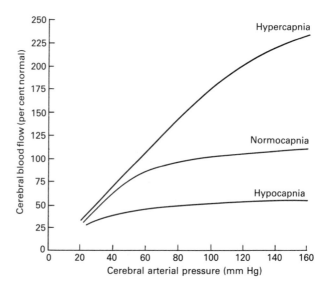

Fig. 39.1. Autoregulation of cerebral blood flow. The flow at normal cerebral
perfusion pressure and normal arterial P_{CO_2} is taken at 100 per cent. Cerebral
perfusion pressure (cerebral arterial pressure minus intracranial pressure) is
5-10 mm Hg less than cerebral arterial pressure. Above a pressure of about 60 mm
Hg the flow is largely independent of pressure. During hypercapnia the
autoregulation is largely lost. During hypocapnia blood flow is only about 50
per cent of the normal value, at all levels of CO_2.

is abolished during hypercapnia; during hypocapnia cerebral blood flow is markedly decreased at all perfusion pressures (Fig. 39.1).

The stimulus for vasodilatation is actually believed to be mediated through the hydrogen ion concentration in the cerebrospinal fluid (see Lassen 1974). Carbon dioxide crosses the blood–brain barrier and reacts with water to form carbonic acid and hence hydrogen ions in the cerebrospinal fluid.

Cerebral blood flow during hypotension

It must first be appreciated that in the upright position cerebral arterial pressure is 15–30 mm Hg lower than that in the aortic arch and the difference is even greater compared with that in a dependent arm (Fig. 39.2). Consciousness starts to be lost when cerebral blood flow falls below about 25 ml/min/100 g, half the normal flow. This level can be reached by severe

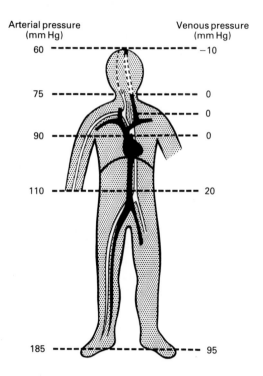

Fig. 39.2. Gravitational effects on arterial and venous blood pressures in erect motionless man. Arterial and venous pressures in the lower part of the body are increased and in the upper part of the body decreased. Note that cerebral arterial pressure is about 15 mm Hg lower than aortic root pressure. Because the brain is enclosed by rigid skull the venous pressures may be below atmospheric. This results in a relatively constant arterial–venous pressure difference in different parts of the brain. (From Hainsworth (1985).)

hypocapnia (P_{CO_2} less than 4 kPa) achieved by hyperventilation, or by cerebral arterial pressure falling below about 40 mm Hg (Fig. 39.1). Note that in the upright position the critical level of cerebral arterial pressure would correspond to a mean brachial arterial pressure of about 70 mm Hg; for example 90/60 mm Hg (mean pressure is approximately diastolic plus 1/3 pulse pressure). Syncope is much less likely to occur when subjects are supine partly because cerebral arterial pressure is then the same as aortic pressure and partly because there is less pooling of blood in dependent veins (cf. Fig. 39.2).

Vasodilatation

According to Poiseuille's equation, if other variables including blood pressure remain constant, an increase in the radius of a vessel would lead to an increase in flow. Indeed, because flow is a function of the fourth power of the radius, a doubling of radius results in a 16-fold increase in flow. Unless there is a response which prevents blood pressure from falling, vasodilatation also results in hypotension. By rearranging Poiseuille's equation, arterial pressure, P, can be seen to be dependent on cardiac output, $\dot{Q}$, and term r, relating to the radius of resistance vessels

$$P \propto \frac{\dot{Q}}{r^4}$$

Thus, the effect of vasodilatation on blood pressure depends on whether the change in r^4 is greater than the change in $\dot{Q}$.

Vasodilatation can be particularly pronounced in skeletal muscle. At rest in a comfortable environment, the cardiac output (typically about 5.5 l/min) is distributed so that less than 20 per cent of it perfuses skeletal muscle even though muscle comprises nearly half the tissue mass. During severe muscular exercise total muscle blood flow may increase from 1 l/min to 20 l/min and it forms the major part of the cardiac output. This intense vasodilatation, however, does not normally lead to a fall in blood pressure but is usually actually associated with a moderate increase in pressure. The main reason for this is that the contracting muscles and increased respiratory activity pump more blood back to the heart, and this increased venous return, together with an increased activity in cardiac sympathetic nerves, increases cardiac output.

The same effect does not occur when there is vasodilatation in the absence of increased muscular activity. Thus administration of vasodilator drugs, such as sodium nitroprusside, or pharmacologically blocking sympathetic vasoconstrictor activity result in vasodilatation with little accompanying increase in cardiac output and this results in a decrease in blood pressure.

Cutaneous vasodilatation occurs in response to heat stress. This is caused partly by a direct effect on the skin blood vessels and partly through a decrease in the discharge of cutaneous sympathetic vasoconstrictor fibres resulting from warming the temperature-regulating centres in the hypothalamus. The range of cutaneous blood flow has been estimated to lie between as little as 20 ml/min for the entire skin during cooling of both skin and body core to as much as 3 l/min during severe heat load (Folkow and Neil 1971). Thermally induced vasodilatation results in a decrease in total vascular resistance and an increased volume of blood in veins, and this may decrease cardiac output and blood pressure and predispose to fainting.

Mechanisms of vasodilatation

The diameter of blood vessels can change in response to neural, chemical, or mechanical influences.

At rest the degree of constriction of both resistance vessels (mainly arterioles) and capacitance vessels (mainly veins) is maintained by a tonic discharge in sympathetic vasoconstrictor (noradrenergic) nerves. A discharge frequency in these nerves of about 10 Hz results in near maximal vasoconstriction. However, at lower discharge frequencies (1–2 Hz) capacitance vessels are relatively more completely constricted than resistance vessels (Fig. 39.3). By determining the responses of resistance and capacitance

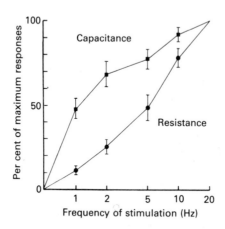

Fig. 39.3. Capacitance and resistance responses of abdominal circulation of anaesthetized dogs to stimulation of splanchnic nerves at various frequencies. Responses expressed as percentages of the changes at 20 Hz. Values are means ± SE from 14 dogs. Note that at 1 Hz the capacitance response was nearly 50 per cent of maximal whereas the resistance response was only about 10 per cent maximal. Above 2 Hz there was little further response of capacitance but larger responses of resistance. (Modified from Karim and Hainsworth (1976).)

to changes in carotid sinus pressure and relating them to the responses in the same animals to direct stimulation of sympathetic nerves, it is possible to infer that changes in carotid sinus pressure over the baroreceptor sensitivity range result in changes in sympathetic efferent discharge frequency between 0 and 5 Hz (Hainsworth and Karim 1976). Furthermore, it was shown that there was no apparent difference in the discharge frequency to resistance and capacitance vessels and this implies that, at most levels of pressure, capacitance vessels are more completely constricted than the resistance vessels. It should be noted that equating reflex responses with those occurring in response to regular stimulation of nerves may be an oversimplification since the spontaneous sympathetic discharge occurs irregularly in bursts (see Chapter 18).

At rest sympathetic nerves are tonically active at a mean frequency of about 1 Hz. Inhibition of this tone results in dilatation of resistance vessels leading to a decrease in vascular resistance. There is also dilatation of capacitance vessels, at least those in the abdominal circulation (see Hainsworth 1986), resulting in less blood returning to the heart and hence a decrease in cardiac output.

Vasodilatation in metabolically active tissues is largely brought about by locally produced chemical vasodilators. These are essentially the products of metabolic activity, so that the flow of blood through muscle, glands, etc. is directly related to their metabolism. Related to this is the phenomenon of autoregulation. This has already been mentioned in relation to the cerebral circulation but it is also observed to varying degrees in many other regions. It is likely that blood flow to most regions is determined by a balance between neurally mediated vasoconstriction and metabolically mediated vasodilatation. Flow is thus normally less than it would be if solely under the influence of metabolic vasodilators. Abrupt removal of the neural vasoconstrictor activity may therefore result in a transient reactive hyperaemia. This is illustrated in Fig. 39.4 in which it can be seen that, during constant pressure perfusion of a dog's hind limb, stimulation of the efferent sympathetic nerves at only 1 Hz decreased the blood flow by about 25 per cent. Immediately after switching off the stimulator, blood flow increased transiently to more than 30 per cent above the steady-state value obtained in absence of stimulation.

In some regions active vasodilatation may occur in response to stimulation of vasodilator nerves. These nerves have been identified in glandular tissue and appear to be peptidergic. In some subprimate species cholinergic sympathetic vasodilator nerves have been identified in skeletal muscle. The existence of these fibres has been demonstrated either by pharmacologically blocking the vasoconstrictor fibres and then stimulating the efferent sympathetic nerves or by stimulating a region in the hypothalamus (the so-called defence area) and observing vasodilatation in skeletal muscle which could be blocked by atropine. In this way evidence of cholinergic sympathetic vasodilator fibres to skeletal muscle has been demonstrated in the cat, dog,

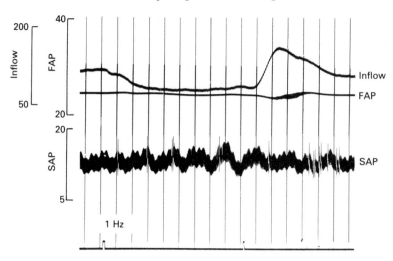

Fig. 39.4. Responses of blood flow, in a dog's hind limb perfused at constant pressure, to electrical stimulation of the lumbar sympathetic trunk. Event marker shows start and end of stimulation. Traces are of flow (ml/min), femoral arterial perfusion pressure (FAP) and systemic arterial blood pressure (SAP) in kPa (1 kPa = 7.5 mm Hg). Note that flow is reduced during period of stimulation and that it overshoots transiently on cessation of the stimulus. (Modified from Hainsworth *et al.* (1983).)

fox, jackal, and mongoose, but not in the rabbit, hare, badger, polecat, or in any of seven species of primate studied (Uvnas, 1966).

Do sympathetic vasodilator nerves occur in man?

It was formerly assumed that man, like the dog and the cat, possesses cholinergic sympathetic vasodilator nerves to his skeletal muscle. The evidence in support of this comes largely from experiments, by Barcroft, Edholm, and Greenfield, on the responses of humans to decreasing circulating blood volume and emotional stress. Barcroft *et al.* (1944) and Barcroft and Edholm (1945) induced fainting by withdrawing blood and applying tourniquets to the thighs. Fainting was immediately preceded by an abrupt increase in forearm blood flow which was prevented by sympathectomy or nerve block. In subjects in whom unilateral sympathectomy had been performed it was noted that the flow in the innervated limb increased to become greater than that in the blocked limb, and this was considered to be evidence of *active* vasodilatation. Blair *et al.* (1959) devised a number of ingenious stressful procedures for medical students, including mental arithmetic, physiology tests, simulated haemorrhage, and offering a dead rabbit's blood and stomach content for drinking! These procedures resulted in muscle vasodilatation.

This was usually smaller following sympathetic blockade or administration of atropine and this led the authors to suggest that the response was mediated by cholinergic nerves.

The evidence against the existence of cholinergic vasodilator nerves in man is more persuasive. First, Uvnas (1966) obtained evidence for these nerves only in some subprimate species and not in any of several primates studied. So their existence in man seems unlikely. Second, the observation that flow in an innervated limb increases transiently to become greater than in a sympathectomized limb does not prove active vasodilatation because it is likely that there would have been reactive hyperaemia following abrupt withdrawal of sympathetic tone. It can be seen from Fig. 39.4 that removal of even a low level of sympathetic efferent activity resulted in an increase in flow which was transiently greater than the steady-state sympathectomized level.

The evidence in support of active cholinergic vasodilatation provided by the administration of atropine is also not conclusive because, although atropine blocks the bradycardia occurring during a vasovagal attack, the fall in blood pressure is not prevented (Lewis 1932). Also, intraarterial atropine failed to block completely the limb vasodilatation in response to stress (Blair et al. 1959). A further elegant piece of evidence against active vasodilatation was provided by Walling and Sundlöf (1982) who recorded activity in efferent sympathetic nerves in two humans during vasovagal fainting. They observed an abrupt cessation of nervous activity with the onset of the hypotension, but there was no suggestion of any increase in other nervous activity which would have been expected if vasodilator nerves had become active.

Bradycardia

In resting subjects, heart rate tends to vary inversely with arterial blood pressure. This is Marey's law and it is an effect of the arterial baroreceptor reflex. In circumstances in which there is a widespread increase in the level of sympathetic activity, such as during exercise, heart rate and blood pressure both increase.

Heart rate is controlled mainly by the activity in the vagus and sympathetic nerves, although it is also influenced by body temperature and the concentrations of various hormones, particularly catecholamines. At rest there is a tonic vagal activity which tends to decrease during inspiration resulting in sinus arrhythmia. Intense vagal activity causes profound bradycardia and can even result in a period of asystole. However, during prolonged vagal stimulation there is usually vagal 'escape' which prevents a potentially dangerous prolonged asystole.

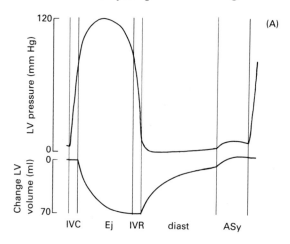

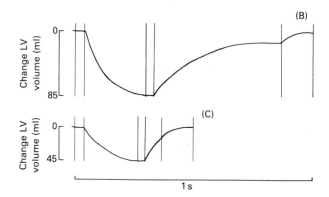

Fig. 39.5. Diagramatic representation of left ventricular (LV) pressures and volumes during the cardiac cycle and the influence of heart rate. IVC, isovolumic contraction phase; Ej, ejection phase; IVR, isovolumic relaxation phase; diast, ventricular and atrial diastole; ASy, atrial systole. (A) shows pressure and volume changes at a heart rate of 80 beats/min (cycle length 0.75 s). Note the rapid ventricular filling during early diastole and the contribution of atrial systole. Stroke volume is 70 ml and cardiac output is 5.6 l/min. (B) shows volume changes at a heart rate of 60 beats/min (cycle length 1.0 s). Diastole is prolonged and there is a period of diastasis during which ventricular filling virtually ceases. Stroke volume increased to 85 ml and cardiac output is only slightly reduced at 5.1 l/min. (C) shows volume changes at a heart rate of 120 beats/min (cycle length 0.5 s). The shortening is mainly at the expense of diastole which is greatly reduced. Atrial systole now makes a major contribution to ventricular filling. Stroke volume decreases to 45 ml and cardiac output remains almost unchanged at 5.4 l/min.

Effect of heart rate on cardiac output

Every student knows the relationship between cardiac output, $\dot{Q}$, heart rate, HR, and stroke volume, SV, to be $\dot{Q} = HR \times SV$. This equation is mathematically unarguable but can be physiologically misleading. It is undeniable that a profound bradycardia with periods of asystole results in a low cardiac output. If a heart is distended, cardiac output is directly proportional to heart rate. However, in resting subjects a change in heart rate between about 60 and 120 beats/min has a relatively small effect on cardiac output and, above about 120 beats/min, output may decrease. The reason for this apparent anomaly is that an increase in rate is offset by a decrease in stroke volume. The main effect of an increase in heart rate could be to *permit* an increase in output to occur. Thus an increase in venous return could not increase cardiac output to the same extent if heart rate remained unchanged, but an increase in rate without an increase in venous return would have little effect. The effect of a change in heart rate on cardiac output is explained by Fig. 39.5. A decrease in heart rate from 80 to 60 beats/min lengthens diastolic filling time and the output per minute is little changed. Similarly, moderate increases in heart rate have only a small effect on cardiac output. However, at very slow heart rates, there would be a prolonged period of diastasis during which filling would cease and so output would fall. At very fast heart rates, although systole is slightly shortened, most of the shortening is at the expense of diastolic filling time and cardiac output again falls.

The effect of a change in heart rate on cardiac output is thus dependent on the rate of venous filling and also on whether it is accompanied by a change in the inotropic state. During exercise, an increase in heart rate is accompanied by a positive inotropic change which, importantly, causes a reduction in the duration of systole thus protecting diastole. Venous filling pressure is high and this results in a large increase in output. On the other hand, during syncope due to hypovolaemia or peripheral vasodilatation, it is likely that venous filling pressure would be low and changes in heart rate would have little effect on cardiac output. This implies that, except in cases in which heart rate is very slow (less than about 40 beats/min), bradycardia is unlikely to make a major contribution to a fall in arterial blood pressure.

Factors predisposing to syncope

In the early part of this chapter, I listed several factors which predisposed to syncope. The cardiac and neural causes of syncope are dealt with in other chapters of this book. However, by far the most common factor predisposing to syncope is a reduction in the return of blood to the heart. Thus fainting almost always occurs during standing, or occasionally sitting, when dependent veins become distended with blood. The effects of posture are enhanced by performing the Valsalva manoeuvre. In this, intrathoracic and intraabdominal pressures are increased by expiring against a resistance or a closed glottis. Initially, the Valsalva results in an increase in arterial blood pressure as the thoracic and abdominal arteries are compressed. After a few seconds, owing to a decreased venous return into the abdomen and thorax due to the high pressures, cardiac output and blood pressure falls and this can lead to syncope. Two clinical manifestations of this are cough syncope and micturition syncope.

Paroxysms of coughing are effectively a Valsalva manoeuvre, but, in addition, there may be reflex vasodilatation from stimulation of airways receptors. If sufficiently intense or prolonged, syncope may result.

Micturition syncope is particularly interesting as many diverse mechanisms seem to operate. Usually the problem occurs when a man stands to micturate after leaving a warm bed. He is vasodilated and therefore peripheral vascular resistance is low. He stands motionless so that the muscle pump mechanism does not operate and the dependent capacitance vessels distend leading to a decrease in venous return. He may have an enlarged prostate and have to perform a Valsalva type of strain. Relief of bladder distension may also result in reflex vasodilatation as the result of a reduced stimulus to bladder stretch receptors (Mary 1989).

The vasovagal syncope

Lewis (1932) described fainting attacks as being vasovagal because they were accompanied by hypotension and bradycardia. He considered that bradycardia usually was not the main cause of the faint since heart rate rarely fell to very low levels (less than 40 beats/min) and the hypotension was little affected by the administration of atropine which prevented the bradycardia. We recently studied two patients who developed profound bradycardia and hypotension during passive head-up tilting. After demand pace-makers had been implanted in these patients, tilting no longer resulted in bradycardia, but both patients still showed almost identical decreases in blood pressure at the same times after tilting.

Barcroft et al. (1944) performed an illuminating study in which they induced fainting in healthy subjects by bleeding and application of tourniquets to the legs. They observed that, before the onset of the faint, heart rate increased and there was also an increase in vascular resistance shown by blood pressure being relatively little changed despite a decrease in cardiac output. During the faint, blood pressure decreased abruptly, accompanied by decreases in heart rate and vascular resistance, but no further fall and perhaps even a small increase in cardiac output. Similar observations, of a fall in vascular resistance but no further fall in cardiac output

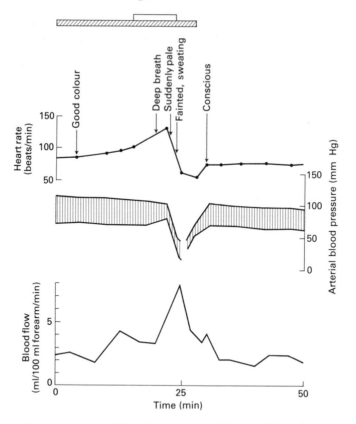

Fig. 39.6. Heart rate, arterial blood pressure, and forearm blood flow in a human subject during a haemorrhagic faint. Shaded bar: venous return impeded by application of tourniquets to both thighs; open bar; venesection. Note that initially blood pressure was relatively well maintained but that heart rate was increased. Then heart rate slowed and blood pressure fell. This was accompanied by an increase in forearm blood flow. (From Barcroft and Edholm (1945).)

during fainting, have also been made by Weissler *et al.* (1957) and Glick and Yu (1963).

Barcroft and Edholm (1945) reported an increase in forearm blood flow during fainting (Fig. 39.6) and suggested that the hypotension was due mainly to dilatation of vessels in skeletal muscle. However, more recent work has suggested that vasodilatation in hypotensive haemorrhage may be more widespread (Vatner and Morita 1987).

Emotional stress leads to increases in heart rate and blood pressure with little change in total vascular resistance. However, if a vasovagal faint occurs, blood pressure, heart rate, and forearm vascular resistance decrease abruptly.

Thus, a vasovagal attack is usually preceded by evidence of increased sympathetic and decreased vagal activity. During this stage blood pressure is maintained or, particularly in emotional faints, increased. The vasovagal attack is characterized by sudden onset of hypotension and bradycardia. The main cause of the hypotension is usually vasodilatation in skeletal muscle and probably elsewhere, due to inhibition of sympathetic vasoconstrictor activity. The bradycardia is usually relatively unimportant because heart rate is seldom greatly slowed and cardiac output does not usually decrease with the onset of the faint. Furthermore, prevention of bradycardia by pacing the heart does not necessarily prevent or even delay syncope.

Possible physiological mechanisms precipitating vasovagal attacks

Although much is known of the factors predisposing to fainting attacks and there have been several analyses of the haemodynamic changes which occur before and during the faint, the mechanism responsible for suddenly switching a response of tachycardia and vasoconstriction to one of bradycardia and vasodilatation remains a matter for speculation. A number of possibilities have been suggested.

An abnormal baroreceptor reflex

Glick and Yu (1963) suggested that the 'trigger' for a vasovagal attack was a transient increase in the stimulation of arterial baroreceptors. This effect might occur in emotional fainting which is accompanied by an initial increase in blood pressure. It is also conceivable that the gain of the baroreceptor reflex might be increased in some circumstances and there is some evidence that angiotensin and vasopressin may act on the central nervous pathways to have this effect (Bishop and Hasser 1987).

In the so-called carotid sinus syndrome, syncope can result from an exaggerated baroreceptor reflex. In the original classical case, syncope was precipitated by pressure on the sinus from a stiff winged collar. Usually, however, the precipitating cause is unknown. Attacks are characterized by bradycardia and hypotension. The bradycardia can be prevented by cardiac pacing or administration of atropine but this may not prevent the fall in blood pressure (Almqvist et al. 1985). The site of the abnormality in the carotid sinus syndrome is unlikely to be in the carotid sinus itself and may be at any site on the reflex arc, including the sinus node. It may be difficult to distinguish from other causes of vasovagal syncope and indeed many patients with unexplained syncope have been shown to have an abnormally sensitive carotid sinus reflex (Wahbha et al. 1989).

Emotional stress

Electrical stimulation of a region within the hypothalamus of anaesthetized cats, the 'defence area', results in increases in heart rate and blood pressure and vasodilatation in skeletal muscle which is blocked by atropine (Eliasson *et al.* 1951). Similar responses were also observed in conscious cats during electrical stimulation of the same area or in response to the application of certain auditory, visual, or cutaneous stimuli (Abrahams *et al.* 1964). This is the 'defence reaction'.

Emotional stress in humans can also result in quite marked cardiovascular changes, including tachycardia, hypertension, and muscle vasodilatation. Barcroft *et al.* (1960) considered that these responses were comparable to the defence reaction in animals. However, in humans the vasodilator responses were little affected by atropine and can be attributed to increases in circulating adrenaline and reduction of vasoconstrictor activity.

In susceptible subjects severe stress can lead to a vasovagal syncope. The tachycardia and hypertension abruptly give way to bradycardia and hypotension. This response does not occur in animals during hypothalamic stimulation.

Stimulation of cardiac receptors

It was shown over 120 years ago by von Bezold and Hirt that intravenous injections of certain chemicals, including veratrum alkaloids, resulted in bradycardia and vasodilatation. Subsequently, Jarisch and later Dawes showed that this reflex could be obtained from stimulation of reflexogenic areas in the heart and particularly those in the left ventricle. The response of bradycardia and hypotension following chemical stimulation of cardiac receptors has become known as the Bezold–Jarisch reflex or the coronary chemoreflex (for references see Hainsworth 1991). The hypotension following chemical stimulation of cardiac afferent nerves may be very profound and can be attributed mainly to dilatation of resistance and capacitance vessels (McGregor *et al.* 1986). The lower part of Fig. 39.7 shows the effects in an anaesthetized dog preparation of injection of veratridine into the blood perfusing the coronary arteries. In addition to an immediate bradycardia, there was a fall in systemic arterial pressure which, during constant flow perfusion, denotes vasodilatation.

Similar responses may also occur in humans following injection of contrast medium into the coronary circulation or during periods of myocardial ischaemia (see Hainsworth 1991). It is generally thought to be unlikely that such a powerful reflex would be elicited only following injections of toxic chemicals or during pathological conditions and there now is evidence that mechanical stimulation of ventricular receptors by physiological changes in pressure also results in vasodilatation (Challenger *et al.* 1987; Tutt *et al.* 1988; Fig. 39.7 top). It has been suggested that unmyelinated ventricular afferent nerves are strongly excited during haemorrhage (Thorén 1987). The proposed mechanism of excitation is an increased force of ventricular contraction, brought about by an increased activity in cardiac sympathetic nerves,

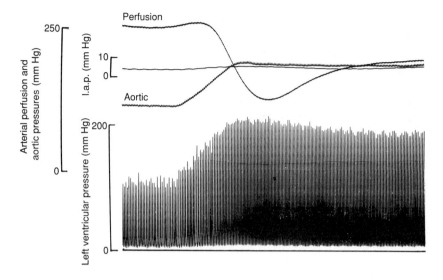

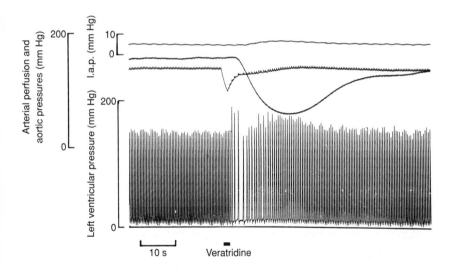

Fig. 39.7. Responses in anaesthetized dog to (top) mechanical and (bottom) chemical stimulation of ventricular receptors. The systemic circulation was perfused at constant flow so that arterial perfusion pressure provides an index of vascular resistance. Traces are of perfusion pressure, left atrial pressure (l.a.p.), aortic root pressure, and left ventricular pressure, all in mm Hg. An increase in aortic root pressure, including coronary arterial and left ventricular pressures, results in vasodilatation, but no change in heart rate. Injection of veratridine (25 μg) into the aortic root results in both vasodilatation and bradycardia.

accompanied by a reduced ventricular filling. In addition to bradycardia and vasodilatation, stimulation of ventricular receptors also results in a reflex relaxation of the stomach and this could explain the feeling of nausea in some patients suffering from myocardial ischaemia.

Initiation of a powerful depressor reflex by stimulation of cardiac ventricular receptors offers a plausible explanation for the vasovagal attack since this is usually preceded by tachycardia, reduced cardiac output, and evidence of increased cardiac sympathetic stimulation. Some recent reports (Almqvist *et al.* 1989; Grubb *et al.* 1991) have noted that the incidence of syncope, in patients during upright tilting, is increased by infusion of isoprenaline. This was attributed to the increased cardiac inotropic state causing increased stimulation of ventricular receptors. This however, may not be the only mechanism whereby isoprenaline provokes syncope as it is also a β_2-adrenoceptor agonist and results in vasodilatation. Abboud (1989) suggested that syncope may result from an abnormal sensitivity of the ventricular receptor reflex in the same way as it is said also to be caused by carotid sinus hypersensitivity. However, the role of ventricular receptors must remain speculative for several reasons. Firstly, relatively few ventricular receptors are excited in this way (Öberg and Thorén 1972) and a recent study showed that the reflex responses to mechanical stimulation of ventricular receptors were not enhanced by sympathetic stimulation (Al-Timman and Hainsworth 1988). Furthermore, if it is a simple reflex effect, it is not clear why it should persist some time after the stimulus has ceased, i.e. the bradycardia and hypotension should immediately remove the stimulus to the receptors. Vatner and Morita (1987) reported that, in unanaesthetized animals during hypotensive haemorrhage, there was a decrease in efferent renal nerve activity which was not prevented by vagal denervation, a procedure which would have blocked afferent activity from cardiac receptors. They also made the interesting observation that blockade of opiate receptors by naloxone, while it did not affect the initial increase in renal nerve activity during non-hypotensive haemorrhage, it did prevent the decrease during hypotensive haemorrhage.

Summary and conclusions

Syncope refers to a transient loss of consciousness when cerebral blood flow is impaired. The critical level of cerebral arterial pressure is about 40 mm Hg and this is reached more readily in the upright subject than when supine. Usually, before the faint there is evidence of an increased activity in the sympathetic nerves. At the onset of a vasovagal attack there is a sudden vasodilatation in skeletal muscle (and probably in other regions) and bradycardia. In most faints the major factor is probably vasodilatation, which results from inhibition of sympathetic vasoconstrictor activity and leads to a decrease in vascular resistance and therefore in blood pressure. However, in some individuals in whom the heart rate decreases below about 40 beats/min bradycardia may also be of some importance.

The mechanism responsible for initiating a vasovagal attack is still unknown. It is likely to be preceded by a decrease in the circulating blood volume, as in postural stress or haemorrhage, and rarely occurs in hypervolaemic individuals, such as those in heart failure. It may also occur in susceptible individuals following emotional stress. Several trigger mechanisms have been proposed. These include stimulation of arterial baroreceptors, the responses to which may be abnormally sensitive, as in the so-called carotid sinus syndrome or as the result of chemical effects on the central nervous pathways. The defence reaction of animals, in which there is tachycardia, hypertension, and muscle vasodilatation in response to hypothalamic stimulation or emotional stress, may have a counterpart in the human. However, in animals this response does not develop into a vasovagal attack. There have also been suggestions that the vasovagal attack may be caused by the Bezold–Jarisch reflex in which stimulation of cardiac ventricular receptors, by powerful contraction on a nearly empty ventricle, may initiate a profound depressor response. However, the evidence on this too is controversial and the mechanism responsible for inducing the vasodilatation and bradycardia still remains to be elucidated.

The physiological advantage to a subject or to the species of a vasovagal attack can only be speculated upon. It is certainly true that the maintenance of an adequate blood flow, particularly to the cerebral circulation, is infinitely more important than the control of arterial blood pressure. Since fainting is much more likely to occur when subjects are upright than when supine, a response that renders a subject supine and thereby assists venous return and cerebral perfusion could be argued to be beneficial. However, there is no evidence that the response has evolved for this purpose, particularly since the actual stimulus is unknown, and it may simply be a coincidental response, the real function of which is concerned with some entirely different purpose.

References

Abboud, F. M. (1989). Ventricular syncope. Is the heart a sensory organ? *New Engl. J. Med.* **320**, 390–2.

Abrahams, V. C., Hilton, S. M., and Zbrozyna, A. W. (1964). The role of active muscle vasodilatation in the alerting stage of the defence reaction. *J. Physiol.* **171**, 189–202.

Almqvist, A., Gornick, C., Benson, D. W. Jr, Dunnigan, A., and Benditt, D. G. (1985). Carotid sinus hypersensitivity: evaluation of the vasodepressor component. *Circulation* **71**, 927–36.

Almqvist, A., Goldenberg, I. E., Milstein, S., Chen, M. Y., Chen, X., Hansen, R., Gornick, C. G., and Benditt, D. G. (1989). Provocation of bradycardia and hypotension by isoproterenol and upright posture in patients with unexplained syncope. *New Engl. J. Med.* **320**, 345–51.

Al-Timman, J. K. A. and Hainsworth, R. (1988). The effects of efferent sympathetic nerve stimulation on reflex vascular responses to changes in ventricular pressure in anaesthetized dogs. *J. Physiol.* **409**, 63P.

Barcroft, H. and Edholm, O. G. (1945). On the vasodilatation in human skeletal muscle during post-haemorrhagic fainting. *J. Physiol.* **104**, 161–75.

Barcroft, H., McMichael, J., and Sharpey-Schafer, E. P. (1944). Posthaemorrhagic fainting. Study by cardiac output and forearm flow. *Lancet* **i**, 489–91.

Barcroft, H., Brod, J., Heijl, Z., Hirsjarvi, E. A., and Kitchen, A. H. (1960). The mechanisms of the vasodilatation in the forearm muscle during stress (mental arithmetic). *Clin. Sci.* **19**, 577–86.

Bishop, V. S. and Hasser, E. M. (1987). Physiological role of ventricular receptors. In *Cardiogenic reflexes* (eds R. Hainsworth, P. N., McWilliam, and D. A. S. G. Mary), pp. 62–73. Oxford University Press, Oxford.

Blair, D. A., Glover, W. E., Greenfield, A. D. M., and Roddie, I. S. (1959). Excitation of cholinergic vasodilator nerves to human skeletal muscles during emotional stress. *J. Physiol.* **148**, 633–47.

Challenger, S., McGregor, K. H., and Hainsworth, R. (1987). Peripheral vascular responses to changes in left ventricular pressure in anaesthetized dogs. *Quart. J. exp. Physiol.* **72**, 271–83.

Eliasson, S., Folkow, B., Lindgren, P., and Uvnas, B. (1951). Activation of sympathetic vasodilator nerves to the skeletal muscles in the cat by hypothalamic stimulation. *Acta physiol. scand.* **23**, 333–51.

Folkow, B. and Neil, E. (1971). *Circulation.* Oxford University Press, Oxford.

Glick, G. and Yu, P. N. (1963). Haemodynamic changes during spontaneous vasovagal reactions. *Am. J. Med.* **34**, 42–50.

Grubb, B. P., Temesy-Armos, P., Hahn, H., and Elliott, L. (1991). Utility of upright tilt-table testing in the evaluation and management of syncope of unknown origin. *Am. J. Med.* **90**, 6–10.

Hainsworth, R. (1985). Arterial blood pressure. In *Hypotensive anaesthesia* (ed. G. E. H. Enderby), pp. 3–29. Churchill Livingstone, Edinburgh.

Hainsworth, R. (1986). Vascular capacitance: its control and importance. *Rev. Physiol. Biochem. Pharmacol.* **105**, 101–73.

Hainsworth, R. (1991). Reflexes from the heart. *Physiol. Rev.* **71**, 617–658.

Hainsworth, R. and Karim, F. (1976). Responses of abdominal vascular capacitance in the anaesthetized dog to changes in carotid sinus pressure. *J. Physiol.* **262**, 659–77.

Hainsworth, R., McGregor, K. H., and Wood, L. M. (1983). Hind-limb vascular-capacitance responses in anaesthetized dogs. *J. Physiol.* **337**, 417–28.

Hainsworth, R., McGregor, K. H., and Ford, R. (1986). Effect of veratridine injected into the aortic root on resistance and capacitance in the abdominal circulation in anaesthetized dogs. *Quart. J. exp. Physiol.* **71**, 589–98.

Karim, F. and Hainsworth, R. (1976). Responses of abdominal vascular capacitance to stimulation of splanchnic nerves. *Am. J. Physiol.* **231**, 434–40.

Lassen, N. A. (1974). Control of cerebral circulation in health and disease. *Circulation Res.* **34**, 749–60.

Lewis, T. (1932). Vasovagal syncope and the carotid sinus mechanism. *Br. med. J.* **1**, 873–6.

Mary, D. A. S. G. (1989). The urinary bladder and cardiovascular reflexes. *Int. J. Cardiol.* **23**, 11–17.

McGregor, K. H., Hainsworth, R., and Ford, R. (1986). Hind-limb vascular responses in anaesthetized dogs to aortic root injections of veratridine. *Quart. J. exp. Physiol.* **71**, 577–87.

Öberg, B. and Thorén, P. (1972). Increased activity in left ventricular receptors during hemorrhage or occlusion of the caval veins in the cat. A possible cause of vasovagal reaction. *Acta physiol. scand.* **85**, 164–73.

Thorén, P. (1987). Depressor reflexes from the heart during severe haemorrhage. In *Cardiogenic reflexes* (ed. R. Hainsworth, P. N. McWilliam, and D. A. S. G. Mary), pp. 389–401. Oxford University Press, Oxford.

Tutt, S. M., McGregor, K. H., and Hainsworth, R. (1988). Reflex vascular responses to changes in left ventricular pressure in anaesthetized dogs. *Quart. J. exp. Physiol.* **73**, 425–31.

Uvnas, B. (1966). Cholinergic vasodilator nerves. *Fed. Proc.* **25**, 1618–22.

Vatner, S. F. and Morita, H. (1987). Biphasic responses of renal nerve activity to haemorrhage in the conscious animal. In *Cardiogenic reflex* (ed. R. Hainsworth, P. N. McWilliam, and D. A. S. G. Mary), pp. 402–10. Oxford University Press, Oxford.

Wahbha, M. M. A. E., Morley, C. A., Al-Shamma, Y. M. H., and Hainsworth, R. (1989). Cardiovascular reflex responses in patients with unexplained syncope. *Clin. Sci.* **77**, 547–53.

Wallin, B. G. and Sundlöf, G. (1982). Sympathetic outflow to muscle during vasovagal syncope. *J. autonom. nerv. system.* **6**, 287–91.

Weissler, A. M., Warren, J. V., Estes, E. H., McIntosh, H. D., and Leonard, J. J. (1957) Vasodepressor syncope. Factors influencing cardiac output. *Circulation* **15**, 875–82.

40. The autonomic nervous system and cardiac dysrhythmias

Nicholas A. Flores and Desmond J. Sheridan

Introduction

The electrical and mechanical functions of the heart are controlled through both the sympathetic and parasympathetic nervous systems which innervate the heart extensively. To achieve the degree of stabilization of cardiac function necessary in a complex, intact organism, regularity of cardiac rhythm is essential. If myocardial contraction and relaxation are altered, changes in cardiac output may follow. Pathological uncompensated reductions in cardiac output and stroke volume may lead to syncope, as discussed in the preceding chapter. The observation in man that syncope may be associated with cardiac electrophysiological changes and arrhythmias (during Adams–Stokes attacks, for example) demonstrates the importance of the maintenance of normal cardiac rhythm. This chapter will outline briefly the mechanisms through which cardiac cellular electrophysiological changes can promote arrhythmogenesis.

Regulation of normal sinus rhythm

Under normal conditions the heart exhibits three main electrophysiological properties which ensure control of the cardiac rhythm, these are: pace-maker activity; ordered conduction; and refractoriness. Changes in these electrophysiological properties and in the responsiveness of myocardial cells to neural and humoral stimulation can result in arrhythmogenesis.

Pace-maker activity

Under normal conditions, the sinus node is the cardiac pace-maker. Other cells which exhibit diastolic depolarization are also potential pace-makers with the capacity to generate action potentials and excite adjacent myocytes. Diastolic depolarization, and thus activity in the sinus node, is regulated by the autonomic nervous system. At the cellular level, depolarization occurs in sinus node cells due to inward currents carried by sodium and calcium ions and a reduced outward potassium current, which together produce an increased intracellular positive charge (depolarization). Once this depolarization reaches a threshold value, action potentials can be initiated and propagated. Sinus node activity controls cardiac rhythm since: (1) not all myocytes are pace-makers; and (2) pace-maker activity occurring in other tissues (the atrioventricular node and His–Purkinje fibres) is such that the rate of diastolic depolarization in these is slower than in the sinus node cells.

Autonomic activity is regulated in the brainstem to allow integration of information from higher cortical centres and the periphery. Sympathetic fibres

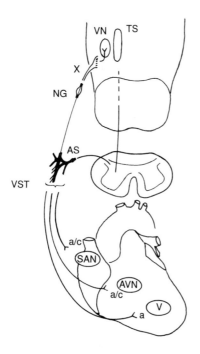

Fig. 40.1. Autonomic neural supply to the heart. Information from the periphery and higher cortical centres is integrated in the tractus solitarius (TS) and influences parasympathetic output from the vagal nucleus (VN) and sympathetic output from the vasomotor centre. Parasympathetic fibres pass in the vagus nerve (X) via the nodose ganglion (NG); sympathetic fibres pass down the inter-mediolateral columns of the spinal cord and emerge through the upper 6–7 thoracic rami communicantes. These pass through the stellate ganglion and ansa subclavia (AS) to join the vagal parasympathetic fibres, forming the vagosympathetic trunk (VST) of mixed nerves which innervate the heart. Sinoatrial (SAN) and atrioventricular (AVN) node cells receive adrenergic (a) and cholinergic (c) fibres, whereas the ventricular myocardium (V) receives predominantly adrenergic fibres.

supply the sinus node, atria, atrioventricular node, ventricles, and coronary arteries; parasympathetic fibres supply the sinus node, atrioventricular node, coronary arteries, ventricles and the atria (but to a lesser extent) (Fig. 40.1). Sympathetic stimulation increases the rate of diastolic depolarization, increasing heart rate, while parasympathetic stimulation produces hyperpolarization (i.e. the transmembrane potential becomes more negative) without changing the rate of diastolic depolarization so that a longer period is needed to reach the threshold for action potential initiation and propagation, effectively reducing heart rate (Fig. 40.2).

Conduction

Co-ordination of atrial and ventricular activation is achieved in the normal heart through the anatomical and physiological properties of the conduction system. The slow-conducting properties of the atrioventricular node protect the ventricles from rapid, disorganized atrial activity but, once the impulse has passed this point, the fast conducting properties of the His–Pukinje fibres ensure rapid, co-ordinated ventricular activation. Uniform ventricular contraction and synchronized depolarization and repolarization throughout the ventricles are the results. Clearly, localized disordered conduction will disturb this and is important in the development of re-entry arrhythmias (Fig. 40.3)

Refractoriness

Once a cardiac myocyte has been depolarized, it is refractory to further stimulation for a specific period of time. In normal cells the refractory

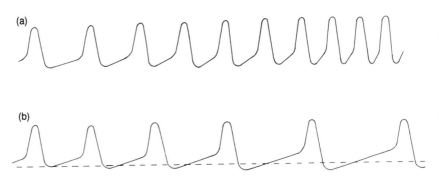

Fig. 40.2. Electrophysiological effects of autonomic neural stimulation of sinus node cells. (a) Sympathetic stimulation increases the rate of diastolic depolarization, allowing the threshold for propagation of an action potential to be reached earlier, increasing heart rate. (b) Parasympathetic stimulation produces a more negative transmembrane potential and, since the rate of depolarization is unchanged, a longer period is required to reach the threshold for propagation of an action potential (shown by the dashed line), reducing heart rate.

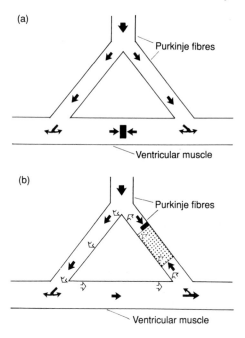

Fig. 40.3. Schematic diagram illustrating how conduction block and changes in refractoriness may contribute to re-entry and arrhythmogenesis. (a) illustrates the normal situation in which the wave of depolarization is conducted through the Purkinje fibres to the ventricular muscle fibres. Re-entry is prevented by the refractoriness of the fibres once stimulated. (b) illustrates how conduction and refractoriness may be altered if conduction is slowed or blocked completely by damage to the fibres (shown by the shaded region). In this situation, anterograde conduction may be blocked, but the impulse may be able to travel in a retrograde direction, re-exciting cells which have overcome their refractory period (shown by the open arrows) and allowing the development of a re-entry circuit which may be resistant to control by higher pace-makers.

period corresponds closely with action potential duration, ensuring rhythmic contraction, an adequate time for ventricular filling, and the orderly spread of activation through the heart. Refractoriness also prevents re-entry, or re-activation of previously activated regions of the heart. Changes in refractoriness of cardiac tissue may, under pathological conditions, allow arrhythmias to occur (Fig. 40.3).

Electrophysiological changes which promote arrhythmogenesis

Changes in pace-maker activity/altered automaticity

From the discussion above, it is clear that changes in the activation of pace-maker cells will change the cardiac rhythm. Sympathetic nerve fibres supply other regions of the heart in addition to the sinus node (Fig. 40.1), so acceleration of other pace-maker sites could also occur during sympathetic nerve stimulation. While uniform autonomic stimulation may not produce an abnormal rhythm, non-uniform stimulation may be arrhythmogenic. Under conditions of localized, focal adrenergic stimulation as may occur during myocardial ischaemia, accelerated pace-maker activity (automaticity) may occur in a ventricular myocyte producing an idioventricular rhythm which may become dominant and potentially propagate into a ventricular arrhythmia.

After-depolarizations

After-depolarizations are oscillations in resting membrane potential which sometimes follow an action potential (Fig. 40.4). If the changes in membrane potential reach threshold, additional action potentials may be triggered, producing ectopic beats and tachycardia. Early after-depolarizations occur before complete repolarization of the action potential (Fig. 40.4(a)), for example, when action potential duration is prolonged (as is found clinically in long QT syndrome or following pharmacological treatment with class 1A or class 3 anti-arrhythmic agents), or by reduction of the repolarizing outward potassium current. Delayed after-depolarizations occur after repolarization of the action potential (Fig. 40.4(b)).

Conduction block and re-entry

If the atrioventricular node fails to conduct sinus node impulses to the His–Purkinje system and ventricles, heart block is said to have occurred. Pace-makers within the ventricles may then become dominant and operate beyond control of the sinus node. If conduction within an area of damaged myocardium is severely disturbed, propagation of the electrical impulse (the wave of depolarization) may be altered so that, by the time activation is completed, the surrounding myocardium may again be excitable, having overcome its refractory period. Under these conditions, re-entry of excitation may occur, followed by arrhythmias (Fig. 40.3). In practice, re-entry does not occur if small areas of non-uniform conduction are present due to the refractoriness of the surrounding tissue.

To understand better the complex interaction between the changes in propagation of the electrical impulse in the heart, with changes in cellular electrophysiology and the onset of ventricular fibrillation affecting the heart as a whole, myocardial mapping studies have been performed (reviewed by Flores and Sheridan 1988). There is now little doubt that ventricular fibrillation is a manifestation of re-entry, probably occurring at several sites in the heart. There is, however, greater uncertainty as to the mechanisms by which it may be initiated: by an ectopic beat or by re-entry of a beat from the sinus node.

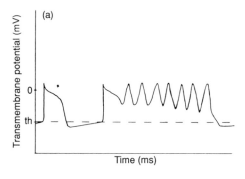

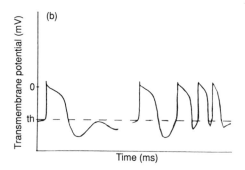

Fig. 40.4. Schematic diagram illustrating how early- and delayed- after-depolarizations produce electrophysiological changes which may contribute to arrhythmogenesis. (a) Early after-depolarizations appear following a normal action potential since repolarization is interrupted by repetitive depolarization of the cell at low membrane potentials. (b) A normal action potential is followed by a transient hyperpolarization and a delayed after-depolarization before stabilizing. If the delayed after-depolarization reaches the threshold voltage (th), extra action potentials may be propagated, but if it fails to reach threshold this will not occur. It may still, however, alter the rate of depolarization towards the threshold and change impulse initiation and conduction.

Arrhythmogenesis and myocardial ischaemia and reperfusion

During ischaemia, metabolic and biochemical changes occur which are associated with rapid and marked changes in cellular electrophysiology. Reduction of coronary blood flow produces a prompt fall in tissue oxygen tension and contraction abnormalities occur within seconds. High-energy phosphate levels (creatine phosphate, ATP) fall rapidly and tissue acidosis develops. Cellular energy metabolism changes from oxidation of free fatty acids to metabolism of glucose. Glycogenolysis is stimulated and potassium ions, lactate, adenosine, and inosine accumulate extracellularly. Accumulation of lipid metabolites (long-chain acyl carnitines and lysophosphoglycerides) also occurs and these have been proposed as having an arrhythmogenic role. These changes have been reviewed and described in detail by Russell (1988).

Cellular electrophysiological changes

During ischaemia, depolarization occurs reducing resting membrane potential and lowering action potential amplitude and upstroke velocity (Penny and Sheridan 1983). Action potential duration also falls quickly during ischaemia. Refractory period follows this, but prolongation occurs initially so that the refractory period is longer than the action potential duration (post-repolarization refractoriness). During the later stages of ischaemia this is reversed and the refractory period may be much less than the action potential duration, so that the close relationship between action potential duration and refractory period is lost (Fig. 40.5). Electrical alternans is a transient phenomenon occurring during early ischaemia in which marked differences in amplitude and duration of alternate action potentials occur (Fig. 40.6). Slowing of impulse conduction through the myocardium also occurs with reductions in action potential upstroke velocity reflecting slowing of transmembrane sodium conductance.

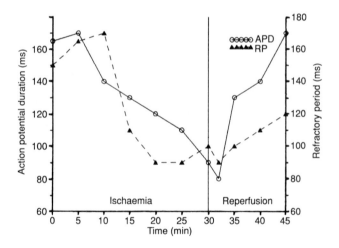

Fig. 40.5. Changes in action potential (APD) and refractory period (RP) during myocardial ischaemia and reperfusion. Prolongation of both parameters occurs initially before they fall rapidly during ischaemia. The normally close relationship between action potential duration and refractory period may then be lost. Reperfusion causes a further transient reduction in action potential duration and refractory period immediately prior to the development of reperfusion arrhythmias and is followed by gradual recovery. (After Penny and Sheridan (1983).)

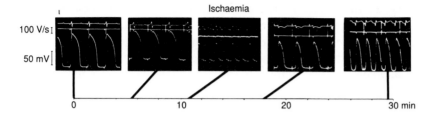

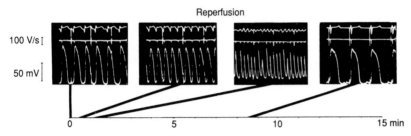

Fig. 40.6. Cellular electrophysiological changes observed during myocardial ischaemia (upper panel) and reperfusion (lower panel) in an isolated guinea-pig heart. In each panel, the upper trace is the ECG recording, the middle trace the recording of upstroke velocity of the action potential, and the lower trace the transmembrane action potential. During ischaemia, depolarization occurs, with reductions in action potential amplitude and duration. At about 10 min of ischaemia, electrical alternans may appear (marked reductions in alternate action potential durations and amplitude) with later recovery prior to the development of ventricular tachycardia. During reperfusion, electrophysiological recovery is rapid. As action potential amplitude and upstroke velocity recover, duration is reduced further before acceleration of ventricular tachycardia occurs and the onset of ventricular fibrillation. (Reproduced with permission from Penny and Sheridan (1983).)

Reperfusion of ischaemic myocardium may lead to further exacerbation of the electrophysiological changes associated with ischaemia. Reperfusion arrhythmias are well-documented experimentally (Flores and Sheridan 1988), and there is some evidence that they may also occur in man, particularly following coronary thrombolysis. The incidence of arrhythmias on reperfusion depends on the duration of the preceding period of ischaemia: arrhythmias do not occur if myocardial damage is slight or so severe as to be irreversible. Similarly, the rate of recovery depends on the rate of reperfusion, with slower recovery and delayed onset of arrhythmias with gradual reperfusion (Penny and Sheridan 1983).

The onset of reperfusion arrhythmias corresponds to recovery of cellular electrophysiology and is rapid. Action potential amplitude and upstroke velocity recover rapidly while action potential duration and refractory period undergo further transient decreases before recovering (Penny and Sheridan 1983). The importance of the combination of reductions in action potential duration and refractoriness occurring while conduction is improving in mediating arrhythmogenesis is apparent from studies which have demonstrated that interventions which are anti-arrhythmic (catecholamine depletion, α-adrenoceptor antagonism, discussed below) prevent the reductions in action potential duration during ischaemia and at the onset of reperfusion. The rapidity of the onset of reperfusion arrhythmias is thought to indicate that they may be caused by wash-out of metabolites accumulated during ischaemia or disinhibition of ischaemia-induced arrhythmogenesis (Nakata *et al.* 1990; Fig. 40.6).

To summarize, disturbances in cardiac cellular electrophysiology (increased automaticity, delayed conduction, reduced or variable refractoriness) increase the susceptibility of the heart to arrhythmias. Changes, which may be of little significance during conditions of normal conduction and refractoriness, may be capable of initiating ventricular fibrillation if these are disturbed when coronary flow is compromised. Severely disturbed conduction may, however, inhibit the development and propagation of arrhythmias.

Mechanisms preventing or promoting arrhythmogenesis during ischaemia

Adrenergic mechanisms

Evidence supporting the role of adrenergic mechanisms in mediating arrhythmias during myocardial ischaemia and reperfusion has been obtained by many groups over the last few years. Adrenergic activity has been shown to be increased in acute myocardial ischaemia and infarction, with release of myocardial catecholamines, increases in plasma and urinary catecholamine levels following infarction, and loss of myocardial noradrenaline (see the reviews by Riemersma 1982 and Sheridan 1982). Surgical or chemical denervation is effective in reducing the incidence of arrhythmias during ischaemia demonstrating further the involvement of adrenergic mechanisms.

Some evidence is available from clinical studies (reviewed by Butrous 1988) that psychological stimuli or stress are able to induce changes in cardiac rhythm. The relative importance of this to the cellular changes which promote arrhythmogenesis has, however, been difficult to define using experimental techniques since experimental stress may not be relevant to, and is unlikely to be the same as ordinary environmental or emotional stress.

α- and β-adrenoceptor stimulation/antagonism

Studies based on adrenoceptor antagonism have attempted to determine the cellular mechanisms through which the sympathetic nervous system mediates

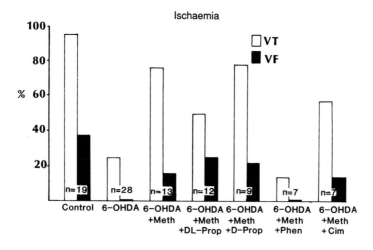

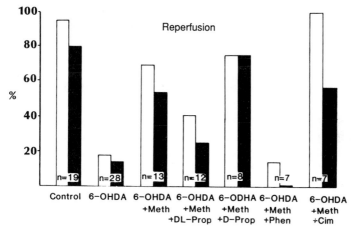

Fig. 40.7.   Percentage incidence of ventricular tachycardia (VT) and ventricular fibrillation (VF) during ischaemia (upper panel) and reperfusion (lower panel) in isolated guinea-pig hearts. Myocardial catecholamine depletion with 6-hydroxydopamine (6-OHDA) reduced arrhythmogenesis during ischaemia and reperfusion, but this was reversed by the α-adrenoceptor agonist methoxamine (meth), independently of β-adrenoceptor antagonism with propranolol (prop) or histamine$_2$-receptor antagonism with cimetidine (cim). Alpha-adrenoceptor antagonism with phentolamine (phen) abolished the arrhythmogenic effect of methoxamine. (Reproduced with permission from Culling *et al.* (1987).)

arrhythmogenesis during myocardial ischaemia and reperfusion. β-adrenoceptor antagonism has been shown to reduce mortality in patients following acute myocardial infarction, but the mechanisms of this effect have not been determined clearly, with variable results in experimental models despite adequate β-adrenoceptor antagonism (Fitzgerald 1982; Flores and

Sheridan 1988). Increases in the numbers of β-adrenoceptors during ischaemia and reperfusion have been reported, but the pathophysiological relevance of these changes remains unclear. In contrast, many groups have demonstrated the involvement of α-adrenoceptors in mediating arrhythmogenesis during experimental myocardial ischaemia and reperfusion (for reviews see Sheridan 1982; Flores and Sheridan 1988). Most studies have demonstrated the effectiveness of α_1-adrenoceptor antagonism in preventing arrhythmogenesis during experimental myocardial ischaemia.

An important observation in understanding the contribution of α-adrenergic mechanisms to enhancing arrhythmogenesis during myocardial ischaemia and reperfusion came from studies in which administration of the α_1-adrenoceptor agonist methoxamine was shown to increase the incidence of ventricular tachycardia and fibrillation in hearts which had been depleted of myocardial catecholamines (Sheridan et al. 1980; Culling et al. 1987). Cellular electrophysiological studies revealed that the mechanisms for this arrhythmogenic effect of α-adrenoceptor stimulation are independent of actions at β-adrenoceptors or histamine$_2$-receptors (Culling et al. 1987, Fig. 40.7) and are independent of changes in blood flow (Sheridan et al. 1980). Furthermore, α-adrenoceptor stimulation enhances the reductions in action potential duration and refractory period occurring during ischaemia and reperfusion which are associated with the arrhythmogenic effect (Culling et al. 1987; Fig. 40.8). The specificity of these mechanisms was confirmed from experiments which demonstrated that α-adrenoceptor antagonists have opposing, anti-arrhythmic actions, attenuating the reductions of action potential duration and refractory period during ischaemia (Penny et al. 1985; Fig. 40.9). Myocardial catecholamine depletion has similar cellular electrophysiological effects and is anti-arrhythmic (Fig. 40.7–40.9; see Flores and Sheridan 1988).

The ability of α-adrenoceptor stimulation to increase arrhythmogenesis during ischaemia by producing specific cellular electrophysiological changes in ischaemic myocardium is in contrast to its effects during normal perfusion when it produces no changes in perfused hearts, but increases action potential duration and refractory period in superfused myocardium (Flores and Sheridan 1988), suggesting that α-adrenoceptor responsiveness may be enhanced during ischaemia. Increases in α-adrenoceptor numbers, which have been reported during ischaemia in some species but not others (Chess-Williams et al. 1990), and observations of increased α-adrenergic responsiveness at the onset of reperfusion support this (Sheridan et al. 1980). Understanding the basis for this increased myocardial sensitivity to α-adrenoceptor agonists is likely to be important in furthering our understanding of the arrhythmogenic effects of ischaemia. In particular, testing of these observations in man is of great importance. Unfortunately, most α-adrenoceptor antagonists that are available for clinical use also act at peripheral sites producing vasodilatation, hypotension, and reduced coronary

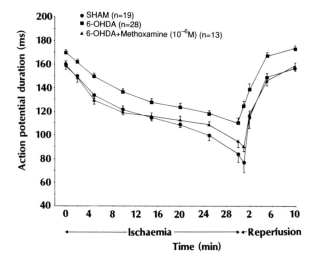

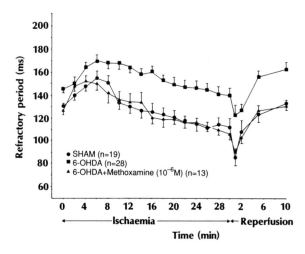

Fig. 40.8. Changes in action potential duration (upper panel) and refractory period (lower panel) during myocardial ischaemia and reperfusion in isolated guinea-pig hearts in the presence of α-adrenoceptor stimulation with methoxamine. Action potential duration was shortened during ischaemia in all groups. Myocardial catecholamine depletion by pre-treatment with 6-hydroxydopamine (6-OHDA) prolonged action potential duration and this effect was maintained throughout the ischaemic period. Perfusion with methoxamine reversed this, restoring values to control. Action potential duration underwent further transient shortening during early reperfusion in control hearts. Catecholamine depletion prevented this, while methoxamine restored this shortening. Similar changes in refractory period were seen. (Reproduced by permission from Culling et al. (1987).)

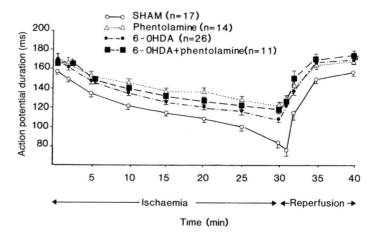

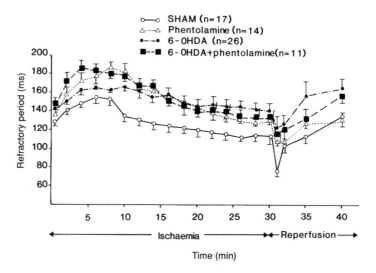

Fig. 40.9. Changes in action potential duration (upper panel) and refractory period (lower panel) during myocardial ischaemia and reperfusion in isolated guinea-pig hearts in the presence of α-adrenoceptor antagonism with phentolamine. Action potential duration was shortened during ischaemia in all groups. Myocardial catecholamine depletion by pre-treatment with 6-hydroxydopamine (6-OHDA) prolonged action potential duration and this effect was maintained throughout the ischaemic period. Perfusion with phentolamine enhanced this effect, increasing action potential duration further. Action potential duration underwent further transient shortening during early reperfusion in control hearts, but catecholamine depletion and phentolamine prevented this. Similar changes in refractory period were seen. (Reproduced with permission from Penny *et al.* (1985).)

perfusion. The availability of novel cardioselective compounds, however, should allow studies to be undertaken in the future in which the ability of α-adrenoceptor antagonists to reduce arrhythmogenesis in man might be investigated.

Parasympathetic mechanisms

The role of parasympathetic mechanisms in altering the arrhythmogenic effects of myocardial ischaemia are less well-established compared with adrenergic mechanisms. Controversy over the effects of vagal stimulation exists for several reasons. Excessive vagal tone may, for example, be anti-arrhythmic due to direct electrophysiological effects or, alternatively, be arrhythmogenic due to the bradycardia induced.

Some experimental evidence (reviewed by Corr *et al.* 1986) is available which suggests that vagal stimulation is able to suppress or abolish ventricular arrhythmias during early ischaemia, but the situation is complicated by reports that during later ischaemia vagal stimulation *increases* arrhythmogenesis by enhancing ventricular automaticity. Conclusive clinical data on this is still lacking. The degree of influence of parasympathetic mechanisms on arrhythmogenesis appears also to depend on the species studied. Experiments in cats have revealed that vagotomy increases the incidence of ventricular fibrillation following coronary artery occlusion, but this is not seen in dogs apparently due to differences in the existing levels of vagal tone and responses between species. Other experimental studies suggest that the effects of parasympathetic mechanisms on arrhythmogenesis may depend on the site of coronary artery occlusion and resultant infarction, and on the amount of time elapsed following the onset of ischaemia. Clinical studies suggest that a similar situation may pertain in man.

Despite some circumstantial evidence of the involvement of the para-sympathetic nervous system in modulating the arrhythmogenic effects of myocardial ischaemia and reperfusion, the situation is far from clear, unlike the contribution of adrenergic mechanisms outlined above. Understanding of the contribution of vagal mechanisms is complicated by observations that any apparently protective effect of vagal stimulation during ischaemia may result primarily from anti-adrenergic effects rather than, or in addition to, any direct myocardial actions. Further work remains to be undertaken to clarify this.

Ionic mechanisms

Changes in the concentration of ions in the extracellular fluid cause alterations in cardiac cellular electrophysiology through changes in the resting membrane potential. Clinical studies have suggested associations between changes in plasma ionic concentrations and vulnerability to arrhythmias. During the early stages of infarction, hypokalaemia is associated with arrhythmogenesis, but the relationship is lost during the later stages of infarction (for a review see Russell 1988). Interpretation of cause and effect is complicated by the fact that hypokalaemia may simply be a manifestation of enhanced adrenergic activity caused by ischaemia, which itself increases arrhythmogenesis. Similar restrictions apply to interpretation of clinical observations of an apparent association between hypomagnesaemia and the incidence of ventricular tachycardia.

Some of the changes occurring during ischaemia are, however, attributable to alterations in the ionic environment. During ischaemia, release of potassium ions occurs rapidly from the ischaemic myocardium. The ratio of intracellular to extracellular concentrations of potassium is one of the main determinants of the resting membrane potential. During ischaemia the inability of energy production to keep pace with energy demands may result in inhibition of the transmembrane $Na^+K^+ATPase$ which acts to maintain the different ionic concentrations inside and outside the cell. Use of ion-selective electrodes has shown that extracellular potassium concentration increases as early as 15 s following coronary artery occlusion, reaching levels of 20 to 30 mmol/l by 60 min (Hirche *et al.* 1982). Increases in extracellular potassium could certainly account for the cellular electrophysiological changes observed during ischaemia (reductions in resting membrane potential, action potential amplitude, upstroke velocity, duration, and delayed conduction.) It is unlikely, however, that potassium accumulation is solely responsible for these changes despite suggestions being made that the early rapid rise in potassium release may be related to the early (class IA) arrhythmias which can occur 2 to 10 min after the onset of ischaemia and the later rise in extracellular potassium concentrations with class IB arrhythmias which usually occur between 12 and 30 min of ischaemia.

By making selective changes in extracellular ionic concentrations under carefully controlled conditions in animals, it is possible to induce electrophysiological changes that can trigger arrhythmias and so investigate the role of the ionic environment and its interaction with adrenergic mechanisms in mediating arrhythmogenesis. Ferrier and Carmeliet (1990) studied the effects of α-adrenoceptor agonists on the transient inward current (I_{ti}), which is reported to be arrhythmogenic, induced by exposure of Purkinje fibres to elevated extracellular Ca^{2+} concentrations or acetylstrophanthidin. These authors reported the most interesting observation that when I_{ti} was induced by acetylstrophanthidin, α-adrenoceptor stimulation inhibited I_{ti} (consistent with an *anti-arrhythmic* effect), yet when I_{ti} was induced by 8 mM Ca^{2+}, α-adrenoceptor stimulation increased the amplitude of I_{ti} (consistent with an *arrhythmogenic*) effect. Thus, α_1-adrenoceptor stimulation can exert pro- or anti-arrhythmic effects depending on the experimental conditions. Other studies have demonstrated the ability of α-adrenoceptor stimulation to promote early after-depolarizations, giving further evidence of the important contribution of α-adrenoceptor-mediated mechanisms to the arrhythmogenic effects of myocardial ischaemia.

Evidence currently available, and reviewed by Heusch (1990), suggests that α_1-adrenoceptor stimulation can lead to increases in cytoplasmic calcium concentrations which could increase Na^+–H^+ exchange through membrane ionic channels. α-adrenoceptor stimulation is thought to be responsible in part for the increase in intracellular calcium which occurs during reperfusion which, in the context of the calcium paradox (readmission of calcium ions), is responsible for cellular uncoupling and other deleterious effects, and could influence arrhythmogenesis during myocardial ischaemia and reperfusion. Mechanisms mediating these changes remain unclear, but the combination of the effects of Na^+–H^+–Ca^{2+} exchange in promoting arrhythmias may be important. The contribution of Na^+–Ca^{2+} exchange mechanisms is also evident from considerations that the arrhythmogenic I_{ti} may be derived from a Na^+–Ca^{2+} exchange current.

Changes in myocardial perfusion during ischaemia

Until recently, coronary vasodilatation was thought to occur during myocardial ischaemia due to metabolic effects induced by the reduction in flow (release of adenosine, reduction in oxygen supply), but evidence is now accumulating that metabolic coronary vasodilatation may compete with α-adrenergic coronary vasoconstriction during ischaemia producing incomplete vasodilatation, i.e. some residual constrictor tone. Heusch (1990) noted that interpretation of experimental results is complicated by apparently different receptor involvement and by observations that α_1-adrenoceptor coronary vasoconstriction is reported to be attenuated by ischaemia, whereas α_2-adrenoceptor coronary vasoconstriction is not, apparently due to the different sensitivities of the receptors to acidosis.

One mechanism that has been proposed to account for the arrhythmogenic effects of α-adrenoceptor stimulation during ischaemia described above is an increase in the severity of the effects of ischaemia due to coronary vasoconstriction. In an early study performed to investigate this (Sheridan et al. 1980), the conclusion was reached that the anti-arrhythmic effect of α-adrenoceptor antagonism was not related to coronary vascular effects and the suggestion offered that α-adrenoceptor stimulation is arrhythmogenic through actions on myocardial α-adrenoceptors. More recent studies, reviewed by Heusch (1990), suggest a complex modulating influence of α-adrenergic mechanisms during reductions in coronary flow, with different effects at different sizes of vessels and in the presence of different degrees of flow reduction. These studies have thus led to renewed interest in the suggestion that α-adrenoceptor-mediated arrhythmogenic effects may be mediated by adverse coronary vasoconstriction and exacerbation of myocardial ischaemia. While α-adrenoceptor-mediated coronary vasoconstriction may be disadvantageous and exacerbate the effects of myocardial ischaemia, the suggestion has never-theless been made that it could *reduce* the effects of ischaemia by preventing a transmural redistribution of flow ('steal') away from the subendocardium.

In contrast to the above findings of α-adrenoceptor-mediated coronary vasoconstriction during ischaemia, a recent study by Kitakaze *et al.* (1989) demonstrated α_2-adrenoceptor-mediated coronary *vasodilatation* in the presence of a severe flow-limiting stenosis and that this is related to the ability of coronary vascular endothelial cells to produce adenosine. The suggestion has been made that α_1-adrenoceptor activity may exert dual effects on vascular tone in ischaemic hearts, producing vasoconstriction of coronary vessels and vasodilatation due to increased adenosine release. The overall response may depend on a balance between these mechanisms. Further work is required to determine the factors which regulate perfusion within ischaemic tissue.

Effects of myocardial stretch

Myocardial mechanical injury and stretch are capable of inducing cardiac cellular electrophysiological effects (e.g. changes in action potential duration and electrical alternans; Lab 1980). Under certain conditions, stretch might also cause delayed after-depolarizations and triggered activity. This has important implications in conditions when the myocardium may be damaged, e.g. during left ventricular hypertrophy (discussed below) or in a ventricular aneurysm.

If the ventricular wall is weakened following a large myocardial infarction, it may stretch during systole, producing an aneurysm, the presence of which is recognized to have a high risk of developing ventricular arrhythmias. Systolic stretching of myocardial cells at the boundary between normal myocardium and the aneurysm may produce depolarizations and so could increase automaticity and alter conduction. Clinical studies have shown that arrhythmias tend to arise from areas bordering the aneurysm rather than from within it, indicating the importance of inhomogeneities between adjacent cells in being able to trigger ventricular arrhythmias. Surgical resection of the aneurysm and adjacent myocardium involved is often effective in suppressing these arrhythmias.

Effects of left ventricular hypertrophy

Left ventricular hypertrophy has been shown to be associated with enhanced susceptibility to arrhythmias and an increased risk of sudden death in man. Cellular electrophysiological changes have been demonstrated during hypertrophy (Taylor *et al.* 1990), including increases in transmembrane inward calcium current, early- and delayed- after-depolarizations and triggered activity, non-uniformly distributed prolongation of action potential duration, and reductions in the amount of electrically effective cell membrane area despite an increase in total membrane area due to cellular enlargement. The result of these differences is that the substrate for re-entrant arrhythmias is produced: prolongation and dispersion of refractoriness together with increased susceptibility to the development of triggered automaticity. This could explain the arrhythmogenic effects of hypertrophy. Further work remains to be done to determine the responses of these hearts to conditions of reduced coronary perfusion, but preliminary results suggest that, during ischaemia in the presence of left ventricular hypertrophy, greater cellular electrophysiological changes occur compared to those seen in normal hearts.

Free radicals

Changes in myocardial and microvascular ultrastructure occurring during ischaemia and reperfusion and the observation of the rapid onset of arrhythmias when reperfusion is initiated have led to the suggestion that readmission of oxygen and production of oxygen-derived free radicals may be important in the initiation of reperfusion-induced arrhythmias. While some evidence is available that anti-oxygen radical interventions can prevent arrhythmogenesis, a recent study reported that restoration of flow and readmission of oxygen are independent determinants of reperfusion-induced arrhythmias and that readmission of oxygen (and production of free radicals) is not required for arrhythmogenesis (Yamada et al. 1990). Thus, other non-specific effects of the anti-oxygen radical agents may be involved in mediating their apparent anti-arrhythmic effect. Oxygen-derived free radicals may, however, be important in acting synergistically with other mechanisms promoting arrhythmias. The ability of oxygen-derived free radicals to influence platelet activation may be of particular importance.

Role of blood-borne factors

The contribution of blood-borne factors (prostanoids, neutrophils, platelets) in exacerbating the effects of myocardial ischaemia has received much attention recently. Studies in man which have demonstrated that inhibition of platelet activation and aggregation can reduce mortality following myocardial infarction indicate the importance of these mechanisms (ISIS-2 1988).

Release of prostanoids occurs during myocardial ischaemia and experimental studies performed over the last ten years have shown that thromboxane A_2 is arrhythmogenic and that prostacyclin is anti-arrhythmic (Coker 1982). The fact that the former agent is involved in promoting platelet aggregation and is released from activated platelets, while the latter agent is secreted from endothelial cells and prevents platelet aggregation indicates the importance of these mechanisms. Other experimental evidence of the involvement of platelets has been obtained: increases in infarct size have been demonstrated in the presence of platelets, together with the ability of antiplatelet interventions to reduce infarct size and arrhythmogenesis (Chakrabarty *et al.* 1991). Preliminary studies indicate that the presence of platelets exacerbates the cellular electrophysiological effects of ischaemia. Further work remains to be done to confirm the relative contribution of factors released from platelets and of platelet accumulation in the microcirculation in mediating the deleterious effects observed. Recent observations in man of release of platelet-activating factor during pacing-induced angina suggest that platelet-mediated changes can occur rapidly. Infusion of platelet-activating factor into anaesthetized rabbits produces a sudden, marked reduction in blood pressure, and ventricular fibrillation follows rapidly (Chakrabarty *et al.* 1991). Platelet-activating factor also has direct myocardial cellular electrophysiological effects during normal perfusion and can increase the incidence of arrhythmias during ischaemia even in the absence of circulating platelets (Flores and Sheridan 1990).

The importance of an intact, undamaged endothelium has been recognized following the discovery of the ability of endothelium-derived relaxing factor (EDRF) to modulate vascular tone and the anti-aggregatory actions of prostacyclin. Recent observations that EDRF is able to prevent platelet aggregation confirm the importance of these mechanisms. Some information is now emerging that there may also be an endothelium-derived hyper-polarizing factor, which is independent of EDRF, and which also controls vascular smooth muscle tone. (Chen *et al.* 1989). Whether this agent is able to affect the electrophysiological properties of myocardial cells directly remains to be determined. The suggestion has also been made that endothelial cells are able to influence vascular tone by regulating production of adenosine (Kitakaze *et al.* 1989).

Other factors

Possible arrhythmogenic effects of histamine have been investigated by some groups since histamine has been shown to prolong atrioventricular conduction (through actions at H_1-receptors) and to increase heart rate and ventricular automaticity (through actions at H_2- receptors). While enhanced sensitivity of ischaemic myocardium to the arrhythmogenic effects of histamine has been demonstrated in some experimental models, evidence of its direct involvement in mediating arrhythmogenesis is not available (reviewed by Flores and Sheridan 1988). Histamine$_2$-receptor antagonism has been shown to have no anti-arrhythmic effects in the isolated, perfused guinea-pig heart, unlike α-adrenoceptor antagonism or myocardial catecholamine depletion (Culling *et al.* 1987).

Following the observation that levels of cyclic adenosine monophosphate (cAMP) increase in the ischaemic heart, interest in its role in generating arrhythmias arose (reviewed by Flores and Sheridan 1988). While several studies showed a close temporal relation between elevation of cAMP levels and arrhythmogenesis during ischaemia, the situation was less clear during reperfusion. More recent studies suggest that electrical instability during reperfusion is not related to increases in cAMP levels and that, under certain conditions, anti-arrhythmic effects may be observed despite elevated tissue levels of cAMP. While cAMP may be involved in mediating some forms of arrhythmias, its importance is less than originally proposed.

Conclusions

Attempts to reduce sudden death in man by using anti-arrhythmic drugs which alter the main determinants of re-entry (conduction and refractoriness) have had limited success. Successful prevention of arrhythmogenesis is more likely to be achieved by preventing or modifying the electrophysiological effects of ischaemia and reperfusion, rather than through preventing the initiation of arrhythmias. The rapid nature of the onset of reperfusion arrhythmias and the ability of the interventions described above to prevent arrhythmias by altering the cellular electrophysiological effects of ischaemia and reperfusion support this.

References

Butrous, G. S. (1988). Autonomic tone modulation of cardiac arrhythmias. In *Clinical aspects of cardiac arrhythmias* (ed. A. J. Camm and D. E. Ward), pp. 49–58. Kluwer Academic Publishers, Dordrecht.

Chakrabarty, S., Thomas, P., and Sheridan, D. J. (1991). Contribution of platelets and platelet activating factor (PAF) to the arrhythmogenic, haemo-dynamic and necrotic effects of acute myocardial ischaemia. *Eur. Heart J.* **22**, 583–9.

Chen, G., Hashitani, H., and Suzuki, H. (1989). Endothelium-dependent relaxation and hyperpolarization of canine coronary artery smooth muscles in relation to the electrogenic Na–K pump. *Br. J. Pharmacol.* **338**, 438–42.

Chess-Williams, R. G., Sheridan, D. J., and Broadley, K. J. (1990). Arrhythmias and α_1-adrenoceptor binding characteristics of the guinea-pig perfused heart during ischaemia and reperfusion. *J. mol. cell. Cardiol.* **22**, 599–606.

Coker, S. J. (1982). Early ventricular arrhythmias arising from acute myocardial ischaemia; possible involvement of prostaglandins and thromboxanes. In *Early arrhythmias resulting from myocardial ischaemia, mechanisms and prevention by drugs* (ed. J. R. Parratt), pp. 219–37. Macmillan, London.

Corr, P. B., Yamada, K. A., and Witkowski, F. X. (1986). Mechanisms controlling cardiac autonomic function and their relation to arrhythmogenesis. In *The heart and cardiovascular system, scientific foundations*, Vol. 2 (ed. H. A. Fozzard, E. Haber, R. B. Jennings, A. M. Katz, and H. E. Morgan) pp. 1343–403. Raven Press, New York.

Culling, W., Penny, W. J., Cunliffe, G., Flores, N. A., and Sheridan, D. J. (1987). Arrhythmogenic and electrophysiological effects of alpha adrenoceptor stimulation during myocardial ischaemia and reperfusion. *J. mol. cell. Cardiol.* **19**, 251–8.

Ferrier, G. R. and Carmeliet, E. (1990). Effects of α-adrenergic agents on transient inward current in rabbit Purkinje fibers. *J. mol. cell. Cardiol.* **22**, 191–200.

Fitzgerald, J. A. (1982). The effects of β-adrenoceptor blocking drugs on early arrhythmias in experimental and clinical myocardial ischaemia. In *Early arrhythmias resulting from myocardial ischaemia, mechanisms and prevention by drugs* (ed. J. R. Parratt), pp. 295–316, Macmillan, London.

Flores, N. A. and Sheridan, D. J. (1988). The electrophysiology of reperfusion-induced arrhythmias following acute myocardial ischaemia. In *Clinical aspects of cardiac arrhythmias* (ed. A. J. Camm and D. E. Ward), pp. 33–48. Kluwer Academic Publishers, Dordrecht.

Flores, N. A. and Sheridan, D. J. (1990). Electrophysiological and arrhythmogenic effects of platelet activating factor during normal perfusion, myocardial ischaemia and reperfusion in the guinea-pig. *Br. J. Pharmacol.* **101**, 734–8.

Heusch, G. (1990). α-adrenergic mechanisms in myocardial ischemia. *Circulation* **81**, 1–13.

Hirche, H., Friedrich, R., Kebbel, U., McDonald, F., and Zylka, V. (1982). Early arrhythmias, myocardial extracellular potassium and pH. In *Early arrhythmias resulting from myocardial ischaemia, mechanisms and prevention by drugs* (ed. J. R. Parratt), pp. 113–24. Macmillan, London.

ISIS-2 (Second International Study of Infarct Survival) Collaborative Group (1988). Randomised trial of intravenous streptokinase, oral aspirin, both, or neither among 17 187 cases of suspected acute myocardial infarction: ISIS-2. *Lancet* **i**, 349–60.

Kitakaze, M., Hori, M., Gotoh, K., Sato, H., Iwakura, K., Kitabatake, A., Inoue, M., and Kamada, T. (1989). Beneficial effects of α_2-adrenoceptor activity on ischemic myocardium during coronary hypoperfusion in dogs. *Circulation Res.* **65**, 1632–45.

Lab, M. J. (1980). Transient depolarisation and action potential alterations following mechanical changes in isolated myocardium. *Cardiovasc. Res.* **14**, 624–37.

Nakata, T., Hearse, D. J., and Curtis, M. J. (1990). Are reperfusion-induced arrhythmias caused by disinhibition of an arrhythmogenic component of ischemia? *J. mol. cell. Cardiol.* **22**, 843–58.

Penny, W. J. and Sheridan, D. J. (1983). Arrhythmias and cellular electrophysiological changes during myocardial ischaemia and reperfusion. *Cardiovasc. Res.* **17**, 363–72.

Penny, W. J., Culling, W., Lewis, M. J., and Sheridan, D. J. (1985). Antiarrhythmic and electrophysiological effects of alpha adrenoceptor blockade during myocardial ischaemia and reperfusion in isolated guinea-pig heart. *J. mol. cell. Cardiol.* **17**, 399–409.

Riemersma, R. A. (1982). Myocardial catecholamine release in acute myocardial ischaemia; relationship to cardiac arrhythmias. In *Early arrhythmias resulting from myocardial ischaemia, mechanisms and prevention by drugs* (ed. J. R. Parratt), pp. 125–38. Macmillan, London.

Russell, D. C. (1988). Metabolic factors in the genesis of ventricular arrhythmias. In *Clinical aspects of cardiac arrhythmias* (ed. A. J. Camm and D. E. Ward), pp. 15–32. Kluwer Academic Publishers, Dordrecht.

Sheridan, D. J. (1982). Myocardial α-adrenoceptors and arrhythmias induced by myocardial ischaemia. In *Early arrhythmias resulting from myocardial ischaemia, mechanisms and prevention by drugs* (ed. J. R. Parratt), pp. 317–28. Macmillan, London.

Sheridan, D. J., Penkoske, P. A., Sobel, B. E., and Corr, P. B. (1980). Alpha adrenergic contributions to dysrhythmia during myocardial ischemia and reperfusion in cats. *J. clin. Invest.* **65**, 161–71.

Taylor, A. L., Winter, R., Thandroyen, F., Murphree, S., Buja, L. M., Eckels, R., Pastor, P., and Kremers, M. (1990). Potentiation of reperfusion-associated ventricular fibrillation by left ventricular hypertrophy. *Circulation Res.* **67**, 501–9.

Yamada, M., Hearse, D. J., and Curtis, M. J. (1990). Reperfusion and readmission of oxygen, pathophysiological relevance of oxygen-derived free radicals to arrhythmogenesis. *Circulation Res.* **67**, 1211–24.

41. Sympathetic neural mechanisms in hypertension

Virend K. Somers and Allyn L. Mark

Introduction

The sympathetic nervous system plays an integral role in circulatory homeostasis. There is accumulating evidence that a relative overactivity of the sympathetic nervous system may be an important aetiological factor in the development and maintenance of arterial hypertension.

This chapter briefly reviews evidence implicating the sympathetic nervous system as a causative factor in hypertension. We will also examine the mechanisms by which increased sympathetic activity induces and maintains elevated levels of arterial pressure, and discuss the possible aetiology of sympathetic overactivity in hypertension, with emphasis on peripheral reflex mechanisms in human hypertension. Lastly, we will explore the effects of humoral agents on the sympathetic nervous system.

The data reviewed are derived mainly from neural and vascular studies in humans with primary and secondary hypertension. Data from recent human studies using techniques such as noradrenaline 'spillover' and microneurography (direct recordings of sympathetic nerve activity in humans) will be emphasized. Because of the scope of the subject and the limited space available, only a few references to the various topics are cited.

Evidence for sympathetic hyperactivity in hypertension

Essential hypertension

Since increases in sympathetic activity can increase either cardiac output or peripheral vascular resistance and thereby increase blood pressure, considerable attention has focused on detecting an abnormally high level of sympathetic activity in patients with hypertension. An early study demonstrated that ganglionic blockade with hexamethonium resulted in greater falls in blood pressure in hypertensive subjects when compared to normals and thus suggested a neurogenic component in hypertension (Doyle and Smirk 1955). This 'neurogenically mediated' hypertension could be explained by either excessive sympathetic activity and/or increased vascular reactivity to the sympathetic neurotransmitter. Egan *et al.* (1987) studied this issue in 24 mild hypertensive patients and 18 normotensive controls. These investigators reported that the hypertensive subjects had elevated levels of arterial plasma noradrenaline. Forearm vasoconstrictor responses to infused noradrenaline were similar in both groups, but α-receptor blockade induced greater reductions in forearm vascular resistance in the hypertensive subjects. The authors concluded that the increased vascular α-adrenergic tone in mild hypertensives is secondary to an increased sympathetic drive and not to increased vascular reactivity. These data, however, did not establish whether the elevated levels of plasma noradrenaline are secondary to increased central sympathetic outflow or to peripheral mechanisms such as facilitated noradrenaline release or an impaired re-uptake of noradrenaline at the adrenergic nerve endings.

A large number of studies in humans have attempted to identify sympathetic overactivity by measurement of plasma (both venous and arterial) catecholamines. These measurements have been made both at rest and during stressors such as mental arithmetic, orthostasis, and exercise. Overall, these studies of plasma catecholamines suggest an increased sympathoadrenal activity in hypertension (Goldstein 1983; Hjemdahl 1988). However, numerous caveats exist in interpreting these data, as discussed by Hjemdahl (1988) and Folkow *et al.* (1983). These include site of measurement (arterial or venous), analytical methods, noradrenaline re-uptake, and the need for regional measurements.

There is a growing body of evidence supporting excessive sympathetic discharge to the kidney in essential hypertension (Oparil 1986). Patients with essential hypertension often have increases in renal vascular resistance, secondary to a functional renal vasoconstriction reversed by infusion of a vasodilator. This renal vasoconstriction appears to be sympathetically mediated. In many hypertensive patients, renal noradrenaline levels are elevated, despite normal plasma venous noradrenaline. Alpha-blockade reverses renal vasoconstriction and increases renal blood flow in hypertensive, but not normotensive humans. Splanchnic neural blockade also increases renal blood flow in hypertensive, but not normotensive humans. This renal vasoconstriction is unlikely to be explained by an increased receptor sensitivity, since renal vascular responsiveness to catecholamines appears to be normal in hypertension.

Using noradrenaline 'spillover' measurements, Esler *et al.* (1986) found that arterial noradrenaline levels and noradrenaline spillover were elevated in hypertensive patients under 60 years of age. This elevation was most marked in the youngest hypertensives (20 to 39 years), and was associated with increased spillover mainly from the heart and kidneys. These data are especially relevant when examined in the context of the 'hyperdynamic circulation' of early human hypertension—increased heart rate, cardiac output, and renal vasoconstriction (Conway 1984).

Microneurography, a method of direct recording of efferent, postganglionic sympathetic nerve traffic to muscle blood vessels by insertion of tungsten microelectrodes into peripheral nerves in humans (Vallbo *et al.* 1979), has added considerably to our understanding of autonomic pathophysiology in hypertension. Microneurographic recordings quantifying resting sympathetic nerve activity to muscle blood vessels in human hypertension have provided conflicting results. Some studies, particularly early studies, reported no increase in muscle sympathetic activity in hypertensive versus normotensive subjects (Wallin and Sundlöf, 1979; Somers *et al.* 1988). In contrast, in a carefully controlled study Anderson *et al.* (1989) found an increased level of muscle sympathetic nerve activity in young hypertensive males. In this study, young normotensive and borderline hypertensive age-matched subjects were studied on low and high salt diets. High salt diet reduced muscle sympathetic nerve activity in both groups. However, borderline hypertensive subjects had a greater muscle sympathetic nerve activity than normotensive subjects on both diets (Fig. 41.1). Studies by Yamada *et al.* (1989) have also provided evidence for higher levels of muscle sympathetic nerve activity in hypertensive as compared to age-matched normotensive humans.

The reasons for the finding of high levels of resting muscle sympathetic nerve activity in hypertensive subjects in some but not all studies are not clear. The variable results are not easily explained by age or differences in the severity of hypertension. In the study by Anderson *et al.* (1989) the hypertensive subjects were heavier than the normotensive controls. Obesity might contribute to increased sympathetic activity as a result of insulin

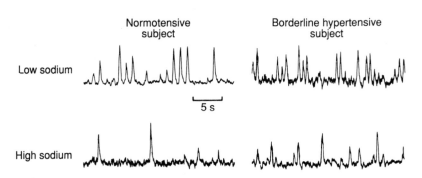

Fig. 41.1. Recordings of muscle sympathetic nerve activity in a normotensive subject and in a borderline hypertensive subject on both low and high sodium diets. Sympathetic nerve activity, which declined from low to high sodium diets, was higher in the borderline hypertensive subject independent of diet. A similar conclusion derived from the summary data on the two groups of subjects. (Reproduced with permission from Anderson *et al.* (1989).)

resistance and hyperinsulinaemia. Studies of cardiopulmonary baroreflexes by Rea and Hamdan (1990) raise the possibility that elevated levels of sympathetic neural drive in mild hypertensives may be partially masked in the supine position owing to a heightened sympathoinhibitory influence of the cardiopulmonary baroreceptors in mild hypertensives. These findings are discussed in greater detail later.

Lastly, important evidence supporting a major role of sympathetic activation in maintaining essential hypertension is the dramatic blood-pressure-lowering effects of sympatholytic agents such as ganglion blockers, alpha methyldopa, clonidine, reserpine, and adrenoceptor blockers. The effects of these agents are fairly specific, and therefore suggest that the sympathetic system is prominently involved in maintaining elevated arterial pressure in hypertension.

Secondary hypertension

The most obvious sympathetic mediated form of secondary hypertension is that due to phaeochromocytoma, where the hypertension is principally due to intermittent release of catecholamines. Sympathetic neural mechanisms may, however, also contribute to chronic mild elevations of blood pressure in patients with phaeochromocytoma due to sustained adrenaline-mediated facilitation of noradrenaline release from peripheral adrenergic nerve terminals.

Heightened sympathetic activation is also a factor in renovascular hypertension. The evidence is described by Oparil (1986) and includes increased levels of plasma and urine noradrenaline and its metabolites in patients with renovascular hypertension. This is not surprising since renovascular hypertension is known to be associated with activation of the renin–angiotensin system which increases sympathetic activity in addition to potentiating the effects of noradrenaline. The importance of sympathetic activity in maintaining renovascular hypertension is further supported by the efficacy of central sympatholytic agents such as clonidine in reducing blood pressure in these patients.

An iatrogenic form of secondary hypertension associated with cyclosporine therapy appears also to involve increased levels of sympathetic nerve activity (SNA). Patients receiving cyclosporine as immunosuppressive therapy have a high incidence of hypertension. This is particularly true of patients receiving cyclosporine after cardiac transplants. Scherrer et al. (1990) have shown an impressive association between direct measurements of sympathetic nerve traffic and hypertension in these patients (Fig. 41.2). Increases in SNA were accompanied by increased vascular resistance. The hypertensive effects of increased SNA in these patients would be potentiated by cyclosporine-mediated augmentation of noradrenaline-induced vasoconstriction. These data, together with evidence in rats of cyclosporine-mediated increases in

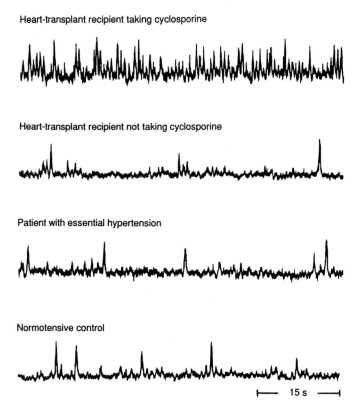

Fig. 42.2. Recordings of muscle sympathetic nerve activity in a heart transplant recipient taking cyclosporine, a heart transplant recipient not taking cyclosporine, a patient with essential hypertension, and a normotensive control subject. The frequency of sympathetic nerve discharge was much higher than normal in the heart transplant recipient on cyclosporine therapy. By comparison, sympathetic activity was normal both in the heart transplant recipient who was not taking cyclosporine and in the patient with essential hypertension.
(Reproduced with permission from Scherrer *et al.* (1990).)

renal SNA and blood pressure prevented by ganglion blockade, provide strong evidence for a causal association between sympathetic activation and cyclosporine-induced hypertension.

Mechanisms by which sympathetic activation may induce and maintain hypertension.

Sympathetic discharge to the heart results in an increase in cardiac output, with positive chronotropic and inotropic effects. In the absence of appropriate reductions in systemic vascular resistance, this increase in cardiac output will result in increased arterial pressure. There is evidence that early hypertension, notably borderline hypertension, is frequently characterized by this 'hyperdynamic' ciculatory state (Julius and Esler 1975). The hyperdynamic circulation of borderline hypertension appears to be largely neurogenic in origin, based on normalization of cardiac output and blood pressure after autonomic blockade.

An increase in sympathetic activity to the peripheral vasculature results in arteriolar vasoconstriction, which serves to raise blood pressure. Furthermore, sympathetic mediated venoconstriction, with consequent central redistribution of blood and increased cardiac output, also acts to increase blood pressure. Borderline hypertensives with hyperkinetic circulations seem to have an increased central blood volume. Borderline hypertensive young men also have a decrease in peripheral venous distensibility which appears to result both from adrenergic mechanisms and structural vascular changes (Takeshita and Mark 1979).

The haemodynamic profiles consistent with sympathetic overactivity appear to be more impressive in early hypertension, as compared to established hypertension, where higher arterial pressures are accompanied by cardiac and vascular smooth muscle hypertrophy, with haemodynamics indicating a normal cardiac output with increased vascular resistance. This suggests a transition from a high-output state of early hypertension to a high-resistance state of established hypertension (Julius and Esler 1975). With the structural vascular changes in established hypertension, including increased vessel wall thickness and decreased lumen diameter, the blood pressure raising effect of a given degree of sympathetic mediated vasoconstriction is magnified.

Increases in renal sympathetic nerve activity may also play an important role in blood pressure elevation. In addition to increasing renal vascular resistance, renal sympathetic activity increases renin release, and increases tubular reabsorption of sodium (DiBona 1989). Consequent expansion of extracellular fluid volume, as well as other effects of sodium retention, will act to raise arterial pressure. Indeed both chronic renal nerve stimulation and intrarenal noradrenaline infusion have been shown to cause hypertension in animal studies.

Even low frequencies of renal sympathetic nerve stimulation, which do not affect renal vascular resistance or glomerular filtration rate, result in increased renal tubular resorption of sodium and water (DiBona 1989). This low level of augmented sympathetic nerve activity attenuates pressure natriuresis, the mechanism whereby an increase in arterial pressure, and hence renal perfusion pressure, act to normalize arterial pressure by an increase in urinary sodium loss. Renal sympathetic activity therefore promotes sodium reabsorption by direct effects on the renal tubules in addition to altering renal haemodynamics.

The renin–angiotensin system and its effects on the kidney may be especially important in a subgroup of patients with 'essential' hypertension.

Hollenberg and Williams (1990) have suggested that abnormalities in the adrenal and renal vascular responses to angiotensin II may account for the elevated blood pressure in about 40 per cent of patients with normal- and high-renin hypertension. This subgroup of salt-sensitive 'non-modulators' exhibits impaired aldosterone and renal blood flow responses to changes in sodium intake. Their adrenal response is set at a level that would be consistent with a high salt diet in a normal individual, while the renal vascular response is set at a level consistent with a low salt diet. Increased salt intake in these patients does not elicit the expected increase in renal blood flow, thus compromising their ability to handle a sodium load. Therapy with angiotensin-converting enzyme inhibitors corrects this abnormal renovascular response to a sodium load. Interestingly, these 'non-modulators' have impressive family histories of hypertension. Even in the normotensive offspring of these hypertensives, subtle abnormalities suggestive of 'non-modulation' have been demonstrated, strongly suggesting a genetic component for this subset of hypertension.

The sympathetic system may also act to initiate or maintain hypertension by trophic effects on the blood vessels (Abboud 1982). This growth-promoting effect appears to be independent of the level of arterial pressure. In stroke-prone hypertensive rats, unilateral superior cervical ganglionectomy reduced the wall-to-lumen ratio of ipsilateral cerebral vessels, despite the fact that perfusion pressure was the same on both sides of the brain (Hart et al. 1980). Noradrenaline, like angiotensin II, can enhance smooth muscle cellular proliferation. These trophic effects on blood vessels are most marked during the early stages of growth. Based on Poiseuille's law, structural changes in blood vessel walls with consequent decreased lumen diameter can have profound functional effects, with an amplification of the vascular resistance change for a given degree of shortening of the smooth muscle—a so-called 'resistance amplifier' (Korner et al. 1989). Korner et al. have suggested that, since the amplification of vascular resistance associated with structural changes in blood vessels can occur early (and precede the onset of hypertension) and since only a slight increase in vessel wall thickness and minimal narrowing of the lumen are necessary to increase vascular resistance, these structural changes may in fact cause the hypertension. This hypothesis needs to be considered against other evidence showing that early hypertension is often associated with increases in cardiac output and a normal total peripheral resistance.

Studies in spontaneously hypertensive rats also suggest a role for the sympathetic nervous system in triggering abnormalities in membrane permeability (Abboud 1982). Noradrenaline reduces the membrane potential of arterial smooth muscle cells, probably by inhibition of the Na^+/K^+ pump, with a resulting increase in passive permeability to cations such as sodium. Transplantation of an artery from a young (but not from an old) normotensive rat into the innervated eye chamber of a hypertensive rat results in membrane permeability abnormalities in cells of the transplanted artery. Denervation of the host anterior eye chamber prevents the development of abnormal membrane permeability. These vascular membrane abnormalities that increase vasoconstrictor responsiveness to noradrenaline and may lead to hypertension probably result from genetically determined sympathetic nerve effects acting in the early stages of growth and development.

Peripheral reflex mechanisms in human hypertension

Arterial baroreflex

Probably the most extensively studied of the possible aetiologies of sympathetic overactivity in hypertension are depressor and pressor autonomic reflexes. The traditional concepts hold, first, that arterial baroreflexes are abnormal in hypertension with a higher threshold for activation and a reduction in sensitivity and, second, that these alterations result from chronic increases in arterial pressure. In recent years, two new concepts have emerged regarding alterations in arterial baroreflexes in hypertension. First, it has been found that Dahl genetically salt-sensitive rats fed a rigorously low salt diet have abnormalities in baroreceptor afferent mechanisms that occur in the absence of an increase in arterial pressure (Mark 1991). This suggests that some alterations in arterial baroreflexes in hypertension could be related to genetic abnormalities that precede and are independent of the increase in arterial pressure. Second, it is now known that abnormalities in baroreflex control of parasympathetic activity (heart rate) do not necessarily predict alterations in baroreflex control of sympathetic nerve activity and vascular resistance. Indeed, there is evidence from both experimental animals and humans that baroreflex control of sympathetic activity, vascular resistance, and arterial pressure may be preserved in early or mild hypertension despite impairment of baroreflex control of heart rate. This dissociation appears to result from a greater central nervous system 'reserve' for maintaining baroreflex control of sympathetic versus parasympathetic activity. Insofar as hypertension is concerned, the baroreflex-mediated sympathetic and vascular resistance responses to blood pressure changes are obviously of greater haemodynamic significance than the heart rate responses.

Cardiopulmonary baroreflex

Borderline hypertensive patients with a family history of hypertension show an augmented increase in sympathetic activity and vascular resistance in

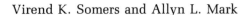

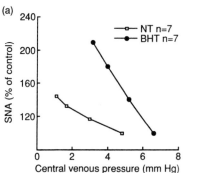

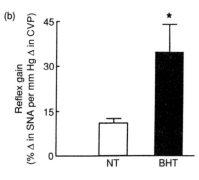

Fig. 41.3. (a) Plot of mean values of central venous pressure (CVP) versus sympathetic nerve activity (SNA) (percentage of control) at rest and during three levels of lower body negative pressure in normotensive (NT) and borderline hypertensive (BHT) subjects. Baseline CVP was higher in BHT, but reductions in CVP produced by lower body negative pressure were similar in both groups. Levels of SNA were greater at each level of CVP in BHT subjects, resulting in a steeper CVP–SNA slope. These findings indicate, first, heightened sympathetic neural drive and, second, an exaggerated cardiopulmonary baroreflex sensitivity in borderline hypertensive subjects. (b) Bar graph showing mean gain of cardiopulmonary baroreflexes in NT and BHT subjects, indicating a significantly greater reflex gain in the borderline hypertensives ($* = P < 0.05$). (Reproduced with permission from Rea and Hamdan (1990).)

response to lower body negative pressure (simulating orthostatic stress; Rea and Hamdan 1990; Fig. 41.3). These findings may help explain the exaggerated diastolic blood pressure increase with upright tilt in borderline hypertension. Importantly, this sympathetic hyperreactivity to non-hypotensive lower body negative pressure occurred despite no detectable abnormality in arterial baroreflex regulation of sympathetic nerve responses to raising and lowering blood pressure. In addition, the augmented sympathetic nerve response to orthostatic stress occurred in the absence of an increased baseline sympathetic activity in the borderline hypertensives in the supine position. Two conclusions emerge from these studies. First, the exaggerated sympathetic response to simulated orthostatic stress suggests that mild hypertensives have a potentiated sympathetic neural drive, but in the supine position this elevated drive is masked by an augmented sympathoinhibitory effect of the cardiopulmonary baroreflex (Fig. 41.4). Subsequent cardiac hypertrophy with attenuation of the augmented sympathoinhibitory effects of the cardiopulmonary baroreceptors may lead to higher sympathetic activity and blood pressure during recumbency (Victor and Morgan 1990). Second, the heightened sympathetic neural drive in mild hypertensives can occur in the absence of impairment of arterial

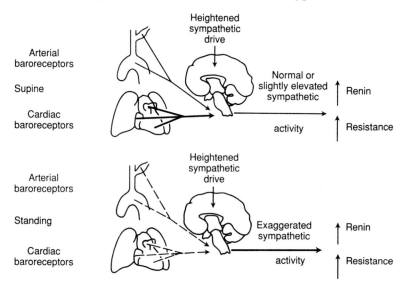

Fig. 41.4. Schematic diagram depicting concept of increased cardiopulmonary baroreflex control of sympathetic nerve activity and heightened central neural drive which may explain the reflex adjustment to changes in posture in mild hypertensives. In the supine position the heightened central neural sympathetic drive is buffered by the increase in cardiopulmonary baroreflex activity, so that sympathetic activity, plasma renin level, and vascular resistance may be normal or only slightly elevated. With standing, however, venous pooling reduces cardiac filling pressures and arterial pressure, thus eliminating the cardiopulmonary baroreflex buffering. Under these conditions, the heightened central neural sympathetic drive is expressed as exaggerated reflex increases in sympathetic nerve activity, plasma renin, and vascular resistance. (Reproduced with permission from Mark (1990).)

baroreflex modulation of sympathetic activity. This strengthens the view that central neural mechanisms may be responsible for enhanced sympathetic nerve activity in early or mild hypertension.

Chemoreflex

The role of the chemoreceptors in determining sympathetic nerve discharge as well as ventilation has recently received considerable attention. Hypoxic stimulation of the peripheral chemoreceptors triggers sympathetic excitation in humans and animals. This chemoreceptor reflex may be exaggerated in spontaneously hypertensive rats (SHR) and hypertensive humans. SHR have a respiratory alkalosis that may result from increased ventilatory drive even during normoxia. These animals also show an increased carotid sinus nerve chemoreceptor discharge in response to hypoxia. Young human hypertensives have an increased inspiratory drive when exposed to hypoxic conditions (Trzebski *et al.* 1982). Sympathetic nerve discharge during hypoxia is also potentiated in borderline hypertensive men (about twice the response seen in age- and weight-matched normotensives; Somers *et al.* 1988). This potentiation is especially marked during voluntary apnoea (about 10-fold the response in normotensives), when the sympathoinhibitory influence of breathing and thoracic afferent activity is eliminated (Fig.41.5 and 41.6). These findings have two important implications. First, heightened resting sympathetic discharge in early hypertension may be explained by an augmented tonic chemoreflex-mediated sympathoexcitation even during normoxia. Second, the strong association between hypertension and sleep apnoea may be explained by chronic sympathoexcitation and consequent blood pressure elevation during sleep, triggered by episodes of hypoxia, hypercapnia, and apnoea. These frequent elevations in sympathetic nerve activity and blood pressure during episodes of sleep apnoea may have functional and structural consequences and may contribute to daytime sympathetic excitation and blood pressure elevation. Increases in plasma adrenaline from hypoxic sympathoadrenal stimulation during sleep apnoea episodes may also contribute significantly to sustained hypertension even during wakefulness, by adrenergic nerve uptake of adrenaline, with

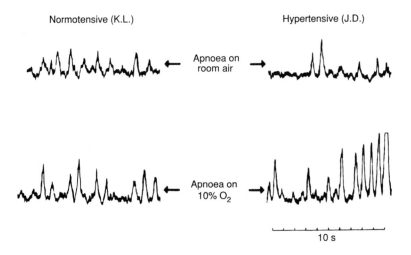

Fig. 41.5. Sympathetic nerve activity during 10 to 15 s of apnoea in a normotensive subject and in a borderline hypertensive subject while breathing room air and while breathing 10 per cent oxygen and 90 per cent nitrogen (hypoxia). During hypoxia the increase in sympathetic nerve activity with apnoea was especially marked in the hypertensive subject. (Reproduced with permission from Somers *et al.* (1988).)

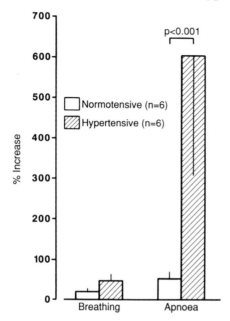

Fig. 41.6. Percentage increases in sympathetic nerve activity during isocapnic hypoxia as compared with room air in six borderline hypertensive and six normotensive subjects (left bars), indicating a greater sympathetic nerve response to hypoxia in borderline hypertensive subjects. With apnoea during hypoxia (right bars), and consequent elimination of the sympathoinhibitory effects of hyperventilation, the potentiated sympathetic nerve response to hypoxia in the borderline hypertensive subjects was especially striking. (Reproduced with permission from Somers *et al.* (1988).)

subsequent facilitation of neural noradrenaline release, as discussed later. Indeed, definitive treatment of sleep apnoea in patients with both sleep apnoea and hypertension frequently results in blood pressure reduction as well.

The sympathetic nervous system may also be important in explaining the increased incidence of ischaemic heart disease, cardiac arrhythmias, and mortality in patients with sleep apnoea. During episodes of sleep apnoea, there are reductions in arterial oxygen levels, elevations in arterial carbon dioxide, and consequent respiratory acidosis. Hypoxia and hypercapnia act synergistically to increase sympathetic nerve activity, with the increase being especially striking during apnoea (elimination of the sympathoinhibitory influence of thoracic afferents; Somers *et al.* 1989). Furthermore, the sympathetic nerve response to hypoxia and apnoea is potentiated in patients with hypertension. Hypertensive patients are also at high risk for sleep apnoea. Thus, repetitive episodes of sleep apnoea with consequent hypoxia, hypercapnia, and acidosis, producing sympathetic activation with resulting increases in plasma catecholamines and blood pressure, may promote cardiac catastrophes such as ischaemia, arrhythmias, and sudden death during sleep. These effects may be magnified in the presence of underlying left ventricular hypertrophy which is known to predispose to ventricular arrhythmias and sudden death.

Environmental stress

Environmental or behavioural factors may be involved in the initiation and maintenance of sympathetic overactivity in hypertension. Mental stress tasks in the laboratory trigger transient elevations in sympathetic activity and blood pressure. Chronic stress may be related to the onset of hypertension in animals. Haemodynamic and catecholamine responses to acute mental stress are more marked in children with a family history of hypertension. Environmental stress increases renal sympathetic nerve activity in SHR and DOCA salt hypertensive, but not WKY rats (DiBona 1989). High salt diet augments the influence of behavioural stress on renal sympathetic nerve activity in SHR. The sympathetic and haemodynamic response to mental stress is able to override the sympathoinhibitory effect of simultaneous baroreceptor stimulation (Anderson *et al.* 1991*b*). Chronic or repetitive stressful stimuli may conceivably result in sustained sympathetic activation and hypertension in susceptible persons. This response may be augmented by the sustained sympathetic neural effects of adrenaline uptake by nerve terminals during stressful stimuli, as discussed next.

Humoral influences on the sympathetic nervous system

Adrenaline

In linking the sympathetic system and hypertension, neural actions of adrenaline have been proposed (Brown and Dollery 1984). Circulating adrenaline is taken up by adrenergic nerve terminals, with subsequent sustained neural release as a cotransmitter with noradrenaline. Neurally released adrenaline stimulates prejunctional β-receptors on adrenergic nerve terminals, thereby facilitating further release of neural noradrenaline. Several studies have reported increased levels of plasma adrenaline in hypertensive patients. Infusion of adrenaline for 6 h can result in a sustained elevation of ambulatory blood pressure for up to 18 h after the infusion (Blankestijn *et al.* 1988). Floras *et al.* (1990) have demonstrated that intraarterial infusion of adrenaline facilitates neurogenic vasoconstriction in borderline hypertensive humans. Tachycardia after adrenaline infusion persists even when plasma adrenaline levels return to normal (Brown and Dollery 1984). Pre-treatment with desipramine, which inhibits neuronal uptake of adrenaline, prevents the tachycardia. Thus, uptake and subsequent release of adrenaline, with facilitation of noradrenaline release at the level of the adrenergic nerve terminals, may contribute to increases in sympathetic activity and reflex responsiveness in hypertensive patients, and to a 'hyperkinetic' circulatory state. It may be that repetitive adrenomedullary stimulation and adrenaline release during stress in subjects prone to developing hypertension could promote a sustained facilitation in neurally released noradrenaline which, over many years, could contribute to sustained hypertension.

Insulin

The importance of insulin in sympathetic activation and hypertension has aroused great interest. Obesity, particularly upper body obesity, is associated with insulin resistance and hyperinsulinaemia. Hypertension is also associated with a state of insulin resistance and hyperinsulinaemia, independent of obesity or diabetes mellitus. Interestingly, the insulin resistance which occurs in obesity and hypertension affects actions of insulin on glucose uptake in skeletal muscle, but actions of insulin on the sympathetic nervous system and the kidney are preserved (Mark 1990). Thus, it has been postulated that the hyperinsulinaemia which occurs in insulin resistance causes renal sodium retention, heightened sympathetic activity, and increased vascular resistance and arterial pressure. Euglycaemic hyperinsulinaemia (insulin $< 400 \,\mu U/m$) results in increases in plasma noradrenaline and modest increases in blood pressure in normotensive humans. Lower levels of insulin (approximately 75 to 150 $\mu U/m$), within the physiological postprandial range, result in increases in muscle sympathetic nerve activity, but produce vasodilatation (not the expected sympathetic vasoconstriction), and do not increase blood pressure in normal humans (Anderson et al. 1991a). Thus, it appears that insulin elicits both pressor (sympathoexcitatory) and depressor (vasodilator) actions. At high levels of plasma insulin, exceeding the physiological range, the pressor effect is predominant. However, with physiological levels in normal humans the sympathoexcitatory and vasodilator actions are balanced and blood pressure does not increase. It is possible that the presence of other factors, such as structural vascular changes, insulin resistance, or genetic predisposition to hypertension, could augment the sympathetic (pressor) action of insulin or attenuate the vasodilator (depressor) action, thereby permitting insulin to produce a sympathetically mediated increase in arterial pressure.

Renin–angiotensin

The interactions between the renin–angiotensin system and the sympathetic nervous system are considerable, and may be especially important in renovascular hypertension and in the 'non-modulator' subset of essential hypertension. Angiotensin II acts on the sympathetic nervous system at the central, ganglionic, and nerve terminal levels, as well as at the adrenal medulla to increase sympathetic nerve activity (Regoli *et al.* 1974). Angiotensin II also facilitates release of noradrenaline, reduces its re-uptake, and sensitizes blood vessels to the effects of noradrenaline. Infusion of exogenous angiotensin II in humans augments sympathetic mediated vasoconstriction (Webb *et al.* 1988). The reductions in sympathetic nerve traffic and heart rate observed when blood pressure is increased by infusions of angiotensin II are significantly less than those seen with equivalent blood pressure elevations using phenylephrine (Matsukawa *et al.* 1988), suggesting that angiotensin II inhibits baroreflex control of both sympathetic activity as well as heart rate in humans. Conversely, angiotensin-converting enzyme inhibition in animals blunts the vascular responses to exogenous noradrenaline as well as to electrical stimulation of the sympathetic nerves. Acute angiotensin-converting enzyme inhibition in hypertensive humans is associated with arterial baroreceptor resetting and facilitation of parasympathetic reflex responsiveness (Zanchetti 1989). These angiotensin–sympathetic-baroreflex interactions may explain the ability of angiotensin-converting enzyme inhibitors to reduce both vascular resistance and blood pressure without any reflex increase in heart rate.

Summary and conclusions

There is clearly a genetic predisposition to essential hypertension, probably polygenic in origin. It is, therefore, unlikely that a single physiological abnormality can explain all cases of hypertension. Many factors, including environmental stressors and diet, may be involved, as exemplified by the so-called 'salt-sensitive subset' of essential hypertension. Further complicating the scenario is that hypertension is itself a dynamic entity, progressing from one haemodynamic and structure/function profile to another, making it difficult to establish whether any isolated finding is a cause or consequence of raised arterial pressure levels. With this magnitude of disease heterogeneity it is not surprising, therefore, that there is some lack of consensus in the literature with regard to the various reflex, cellular, and other abnormalities that have been described. It is possible that the genesis and maintenance of hypertension is both polygenic and multifactorial, with different abnormalities exerting different degrees of influence in various subsets of essential hypertension.

The weight of evidence, though not unequivocal, strongly suggests that sympathetic overactivity is important in the aetiology and maintenance of hypertension. This appears to be especially true for the early stages of hypertension. In the later stages of hypertension, the sympathetic nervous system may continue to be important in augmenting the vascular and myocardial dysfunction and structural damage that ensue from chronic elevations in arterial pressure.

Acknowledgements

The research of the authors and their colleagues which is described in this review was supported by grants HL44546, HL14388, HL24962 from the National Heart, Lung, and Blood Institute; by grant RR59 from the General Clinical Research Centers Program, Division of Research Resources, National Institutes of Health; and by research funds from the Department of Veterans Affairs. The authors thank Nancy Davin for superb secretarial assistance.

References

Abboud, F. M. (1982). The sympathetic system in hypertension: State-of-the-art review. *Hypertension* **4**(suppl.2), II 208–25.
Anderson, E. A., Sinkey, C. A., Lawton, W. J., and Mark, A. L. (1989). Elevated sympathetic nerve activity in borderline hypertensive humans: Evidence from direct intraneural recordings. *Hypertension* **14**, 177–3.
Anderson, E. A., Hoffman, R. P., Balon, T. W., Sinkey, C. A., and Mark, A. L. (1991*a*). Hyperinsulinemia produces both sympathetic neural activation and vasodilation in normal humans. *J. clin. Invest.* **87**, 2246–52.
Anderson, E. A., Sinkey, C. A., and Mark, A. L. (1991*b*). Mental stress increases sympathetic nerve activity during sustained baroreceoptor stimulation in humans. *Hypertension* **17**, III 43–9.
Blankestijn, P. J., Man in't Veld, A. J., Tulen, J., van den Meiracker, A. H., Boomsma, F., Derkx, F. H. M., Moleman, P., Ritsema van Eck, H. J., Mulder, P., Lamberts, S. W. J., and Schalekamp, M. A. D. H. (1988). Twenty-four hour pressor effect of infused adrenaline in normotensive subjects: a randomized controlled double-blind cross-over study. *J. Hypertension* **6**(suppl.4), S562–4.
Brown, M. J. and Dollery, C. T. (1984). Adrenaline and hypertension. *Clin. exp. Hypertension—Theory Practice* **A6**(1&2) and 539–49.
Conway, J. (1984). Hemodynamic aspects of essential hypertension in humans. *Physiol. Rev.* **64**, 617–59.
DiBona, G. F. (1989). Sympathetic nervous system influences on the kidney: role in hypertension *Am. J. Hypertension* **2**(suppl.), 119S–24S.
Doyle, A. E. and Smirk, F. H. (1955). The neurogenic component in hypertension. *Circulation* **12**, 543–52.
Egan, B., Panis, R., Hinderliter, A., Schork, N., and Julius, S. (1987). Mechanism of increased alpha adrenergic vasoconstriction in human essential hypertension. *J. clin. Invest.* **80**, 812–17.
Esler, M., Jennings, G., Biviano, B., Lambert, G., and Hasking, G. (1986). Mechanism of elevated plasma noradrenaline in the course of essential hypertension. *J. Cardiovasc. Pharmacol.* **8**(suppl.5), S39–43.
Floras, J. S., Aylward, P. E., Mark, A. L., and Abboud, F. M. (1990). Adrenaline facilitates neurogenic vasoconstriction in borderline hypertensive subjects. *J. Hypertension* **8**, 443–8.

Folkow, B., DiBona, G. F., Hjemdahl, P., Thorén, P., and Wallin, B. G. (1983). Measurements of plasma norepinephrine concentrations in human primary hypertension: A word of caution on their applicability for assessing neurogenic contributions. *Hypertension* **5**, 399–403

Goldstein, D. S. (1983). Plasma catecholamine and essential hypertension: An analytical review. *Hypertension* **5**, 86–99.

Hart, M. N., Heistad, D. D., and Brody, M. J. (1980). Effect of chronic hypertension and sympathetic denervation on wall/lumen ratio of cerebral vessels. *Hypertension* **2**, 419–23.

Hjemdahl, P. (1988). Plasma catecholamines as markers for sympatho-adrenal activity in human primary hypertension. *Pharmacol. Toxicol.* (suppl.I), 27–31.

Hollenberg, N. K. and Williams, G. H. (1990). Abnormal renal function, sodium-volume homeostasis, and renin system behaviour in normal-renin essential hypertension. In *Hypertension pathophysiology diagnosis and mangement* (ed. J. H Laragh and B. M. Brenner), pp. 1349–70 Raven Press, New York.

Julius, S. and Esler, M. (1975). Autonomic nervous cardiovascular regulation in borderline hypertension. *Am. J. Cardiol.* **36**, 685–96.

Korner, P. I., Bobik, A., Angus, J. A., Adams, M. A., and Friberg, P. (1989). Resistance control in hypertension. *J. Hypertension* **7**(suppl.4), S125–34.

Mark, A. L. (1990). Regulation of sympathetic nerve activity in mild human hypertension. *J. Hypertension* **8**(suppl.7), S67–75.

Mark, A. L. (1991). Sympathetic neural contribution to salt induced hypertension in Dahl rats. *Hypertension* **17**(suppl. 1), 186–90.

Matsukawa, T., Gotoh, E., Miyajima, E., Yamada, Y., Shionoiri, H., Tockikubo, O., and Ishii, M. (1988). Angiotensin II inhibits baroreflex control of muscle sympathetic nerve activity and the heart rate in patients with essential hypertension. *J. Hypertension* **6**(suppl. 4), S501–4.

Oparil, S. (1986) The sympathetic nervous system in clinical and experimental hypertension. *Kidney Int.* **30**, 4437–52.

Rea, R. F. and Hamdan, M. (1990). Baroreflex control of muscle sympathetic nerve activity in borderline hypertension. *Circulation* **82**, 856–62.

Regoli, D., Park, W. K., and Rioux, F. (1974). Pharmacology of angiotensin *Pharmacol. Rev.* **26**, 69–123.

Scherrer, U., Vissing, S. F., Morgan, B. J., Rollins, J. A., Tindall, R. S. A., Ring, A., Hanson, P., Mohanty, P. K., and Victor, R. G. (1990). Cyclosporine-induced sympathetic activation and hypertension after heart transplantation. *New. Engl. J. Med.* **323**, 693–9.

Somers, V. K., Mark, A. L., and Abboud, F. M. (1988). Potentiation of sympathetic nerve responses to hypoxia in borderline hypertensive subjects. *Hypertension* **11**, 608–12.

Somers, V. K., Mark A. L., Zavala, D. C., and Abboud, F. M. (1989). Contrasting effects of hypoxia and hypercapnia on ventilation and sympathetic activity in humans. *J. Appl. Physiol.* **67**, 2101–6.

Takeshita, A. and Mark, A. L. (1979). Decreased venous distensibility in borderline hypertension. *Hypertension* **1**, 202–6.

Trzebski, A., Tafil, M., Zoltowski, M., and Przybylski, J. (1982). Increased sensitivity of the arterial chemoreceptor drive in young men with mild hypertension. *Cardiovasc. Res.* **16**, 163–72.

Vallbo, A. B., Hagbarth, K. E., Torebjörk, H. E., and Wallin, B. G. (1979). Somatosensory, proprioceptive and sympathetic activity in human peripheral nerves. *Physiol. Rev.* **59**, 919–57.

Victor, R. G. and Morgan, B. J. (1990). Baroreceptors and hypertension. *Circulation* **82**(3), 1057–9.

Wallin, B. G. and Sundlöf, G. (1979). A quantative study of muscle nerve sympathetic activity in resting normotensive and hypertensive subjects. *Hypertension* **1**, 67–77.

Webb, D. J., Seidelin, P. H., Benjamin N., Collier, J. G., and Struthers, A. D. (1988). Sympathetically mediated vasoconstriction is augmented by angiotensin II in man. *J. Hypertension* **6**(suppl.4), S542–3.

Yamada Y., Miyajima, E., Tochikubo, O., Matsukawa, T., and Ishii, M. (1989). Age-related changes in muscle sympathetic nerve activity in essential hypertension. *Hypertension* **13**, 870–7.

Zanchetti, A. (1989). The clinical role of angiotensin converting enzyme inhibitors in antihypertensive therapy in the 1990s *J. Hypertension* **7**(suppl.5), S37–40.

42. Cardiac failure and the autonomic nervous system

Gary S. Francis and Jay N. Cohn

Introduction

Congestive heart failure is a clinical syndrome complicating the course of most forms of heart disease and characterized in its extreme form by circulatory congestion and reduced flow to organ systems. Ventricular systolic and/or diastolic function are impaired in this syndrome, and this myocardial dysfunction has remained the primary focus of attention of physiologists and cardiologists for many years. More recently, interest has been directed to abnormalities of the peripheral circulation and to activation of various neuroendocrine systems, particularly the sympathetic nervous system. Chronic activation of the sympathetic nervous system and its altered responsiveness may contribute importantly to the symptoms, signs, and natural history of heart failure.

It has been apparent for more than 40 years that patients with heart failure have a defect in autonomic nervous system control as manifested by limited activation of the sympathetic nervous system in response to the upright posture (Brigden and Sharpey-Schafer 1950). A variety of other reflex control mechanisms also appears to be impaired (Hirsch *et al.* 1987). Disturbances in both the sympathetic and parasympathetic nervous systems can be demonstrated. The extent of autonomic dysfunction tends to parallel the clinical haemodynamic severity of heart failure (Olivari *et al.* 1983).

The past decade has been a period of intense research activity in neuro-hormonal control mechanisms in congestive heart failure, with studies focusing on sympathetic nervous system activity at rest and in response to various stimuli (e.g. dynamic exercise, upright tilt, lower body negative pressure, acute vasodilatation; Hirsch *et al.* 1987). Demonstrated abnormalities in such responses appear to be partially reversed by pharmacological interventions such as angiotensin-converting enzymme inhibitors (Cody *et al.* 1982). The ultimate treatment for severe heart failure, heart transplantation, also tends to reverse reflex control abnormalities (Levine *et al.* 1986; Ellenbogen *et al.* 1989), although transplant patients may continue to demonstrate some disturbances in autonomic function.

The purpose of this chapter is to review the evidence for disturbances in autonomic control mechanisms common to the syndrome of congestive heart failure, and to strengthen our understanding as to how these abnormalities contribute to the pathophysiology of this complex syndrome.

Myocardial β-adrenoceptors

The membrane-bound β-adrenoceptor–G protein–adenylate cyclase complex is a powerful regulator of cardiac contractility in both the non-failing and failing heart (Fig. 42.1). The β_1- and β_2-adrenergic cell surface membrane receptors, parts of which protrude into the extracellular space, interact with a number of messengers, including the neurotransmitter noradrenaline (NA).

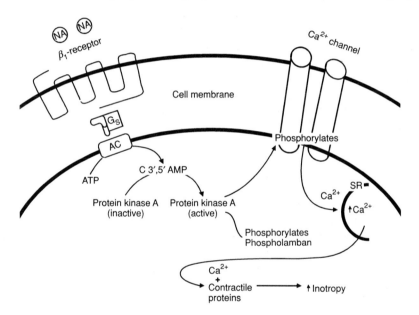

Fig. 42.1. The membrane bound β-adrenergic receptor-G protein-adenylate cyclase complex. The signal (i.e. noradrenaline) engages the membrane bound β_1-receptor, which is coupled to a guanine nucleotide regulatory protein (G_s protein). The G_s protein dissociates from the receptor and activates the enzyme adenylate cyclase (AC). Adenosine triphosphate (ATP) is converted to c 3', 5' AMP, which in turn catalyses inactive protein kinase A to active protein kinase A (PKA). PKA then phosphorylates a number of highly specialized proteins, including membrane-bound calcium channels to allow the influx of Ca^{2+} into the cell. Ca^{2+} is transported into the intracellular Ca^{2+} storage depots called sarcoplasmic reticulae (SR). The SR then provides Ca^{2+} for interaction with contractile proteins. Contraction of the myofilaments is dependent on phosphorylation by PKA of phospholamban, a specialized protein.

By coupling to stimulatory guanine-nucleotide-binding proteins (G_s proteins), the membrane β-adrenoceptors mediate stimulation of adenylate cyclase. Cyclic adenosine monophosphate (cAMP) is generated from adenosine triphosphate (ATP) via adenylate cyclase, and cAMP in turn catalyses a number of phosphorylation reactions mediated by protein kinase A. These reactions include phosphorylation of calcium channels, leading to a greater increase in calcium influx, and phosphorylation of phospholamban, leading to enhanced calcium uptake in the sarcoplasmic reticulum and subsequent augmented release of calcium to the myofilaments. The net result is an increase in myocardial contractility.

The non-failing human heart primarily relies on β_1-adrenoceptors. Approximately 80 per cent of the total pool of β-receptors are of the β_1 variety. β_2-adrenoceptors generate relatively little cAMP.

The cDNA for the human β_1-receptor has been cloned, and its primary amino acid structure has been elucidated. In 1982 Bristow and colleagues reported that myocardial β-adrenoceptors measured in failing human ventricles were markedly subsensitive to stimulation by the non-selective agonist isoproterenol. This alteration of the inotropic response appeared to be explicable by a decrease in the total pool of membrane-bound β-adrenoceptors as assessed by maximal [^{3}H]-dihydroalprenolol binding. These authors demonstrated a highly significant reduction in isoproterenol-stimulated adenylate cyclase activity in the left ventricles of hearts removed from patients about to undergo heart transplantation (Fig. 42.2). Later studies from this same group demonstrated that 'down-regulation' of the total β-receptor population appears to begin early in mild heart failure, with some hearts showing a 60 to 70 per cent reduction in β_1-receptor density when heart failure was more advanced. Of interest, papillary muscles from these failing hearts still responded normally with a positive inotropic response to calcium, thus implying that the primary lesion is reduced β-adrenoceptor density and/or receptor uncoupling rather than contractile protein deficiency. Since β_2-receptor density remains unchanged in the failing heart, the selective loss of β_1-receptors leads to a change in β_1/β_2 subtype ratio from approximately 80:20 to 60:40 in failing hearts. However, despite increased membrane density, the β_2-receptor is 'uncoupled' to some extent in the failing heart. This β_2-uncoupling may be related to increased Gi protein activity, which inhibits the stimulation of cAMP.

It is likely that more than one mechanism is responsible for the down-regulation of β_1-adrenoceptors that occurs in heart failure. Although the failing myocardium is depleted of NA, cardiac-derived NA (as measured from the coronary sinus) is increased in heart failure. There may also be a decrease in NA uptake by cardiac sympathetic nerves. Increased local concentration of NA may thereby reduce the density of membrane-bound β_1-receptors, reducing the sensitivity of the myocardium to NA. However, it is difficult to reconcile increased local concentration of NA when the myocardium is

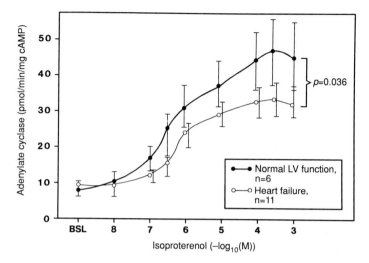

Fig. 42.2.   The influence of L-isoproterenol of myocardial tissue isolated from the left ventricles (LV) of patients with severe congestive heart failure who later received a heart transplant (open circles) and from normal hearts of potential heart donors (closed circles). The failing myocardial tissue is unable to generate a normal amount of adenylate cyclase in response to L-isoproterenol. BSL: Baseline (Taken with permission from Bristow *et al.* (1982).)

known to be depleted of NA. The precise mechanism of β_1-receptor density 'down-regulation' remains unclear, but it appears to be a reversible phenomenon, as treatment with the semi-selective β-blocking agent metoprolol can restore both the β_1-receptor density and the responsiveness to the β_1-agonist dobutamine. The reduction in myocardial membrane-bound β_1-receptors is a marker of the adrenergic compensatory process, but it also could play a direct role in the pathophysiology of heart failure by interfering with the myocardial response to increased workloads.

Plasma noradrenaline levels measured at rest

The radioenzymatic technique of measuring plasma NA levels was an important step in bringing to the bedside a rapid and precise method of detecting heightened 'sympathetic activity' in patients with heart failure. It now seems clear that the sympathetic nervous system is activated progressively as the signs and symptoms increase over time. Patients with left ventricular dysfunction (ejection fraction ≤ 35 per cent) without overt signs and syptoms of heart failure have increased levels of plasma NA as well as increased levels of atrial natriuretic factor and arginine vasopressin (Francis *et al.* 1990). In general, those patients with more advanced heart failure have the greatest increment in plasma NA. The normal resting value of NA is age-dependent and is generally in the range of 150–300 pg/ml. Patients with congestive heart failure have values of plasma NA in the range of 300 to 3000 pg/ml, but typically average about 500–600 pg/ml.

The cause of the increase in plasma NA in patients with congestive heart failure is poorly understood. The sympathetic nervous system and renin–angiotensin system are likely activated in a presumed attempt to maintain circulatory homeostasis in the face of a falling cardiac output (Francis *et al.* 1984), but the actual signal and how it is processed have remained elusive. Directly measured sympathetic nerve 'traffic' using a microneurographic technique has been found to be increased in the peroneal nerve of patients with heart failure (Leimbach *et al.* 1986). The correlation between directly measured nerve traffic and plasma NA is quite good, suggesting that plasma NA is a reasonable index of generalized sympathetic activity in the context of heart failure. Using tritiated NA, Hasking and colleagues (1986) have demonstrated that both 'spillover' from sympathetic neurons and delayed

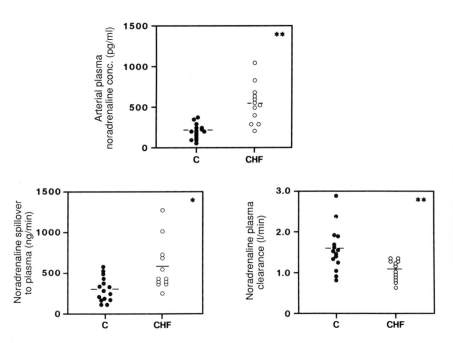

Fig. 42.3. Plasma noradrenaline concentration and its determinants in subjects with and without congestive heart failure (CHF). $*p < 0.02$; $**p < 0.002$. Using radioactive tracer techniques, patients with CHF demonstrate enhanced 'spillover' of NA from synaptic clefts into plasma and reduced clearance of NA from the circulation. Both mechanisms could contribute to increased plasma concentrations of NA in patients with CHF. C, controls. (Taken with permission from Hasking *et al.* (1986).)

clearance from the circulation are important contributors to increased levels of NA in patients with heart failure (Fig. 42.3). The correlation between resting levels of NA and haemodynamic measurements such as cardiac output, systemic vascular resistance, and blood pressure are rather modest. Moreover, plasma NA correlates only poorly with plasma renin activity and arginine vasopressin, thus suggesting that these neurohormones are under separate control mechanisms.

The parasympathetic nervous system is also abnormal in patients with heart disease (Eckberg *et al.* 1971). For any given increase in blood pressure, there is less than the usual degree of heart rate slowing. Moreover, patients with heart failure demonstrate less respiratory variation in heart rate than healthy control subjects. The cause of this relative withdrawal of vagal tone is unclear, but the reduced variation in heart rate may have prognostic significance. Of interest, the variation in R–R interval is improved, but not normalized, following orthotopic heart transplantation (Sands *et al.* 1989).

Direct recordings of efferent sympathetic nerve activity from peripheral nerves in intact human subjects have been made possible by the technique of microneurography, originally developed by Valbo and colleagues (1979). Recent studies by Ferguson *et al.* (1990) noted that the marked increase in microneurographically measured sympathetic nerve activity in patients with heart failure was significantly and inversely correlated with left ventricular stroke work index ($r = -0.86$) and positively correlated with left-sided cardiac filling pressures ($r = 0.82$). There was no correlation between sympathetic activity and left ventricular ejection fraction or mean arterial pressure. Similarly to the observations of Levine and associates (1982) using plasma NA, Ferguson *et al.* (1990) demonstrated a correlation between cardiac performance and microneurographic efferent sympathetic nerve activity in patients with moderate-to-severe heart failure. The correlation between resting efferent nerve activity and resting levels of plasma NA was 0.72 in the Ferguson study. Plasma NA or directly measured nerve activity can separate mildly ill patients from those with severe disease, but these measurements do not clearly discriminate between patients with intermediate forms of heart failure, i.e. between New York Heart Association functional classes II and III.

In 1984 Cohn *et al.* reported that plasma NA levels provide a better guide to prognosis in patients with heart failure than other commonly measured indices of cardiac performance. In this study the plasma NA was the best independent prognostic variable among several haemodynamic and biochemical measurements as determined by multivariate regression analyses of survival times. An update of this analysis (Rector *et al.* 1987) indicated that a cut-off value of 600 pg/ml provides the most prognostic information (Fig. 42.4). The idea of using plasma NA to determine prognosis has been very valuable when evaluating patients for heart transplantation, where conventional haemodynamic measurements, such as ejection fraction, cardiac output, and left

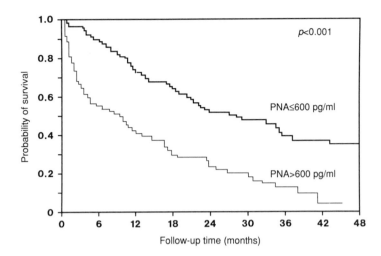

Fig. 42.4. The relationship between probability of survival and plasma adrenaline (PNA) in 217 patients with congestive heart failure. A cut-off value of 600 pg/ml provides the most prognostic information as determined by multivariate regression analysis of survival times. (Taken with permission from Rector *et al.* (1987).)

ventricular filling pressure, are uniformly abnormal and therefore not discriminatory. A markedly increased plasma NA level (i.e. $>600\,\text{pg/ml}$) is rather consistently associated with a poor prognosis.

Plasma NA levels measured during exercise

Early studies using a fluorometric technique to measure plasma NA in patients with heart failure demonstrated a greater than normal augmentation during exercise. However, careful analysis of these data indicates that patients simply stopped exercising sooner and achieved a peak total body oxygen consumption at an earlier point in time. Francis and colleagues (1982), using the more sensitive radioenzymatic technique to measure plasma NA, confirmed the finding of early augmentation of sympathetic nervous system activity during exercise in patients with heart failure (Fig. 42.5). It is apparent from both of these studies that patients with heart failure and normal control subjects were not exercising in the same physiological framework. At relatively mild workloads patients with heart failure might have already become exhausted and achieved their peak oxygen consumption, whereas control subjects were still exercising well below their anaerobic threshold.

To normalize the data so that both patients and control subjects could be compared in the same physiological framework, Francis *et al.* (1985)

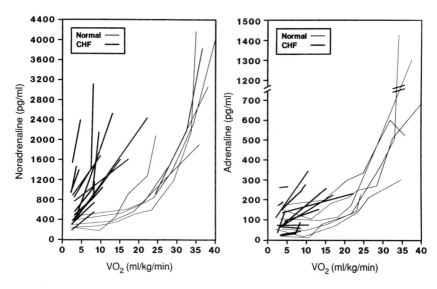

Fig. 42.5. Plasma noradrenaline response to exercise during graded bicycle ergometry is shown in thin lines for normal subjects and in thick lines for patients with congestive heart failure (CHF). VO$_2$, total body oxygen consumption. (Taken with permission from Francis *et al.* (1982).)

performed progressive bicycle ergometry and sequential plasma NA measurements at each stage of exercise. For identical levels of exercise (defined as the percentage of peak VO$_2$), patients with heart failure demonstrated an attenuation of the NA response as measured by a significantly flatter plasma NA upward curve during exercise (Fig. 42.6). However, a subsequent study by Hasking and colleagues (1988) using titriated NA kinetics demonstrated increased 'spillover' of NA during exercise in patients with heart failure compared with control subjects. The variance of these studies may have to do with differences in patient populations, techniques, etc. What remains clear is that patients with heart failure demonstrate an abnormality of the sympathetic nervous system during exercise. Such patients show an early abrupt rise in plasma NA accompanied by an inability to mount a normal heart rate response and a failure to reduce peripheral vascular resistance to the same extent as normals. It is possible that these abnormalities contribute to their inability to perform a high level of physical activity.

Disturbed baroreceptor function

Cardiopulmonary receptors located in the heart and lungs and baroreceptors in the great vessels normally respond to changes in pressure and volume by altering the activity of the sympathetic and parasympathetic nervous systems.

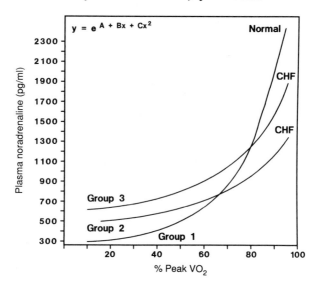

Fig. 42.6. The plasma noradrenaline response to dynamic upright exercise is plotted as a function of relative work intensity, expressed by per cent peak oxygen uptake (% peak VO_2). There is no difference in slope between group 2 (mild heart failure) and group 3 (severe heart failure). Group 1 (normal) has a steeper slope than that in groups 2 and 3 ($p = 0.002$), indicating that, at relative work intensities, normal subjects have augmented sympathetic drive. (Taken with permission from Francis *et al.* (1985).)

In humans, heart failure is associated with abnormal autonomic responses, but the precise mechanisms underlying these abnormalities have not been completely defined. Many clinical studies have demonstrated that patients with heart failure have altered peripheral vascular and neuroendocrine responses to postural changes and orthostatic stress. Such patients demonstrate a failure to increase plasma NA (and peripheral vascular constriction) in response to a decrease in cardiac filling pressures (so-called 'unloading' of cardiopulmonary baroreceptors) (Fig. 42.7). Occasionally, there is even a paradoxical vasodilatory response to such orthostatic stress. While normal subjects develop marked increases in sympathetic neural activity during modest nitroprusside-induced decreases in arterial and cardiac filling pressures, this response is significantly blunted in patients with heart failure (Fig. 42.8). The prognosis of patients with heart failure is poorer when they fail to activate the sympathetic nervous system during nitroprusside-induced vasodilatation (Fig. 42.9).

Patients with heart failure also have a reduced tachycardia response to blood loss. Lowering of blood pressure by the technique of lower body negative pressure to 'unload' low-pressure cardiopulmonary baroreceptors

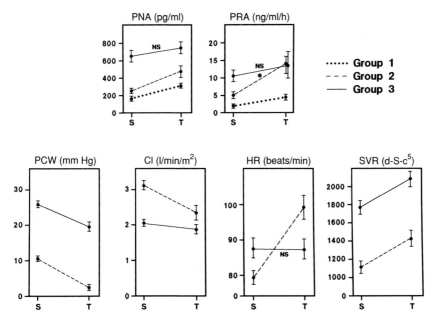

Fig. 42.7. Measurements of plasma noradrenaline (PNA) and plasma renin activity (PRA) during supine rest (S) and 60° orthostatic tilt (T) in normal subjects (group 1), patients with symptoms of heart failure but normal resting haemodynamics (group 2), and patients with heart failure and abnormal resting haemodynamics (group 3). The haemodynamic responses to tilt for groups 2 and 3 are shown in the lower panel. Pulmonary capillary wedge pressure (PCW), cardiac index (CI), and systemic vascular resistance (SVR) all changed significantly. Heart rate (HR) increased significantly in group 2, but did not change in group 3. (Taken with permission from Levine *et al.* (1983).)

fails to cause the expected increase in peripheral vasoconstriction (Fig. 42.10; Ferguson *et al.* 1984). These observations support the hypothesis that an impairment of cardiopulmonary baroreflex mechanisms is at least one of the primary abnormalities responsible for the abnormal othostatic responses observed in patients with heart failure. The abnormal response to upright tilt can be improved with therapy (angiotensin-converting enzyme inhibitors) (Cody *et al.* 1982) and the blunted heart-rate lowering response to pressor activity is rapidly normalized following cardiac transplantation (Ellenbogen *et al.* 1989), suggesting that these are 'functional' disturbances rather than due to structural abnormalities. Ferguson and colleagues (1989) have reported that acute digitalization can reduce microneurographically measured efferent sympathetic nerve activity in patients with heart failure and tends to normalize the response to lower body negative pressure. Evidence that the sympatho-inhibitory effect of digitalis is not solely related to reflex sympathetic withdrawal secondary to improved cardiac output was provided by a lack of

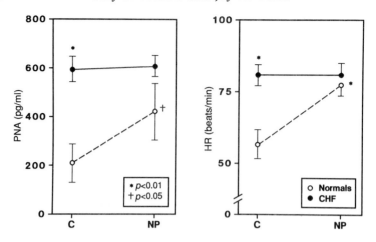

Fig. 42.8. Response of plasma noradrenaline (PNA) and heart rate (HR) to nitroprusside infusion (NP) in 5 normal subjects (closed circles) and 46 patients with congestive heart failure (CHF) (open circles). Symbols above the control columns (C) indicate significant difference between normal subjects and patients with congestive heart failure; symbols in NP columns indicate significant changes from control during nitroprusside infusion. *p (probability) <0.01; †p<0.05. Mean values ± standard error of the mean are shown. (Taken with permission from Olivari *et al.* (1983).)

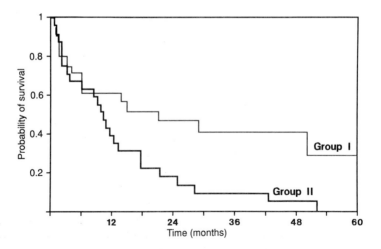

Fig. 42.9. Wilcoxon life table analysis of 21 patients in group I and 25 in group II. Group I and group II denote patients with and without a rise in plasma noradrenaline, respectively, during nitroprusside infusion. (Taken with permission from Olivari *et al.* (1983).)

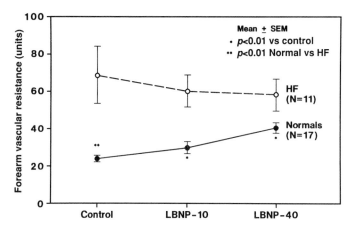

Fig. 42.10. Responses of normal subjects and patients with heart failure (HF) to unloading (deactivation) of baroreceptors with orthostatic stress produced by lower body negative pressure (LBNP) at – 10 mm Hg (LBNP, – 10) and at – 40 mm Hg (LBNP, – 40). Control forearm vascular resistance (venous occlusion plethysmography) was significantly higher in the heart failure patients than in the normal subjects. Normal subjects developed significant forearm vasoconstriction during LBNP (manifested by an increase in forearm vascular resistance). In contrast, patients with heart failure failed to vasoconstrict and tended to experience paradoxical vasodilation during LBNP. (Taken with permission from Ferguson *et al.* (1984).)

directly measured sympathoinhibition with dobutamine, a powerful positive inotropic agent (Feguson *et al.* 1989). It is possible that digitalis acutely sensitizes tonically active cardiac and arterial baroreceptors, thereby improving their response to changes in pressure and volume.

One of the hallmarks of congestive heart failure is chronically elevated sympathetic nervous system activity. It is possible that abnormalities of baroreflex control contribute to the heightened sympathetic drive (Fig. 42.11; Hirsch *et al.* 1987). Baroreceptors are sensory endings that normally respond to changes in mechanical deformation. Using the canine pacing model of low cardiac output heart failure, Dibner-Dunlap and Thames (1989) have recorded from baroreceptor fibres and found the sensitivity of these receptors to be diminished. Dogs with chronic heart failure induced by an aorto-caval fistula also demonstrate a reduced neural discharge rate from left atrial receptors during volume expansion. There appears to be a defect in transduction of the pressure stimulus, such that there is reduced baroreceptor input for any given arterial pressure. Preliminary studies suggest that this defect may be caused by cellular alterations in Na^+–K^+ pump activity, since this attenuation in sensitivity is partially reversed by ouabain, a digitalis-like drug that blocks Na^+–K^+ ATPase action.

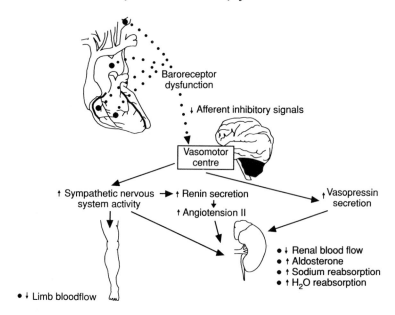

Fig. 42.11. Relationship of abnormal baroreceptor function to neurohormonal activation and regional blood flow in congestive heart failure. Increases in atrial and ventricular filling pressures and increased mean arterial or pulse pressure normally stimulate cardiopulmonary and arterial baroreceptors. Baroreceptor activation sends inhibitory signals to the medullary vasomotor centre, with suppression of sympathetic efferent activity and increased vagal efferent activity (not shown). Baroreflex inhibition is blunted in heart failure, with consequent increased activation of sympathetic and renin–angiotensin systems, and with increased neurohypophyseal release of vasopressin. Limb and renal vasoconstriction ensue, as well as renal retention of sodium and water. (Taken with permission from Hirsch *et al.* (1987).)

Impaired baroreflex abnormalities may contribute to the pathophysiology of heart failure by increasing sympathetic nervous system activity (in itself a likely detrimental finding), by causing a suboptimal heart rate response to changes in blood pressure, and by causing an inappropriate response to orthostatic stress. Attenuation of cardiopulmonary and arterial baroreceptor function may also contribute to renal vasoconstriction, and thereby enhance sodium and water retention. Baroreceptor dysfunction may also promote activation of the renin–angiotensin system and the release of arginine vasopressin, and can be associated with dilutional hyponatraemia. It may not be coincidental that two of the principal markers for an unfavourable prognosis in patients with heart failure—increased plasma NA concentration and hyponatraemia—share baroreceptor dysfunction as a common theme.

Autonomic dysfunction following cardiac transplantation

Following heart transplantation there is usually normalization of resting plasma NA levels and reversal of some but not all baroreceptor reflex abnormalities. However, disturbances in sensitivity to catecholamines persist and cardiopulmonary baroreflex control of forearm vascular resistance remains impaired. Experimental chronic denervation in dogs results in 'up-regulation' of β-adrenoceptors and 'down-regulation' of muscarinic receptors. A 'supersensitivity' to catecholamines develops. The major mechanism of denervation supersensitivity to NA appears to involve lack of neuronal NA reuptake. Despite animal data to the contrary, recent data from human orthotopic cardiac allografts indicate that myocardial β-adrenergic receptors are not increased. Moreover, there is no direct evidence of β-receptor-mediated supersensitivity of post-synaptic origin in patients. The β-adrenergic supersensitivity is likely presynaptic in origin.

Patients with heart transplants generally exhibit a relative resting tachycardia (90–110 beats per minute) and demonstrate little or no increase in heart rate within 30 seconds of standing up. There is also a characteristic delayed rate of acceleration during dynamic and isometric exercise, and also a delayed deceleration at the end of exercise. Carotid sinus massage and the Valsalva manoeuvre do not affect the heart rate in the donor heart. Of interest, heart-transplant patients do demonstrate a marked tachycardia (130–140 beats per minute) in response to fever (Francis and Cohn, personal observations).

There has been a general consensus that the human donor heart is not reinnervated. Histochemical studies have failed to demonstrate reinnervation beyond the suture line following transplantation. In contrast with humans, the transplanted hearts of experimental animals have been shown to exhibit functional extrinsic reinnervation. The distinction between reinnervation in humans and animals may represent either a species difference or variations between allografts and autografts, since many of the animal experiments involved autotransplantation. Following human heart transplantation, myocardial catecholamines are undetectable in tissue biopsies up to five years, indicating that, at least soon after transplantation, the adrenergic responses of these hearts probably depend mainly on variations in plasma catecholamines or presynaptic supersensitivity.

Recent evidence now suggests that some patients have functional reinnervation developing 2 or more years following heart transplantation. Wilson and colleagues (1991) have demonstrated clear increases in NA flowing from the coronary sinus of orthotopically transplanted human hearts when tyramine is given systematically or directly into the coronary arteries. Tyramine is known to displace NA from sympathetic neurons, and should increase NA efflux only if there is functional reinnervation. Moreover, evidence is now accumulating that functional reinnervation may occur in a minority of heterotopic allografts. A recent study identified one case out of nine in which electrocardiographic and indirect clinical evidence of functional reinnervation was obtained 33 months after orthotopic cardiac transplantation. We have seen occasional patients with orthotopic cardiac transplantation who have developed severe coronary artery disease and classic angina pectoris, although, typically, coronary disease remains clinically silent in the transplant population.

In summary, heart transplant and heart–lung transplant will reverse some of the autonomic deficiencies observed in preceeding severe heart failure, but patients may continue to demonstrate some autonomic abnormalities including presynaptic supersensitivity to catecholamines, a blunted response to upright posture and exercise, and reduced heart rate variation. These persistent abnormalities do not keep them from leading a nearly normal lifestyle. Although mainly dependent soon after transplantation on circulating catecholamines, new data are emerging suggesting that reinnervation occurs in some cases.

Role of the autonomic nervous system in the clinical syndrome

Still unresolved is whether the protean abnormalities in afferent and efferent sympathetic nervous system function in heart failure are fundamental to the clinical manifestations of the syndrome or are merely epiphenomena indicative of the severity of the physiological derangement. It is clear that at least some of the clinical signs—tachycardia, cool extremities, diaphoresis—are at least in part due to sympathetic activation. Other manifestations—renal sodium conservation, ventricular arrhythmia—are probably aggravated by the sympathetic nervous system. Other important complications of the disease— exercise intolerance, sudden death, ventricular hypertrophy and remodelling, atrial fibrillation, renin stimulation, etc.—could be in part related to autonomic dysfunction but the evidence for this relationship is not yet persuasive.

Attempts to block the enhanced sympathetic nervous system activity represent an interesting and provocative approach to long-term therapy of heart failure. α-adrenoceptor blockade, as a means of producing systemic vasodilation, exerts a favourable acute haemodynamic effect but no evidence for long-term efficacy. β-adrenoceptor blockade appears in limited preliminary studies to exert a long-term favourable effect in at least some patients with dilated cardiomyopathy. The mechanism of this possible favourable response remains to be determined. Only by mechanistic studies with more selective inhibitors of autonomic dysfunction will it be possible to establish more precisely the role of neuroendocrine abnormalities in the natural history of heart failure.

References

Brigden, W. and Sharpey-Schafer, E. P. (1950). Postural changes in peripheral blood flow in cases with left heart failure. *Clin. Sci.* **9**, 93–100.

Bristow, M. R., Ginsburg, R., Minobe, W., Cubicciotti, R. S., Sageman, W. S., Lurie, K., Billingham, M. E., Harrison, D. C., and Stinson, E. B. (1982). Decreased catecholamine sensitivity and β-adrenergic-receptor density in failing human hearts. *New Engl. J. Med.* **307**, 205–11.

Cody, R. J., Kenneth, W. F., Kluger, J., and Laragh, J. H. (1982). Mechanisms governing the postural response and baroreceptor abnormalities in chronic congestive heart failure: effect of acute long-term converting-enzyme inhibition. *Circulation* **66** (1), 135–42.

Cohn, J. N., Levine, T. B., Olivari, M. T., Garberg, V., Lura, D., Francis, G. S., Simon, A. B., and Rector, T. (1984). Plasma norepinephrine as a guide to prognosis in patients with chronic congestive heart failure. *New Engl. J. Med.* **311**, 819–23.

Dibner-Dunlap, M. E. and Thames, M. D. (1989). Reflex control of renal sympathetic nerve activity is preserved in heart failure despite reduced arterial baroreceptor sensitivity. *Circulation Res.* **65**, 1526–35.

Eckberg, D. L., Drabinsky, M., and Braunwald, E. (1971). Defective cardiac parasympathetic control in patients with heart disease. *New Engl. J. Med.* **265**, 877–83.

Ellenbogen, K. A., Mohanty, P. K., Szentpetery, S., and Thames, M. D. (1989). Arterial baroreflex abnormalities in heart failure: reversal after orthotopic cardiac transplantation. *Circulation* **79**, 51–8.

Ferguson, D. W., Abboud, F. M., and Mark, A. L. (1984). Selective impairment of baroreflex mediated vasoconstrictor responses in patients with ventricular dysfunction. *Circulation* **69**, 451–60.

Ferguson, D. W., Berg, W. J., Sanders, J. S., Roach, P. J., Kempf, J. S., and Kienzle, M. G. (1989). Sympathoinhibitory responses to digitalis glycosides in heart failure patients. *Circulation* **80**, 65–77.

Ferguson, D. W., Berg, W. J., Sanders, J. S., and Kempf, S. J. (1990). Clinical and hemodynamic correlates of sympathetic nerve activity in normal humans and patients with heart failure: Evidence from direct microneurographic recordings. *J. Am. Coll. Cardiol.* **16**, 1125–34.

Francis, G. S., Goldsmith, S. R., Ziesche, S. M., and Cohn, J. N. (1982). Response of plasma norepinephrine and epinephrine to dynamic exercise in patients with congestive heart failure. *Am. J. Cardiol.* **49**, 1152–6.

Francis, G. S., Goldsmith, S. R., Levine, T. B., Olivari, M. T., and Cohn, J. N. (1984). The neurohumoral axis in congestive heart failure. *Ann. intern. Med.* **101**, 370–7.

Francis, G. S., Goldsmith, S. R., Ziesche, S., Nakajima, H., and Cohn, J. N. (1985). Relative attenuation of sympathetic drive during exercise in patients with congestive heart failure. *J. Am. Coll. Cardiol.* **5**, 832–9.

Francis, G. S., Benedict, C., Johnstone, D. E., Kirlin, P. C., Nicklas, J., Liang, C., Kubo, S. H., Rudin-Toretsky, E., and Yusuf, S. (1990). Comparison of neuroendocrine activation in patients with left ventricular dysfunction with and without congestive heart failure. *Circulation* **82**, 1724–9.

Hasking, G. J., Esler, M. D., Jennings, G. L., Burton, D., and Korner, P. I. (1986). Norepinephrine spillover to plasma in patients with congestive heart failure: evidence of increased overall and cardiorenal sympathetic nervous activity. *Circulation* **73**(4), 615–21.

Hasking, G. J., Esler, M. D., Jennings, G. L., Dewar, E., and Lambert, G. (1988). Norepinephrine spillover to plasma during steady-state supine bicycle exercise. *Circulation* **78**(3), 1–7.

Hirsch, A. T., Dzau, V. J., and Creager, M. A. (1987). Baroreceptor function in congestive heart failure: effect on neurohumoral activation and regional fascular resistance. *Circulation* **75**(suppl. IV), IV36–48.

Leimbach, W. N., Wallin, G., Victor, R. G., Aylward, P. E., Sundlof, G., and Mark, A. L. (1986). Direct evidence from intraneural recordings for increased central sympathetic outflow in patients with heart failure. *Circulation* **73**, 913–19.

Levine, T. B., Francis, G. S., Goldsmith, S. R., Simon, A. B., and Cohn, J. N. (1982). Activity of the sympathetic nervous system and renin–angiotensin system assessed by plasma hormone levels and their relation to hemodynamic abnormalities in congestive heart failure. *Am. J. Cardiol.* **49**, 1659–66.

Levine, T. B., Olivari, M. T., and Cohn, J. N. (1986). Effects of orthotopic heart transplantation on sympathetic control mechanisms in congestive heart failure. *Am. J. Cardiol.* **58**, 1035–40.

Olivari, M. T., Levine, B., and Cohn, J. N. (1983). Abnormal neurohumoral response to nitroprusside infusion in congestive heart failure. *J. Am. Coll. Cardiol.* **2**(3), 411–17.

Rector, T. S., Olivari, M. T., Levine, T. B., Francis, G. S., and Cohn, J. N. (1987). Predicting survival for an individual with congestive heart failure using the plasma norepinephrine concentration. *Am. Heart J.* **114**, 148–52.

Sands, K. E. F., Appel, M. L., Lilly, L. S., Schoen, F. J., Mudge, G. H., Jr, and Cohen, R. J. (1989). Power spectrum analysis of heart rate variability in human cardiac transplant recipients. *Circulation* **79**, 76–82.

Valbo, A. B., Hagbarth, K. E., Torebjork, H. E., and Wallin, B. G. (1979). Somatosensory, proprioceptive, and sympathetic activity in human peripheral nerves. *Physiol. Rev.* **59**, 919–67.

Wilson, R. F., Christensen, B. V., Simon, A., Olivari, M. T., White, C. W., and Laxson, D. D. (1991). Evidence for structural sympathetic reinnervation after orthotopic cardiac transplantation in humans. *Circulation* **83**, 1210–20.

43. Autonomic disturbances in spinal cord lesions

Christopher J. Mathias and Hans L. Frankel

Introduction

The integrity of the spinal cord is of particular importance to the normal functioning of the autonomic nervous system, as the entire sympathetic outflow (from T1 to L2/3) and a proportion of the parasympathetic outflow (the sacral parasympathetic) traverse and synapse in the spinal cord before they supply their target organs. In patients with spinal cord injuries there are therefore varying degrees of autonomic involvement, depending upon the site and extent of the lesion. In patients with cervical cord transection, if complete, the entire sympathetic and sacral parasympathetic outflow is separated from cerebral control. This results in a variety of abnormalities affecting the cardiovascular, thermoregulatory, gastrointestinal, urinary, and reproductive systems. In patients with transection, which is common after traumatic injuries to the spinal cord, despite destruction of one or more segments the distal portion of the spinal cord often retains function, although independently of the brain. This results, in certain situations, in additional autonomic abnormalities. This chapter will concentrate on patients with cervical and high thoracic spinal cord lesions, as these patients often have major clinical problems resulting from autonomic dysfunction.

Recently injured versus chronically injured

There are differences between the autonomic problems affecting recently and chronically injuried patients following a spinal lesion. Soon after transection of the spinal cord there is initially a transient state of hypoexcitability of the isolated cord, described as 'spinal shock'. This is partially analogous to cerebral shock, as observed in the early stages after a hemisphere lesion. In spinal shock there is flaccid paralysis of the muscles, with lack of tendon reflexes. Spinal autonomic function is also impaired; the urinary bladder and large bowel are usually atonic, there is dilatation of blood vessels particularly in the skin, and spinal autonomic reflexes cannot be elicited. This stage of spinal cord depression may last from a few days to a few weeks, after which isolated activity of the spinal cord usually returns. This heralds the onset of a different range of autonomic abnormalities, which are often the result of autonomic reflex activity at a spinal level, without the normal control from higher centres in the brain.

The biochemical and molecular basis of spinal shock is not known. A range of possibilities has been proposed over the years, ranging from alterations in monoamine and neuropeptide transmitters, to abnormalities involving free oxygen radicals, lipid peroxidation, and calcium ions. Previously promising work in animals using the opiate antagonist, naloxone, and the endogenous antagonist, thyrotrophin-releasing hormone, have not been fulfilled in man. More recently, however, some benefit has been shown with methyl-prednisolone (Bracken *et al.* 1990) raising a number of possibilities which include the deleterious effects of lipid peroxidation and hydrolysis, and breakdown of cell membranes. This is, however, more likely to be related to neuronal damage and its prevention, rather than to the understanding of the mechanisms of spinal shock. The reversal of the processes causing spinal shock is of clinical importance, as a reduction in skeletal muscle flaccidity and neural activation of the vasculature is probably beneficial in preventing deep venous thrombosis; furthermore, postural hypotension which occurs in the early stages is less likely to be a problem and the return of activity to the bladder and bowel helps speed up the overall rehabilitation process.

The descriptions below largely relate to the chronic stage of spinal cord injuries, unless specifically stated. They will apply to both tetraplegics and high thoracic spinal cord lesions, unless otherwise indicated.

The cardiovascular system

Basal blood pressure and heart rate

The recently injured

The basal supine blood pressure in recently injured tetraplegics in spinal shock is usually lower than normal, and this applies particularly to the diastolic blood pressure (57 mm Hg in tetraplegics and 82 mm Hg in normal subjects; Mathias *et al.* 1979*a*). The extent and the duration of the hypotension varies, as it is dependent upon a number of factors including complicating trauma and drug therapy. In animal studies, cervical or high thoracic transection often results in an initial hypertensive phase of only a few minutes in duration. This is thought to be related to increased sympathoadrenal activation, although plasma noradrenaline levels may remain elevated for hours. In man, observations immediately after transection are limited. Cardiovascular and neurohormonal measurements from the second day after injury indicate a low basal blood pressure and low levels of both plasma noradrenaline and adrenaline (Fig. 43.1). It is likely that the level of blood pressure is

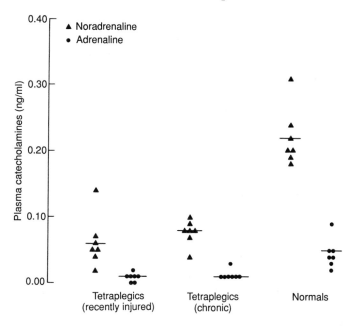

Fig. 43.1. Resting levels of plasma noradrenaline and adrenaline in recently injured tetraplegics in spinal shock, in chronic tetraplegics, and in normal age-matched subjects. The horizontal bar indicates the mean value. Basal catecholamines in both recently injured and chronic tetraplegics are approximately 35 per cent of normal levels. (From Mathias *et al.* (1979*a*).)

secondary to the marked diminution in sympathetic nervous activity, which is recognized as normally accounting for about 20 per cent of vascular tone. It is unlikely that skeletal muscle paralysis alone contributes, as patients with tetraplegia due to poliomyelitis often have normal or even higher levels of blood pressure.

In recently injured tetraplegics in spinal shock the basal heart rate is usually below 100 beats/min, unlike in patients with low spinal cord injuries in whom the heart rate is often higher. This is probably due to a reduction in neural and hormonal sympathetic mediated chronotropic influences in the tetraplegics. The efferent cardiac parasympathetic pathways, however, are intact and the absence of sympathetic activation may predispose susceptible patients to vagal overactivity. This may result in bradycardia and cardiac arrest, as has been noted during tracheal stimulation.

The chronically injured

In the chronic stage, the basal level of both systolic and diastolic blood pressure in high lesions is lower than in normal subjects (Fig. 43.2; Frankel *et al.* 1972; Mathias *et al.* 1976*a*). Basal levels of plasma noradrenaline and adrenaline

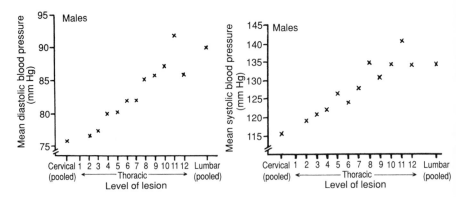

Fig. 43.2. Relationship between systolic and diastolic blood pressure in male patients with spinal cord lesions at differing levels. Tetraplegics have the lowest resting blood pressure. (From Frankel *et al.* (1972).)

in tetraplegics, in the absence of stimulation from below the lesion, remain low as in the stage of spinal shock, reflecting absent tonic supraspinal sympathetic impulses and diminished peripheral sympathetic activity. This has been confirmed in tetraplegics using sensitive techniques of microneurography to detect skin and muscle sympathetic nerve activity (Stjernberg *et al.* 1986). Patients with spinal cord injury, however, are prone to renal damage and renal failure which may account for sustained hypertension in some.

In the absence of adequate resting sympathetic tone a number of secondary mechanisms, particularly hormonal, attempt to compensate for and help maintain blood pressure. An important component is the renin–angiotensin--aldosterone system, which through the direct pressor effects of angiotensin II and the salt-retaining effects of aldosterone helps raise blood pressure. This is particularly evident when drugs which interfere with the system are used; the angiotensin-converting enzyme inhibitor, captopril, substantially lowers supine blood pressure in tetraplegics. Even small doses of diuretics, which cause salt loss and lower intravascular fluid volume, may cause a catastrophic fall in supine blood pressure. A low salt diet lowers blood pressure, despite the ability of tetraplegics to reduce salt excretion as do normal subjects (Sutters *et al.* 1991). In tetraplegics recumbency itself may induce a diuresis but not a natriuresis. This differs from patients with primary autonomic failure, in whom recumbency causes both diuresis and natriuresis (Kooner *et al.* 1987); these patients also have nocturnal polyuria (Chapter 14). The difference may relate to the ability of the tetraplegics to mount an adequate hormonal response to oppose natriuresis, unlike the autonomic failure patients in whom these responses are often muted (Chapter 10). These observations have practical importance, as a period of recumbency in high

Table 43.1. Clinical manifestations of postural hypotension

Giddiness, buzzing, and ringing in ears
Blurring, greying out, and loss of vision
Tingling in hands
Facial pallor
Syncope
Hypotension and elevation in heart rate
Bradycardia may occasionally occur
Venous pooling and cyanotic discoloration of lower limbs
Reduced urine secretion

---

spinal lesions will often result in accentuation of postural hypotension. Head-up tilt may help prevent this problem, although its value has not been formally evaluated.

In chronic high lesions the basal heart rate may be only marginally lower than, or no different from, that in normal subjects. This suggests a major role for the vagus in the control of heart rate. This is further emphasized by the changes in heart rate which occur when baroreceptor afferents are influenced either by a rise or a fall in blood pressure, which results in reciprocal changes in vagal efferent activity.

Cardiovascular responses to physiological stimuli

In tetraplegics the brain is functionally separated from the peripheral sympathetic nervous system. This may cause a number of abnormalities, when cardiovascular responses are the result of cerebral initiation or modulation. Depending on the level and extent of the lesion, there are varying disturbances.

Postural change

Patients with high spinal cord lesions are prone to hypotension, which commonly occurs during postural change from the horizontal to the upright position. This occurs in both recently injured patients in spinal shock and in chronically injured patients, especially in the early stages during rehabilitation. Their mobility, even in a wheelchair, can be considerably impeded. The fall in blood pressure is accompanied by symptoms mainly related to diminished cerebral perfusion (Table 43.1). The symptoms can vary in nature and intensity and are not necessarily related to the degree of hypotension.

During head-up postural change, as on a tilt table, there is usually an immediate fall in both systolic and diastolic blood pressure. The pressure may fall to extremely low levels, but there is usually no loss of consciousness except in recently injured tetraplegics or in chronic tetraplegics following a period of recumbency. This tolerance to a low cerebral perfusion pressure is similar to that of patients with chronic autonomic failure, who are also

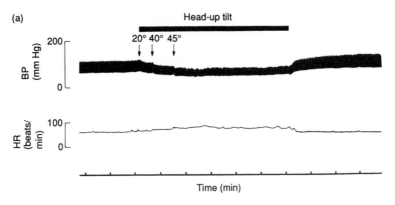

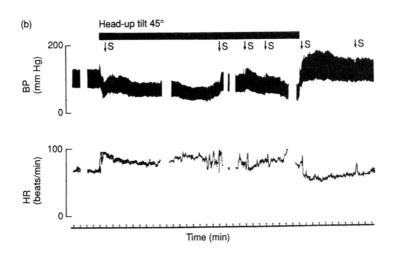

Fig. 43.3. (a) Blood pressure (BP) and heart rate (HR) in a tetraplegic patient before and after head-up tilt, in the early stages of rehabilitation, where there were few muscle spasms and minimal autonomic dysreflexia. (From Frankel and Mathias (1976).) (b) Blood pressure (BP) and heart rate (HR) in a tetraplegic patient before, during, and after head-up tilt to 45°. Blood pressure promptly falls but with partial recovery, which in this case is linked to skeletal muscle spasms (S) inducing spinal sympathetic activity. Some of the later oscillations may be due to the rise in plasma renin, which was measured where there are interruptions in the intraarterial record. In the later phases of tilt, skeletal muscle spasms occur more frequently, and further elevate the blood pressure. On return to the horizontal, blood pressure rises rapidly above the previous level, and then slowly returns to the horizontal. Heart rate usually moves in the opposite direction, except during muscle spasms, where there is an increase. (From Mathias and Frankel (1988).)

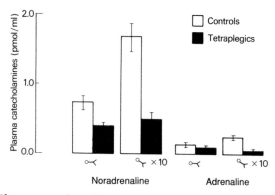

Fig. 43.4. Plasma noradrenaline and adrenaline levels in controls (normal subjects) and chronic tetraplegic patients at rest and during head-up tilt to 45° for 10 min. There is a rise in plasma noradrenaline in the control subjects but little change in the tetraplegics. The bars indicate ± SEM.

able to autoregulate their cerebral circulation despite an extremely low perfusion blood pressure (Chapter 33). The precise mechanisms responsible for this are unclear.

Following the initial fall in blood pressure, the subsequent responses vary. In some patients, especially in the early stages, blood pressure continues to fall (Fig. 43.3(a)). There is no rise in levels of plasma noradrenaline in the early phases following head-up postural change (Fig. 43.4), consistent with the inability of these patients to reflexly increase sympathetic nervous activity in response to postural change, as occurs normally. In many chronically injured patients, however, if tilt is prolonged, the blood pressure tends to partly recover, often with oscillations (Fig. 43.4(b)). This recovery may be related to activation of the renin–angiotensin–aldosterone system. The release of renin appears to be independent of sympathetic stimulation and may be secondary to renal baroreceptor stimulation from the fall in renal perfusion pressure (Fig. 43.5(a)). Renin results in the formation of the peptide angiotensin II, which has powerful direct vasoconstrictor effects, may facilitate peripheral noradrenaline release and activity, and also stimulates the release of aldosterone from the adrenal cortex (Fig. 43.5(b)). The salt- and water-retaining effects of aldosterone have slower but important effects in increasing intravascular volume. These actions of the renin–angiotensin–aldosterone system help raise blood pressure. A further mechanism contributing to blood pressure recovery during tilt is the activation of spinal reflexes either from stimulation of the skin, the skeletal muscles, or the viscera. This is more likely to account for the reduction in peripheral blood flow and rise in occluded venous pressure observed during head-up tilt in tetraplegics than the spinal postural reflexes that were previously proposed. Local sympathetic reflexes (veno-arteriolar reflexes) also

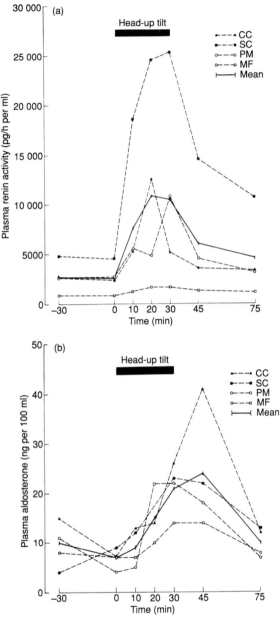

Fig. 43.5. (a) Plasma renin activity levels in four chronic tetraplegic patients before, during, and after head-up tilt to 45°. In three patients there was pronounced hypotension and a marked rise in plasma renin activity levels. Patient MF had minimal changes in blood pressure during head-up tilt and the smallest rise in plasma renin activity. (From Mathias *et al.* (1975).) (b) Plasma aldosterone levels before, during, and after head-up tilt to 45° in the same four

appear to operate in high lesions during postural change (Skagen and Henriksen 1986).

During head-up postural change the fall in blood pressure is accompanied by a reduction in central venous pressure, stroke volume, and cardiac output, which is probably the result of venous pooling, diminished venous return, and the inability to increase sympathetic cardiac inotropic activity. Venous pooling often causes cyanotic discoloration of the legs and may account for ankle oedema, as observed in high lesions in wheelchairs. Urine volume is usually reduced, often to extremely low levels, which occasionally raises the question of whether there may be obstruction to the urinary outflow tract. Oliguria may be due to a combination of causes; these include a fall in blood pressure, thus reducing renal plasma flow and glomerular filtration rate, and an elevation in levels of the antidiuretic hormone, vasopressin. In high spinal lesions there is an exaggerated rise in vasopressin levels during head-up tilt as compared to that in normal subjects (Chapter 19).

During head-up postural change there is often a rapid rise in heart rate, which is inversely related to the fall in blood pressure. This is likely to be due to withdrawal of vagal tone in response to unloading of baroreceptor afferents, as it is markedly attenuated although not abolished by atropine. Propranolol also reduces the heart rate rise during tilt, suggesting that β-adrenoceptor stimulation also partially contributes. In the majority of patients, heart rate does not usually rise above 100 beats/min even during a marked fall in blood pressure. This is therefore different from the situation in patients with an intact sympathetic nervous system, who are in 'shock' with a similarly low level of blood pressure. The inability of patients with high lesions to adequately increase both sympathetic nervous activity and adrenal secretion in response to hypotension results in diminished adrenoceptor stimulation of the heart rate. This may further account for why the majority of tetraplegics, despite the fall in blood pressure, do not exhibit abnormalities in cardiac rhythm. When this occasionally occurs it may be the result of impaired coronary perfusion especially in patients with co-existent coronary artery disease.

The clinical problems resulting from postural hypotension in high spinal lesions are not usually as severe and prolonged as those in patients with primary autonomic failure. Postural hypotension may, however, be particularly severe in the early stages of rehabilitation or following prolonged recumbency. Clinical observations indicate that the symptoms of postural hypotension are often diminished with frequent postural change to the head-up position, along with elevation of the head end of the bed at night. The activation of the renin–angiotensin–aldosterone axis, with both early and longer acting effects resulting from vasoconstriction and plasma volume

---

Fig. 43.5. *(continued)* patients as in (a). The rise in plasma aldosterone levels is later in timing to that of plasma renin activity. (From Mathias *et al.* (1975).)

expansion, probably helps buffer the fall in blood pressure during head-up postural change. Another possibility is that the changes improve further the ability of high spinal patients to autoregulate their cerebral blood flow, which they can often do at considerably lower perfusion pressures than normal subjects. Whether changes in other circulating and locally produced hormones acting on the cerebral vasculature also contribute is not known.

A variety of physical methods have been used to prevent postural hypotension; these include abdominal binders and thigh cuffs, which prevent venous pooling, and may help some patients. Activation of spinal sympathetic reflexes, by induction of muscle spasms or tapping of the anterior abdominal wall suprapubically to activate the urinary bladder, are of value in some patients presumably by causing autonomic dysreflexia and thus elevating blood pressure.

There is a range of drugs, as used in patients with autonomic failure (Chapter 33), which may alleviate postural hypotension in high spinal cord lesions. Such spinal patients, unlike patients with autonomic failure, are, however, prone to paroxysms of hypertension, which may be severe and exacerbated by such drugs. Their use, however, may be necessary for limited periods, when postural hypotension is a particular problem, as in the early stages of rehabilitation and after prolonged recumbency. Ephedrine in a dose of 15 mg half an hour before postural change is often of value. Its ability to act directly on adrenoceptors and indirectly by releasing noradrenaline is probably the basis of its efficacy. Dihydroergotamine and other α-adrenoceptor agonists may have a role, especially if they have short-lived effects. Indomethacin, a prostaglandin synthetase inhibitor, also elevates basal blood pressure and reduces the blood pressure fall during postural change but has potential side-effects. In the majority of patients, however, drugs are not needed.

Valsalva manoeuvre

In high spinal lesions the responses to the Valsalva manoeuvre are abnormal because the baroreceptor reflex is impaired due to the disruption of sympathetic efferent pathways through the cervical and thoracic spinal cord. When intrathoracic pressure is elevated there is a fall in blood pressure, despite a fairly modest increase in intrathoracic pressure, which is often difficult to achieve and maintain because of the inability to activate intercostal muscles (Fig. 43.6). There is no recovery in blood pressure while the intrathoracic pressure is elevated. Heart rate rises with the fall in blood pressure because the cardiac vagi respond to the fall in blood pressure. On reducing the elevated intrathoracic pressure, there is a gradual recovery of blood pressure with a reduction in heart rate that does not fall below the basal level.

The blood pressure may fall to extremely low levels during the Valsalva manoeuvre if intrathoracic pressure is elevated to 20 or 30 mm Hg, as demonstrated in a tetraplegic who suffered severe dizziness while singing, which raised her intrathoracic pressure (van Lieshout et al. 1991). This ability

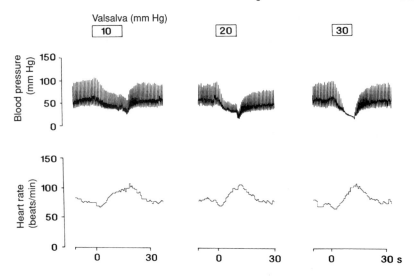

Fig. 43.6. Blood pressure and heart rate responses to the Valsalva manoeuvre in a tetraplegic patient. With increasing degrees of intrathoracic pressure there is a progressively greater fall in blood pressure in phase II. There is virtually no blood pressure recording when intrathoracic pressure is raised to 30 mm Hg. Blood pressure has been measured non-invasively with the Finapres. (van Lieshout *et al.* (1991).)

to lower blood pressure has also been used to the benefit of patients, to prevent hypertension during urological surgery by increasing positive pressure during assisted ventilation (Welply *et al.* 1975).

Pressor stimuli originating above the lesion

Pressor stimuli dependent on sympathetic activation that either originate in, or are modulated by, the brain do not raise blood pressure in patients with complete cervical cord transection. Stimuli such as mental arithmetic, a loud noise, and cutaneous stimulation by either pain or cold in areas above the lesion have no effect in tetraplegics, unlike in normal subjects in whom they elevate blood pressure. The lack of response to these stimuli provides evidence of severance of sympathetic pathways descending within the cervical spinal cord.

Pressor stimuli originating below the lesion—'autonomic dysreflexia'

The reverse, an exaggerated rise in blood pressure, occurs in high spinal lesions when stimuli originate below the level of the lesion. Stimulation of the skin, abdominal and pelvic viscera, or skeletal muscles, can cause a paroxysmal rise in blood pressure (Fig. 43.7), which is usually accompanied by a fall in heart rate because of increased vagal activity. In recently injured tetraplegics

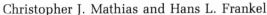

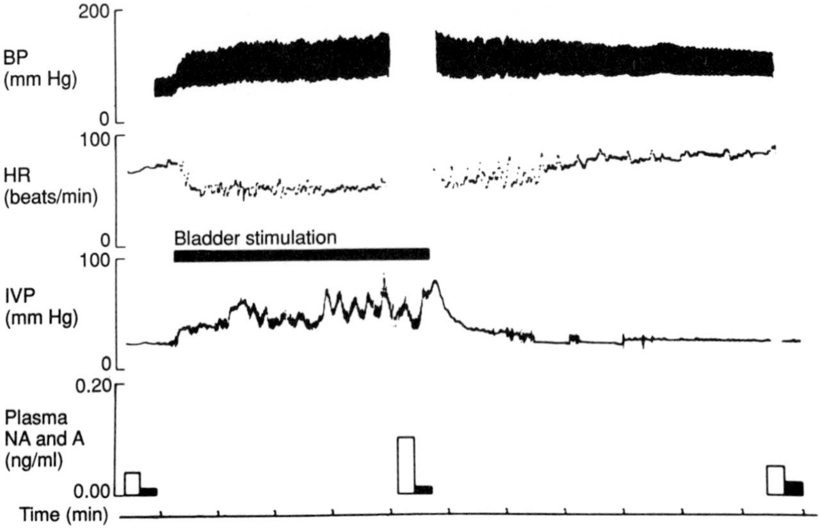

Fig. 43.7. Blood pressure (BP), heart rate (HR), intravesical pressure (IVP), and plasma noradrenaline (NA, filled squares) and adrenaline (A, filled circles) levels in a tetraplegic patient before, during, and after bladder stimulation induced by suprapubic percussion of the anterior abdominal wall. The rise in BP is accompanied by a fall in heart rate as a result of increased vagal activity in response to the rise in blood pressure. Plasma NA (open bars), but not A (filled bars), levels rise, suggesting an increase in sympathetic neural activity independently of adrenomedullary activation. (From Mathias and Frankel (1986).)

in spinal shock there is often no change in blood pressure or heart rate during such stimulation (Fig. 43.8). This differs markedly from the chronic stage when there is increased activity in a number of target organs supplied by the sympathetic and parasympathetic nerves. These effects, in combination, contribute to the syndrome of autonomic dysreflexia (Table 43.2). Detailed observations were made by Head and Riddoch (1917) who described sweating around and above the level of the lesion, with evacuation of the urinary bladder and rectum, penile erection, and seminal fluid emission together with skeletal muscle spasms—components of the 'mass reflex' in response to cutaneous stimulation below the lesion or during bladder and bowel evacuation. The cardiovascular changes, however, were not described until 1947, when Guttmann and Whitteridge reported their observations during urinary bladder stimulation.

The cardiovascular responses to stimuli below the lesion include a rise in both systolic and diastolic blood pressure. There is a marked reduction in peripheral blood flow (Fig. 43.9) which may result in cold limbs, thus accounting for one of the original terms used to describe autonomic dysreflexia, poikilothermia spinalis. In addition to constriction of resistance

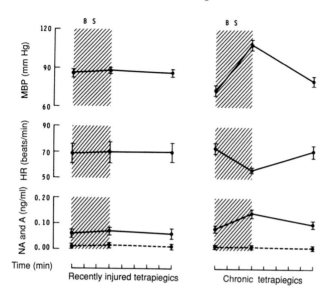

Fig. 43.8. Average levels of mean blood pressure (MBP), heart rate (HR), and plasma noradrenaline (NA, continuous line) and adrenaline (A, interrupted line) in recently injured and chronic tetraplegics, before, during, and after bladder stimulation (BS). The bars indicate ± SEM. No changes occur in the recently injured tetraplegics, unlike the chronic tetraplegics in whom MBP and plasma NA levels rise and HR falls. There are no changes in plasma A levels. (From Mathias *et al.* (1979a).)

Table 43.2.   Clinical manifestations of autonomic dysreflexia

Paraesthesiae in neck, shoulders, and arms
Fullness in head
Hot ears
Throbbing headache especially in the occipital and frontal
 regions
Tightness in chest and dyspnoea
Hypertension and bradycardia
Occasionally cardiac dysrythmias
Pupillary dilatation
Above lesion—pallor initially, followed by flushing of face
 and neck and sweating in areas above and around the
 lesion
Below lesion—cold peripheries; piloerection
Contraction of urinary bladder and large bowel*
Penile erection and seminal fluid emission*

*May occur as part of the 'mass reflex'.

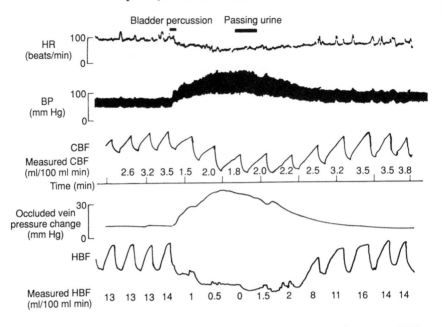

Fig. 43.9. The effects of bladder percussion and micturition on heart rate (HR), blood pressure (BP), calf blood flow (CBF), occluded vein pressure, and hand blood flow (HBF) in a chronic tetraplegic with a physiologically complete transection of the cervical spinal cord. The rise in blood pressure is accompanied by a fall in heart rate (after an initial transient rise), a marked reduction in both calf and hand blood flow, and a rise in occluded vein pressure. (From Corbett *et al.* (1971).)

vessels, there is also a rise in occluded venous pressure indicating contraction in capacitance vessels. There is an elevation in both stroke volume and cardiac output, suggestive of activation of spinal cardiac reflexes. These changes occur soon after stimulation, the rapidity indicating that they are of neurogenic origin and likely to be due to reflex sympathetic activity through the isolated spinal cord. Biochemical evidence of increased sympathoneural activity has been obtained from levels of plasma noradrenaline, which are closely correlated with the blood pressure changes (Fig. 43.10(a), (b)). Plasma adrenaline levels do not change, indicating that adrenomedullary secretion does not contribute to the elevation in blood pressure. However, plasma noradrenaline levels, even at the height of hypertension and despite their increasing by two- or threefold, are only moderately above the resting basal levels of normal subjects. This differs markedly from the extremely high levels of plasma catecholamines often found in patients with a phaeochromocytoma (Chapter 14). Levels of plasma dopamine β-hydroxylase, the enzyme released with noradrenaline from sympathetic nerve terminals and considered to be an even better marker of sympathetic nerve activity, rise slowly during short-lived stimuli such as bladder stimulation, and continue to rise even after cessation of the stimulus, unlike plasma noradrenaline levels (Mathias *et al.* 1976*b*; Fig. 43.10(a)–(c)). This is probably due to a combination of reasons, which include the longer half-life of dopamine β-hydroxylase in plasma and a slower entry into the circulation than noradrenaline. Because of its larger molecular weight its entry is probably through lymphatic channels rather than through diffusion through vessel walls. There is no relationship between the elevation in blood pressure and plasma dopamine β-hydroxylase levels (Fig. 43.10(d)). During autonomic dysreflexia, levels of other vasoconstrictor substances in plasma, such as renin (and by inference angiotensin II levels), remain unchanged or fall. Whether levels of other vasoconstrictor peptides such as neuropeptide Y and endothelin rise is not known. These are, however, more likely to play a local role than through circulating levels. Potential vasodilator substances, such as levels of plasma prostaglandin E-2 rise. This may occur either as a result of sympathetic stimulation or in response to the elevation in blood pressure.

The rise in blood pressure and the widespread involvement of the vasculature below the lesion, despite a modest and often localized stimulus only involving a few segments, suggest the spread of neuronal impulses intraspinally and/or extraspinally. In tetraplegics, microneurography studies indicate only a moderate and transient rise in muscle sympathetic nerve activity during autonomic dysreflexia (Stjernberg *et al.* 1986) with no association between the cardiac cycle and muscle sympathetic nerve discharge as occurs normally (Fig. 43.11). The result of these neurophysiological studies, in conjunction with the neurohormonal observations, indicate that the term autonomic hyperreflexia is erroneous and should not be used. There is, however, evidence of hyperactivity of target organs innervated by the autonomic nervous system. The exaggerated blood pressure response to various stimuli suggests supersensitivity of adrenoceptors, or that other mechanisms are responsible for the enhanced vascular response. Increased pressor responses to stimuli do not occur in patients with lesions below the fifth thoracic segment (Fig. 43.12), indicating that the sympathetic neural outflow above that level is of major importance in blood pressure homeostasis. It is likely that in the lesions below T5 there is sparing of the neural control of the large splanchnic circulatory bed. In high lesions stimuli causing autonomic dysreflexia unmask primary cutaneovascular, viscerovascular, and somatovascular reflexes; these primary effects appear to be modulated by the brain in both normal subjects and in patients with lesions below T5, thus preventing hypertension.

In high lesions, the heart rate may rise transiently with the elevation in blood pressure, presumably because of sympathetic stimulation of the heart as a result of spinal cardiac reflexes. There is usually a subsequent fall in heart rate because of stimulation of sinoaortic baroreceptors and increased

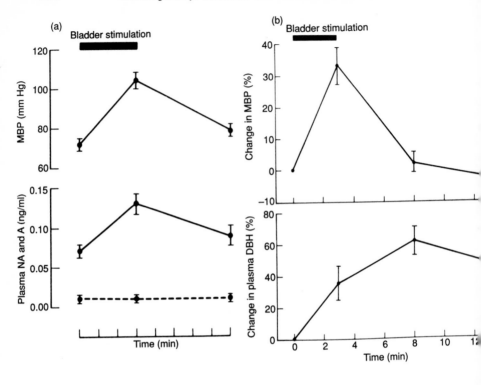

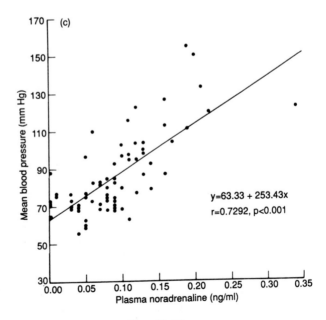

Fig. 43.10.

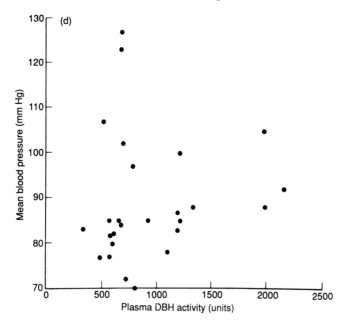

Fig. 43.10.   (a), (b) The changes in mean blood pressure (MBP) in tetraplegic patients before, during, and after bladder stimulation. (a) The changes in plasma noradrenaline (NA, continuous line) and adrenaline (A, dashed line) levels. Noradrenaline levels rise with the blood pressure and fall as the pressor effects wane. There is no change in plasma adrenaline levels. (b) Levels of plasma dopamine β-hydroxylase (DBH) rise slowly and remain elevated for a longer period. The bars indicate $\pm$ SEM. (c) There is a strong relationship between mean blood pressure and plasma noradrenaline levels, which is not so for (d) plasma dopamine β-hydroxylase. In short-term studies, in particular, plasma noradrenaline levels appear to be a better indicator of sympathoneural activation than plasma dopamine β-hydroxylase levels. (From Mathias (1976a).)

vagal efferent activity. This may help dampen the rise in blood pressure during autonomic dysreflexia, as parasympathetic blockade with atropine or other anticholinergic agents can prevent this reflexly induced fall in heart rate and often result in an even greater rise in blood pressure. During autonomic dysreflexia there is often facial vasodilatation accompanied by sweating, which may be profuse above the level of the lesion (Fig. 43.13). Sweating below the level of the lesion may be minimal. The precise mechanisms responsible are not known.

Autonomic dysreflexia is of clinical relevance. Mild episodes probably occur intermittently through the day and are of little consequence. When prolonged, however, they cause considerable morbidity, as a result of excessive sweating

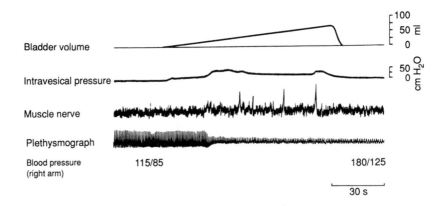

Fig. 43.11. Mean voltage neurogram record of sympathetic activity in a peroneal muscle nerve fascicle obtained while filling the urinary bladder with carbon dioxide (CO_2) at 50 cm^3/min in a patient with a C5 lesion. There is an increase in intravesical volume and pressure associated with marked cutaneous vasoconstriction, as indicated by the photoelectric pulse plethysmograph. Blood pressure is markedly elevated despite only a moderate increase in sympathetic nerve activity. (From Stjernberg *et al.* (1986).)

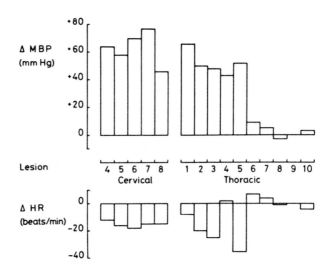

Fig. 43.12. Changes in mean blood pressure (Δ MBP) and heart rate (Δ HR) in patients with spinal cord lesions at different levels (cervical and thoracic) after bladder stimulation induced by suprapubic percussion of the anterior abdominal wall. In the cervical and high thoracic lesions there is a marked elevation in blood pressure and a fall in heart rate. In patients with lesions below T5 there are minimal cardiovascular changes. (From Mathias and Frankel (1986).)

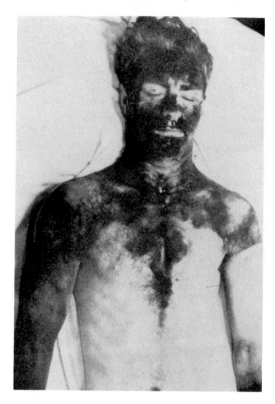

Fig. 43.13. Distribution of sweating, indicated by darker areas covered by quini-zarine dye, in a tetraplegic patient during bladder distension. The band over the left arm indicates the site of the sphygmomanometer cuff. (From Guttmann (1976).)

over the head and neck, and a throbbing headache. The latter is often, but not always, related to the level of blood pressure and may be dependent on distension of pain-sensitive cranial blood vessels. With recurrent episodes of dysreflexia, headache may be particularly severe despite later, but only modest elevations in blood pressure. This may be due to increased sensitivity of afferent nerves on blood vessels caused by the formation or release of substances which include substance P, calcitonin gene-related peptide, and prostaglandins. Other complications of the vasospasm and hypertension accompanying autonomic dysreflexia include myocardial failure and neurological deficits such as epileptic seizures, visual defects, and cerebral haemorrhage. These may result in extensive and permanent neurological deficits or death. Whether these cardiovascular abnormalities may become an even greater problem as the life expectancy of these patients increases and they become more vulnerable to cardiovascular and cerebrovascular damage remains to be determined.

Table 43.3. Causes of autonomic dysreflexia

Abdominal or pelvic visceral stimulation

Ureter
  Calculus

Urinary bladder
  Distension by blocked catheter or discoordinated bladder
    infection
  Irritation by calculus, catheter, or bladder washout

Rectum and anus
  Enemata
  Faecal retention
  Anal fissure

Gastrointestinal organs
  Gastric dilatation
  Gastric ulceration
  Cholecystitis or cholelithiasis

Uterus
  Contraction during pregnancy
  Menstruation, occasionally

Cutaneous stimulation

Pressure sores
Infected ingrowing toenails
Burns

Skeletal Muscle Spasms

Especially in limbs with contractures

Miscellaneous

  Intrathecal neostigmine
  Electro-ejaculatory procedures
  Ejaculation
  Vaginal dilatation
  Urethra–insertion of catheter or abscess
  Fractures of bones

The management of autonomic dysreflexia is of considerable importance. The key factor is prevention. It is necessary to determine the provoking cause and rectify it (Table 43.3). To lower blood pressure rapidly, head-up tilt (which causes venous pooling) may be initially used. A range of drugs are helpful, and their actions are related to the postulated mechanisms responsible for autonomic dysreflexia (Table 43.4). Preventing afferent stimulation, for

Table 43.4.   Some of the drugs used in the management of autonomic dysreflexia classified according to their major site of action on the reflex arc and target organs

Afferent		Topical lignocaine
Spinal cord		Clonidine*
		Reserpine*
		Spinal anaesthetics
Efferent	Sympathetic ganglia	Hexamethonium
	Sympathetic nerve terminals	Guanethidine
	α-adrenoceptors	Phenoxybenzamine
Target organs	Blood vessels	Glyceryl trinitrate
		Nifedipine
	Sweat glands	Probanthine

*Clonidine and reserpine have multiple effects some of which are peripheral.

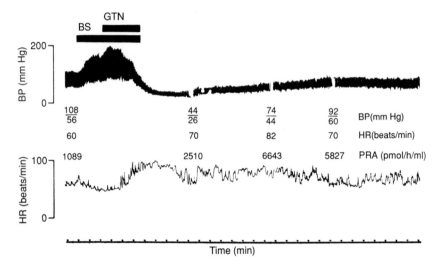

Fig. 43.14.   Blood pressure (BP) and heart rate (HR) in a tetraplegic in the supine position before, during, and after bladder stimulation (BS) by suprapubic percussion of the anterior abdominal wall, which induces hypertension. Sublingual glyceryl trinitrate (GTN) (0.5 mg for 3.5 min) rapidly reverses the hypertension, elevates the heart rate, and then causes substantial hypotension. Levels of plasma renin activity (PRA) rise as a result of the fall in blood pressure. (From Mathias and Frankel (1988).)

instance by the use of a local anaesthetic, such as lignocaine in the urinary bladder, can be effective. Drugs which act partially (reserpine) or entirely (spinal anaesthetics) on the spinal cord are particularly useful especially in severe episodes of dysreflexia. The ganglionic blocker, hexamethonium, was successfully used in the past but, like other drugs which reduce sympathetic efferent activity, is likely to cause profound postural hypotension. The α_2-adrenoceptor agonist, clonidine, does not lower supine blood pressure but reduces hypertension during autonomic dysreflexia (Mathias *et al.* 1979c). Drugs acting directly on blood vessels, such as glyceryl trinitrate, or calcium channel blockers, such as nifedipine, are also effective and have the advantage of being given sublingually. They also have the potential to cause severe hypotension (Fig. 43.14).

The α-adrenoceptor blockers, which theoretically should be highly effective in autonomic dysreflexia, are not entirely successful in preventing hypertension. Phenoxybenzamine and prazosin may be useful in autonomic dysreflexia due to bladder outflow obstruction, as they relax the smooth muscle of the urinary sphincter. α-adrenoceptor blockers like phentolamine may not prevent the paroxysmal surges in blood pressure during autonomic dysreflexia (Fig. 43.15). The reasons for this are unclear, but could include inadequate entry and disposition of the α-blocker to postsynaptic sites, thus enabling the transsynaptic actions of noradrenaline to continue. Furthermore,

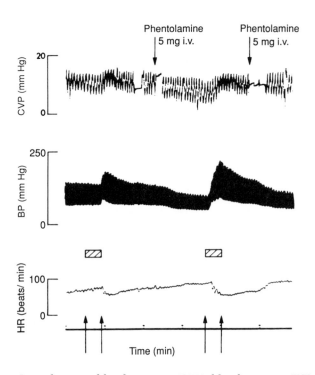

Fig. 43.15. Central venous blood pressure (CVP), blood pressure (BP), and heart rate (HR) in a tetraplegic patient undergoing electroejaculation, with stimuli given per rectum over the seminal vesicles during the times indicated by arrows and hatched areas. The α-adrenoceptor blocker phentolamine did not suppress the paroxysmal rise in blood pressure during stimulation, even when reassessed (not shown here) after 10 mg was administered.

during autonomic dysreflexia there also may be secretion from sympathetic nerve endings of non-adrenergic substances, such as neuropeptide Y or adenosine triphosphate (ATP) which may cause vasoconstriction, not affected by α-adrenoceptor blockers. Preventing release, or depleting tissue levels of such substances may explain the greater benefit provided by drugs such as reserpine and guanethidine in severe cases of dysreflexia, when other agents have failed.

In some patients, autonomic dysreflexia may be a major and recurring problem because of difficulty in either defining or resolving the precipitating cause. More unusual examples of the former are gastric ulceration or cholecystitis, which are difficult to detect because of lack of pain. A more common example, which may, however, also be missed, is an anal fissure. Despite recognizing the cause, it may be extremely difficult to resolve problems which include severe skeletal muscle spasms or recurrent urinary bladder infection. Long-term drug therapy for autonomic dysreflexia in such patients is often only partially successful and may result in undesirable

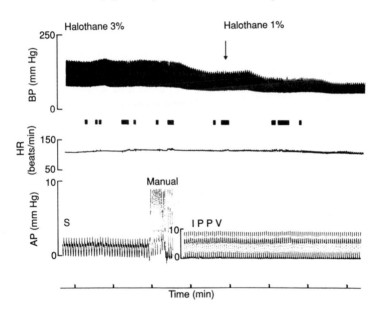

Fig. 43.16. Changes in blood pressure (BP) and heart rate (HR) of a chronic tetraplegic patient undergoing transurethral resection. The dark blocks indicate where resection and diathermy were performed. Airway pressure (AP) is also indicated when the patient was breathing spontaneously, was manually ventilated, and on intermittent positive pressure ventilation (IPPV). The blood pressure has been satisfactorily controlled on 3 per cent halothane. Increasing airway pressure reduces blood pressure and enables the use of a lower concentration of halothane (1 per cent), which successfully maintains the blood pressure during operative procedures which would otherwise greatly elevate it. (From Welply *et al.* (1975).)

side-effects. In severe cases, surgical procedures on the spinal cord, such as rhizotomy and cordotomy, or peripheral procedures, such as sacral and hypogastric neurotomy, may need to be considered. Non-surgical approaches, such as subarachnoid block with alcohol or phenol, have also been utilized. These procedures, however, usually abolish spinal reflex activity and result in flaccidity of skeletal muscles, and bladder and bowel atony, with their attendant disadvantages.

Autonomic dysreflexia can be a particular problem during surgery, especially if either the urinary bladder or the large bowel is involved. In these patients either spinal anaesthesia or a general anaesthetic, such as halothane, along with an increase in positive pressure ventilation, is often successful in controlling the hypertension (Fig. 43.16). Short-acting ganglionic blockers, such as trimethaphan, have been successfully used during surgery. The management of autonomic dysreflexia during pregnancy is discussed later.

Tracheal stimulation and intubation

Recently injured tetraplegics with high cervical lesions involving spinal segments that supply the phrenic nerves are dependent on artificial respiration because of diaphragmatic paralysis. In these patients bradycardia and cardiac arrest may occur during tracheal suction, especially when they are hypoxic (Fig. 43.17). The bradycardia is effectively prevented by atropine, which confirms the role of vagal efferent pathways in the response. The mechanisms by which tracheal suction and hypoxia contribute to bradycardia in these patients are outlined in Table 43.5. These stimuli activate vagal and glossopharyngeal afferents that increase vagal efferent activity. This is opposed by a number of factors which includes the pulmonary inflation vagal reflex, which normally raises heart rate, as is observed in spontaneously breathing tetraplegics when exposed either to hypoxia or to tracheal suction (Fig. 43.18). Other factors include the inability to activate sympathetic nerves, which are normally stimulated by tracheal suction or hypoxia.

The management of bradycardia and cardiac arrest during tracheal suction is directly related to knowledge of the mechanisms involved. Reconnecting the patient to the respirator will activate the pulmonary inflation vagal reflex, and the addition of oxygen will reverse hypoxia. External cardiac massage may be needed along with intravenous atropine. Precipitant factors often include respiratory infection and pulmonary emboli. Both cause hypoxia, which initially may be difficult to reverse. Such patients may need maintenance atropine, in a dose of 0.3 or 0.6 mg either subcutaneously or intramuscularly at 4-hourly intervals. Parasympathomimetic agents such as neostigmine and carbachol, which reverse bladder and bowel atony in spinal shock, should be avoided or used with caution. Heart rate may be increased also by the use of β_1-adrenoceptor agonists, but drugs such as isoprenaline also have actions on vasodilatatory β_2-adrenoceptors which

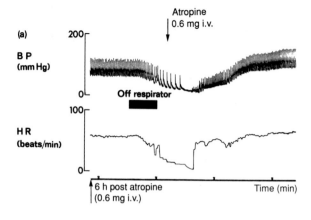

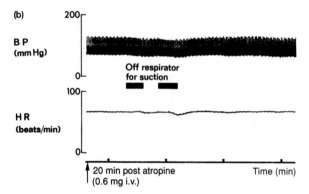

Fig. 43.17. (a) The effect of disconnecting the respirator (as required for aspirating the airways) on the blood pressure (BP) and heart rate (HR) of a recently injured tetraplegic patient (C4/5 lesion) in spinal shock, 6 h after the last dose of intravenous atropine. Sinus bradycardia and cardiac arrest (also observed on the electrocardiograph) were reversed by reconnection, intravenous atropine, and external cardiac massage. (From Frankel *et al.* (1975).) (b) The effect of tracheal suction, 20 min after atrophine. Disconnection from the respirator and tracheal suction did not lower either heart rate or blood pressure. (From Mathias (1976*b*).)

may lower blood pressure further, as in chronic tetraplegics (Chapter 14). Temporary demand pace-makers have also been used.

In chronic tetraplegics, bradycardia and cardiac arrest may also occur when the trachea is stimulated while respiration is prevented, despite the potential presence of opposing sympathetic cardiac reflexes operating at a spinal level. This may occur during endotracheal intubation after the use of skeletal muscle relaxants such as suxamethonium (Fig. 43.19). The mechanisms of this vagal reflex appear similar to those described in recently injured

Table 43.5.   The major mechanisms contributing to bradycardia and cardiac arrest in recently injured tetraplegics in spinal shock during tracheal suction and hypoxia.

	Tracheal suction	Hypoxia
Normal	Increased sympathetic nervous activity causes tachycardia and raises blood pressure	Bradycardia is the primary response opposed by the pulmonary (inflation) vagal reflex, resulting in tachycardia
Tetraplegics	No increase in sympathetic nervous activity, therefore no rise in heart rate or blood pressure. Vagal afferent stimulation may lead to unopposed vagal efferent activity	The primary response, bradycardia, is not opposed by the pulmonary (inflation) vagal reflex, because of disconnection from respirator or 'fixed' respiratory rate

↘   ↙

Increased vagal cardiac tone

↓

Bradycardia and cardiac arrest

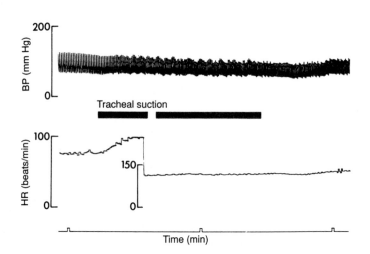

Fig. 43.18.   Effect of tracheal suction on blood pressure (BP) and heart rate (HR) of a chronic tetraplegic patient 7 months after injury when he had recovered spontaneous respiration and isolated reflex spinal cord sympathetic activity. Tracheal suction performed through an indwelling tracheostomy tube caused hyperventilation, tachycardia, and a fall in blood pressure. The heart rate scale alters as shown. (From Mathias (1976*b*).)

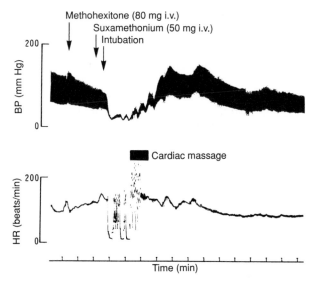

Fig. 43.19. The effect of endotracheal intubation on blood pressure (BP) and heart rate (HR) of a chronic tetraplegic patient being anaesthetized for urological surgery. Intubation was followed by cardiac arrest which was reversed by oxygen and external cardiac massage. (From Welply *et al.* (1975).)

tetraplegics, with afferent vagal stimulation causing an increase in vagal efferent activity that is not opposed by the pulmonary inflation reflex because of respiratory paralysis. An important practical point is to administer an adequate amount of atropine prior to intubation, especially in patients who are at greater risk from autonomic dysreflexia and increased cardiac vagal activity, such as during urological surgery.

Food ingestion

In tetraplegics, unlike patients with chronic primary autonomic failure (Chapter 26), ingestion of either a balanced meal, an equivalent liquid meal, or an isocaloric solution of glucose does not result in a substantial fall in supine blood pressure. The modest fall in blood pressure is accompanied by an elevation in heart rate. Levels of forearm venous plasma noradrenaline do not change, excluding a generalized increase in sympathetic nerve activity. The mechanisms responsible for preventing a substantial fall in blood pressure in tetraplegics are unclear; these could include the stimulation of reflexes from the gastrointestinal tract and mesentery (Chapter 26).

Hypoglycaemia

In normal man, hypoglycaemia results in a marked rise in plasma adrenaline levels and a modest rise in plasma noradrenaline levels. The clinical manifestations include anxiety, tremulousness, hunger, sweating, and tachycardia. There is little change in mean blood pressure as systolic blood pressure often rises and there is a small fall in diastolic blood pressure. Microneurography studies indicate that both muscle and skin sympathetic nerve activity increase during insulin hypoglycaemia, indicating that the response in normal man is not entirely due to adrenal stimulation and release of adrenaline (Fagius *et al.* 1986). Similar or even greater increases in integrated muscle sympathetic nerve activity occur in adrenalectomized patients, in whom there is no rise in plasma adrenaline levels (Fagius *et al.* 1986).

In tetraplegics, insulin-induced hypoglycaemia does not raise levels of plasma adrenaline or noradrenaline (Fig. 43.20). There is a fall in systolic blood pressure, along with a rise in heart rate. There are no symptoms of hypoglycaemia except for sedation, which is readily reversed with intravenous hypertonic glucose. If rapidly injected, however, this may cause a marked fall in blood pressure, as has been observed in patients with primary autonomic failure. The symptoms accompanying hypoglycaemia in normal man, therefore, appear to be largely dependent upon an elevation in

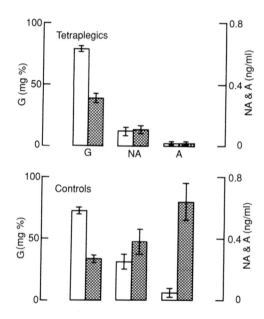

Fig. 43.20. Levels of blood glucose (G), plasma noradrenaline (NA), and adrenaline (A) before (blank histograms) and during (hatched histograms) insulin-induced hypoglycaemia in chronic tetraplegics (upper panel) and normal subjects (controls, lower panel). In the controls hypoglycaemia caused a small rise in plasma noradrenaline and a marked elevation in plasma adrenaline levels. A similar degree of hypoglycaemia did not change the low plasma noradrenaline and adrenaline levels in the tetraplegics. The bars indicate ± SEM. (From Mathias *et al.* (1979*b*).)

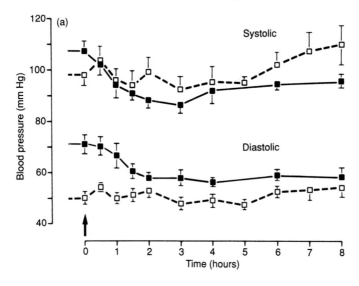

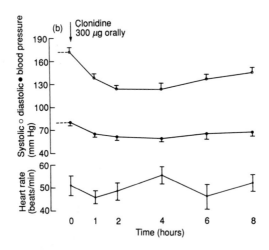

Fig. 43.21. (a) The effect of 300 µg of oral clonidine (↑) on systolic and diastolic blood pressure of normal subjects (filled squares, continuous line) and chronic tetraplegics (open squares, dashed line). There is a substantial fall in both systolic and diastolic blood pressure in the normal subjects but no fall in blood pressure in the tetraplegics. The bars indicate ± SEM. (From Reid *et al.* (1977).) (b) Systolic and diastolic blood pressure and heart rate recorded at the end of 3 min of bladder stimulation in a group of chronic tetraplegics before and after 300 µg of clonidine. There is a marked attenuation of the pressor response with the largest reductions in the second and fourth hours. Effects persist even 8 hours after clonidine. The bars indicate ± SEM.

adrenaline levels and intact sympathetic nervous pathways. In tetraplegics and high thoracic lesions, the lack of warning signs accompanying neuro-glycopenia are similar to observations made in some patients with diabetes mellitus and complicating autonomic neuropathy, or patients on non-selective β-adrenergic blockers.

Cardiovascular responses to pharmacological stimuli

Centrally acting agents—clonidine

Clonidine is an α_2-adrenoceptor agonist which has a number of actions that include cerebral effects, predominantly on the brainstem. In normal man this results in a withdrawal of sympathetic tone and a fall in blood pressure. Effects on the medullary vagal centres result in a fall in heart rate. In patients with tetraplegia, intravenous clonidine (approximately $150 \mu g$) transiently raises blood pressure, consistent with its peripheral agonist effects on postsynaptic α_1 and α_2 adrenoceptors. Neither intravenous nor oral clonidine ($300 \mu g$) lowers supine basal levels of blood pressure in tetraplegics (Fig. 43.21(a)) because of the disruption of descending sympathetic pathways. The heart rate, however, falls, in keeping with its vagal effects. Clonidine has additional effects, either on sympathetic neurons within the spinal cord or on peripheral presynaptic α_2 adrenoceptors which inhibit noradrenaline release. These may explain its partial ability to prevent hypertension during autonomic dysreflexia, as demonstrated during bladder stimulation (Fig. 43.2 (b); Mathias *et al.* 1979*c*). Clonidine is also able to reduce skeletal muscle spasms (Maynard 1986). These actions may explain its value in the management of autonomic dysreflexia in high spinal cord lesions.

Peripherally acting vasopressor agents

An increased pressor response to intravenously infused noradrenaline occurs in both recently injured and chronic tetraplegics (Fig. 43.22). This was originally considered to be a clinical manifestation of denervation hypersensitivity, as relating to Canon's law that denervated organs are supersensitive to their neurotransmitter. In classical denervation hyper-sensitivity, however, impairment of function of postganglionic sympathetic nerve terminals results in reduction in the neuronal uptake of noradrenaline. This inability to clear noradrenaline increases its synaptic concentration and results in a greater target organ response. In tetraplegics, however, there is histochemical evidence of intact adrenergic nerve terminals (Norberg and Normell 1974) and functional evidence, during autonomic dysreflexia, of the integrity of postganglionic sympathetic nerves. Circulating levels of noradrenaline in tetraplegics and normal subjects are similar after identical intravenous infusions of noradrenaline, although the pressor responses are markedly different (Mathias *et al.* 1976*c*). Impaired clearance and higher levels

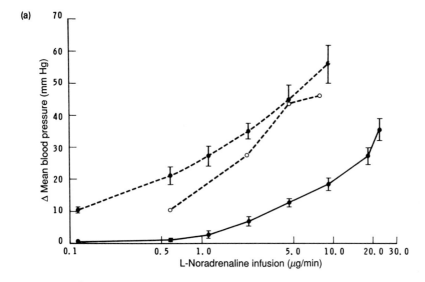

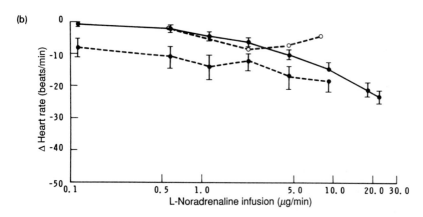

Fig. 43.22. Changes (Δ) in average mean blood pressure and heart rate during different dose infusion rates of noradrenaline in three recently injured tetraplegics (open circles, dashed line), five chronic tetraplegics (filled circles, dashed line), and 10 control subjects (filled circle, continuous line). The bars indicate ± SEM. There is an enhanced pressor response to noradrenaline in both groups of tetraplegics over the entire dose range studied. (From Mathias *et al.* (1976c; 1979a).)

of noradrenaline in classical denervation supersensitivity do not appear to account for the increased pressor responses in tetraplegics.

The lesion in tetraplegics and high thoracic lesions is effectively preganglionic, which is more proximal to the experimental lesions of immediately preganglionic nerves that can also cause an enhanced response to noradrenaline (decentralization hypersensitivity). This is thought to be due to an increase in receptor population, an improvement of the functional link between receptor activation and the final response, or both factors. Although tetraplegics have a low background level of sympathetic activity this is punctuated by repeated episodes of autonomic dysreflexia, which ensure that sympathetic nerve terminals and receptors and target organs are intermittently kept active and stimulated. There is indirect evidence, based on *in vitro* studies of platelet α_2 adrenoceptor binding, that tetraplegics have a normal population of α-adrenoceptors (Davies *et al.* 1982). Microneurography studies, however, indicate a modest increase in muscle sympathetic nerve activity during autonomic dysreflexia when there is a pronounced vascular response (Stjernbeg *et al.* 1986), suggesting that decentralization supersensitivity, for reasons that are currently unclear, may contribute to the enhanced pressor response to noradrenaline.

A further possibility includes the impairment of baroreflex pathways which descend through the cervical spinal cord and are normally concerned with buffering a rise in blood pressure. This would explain the elevated pressor response during autonomic dysreflexia and the clearly defined relationship between these hypertensive responses and the segmental level of the lesion at T5. In normal subjects it is likely that, despite a substantial rise in sympathoneural activity induced by a range of stimuli, blood pressure is maintained at near normal levels by baroreflexes, partly through the vagal efferents and predominantly by descending nerve tracts within the spinal cord, which selectively inhibit sympathetic vasoconstrictor activity and may even cause vasodilatation by mechanisms that are yet to be clearly defined in man. The only intact efferent component of the baroreflex pathways in tetraplegics is the vagal outflow; this slows the heart but is clearly inadequate in controlling the rise in blood pressure during autonomic dysreflexia. It is possible, therefore, that the absence of blood pressure restraining reflexes descending through the cervical and upper thoracic spinal cord down to the level of T5 may be a major factor accounting for the enhanced pressor responses to noradrenaline. This may also explain the observations that exaggerated pressor responses are not specific to α-adrenoceptor agonists but occur in response to agents with different structures and properties ranging from phenylephrine, to prostaglandin F2α, and angiotensin II. The low circulating levels of adrenaline and noradrenaline may not be major contributory factors, as there is a similar degree of pressor sensitivity to angiotensin II (Fig. 43.23), despite normal or elevated circulating levels of renin and angiotensin II. This argues strongly against receptor upregulation alone being a factor.

The enhanced responses to pressor agents are of clinical importance, as the 5 to 10-fold increase in sensitivity should be borne in mind if drugs with pressor actions are used in high spinal lesions.

Peripherally acting vasodepressor agents
Enhanced depressor responses to a range of vasodilatory substances also occur

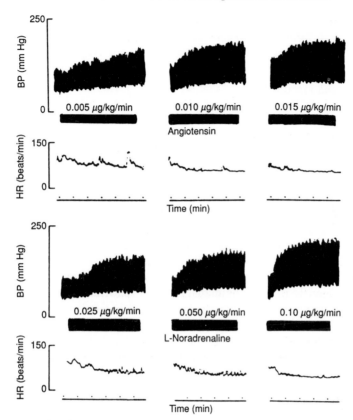

Fig. 43.23. Blood pressure (BP) and heart rate (HR) effects of different dose infusion rates of angiotensin II (upper panels) and L-noradrenaline (lower panels) given intravenously to a chronic tetraplegic patient. These doses of angiotensin II and noradrenaline cause only small blood pressure changes in normal subjects. (From Mathias and Frankel (1986).)

in high spinal cord lesions. Bolus injections and intravenous infusion of isoprenaline lower blood pressure substantially (Chapter 14). Indirect evidence from *in vitro* β-adrenoceptor binding studies on lymphocytes exclude up-regulation of these receptors. In high lesions isoprenaline will stimulate both β_1- and β_2-adrenoceptors; it is likely that stimulation of the latter causes vasodilatation which would normally stimulate the baroreflex pathways, increase sympathetic activity, and prevent a substantial fall in blood pressure. This would not occur in high lesions and may account for the fall in blood pressure. The increase in heart rate, which is often exaggerated, is likely to be a combination of the vagal response to the fall in blood pressure and the direct β_1 effects of isoprenaline.

Enhanced vasodepressor responses occur to a variety of drugs including intravenous prostaglandin E2 and sublingual glyceryl trinitrate. The latter may be used to advantage in high lesions, as it can be readily taken and can substantially lower blood pressure in autonomic dysreflexia. The risk of extreme hypotension should be kept in mind (Fig. 43.14).

Cutaneous circulation

The skin is innervated by the sympathetic nervous system and changes may occur both in recently injured and in chronic tetraplegics. Soon after injury there is often vasodilatation in the periphery, as the skin below the level of the lesion is often warmer and veins appear dilated. It is not clear if this may lead to extravasation of fluid into subcutaneous tissue and contribute to skin breakdown and pressure sores, which is a major problem in recently injured patients. The vasodilatation may also involve mucosal tissues such as the nose, and result in nasal congestion, a problem seen in patients with high lesions who often have to breathe through their mouth. This has been referred to as Guttmann's sign, and is similar to the nasal vasodilatation after α-adrenoceptor blockade induced by either phenoxybenzamine or guanethidine, both previously used in the management of patients with hypertension.

The cutaneous responses to the Lewis or triple response and to histamine vary in the different stages. In the stage of spinal shock, responses above and below the lesion are similar (Guttmann 1976). This differs from the later phases with return of isolated spinal cord reflex activity, when stimulation of skin below the lesion results in cutaneous vasoconstriction, leading to skin pallor which may last for a prolonged period—hence the term 'dermatographia alba', as compared to 'dermatographia rubra' in the stage of spinal shock. In chronic high lesions, during autonomic dysreflexia there may be marked constriction of cutaneous blood vessels (causing cold peripheries; poikilothermia spinalis) and activation of piloerector muscles (causing goose skin and pimples; cutis anserina) below the level of the lesion.

Thermoregulation

The autonomic nervous system plays an important role in the regulation of body temperature, which may be seriously deranged in tetraplegics.

Hypothermia

On exposure to cold a number of mechanisms are activated, which are dependent initially on appreciation of the temperature change and then on the ability to increase heat production and gain. Cold appreciation is dependent upon activation of both cutaneous and also central temperature receptors, which may explain why tetraplegics, although they have only a limited area of intact sensation, can still detect body cooling.

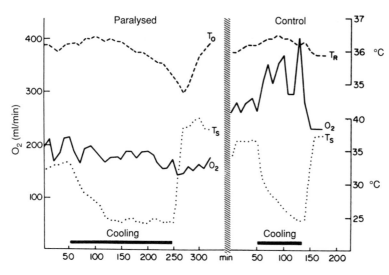

Fig. 43.24. The effect of body cooling on oesophageal (T_o), rectal (T_r), and skin (T_s) temperature and oxygen consumption (O_2) of a severely paralysed patient with poliomyelitis and a normal subject (control). The lack of shivering in the patient causes no rise in oxygen consumption and heat production which leads to a fall in central temperature, unlike the normal subject. (From Johnson and Spalding 1963).

One of the major mechanisms responsible for heat production is shivering thermogenesis, which depends upon activation of skeletal muscles and shivering. In tetraplegics and those with high thoracic spinal cord lesions, a major proportion of skeletal muscle mass is not directly under voluntary control; this is a particular problem in spinal shock when there is skeletal muscle flaccidity. Hypothermia may therefore readily occur in such patients, as it does in other groups without autonomic lesions who have extensive paralysis either due to drugs or to poliomyelitis (Fig. 43.24). Tetraplegics and those with high thoracic lesions have the ability to shiver in innervated areas as the body temperature falls, but this often results only in a small increase in metabolism, which, dependent upon the external temperature, may be inadequate for body temperature homeostasis. An additional problem in recently injured tetraplegics in spinal shock is cutaneous vasodilatation, and the inability to appropriately vasoconstrict. This enhances heat loss, lowers body temperature further, and can be a particular problem in causing hypothermia especially in temperate climates (Fig. 43.25). A low-reading rectal thermometer is essential in the assessment and management of hypothermia. The patient should be warmed externally, with care taken to prevent skin damage, and internally, using warm drinks or infusion of warm saline. Drugs (including alcohol), which cause cutaneous vasodilatation and increase heat loss should therefore be strictly avoided.

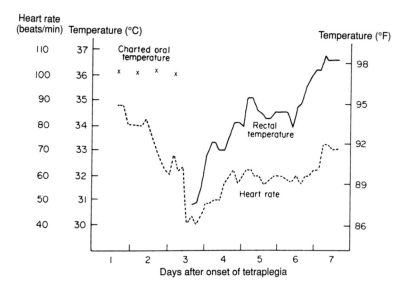

Fig. 43.25. Fall in central temperature (measured as rectal temperature) and heart rate in a recently injured tetraplegic in a temperate climate. Hypothermia is best monitored with a low-reading rectal thermometer and, as indicated, may be missed if oral temperature is recorded. (From Pledger (1962).)

Hyperthermia

Hyperthermia, may occur particularly in tetraplegics and high spinal cord lesions when environmental temperature is elevated, or in response to infection. Heat loss is dependent on two major mechanisms, vasodilatation and sweating, both of which are impaired in spinal lesions. Vasodilatation normally occurs during warming, and is dependent on a rise in central temperature. It may occur passively, as a result of withdrawal of sympathetic vasoconstrictor tone, or actively. Both components are dependent on neural pathways within the cervical spinal cord, which are involved in high spinal cord lesions (Fig. 43.26). Vasodilatation may also occur following application of radiant or local heat to tetraplegics; this is more likely to be a direct effect than due to reflexes via the isolated spinal cord.

Sweating normally causes heat loss by evaporation, and is dependent upon a rise in central temperature and activation of sudomotor fibres within the sympathetic nervous system. Thermoregulatory sweating in large areas below the lesion is impaired in high spinal lesions, and is a further reason for their being prone to hyperthermia.

The maintenance of a suitable environmental temperature is of importance in the prevention of hyperthermia in high spinal lesions. When hyperthermia occurs, cooling with the aid of tepid sponging and increased air flow with

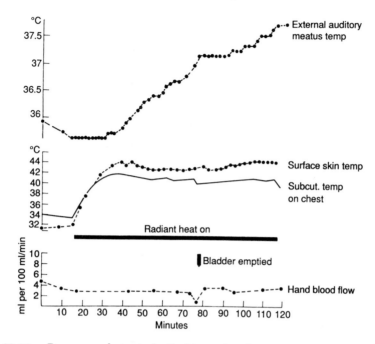

Fig. 43.26. Pronounced rise in both skin and oral temperature (measured as external auditory meatus temperature) during application of radiant heat to the trunk of a tetraplegic patient. Hand blood flow does not rise indicating lack of vasodilatation, as would normally occur during an elevation in temperature. (From Johnson (1965).)

a fan accelerates heat loss by a combination of evaporation, conduction, and convection. In severe cases, ice-cooled saline by intravenous infusion or urinary bladder irrigation and, in extreme cases, immersion of the whole body in an ice bath may be necessary. In hyperpyrexia associated with infection, drugs such as aspirin and paracetamol appear to be effective in lowering body temperature. The mechanisms by which they do this are unclear. Chlorpromazine is also effective, but has the potential to induce hypotension.

Gastrointestinal system

The autonomic nervous system richly innervates the gastrointestinal tract which is often affected especially in the early stages after spinal cord lesions.

Upper gastrointestinal bleeding

There is a high incidence of upper gastrointestinal bleeding in the early stages following spinal cord injury. The incidence is greater in those with higher lesions. It is often unrelated to a previous history of peptic ulceration and may not be related to concomitant drug therapy, such as dexamethasone and analgesics. In such patients there is evidence of increased vagal activity, which may cause hyperacidity, along with high gastrin levels which may furthermore contribute to gastric hypersecretion and ulceration.

The lesions may be either patchy or extensive and affect the oesophagus, stomach, or the duodenum. Erosions and ulceration may occur. Abdominal pain is usually absent. Shoulder-tip pain, accentuated by abdominal palpation, may indicate perforation. Haematemesis or melaena may occur. Fibre-optic endoscopy is probably the investigation of choice, the major limitation being the restriction to cervical spine mobility. Atropine may be needed to prevent vagal reflexes and bradycardia. The management consists of the administration of H2 receptor antagonists (such as cimetidine or ranitidine), antacids, and fluid and blood replacement where relevant. The role of newer drugs such as omeprazole and orally active prostaglandin analogues, has not been clearly defined. Surgery may occasionally be needed.

Paralytic ileus

This often occurs in spinal shock and may be accompanied by gastric dilatation. The mechanisms remain unclear as the motor innervation of the stomach and small intestines is by the vagus nerves, which are intact and often hyperactive in this phase. Paralytic ileus usually occurs a few days after injury and may be induced by solid food, which should therefore be avoided in the immediate period following a cervical or high thoracic spinal cord injury.

Paralytic ileus results in meteorism which is a particular problem as it interferes with the movement of the diaphragm, often the only major functional muscle of respiration in these patients. It may be particularly prolonged in patients with intercurrent infection. The management consists of gastrointestinal aspiration to prevent further dilatation, the administration of intravenous fluids, and, if necessary, intravenous alimentation. Parasympathomimetic agents such as neostigmine are occasionally used to activate the bowel but carry the risk of potentiating bradycardia and cardiac arrest, especially in patients with high cervical lesions on artificial respiration. The dopamine antagonist, metoclopramide, which enhances gastric emptying, may be of value in some cases. It may be that newer drugs that increase gastrointestinal motility, such as the prodrug, cisapride, and the cholecystokinin antagonist, loxeglumide, will be of value. Once spinal shock has subsided small intestine function often returns to normal. Tetraplegics and high thoracic lesions are, however, prone to paralytic ileus even in the chronic stage, especially after undergoing general anaesthesia and abdominal surgery.

Large bowel dysfunction

In spinal shock, paralysis of the sacral parasympathetic results in atony of the colon and rectum. Voluntary or reflexly induced defecation does not occur and this results in faecal retention. Digital evacuation is often necessary in the early stages.

After the stage of spinal shock, autonomous function of the lower bowel returns and is regulated at a spinal level, as it is abolished by intrathecal block with alcohol (Guttmann 1976). The stimulus to bowel activity appears to be increased volume and distension, which then causes relaxation of the external anal sphincter and evacuation of contents. This stimulus is utilized in the reconditioning of lower bowel function. The diet should therefore include high residue foods together with mild laxatives and stool softeners, to ensure regular bowel evacuation. This is an important part of the management, as regular bowel movement prevents faecal retention which predisposes patients with high lesions to autonomic dysreflexia for a variety of reasons. These include distension of the lower bowel and the predisposition to haemorrhoids and anal fissures.

The urinary system

Function of the urinary bladder is dependent upon higher centres in the brain and the sympathetic and parasympathetic nerves and is therefore affected in varying degrees in patients with spinal cord lesions. In the chronic stage complications to the ureters and kidneys, such as infection, calculi, urinary reflux, hydroureters, and hydronephrosis, may lead to renal damage resulting in chronic renal failure, which largely stems from this basic dysfunction.

In spinal shock there is usually complete paralysis of bladder function with retention of urine followed by distension and urinary overflow after excessive intravesical pressure has developed. This should be avoided, as it often impedes functional return of detrusor muscle activity once spinal shock has subsided. Bladder paralysis is invariable in most adult Europeans, but does not usually occur in children and adult Afro-Caribbeans. The management in spinal shock consists of drainage using an indwelling catheter, or preferably intermittent catheterization which causes fewer complications.

With the return of parasympathetic activity within the isolated sacral cord there is detrusor muscle contraction which occurs in response to filling of the urinary bladder or following stimuli such as tapping of the anterior abdominal wall suprapubically. This is the automatic reflex bladder, or neurogenic bladder. During detrusor contraction there is a need for simultaneous relaxation of the sphincters and pelvic floor to allow the free passage of urine. Training is needed to achieve co-ordination of these components of bladder function and, if this is successful, male patients may be catheter-free, using a condom and receptacle to collect urine. In some patients, however, detrusor contraction is not accompanied by simultaneous relaxation of the bladder outlet, and in high lesions, the resultant discoordinated bladder can cause marked autonomic dysreflexia. Retained urine often results in infection, which can involve the kidneys, especially when there is retrograde pressure in the urinary tract. In such patients an indwelling catheter or urological surgery is needed to relieve the functional obstruction. The α-adrenoceptor blockers, phenoxybenzamine and prazosin, may be of value in some patients as the bladder outlet is relaxed. In low lesions there may be a flaccid bladder even in the chronic stage. Manual compression using Crede's manoeuvre is needed to ensure complete emptying, along with the other aids for urine collection.

In female patients, the bladder can be trained to empty in response to distension and external stimuli. Because of the lack of suitable collecting systems, there may be incontinence which is often not helped by an indwelling catheter. In some, an ileal conduit may be the most practical outcome.

Reproductive system

In the male reproducion and sexual function is dependent on the interrelationship between parasympathetic and sympathetic nerve function and is therefore usually impaired. Few changes occur in the female with spinal cord injuries.

The male

Penile erection is dependent largely upon the sacral parasympathetic nerves with ejaculation dependent upon the sympathetic nerves. In spinal shock there is an absence of both erectile and ejaculatory function. In some patients, however, passive penile enlargement and priapism may occur, probably due to paralytic dilatation resulting in engorgement of the corpora cavernosa. Following the return of isolated spinal cord reflex activity, penile erection may occur if the glans penis is stimulated, or as part of autonomic dysreflexia. Ejaculation, however, seldom occurs per urethra and is usually retrograde, as the associated contraction of muscles at the bladder neck which prevents seminal fluid flowing back into the bladder does not usually occur. In spinal cord injuries, therefore, procreation in the male is largely dependent on the collection of seminal fluid for artificial insemination. The original technique involved intrathecal neostigmine (Guttmann 1976) which caused skeletal muscle depression followed by penile erection and ejaculation. In high lesions, side-effects such as vomiting and severe autonomic dysreflexia often occurred and in one patient this resulted in cerebral haemorrhage and death. The technique of electro-ejaculation is now used, although this may also result in severe hypertension, and careful monitoring of blood pressure is necessary in those with high lesions, especially when seminal emission occurs. Many of the drugs that are often used to lower blood pressure in autonomic dysreflexia are not the ideal ones to use during such procedures as they interrupt sympathetic pathways and have the potential to interfere with ejaculation.

The female

In women transient disruption of the menstrual cycle is often observed after spinal lesions, as occurs during other traumatic conditions or illnesses. There is usually a return to normal menstrual periods within a year. Successful pregnancies have been reported in both tetraplegics and paraplegics. In those with high lesions a particular problem is severe autonomic dysreflexia and paroxysmal hypertension (Fig. 43.27) which may be accompanied by cardiac dysrhythmias especially during uterine contractions. Such patients are particularly prone to epileptic seizures and cerebral haemorrhage and it is essential to lower their blood pressure. Anticonvulsants such as phenytoin may be needed. Spinal anaesthesia appears to be a satisfactory method of

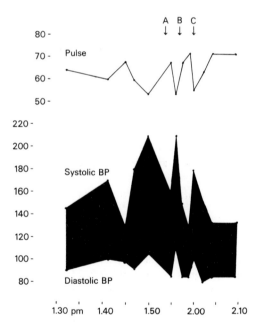

Fig. 43.27. Blood pressure and pulse rate in a paraplegic patient with a high thoracic lesion (T5) during (A) application of forceps, (B) completion of delivery, and (C) placental delivery. The hypertension is closely followed by bradycardia. (From Guttmann *et al.* (1965).)

preventing the hypertension without interfering with uterine contraction. This often allows progression of a normal delivery and avoids a Caesarean section.

References

Bracken, M. B., Shepard, M. J., Collins, W. F. Holford, T. R., Young, W., Baskin, D. S., Eisenberg, H. M., Flamm, E., Leo-Summers, L., Maroon, J., Marshall, L. F., Perot, P. L., Piepmeier, J., Sonntag, V. K. H., Wagner, F. C., Wilberger, J. E., and Winn, H. R. (1990) A randomized, controlled trial of methylprednisolone or naloxone in the treatment of acute spinal-cord injury. *New Engl. J. Med.* **322**, 1405–11.

Corbett, J. L., Frankel, H. L., and Harris, P. J. (1971). Cardio-vascular reflex responses to cutaneous and visceral stimuli in spinal man. *J. Physiol.* **215**, 395.

Davies, I. B., Mathias, C. J., Sudera, D., and Sever, P. S. (1982). Agonist regulation of alpha-adrenergic receptor responses in man. *J. Cardiovasc. Pharmacol.* **4**, s139–44.

Fagius, J., Niklasson, F., and Bern, E. C. (1986). Sympathetic outflow in human muscle nerves increases during hypoglycaemia. *Diabetes* **35**, 1124–9.

Frankel, H. L. and Mathias, C. J. (1976). The cardiovascular system in paraplegia and tetraplegia. In *Handbook of clinical neurology,* Vol. 26. *Injuries of the spine and spinal cord,* Part II (ed. P. J. Vinken and G. W. Bruyn), pp. 313–33. North-Holland, Amsterdam.

Frankel, H. L., Michaelis, L. S., Golding, D. R., and Beral, V. (1972). The blood pressure in paraplegia-1. *Paraplegia* **10**, 193–8.

Frankel, H. L., Mathias, C. J., and Spalding, J. M. K. (1975). Mechanisms of reflex cardiac arrest in tetraplegic patients. *Lancet* **ii**, 1183–5.

Guttmann, L. (1976). *Spinal cord injuries. Comprehensive management and research* (2nd edn). Blackwell Scientific, Oxford.

Guttmann, L. and Whitteridge, D. (1947). Effects of bladder distension on autonomic mechanisms after spinal cord injury. *Brain* **70**, 361–404.

Guttmann, L., Frankel, H. L, and Paeslack, V. (1965). Cardiac irregularities during labour in paraplegic women. *Paraplegia* **3**, 144–51.

Head, H. and Riddoch, G. (1917). The autonomic bladder, excessive sweating and some other reflex conditions in gross injuries of the spinal cord. *Brain* **40**, 188–263.

Johnson, R. H. (1965). Neurological studies in temperature regulation. *Ann. Roy. Coll. Surg.* **36**, 339–52.

Johnson, R. H. and Spalding, J. M. K. (1963). Whole body metabolism of a paralysed man during surface cooling. *J. Physiol.* **166**, 24P.

Kooner, J. S, da Costa, D. F., Frankel, H. L., Bannister, R., Peart, W. S., and Mathias, C. J. (1987). Recumbency induces hypertension, diuresis and natriuresis in autonomic failure, but diuresis alone in tetraplegia. *J. Hypertension* **5**(suppl.5), 327–9.

Mathias, C. J. (1976a). Neurological disturbances of the cardiovascular system. D. Phil. thesis, University of Oxford.

Mathias, C. J. (1976b). Bradycardia and cardiac arrest during tracheal suction—mechanisms in tetraplegic patients. *Eur. J. intensive care Med.* **2**, 147–56.

Mathias, C. J. and Frankel, H. L (1986). The neurological and hormonal control of blood vessels and heart in spinal man. *J. autonom. nerv. Syst.* (suppl.) 457–64.

Mathias, C. J. and Frankel, H. L (1988). Cardiovascular control in spinal man. *Ann. Rev. Physiol.* **50**, 577–92.

Mathias, C. J., Christensen, N. J., Corbett, J. L., Frankel, H. L., Goodwin, T. J., and Peart, W. S. (1975). Plasma catecholamines, plasma renin activity and plasma aldosterone in tetraplegic man, horizontal and tilted. *Clin. Sci. mol. Med.* **49**, 291–9.

Mathias, C. J., Christensen, N. J., Corbett, J. L., Frankel, H. L., and Spalding, J. M. K. (1976a). Plasma catecholamines during paroxysmal neurogenic hypertension in quadriplegic man. *Circulation Res.* **39**, 204–8.

Mathias, C. J., Smith, A. D., Frankel, H. L., and Spalding, J. M. K. (1976b). Release of dopamine B-hydroxylase during hypertension from sympathetic over-activity in man. *Cardiovascular Res.* **10**, 176–81.

Mathias, C. J., Frankel, H. L., Christensen, N. J., and Spalding, J. M. K. (1976c). Enhanced pressor response to noradrenaline in patients with cervical spinal cord transection. *Brain* **99**, 757–70.

Mathias, C. J., Christensen, N. J., Frankel, H. L., and Spalding, J. M. K. (1979a). Cardiovascular control in recently injured tetraplegics in spinal shock. *Quart. J. Med.*, NS **48**, 273–87.

Mathias, C. J., Frankel, H. L., Turner, R. C., and Christensen, J. N. (1979b). Physiological responses to insulin hypoglycaemia in spinal man. *Paraplegia* **17**, 319–26.

Mathias, C. J., Reid, J. L., Wing, L. M. H., Frankel, H. L., and Christensen, N. J.(1979c). Antihypertensive effects of clonidine in tetraplegic subjects devoid of central sympathetic control. *Clin. Sci.* **57**, 425–8s.

Maynard, F. M. (1986). Early clinical experience with clonidine in spinal spasticity. *Paraplegia* **24**, 175–82.

Norberg, K. A. and Normell, L. A. (1974). Histochemical demonstration of sympathetic adrenergic denervation in human skin. *Acta neurol. scand,* **50**, 261.

Pledger, H. G. (1962). Disorders of temperature regulation in acute traumatic paraplegia. *J. Bone Joint Surg.* **44B**, 110–13.

Reid, J. L. Wing, L. M. H., Mathias, C. J., Frankel, H. L., and Neill, E. (1977). The central hypotensive effect of clonidine: studies in tetraplegic subjects. *Clin. Pharmacol. Therapeut.* **21**, 375–81.

Skagen, K. and Henriksen, O. (1986). Local and central sympathetic vasoconstrictor reflexes in human limbs during orthostatic stress. In *The sympatho-adrenal system. Physiology and pathophysiology* (ed. N. J. Christensen, O. Henriksen, and N. A. Lassen), pp. 83–94. Munksgaard, Copenhagen.

Stjernberg, L., Blumberg, H., and Wallin, B. G. (1986). Sympathetic activity in man after spinal cord injury: outflow to muscle below the lesion. *Brain* **109**, 695–715.

Sutters, M., Wakefield, C., Appleyard, M., O'Neil, R., Frankel, H. L., Mathias, C. J., and Peart, W. S. (1991). Body fluid homeostasis during salt restriction in tetraplegic man. *Clin. autonom. Res.* **1**, 89.

van Lieshout, J. J., Imholz, B. P. M., Wesseling, K. H., Speelman, J. D., and Wieling, W. (1991). Singing-induced hypotension: a complication of high spinal cord lesion. *Netherlands J. Med.* **38**, 75–9.

Welply, N. C., Mathias, C. J., and Frankel, H. L. (1975). Circulatory reflexes in tetraplegics during artificial ventilation and general anaesthesia. *Paraplegia* **13**, 172–82.

44. Ageing and the autonomic nervous system

Ralph H. Johnson

Introduction

As the clinician observes the world's stage and the seven ages of man which are the acts of each man's play, he can be led, like Shakespeare, to conclude that the final act is one 'sans teeth, sans eyes, sans taste, sans everything'. The student of the autonomic nervous system, however, finds many surprises. As age advances, homeostasis remains active and physiological stresses receive their usual autonomic responses although their efficiency may be reduced. Paradoxes abound. The arterial blood pressure rises with age. Blood catecholamines, particularly noradrenaline, are elevated compared with concentrations found at younger ages, but it is not clear that the raised blood pressure is in response to this. It is in youth that rapid standing leads to sudden syncope, whereas older people can stand with no such response and yet their baroreflexes are apparently less active. The sensitivity of the carotid sinus may increase with ageing and its sudden stimulation may lead to unconsciousness and even death.

Thus autonomic function appears to be modified by age but its failure is not a necessary attribute of ageing. Those who suffer autonomic dysfunction are therefore abnormal, the cause being frequently obvious (Collins 1983), but sometimes none can be found. This review will consider the two major functions of thermoregulation and blood pressure regulation and situations in old age in which they are disordered. The effects of ageing upon autonomic function have been reviewed by Johnson and Spalding (1974) and Johnson *et al.* (1984).

Temperature regulation

Physiological changes with ageing

In old age, central body temperature remains relatively stable in spite of large variations in environmental temperature and it has one of the smallest coefficients of variation found in bodily functions. Body temperature exhibits circadian rhythm, the temperature being lowest in the early morning and highest in the late evening, and this rhythm takes several days to adjust if the usual rhythm of sleeping and waking is altered by shift work or by travelling to another part of the globe. Temperature regulation depends upon the balance of heat production and heat loss, and little is known about the central controlling mechanisms in the hypothalamus, although changes in heat loss mechanisms, in particular, have been studied in relation to ageing. It is probable that the ability to produce heat by shivering reduces with ageing with a reduction of muscle bulk. Heat loss mechanisms may also be affected by ageing. It has been shown that, in aged subjects, the temperature threshold for sweating is higher and that, with a given heat stress, the sweat rate is lower in elderly people. It appears that the reduced response and elevated threshold may be more pronounced in aged females but there is considerable variability in different subjects and different body sites (Foster *et al.* 1976). The responses are most reduced over the forehead and limbs and over the trunk and some subjects, particularly women, fail to sweat at all with a central temperature of up to 38°C. There is also delayed development of vasodilatation in some elderly subjects, as discussed below. It is not clear, however, whether deficient responses reflect a reduction in active sweat glands or deterioration in vasomotor function on the one hand or incipient autonomic failure. The significantly higher core temperature threshold required for sweating is, however, an indication of an ageing effect on thermoregulatory mechanisms.

Hyperthermia

Although deaths in elderly people are more frequent during heat waves, the causes are chiefly ischaemic heart disease or cerebrovascular disease. The reduced ability to sweat, however, may result in hyperthermia and this may predispose to other problems even though it has not been demonstrated to be a specific cause of death in itself. As with sweating, it has been observed that a greater rise in core temperature is necessary to induce maximum vasodilatation in elderly subjects. However, in another study, it was found that the degree of vasodilatation was the same in elderly people as in young controls. Once sweating is initiated, some observers have found that there is no further rise in core temperature in either elderly people or younger age groups. It must be concluded that hyperthermia is induced more rapidly in old people and that it is usually the rate of change which is dangerous rather than the core temperature itself.

Hypothermia

A wide range of disorders may contribute to the development of hypothermia (Table 44.1). It is usually defined as present when the core temperature is

Table 44.1. Causes of hypothermia

Hypothydroidism, hypopituitarism

Cold exposure

Drugs (particularly psychotropic drugs)

Ethanol

Neurological disease

Cerebrovascular disease
Parkinson's disease
Corpus callosum agenesis
Hypothalamic lesions
    Tumour
    Vascular
    Wernicke's encephalopathy
    Diencephalic epilepsy
    Idiopathic
Spinal cord lesions
    Paraplegia
    Tetraplegia

In association with general debility

    e.g. blood dyscrasias

---

below 35°C. Although hypothermia is usually provoked in these disorders by exposure to cold, it is possible for it to occur in some disorders under normal environmental conditions, for example, in hypothyroidism, with hypothalamic lesions, and with high spinal cord lesions. Lack of mobility due to a cerebrovascular accident or a fall from which the patient cannot get up may be a contributory factor, particularly if the floor is cold. One of the chief problems is that of recognition and a low-reading thermometer should be in routine use with elderly patients. Rectal temperature is usually more reliable than oral temperature in patients with hypothermia. There may be a history of progressive mental deterioration over days, and the degree of mental confusion is related to the level of temperature. Consciousness is usually severely impaired when the central temperature falls below 32°C.

Hypothermia has been found frequently in elderly people during cold winters, and has been recorded as a cause of death during cold periods, but even so it may be unrecognized. Although it may be associated with one of the pathological conditions shown in Table 44.1, and provoked by exposure to cold, it does appear that there may be failure of normal thermoregulation in some elderly people without evidence of overt disease. Elderly survivors from accidental hypothermia and elderly controls in whom hypothermia had not been known to occur were examined during

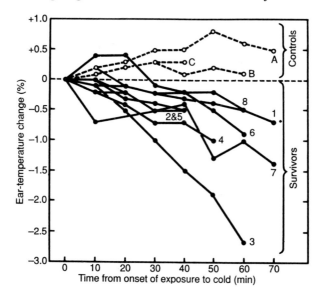

Fig. 44.1. The effect on central (external auditory meatus) temperature of exposure to cold (air fanned over the naked body) in three elderly control subjects (A, B, and C) and in eight survivors from hypothermia of the elderly. In the control subjects, exposure to cold caused a slight rise in central temperature (as occurs in normal young subjects), but in the survivors from hypothermia there was a fall in central temperature, indicating a failure of normal body temperature control. (Taken with permission from Macmillan *et al.* (1967).)

thermoregulatory tests (Macmillan *et al.* 1967). The survivors' resting central temperature was low and when they were exposed to cold, it fell progressively and abnormally compared with the controls (Fig. 44.1). This was due to impairment of heat production mechanisms and a failure to control heat loss. In some of the subjects the studies were carried out as long as 3 years after the episode of hypothermia which had been recorded. It must be concluded that survivors from accidental hypothermia of the elderly may be at risk from another episode of hypothermia, even if exposed to moderate cold.

It has been shown that vasodilatation in the hand only develops in normal subjects when the central body temperature is greater than 36.5°C (Cooper *et al.* 1964). However, in elderly subjects who had survived accidental hypothermia, there was obvious reflex vasodilatation below this core temperature in response to trunk warming. It appears likely that this derangement of thermoregulation is a cause, rather than effect, of the episode(s) of accidental hypothermia, although it may contribute to it. This abnormality has been studied in detail in a group of these patients (Johnson and Park 1973) and, although circulatory control of arterial blood pressure

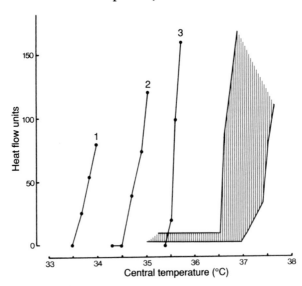

Fig. 44.2. Heat elimination from an index finger (galvanometer units) during radiant heating of the trunk in three patients (1, 2, 3) who have previously suffered from episodes of accidental hypothermia. The horizontal axis indicates the central temperature (external auditory meatus) at which the change in heat elimination occurred. The hatched area indicates the normal range described by Cooper *et al.* (1964). Reflex vasodilatation occurred at an unusually low central temperature, below 36.5°C. (Taken with permission from Johnson and Park (1973).

was apparently normal, orthostatic hypotension not being present, patients who had suffered episodes of accidental hypothermia were found to have vascular reflexes active at abnormally low central temperatures (Fig. 44.2). Although reflex shivering could be initiated in these subjects, it was not initiated by a fall in central temperature (Fig. 44.3). The reflex pathways for thermoregulation in man subserving vasodilatation and shivering, therefore, have a separate integrity which is physiologically independent of central thermoregulatory mechanisms (Fig. 44.4).

Normal thermoregulation depends upon controlling mechanisms in the hypothalamus which inhibit reflex vasodilatation in normal subjects when the central temperature is below 36.5°C. The reflex is active below this temperature if the hypothalamus is non-functioning and its pathway is therefore subthalamic. Blood pressure regulation on the other hand, is independent of the hypothalamus so that blood pressure regulation is normal in patients with hypothalamic damage.

Another reflex which was present in these individuals was the ventilatory stimulation which occurs on exposure to cold, independent of change in metabolism. In those subjects with abnormal thermoregulation, increased ventilation could be obtained, which is in keeping with its reflex mediation

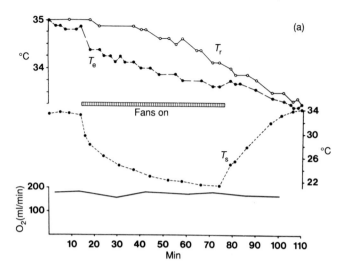

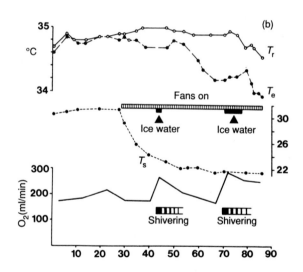

Fig. 44.3.   Shivering and oxygen consumption in a patient who has previously suffered from an episode of accidental hypothermia. T_r, Rectal temperature; T_e, external auditory meatus temperature; T_s, surface skin temperature on the trunk (one point). (a) During trunk cooling by fans (hatched bar) no shivering or rise of oxygen consumption occurred in spite of considerable fall of central temperature. (b) During fan cooling with addition of immersion of the feet in cold water (solid bars) shivering occurred during skin cooling with cold water.
(Taken with permission from Johnson and Park (1973).)

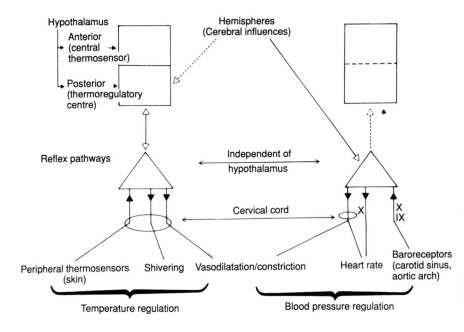

Fig. 44.4. Diagram of thermoregulatory and blood pressure reflexes in relation to the hypothalamus. Reflex pathways for sweating and vasomotor control, and also blood pressure control are physiologically independent of the hypothalamus, but in normal subjects thermoregulatory reflexes are dependent upon the thermoregulatory centre in the hypothalamus. If the hypothalamus is inactive the reflexes subserving thermoregulation may still be active and can operate at abnormally low central temperatures. Afferent information from the baroreflexes influences vasopressin release from the hypothalamus (shown by* in this diagram). (Taken with permission from Johnson *et al.* (1990).)

at a midbrain level or below, independent of hypothalamic function (Keatinge and Nadel 1965). These findings in elderly patients, suggesting that hypothalamic dysfunction contributes to accidental hypothermia in some elderly patients at least, is in keeping with the pathophysiological observations observed in patients with hypothalamic tumours (Johnson *et al.* 1990).

Hypothermia is a clinical complication requiring active management. External rewarming may be adequate but this may result in mobilization of intensely cold peripheral blood so that core temperature falls even further at the start of rewarming. Other more heroic methods, including the use of warm intravenous fluids or extracorporeal warming by peritoneal dialysis, gastric lavage, or cardiopulmonary bypass, should be considered in patients who are apparently dead, but found under circumstances suggesting accidental hypothermia (Keatinge 1991). Hyperkalaemia may be a marker for

Table 44.2. Tests of autonomic nervous system function affected by age in up to 76 patients aged 5–85 years

Test	Number of subjects			Age (years) Median, range	Effect of age	Relation to age*				
	Total	Male	Female			r	p	a	b	Sy/x
Valsalva ratio	76	32	44	35, 5–85	Linear decrease	−0.55	<0.001	2.28	−0.006	1.21
Sinus arrhythmia (beats/min)	72	28	44	35, 5–85	Linear decrease	−0.67	<0.001	41.7	−0.34	8.6
E:I ratio	72	28	44	35, 5–85	Linear decrease	−0.73	<0.001	1.53	−0.004	1.10
30:15 ratio	71	28	43	36, 5–85	Linear decrease	−0.43	<0.001	1.40	−0.003	1.14
Resting heart rate (beats/min)	70	27	43	35, 5–85	Quadratic	0.41†	0.003	90.3	−0.97	10.5
Change in heart rate with tilting (beats/min)	70	27	43	35, 5–85	Linear decrease	−0.35	0.003	16.6	−0.11	7.0
Supine plasma noradrenaline levels (nm/l)	55	20	35	42, 15–85	Linear increase	0.56	<0.001	0.91	0.01	1.57
Baroreceptor sensitivity (mm Hg/ms)	21	10	11	47, 24–82	Linear decrease‡	−0.82	<0.001	44.26	−0.39	1.72
Valsalva systolic overshoot (mm Hg)	21	10	11	47, 24–82	Linear decrease	−0.54	0.01	71.0	−0.14	1.56

Taken with permission from Ingall et al. 1990.
*Relation to age is determined by a regression equation: r, correlation coefficient; a intercept; b slope of regression line; Sy/x, standard deviation of residuals.
†Multiple correlation coefficient of quadratic regression.
‡Significant linear decrease seen with both males and females. After controlling for the effect of age, the baroreceptor sensitivity for females was significantly lower than that for males ($p = 0.01$).

Table 44.3. Tests of autonomic nervous system function not affected by age in 70 patients aged 5–85 years

Test	Number of subjects			Age (years) Median, range	Relation to age		Mean ± SD
	Total	Male	Female		r	p	
Change in systolic blood pressure with tilting (mm Hg)	70	27	43	35, 5–85	0.18	>0.05	−3.0 ± 11.6
Change in diastolic blood pressure with tilting (mm Hg)	70	27	43	35, 5–85	0.07	>0.05	1.7 ± 6.7
Change in diastolic blood pressure with isometric exercise (mm Hg)	66	26	40	36, 13–85	0.005	>0.05	33.5 ± 13.3
Percentage increase in plasma NA* with tilting	54	20	34	44.5, 15–85	0.06	>0.05	83.4 ± 43.6

Taken with permission from Ingall *et al.* (1990).
*NA, noradrenaline

non-recoverable hypothermia. The main aim of therapy, however, is to achieve rewarming without associated arterial hypotension: metabolic intervention is rarely necessary.

Cardiovascular control

Physiological changes with ageing

The normal range of arterial blood pressure between the systolic and diastolic pressures increases with age. Elderly subjects without disease may therefore have systolic pressures which would be unacceptable in younger people. The effect of ageing on diastolic pressure is much less clear and, after the age of 70 years, some workers have found that diastolic pressure does not significantly increase. Noradrenaline levels increase with age in normal subjects (Young *et al.* 1980), largely due to decreased clearance (Esler *et al.* 1981). Just as in essential hypertension, it is not clear that the raised noradrenaline concentrations are actually responsible for the raised blood pressure, as receptor responses to noradrenaline must also be considered. There is an age-related decline in responsiveness of heart rate, forearm blood flow, and renin to isoprenaline infusion in old age, suggesting diminished β-adrenoceptor responsiveness. The response of cyclic adenosine monophosphate in lymphocytes is also reduced in line with this possibility. These changes could be related to the raised noradrenaline levels, either as cause or effect. It also appears that α-adrenoceptor responsiveness declines with age.

When autonomic function studies are carried out in healthy subjects over a wide age range it is tests of vagal function which predominantly show age-related changes. A study of patients up to the age of 85 years showed that changes in Valsalva's ratio, the heart rate responses to deep breathing and standing, and baroreceptor sensitivity have a negative linear relationship to age as described in Table 44.2 (Ingall *et al.* 1990). Resting heart rate has a different relationship, being greater in children and in elderly subjects than in young adults and those in middle life. Tests of sympathetic function, including blood pressure and plasma noradrenaline responses to tilting and the blood pressure response to isometric exercise, showed no relationship to ageing (Table 44.3), although some authors have found greater falls in blood pressure on standing or with body tilting as age increases. In those tests which assess both parasympathetic (vagal) and sympathetic function, for example, heart rate change with body tilting and the overshoot of diastolic blood pressure in the recovery phase of Valsalva's manoeuvre, the responses are related negatively to age (i.e. as age increases, responses decline). Ingall and his colleagues discussed the difference found in various previous studies but generally they are consistent with their results (Tables 44.2 and 44.3).

The differences in the responses to change in posture in various studies may be related to the physiological differences in response to body tilting compared with standing. The absence of an age-related effect in the studies on sympathetic cardiovascular function may in part be due to a lack of sensitivity of these particular tests because there is a difference in the vasomotor response to cooling with ageing and also differences in sweating function, as previously described. There is also diminution of autonomic activity related to pupillary function in the eye as age advances.

Neuropathological studies have shown that there is a decrease in the number of nerve cells in intermediolateral cell columns of the spinal cord and in sympathetic ganglia as age advances, which is constant with change in sympathetic function. It is nevertheless noteworthy that standard tests of cardiovascular sympathetic function show no age-related changes in relation to sympathetic activity as already noted.

There continues to be considerable interest in the changes in vascular regulation with ageing. The National Institutes of Health have drawn together a list of many problems requiring study. They emphasize the importance of standardized evaluation methods in any future studies of elderly people (Horan *et al.* 1986).

Carotid sinus hypersensitivity

As described in the previous section, as people get older, baroreflexes become less sensitive. Paradoxically, in many elderly people the carotid sinus becomes hypersensitive to external manipulation and only mild stimulation may result in bradycardia and development of hypotension (Mankikar and Clark 1975; see also Chapter 39). The bradycardia results from increased reflex vagal activity an the hypotension may be in part due to this and also to concomitant vasodilatation due to sympathetic changes. This was regarded as a relatively rare condition but, more recently, it has been shown to be present in around 14 per cent of elderly people in one series (Murphy *et al.* 1986). It may lead to syncope, 'carotid sinus syncope', preceded by involuntary movements, mental confusion, and sometimes focal disturbances as a result of impaired cerebral blood supply, perhaps associated with concomitant cerebrovascular disease. This condition may be provoked by turning the head to one side or by pressure on the neck on hyperflexing or extending the neck. It is probable that the hypersensitivity results from a change in structure in the artery walls rather than because carotid artery occlusion occurs. It may be that change in vascular rigidity makes the baroreceptors hypersensitive to deformation whereas they are generally less sensitive to change of blood pressure intramurally. This particular form of arrhythmia has frequently been unrecognized: it should be considered in any elderly person who suffers from symptoms such as attacks of loss of consciousness that could arise from it. Baroreceptor activity also influences vasopressin release and it could be that elderly people have altered vasopressin responses, perhaps contributing to the development of oedema or hyponatraemia in elderly people: this possibility requires further study.

Orthostatic hypotension

Orthostatic hypotension occurs frequently in elderly people. The diagnosis depends upon the postural fall of blood pressure being greater than that found in normal subjects. This is usually defined as a fall of more than 20 mm Hg in systolic blood pressure or more than 10 mm Hg in diastolic pressure. The proportion of elderly people in whom falls of this extent have been found ranges from 10 to 20 per cent of all people over the age of 65 years, when in institutional care. The proportion is lower in elderly subjects living in the community but an overall prevalence of about 10 per cent is likely. In order to compare observations between patients and between different studies, it is essential that they are examined under standard conditions of change of posture. The patient should be lying supine for at least 20 min and should then stand on his or her own accord. The blood pressure should then be taken 2 and 5 min after standing.

Orthostatic hypotension occurs with a wide range of well recognized syndromes associated with autonomic dysfunction as described extensively in this volume. Numerous drugs have orthostatic hypotension as a side-effect (Table 44.4), particularly antihypertensive drugs, including recently introduced agents such as calcium channel blocking agents and angiotensin-converting enzyme inhibitors. Diuretics also precipitate hypotension and a number of drugs used in psychiatric management are particularly prone to this complication. In clinical disorders in which there is an association with orthostatic hypotension, it is convenient to consider the part of the baroreflex affected. The lesion may be on the afferent side of the arc, in some it may be central, in the brainstem, or it may be in efferent pathways in the spinal cord or peripheral nerves (Table 44.5). Among chronic neurological disorders which occur in elderly subjects rather than younger age groups are pure autonomic failure (formerly known as idiopathic orthostatic hypotension) and multiple system atrophy (MSA) in which there is neuronal loss in intermediolateral columns of the spinal cord, the site of sympathetic preganglionic cell bodies. Other disorders in which orthostatic hypotension occurs particularly in the elderly, are Parkinson's disease, diabetes mellitus, and chronic alcoholism. It may rarely be found as a complication of pernicious anaemia and improvement takes place with treatment with vitamin B_{12} (Eisenhofer et al. 1982).

Orthostatic hypotension without a
definite neurological association

Orthostatic hypotension occurs in many elderly people even when they are not receiving drugs with a hypotensive side-effect and have no obvious disease

Table 44.4.   Some drugs which may produce orthostatic hypotension

---

Antihypertensive agents, particularly

Calcium channel blocking agents
Angiotensin converting enzyme inhibitors
Adrenergic nerve blocking agents
α-adrenoceptor blocking drugs

Thiazides and other diuretics

Psychotherapeutic drugs

Phenothiazines
Tricyclic antidepressants
Butyrophenones
Barbiturates

Antiparkinsonian drugs

L-dopa
Bromocriptine

Ethanol

Cannabis

---

in which orthostatic hypotension may be a complication. Their blood pressure falls are frequently less dramatic than those observed in patients with overt neurological disease. In a study in 1965, it appeared possible that some of the elderly patients with orthostatic hypotension suffered from cerebrovascular disease (Johnson *et al.* 1965). However, part of the evidence depended upon the absence of the normal vasoconstrictor response to Valsalva's manoeuvre and it is now clear that this becomes blunted with ageing. Subsequently, it was shown that a number of non-neurological causes may contribute to orthostatic hypotension, including the presence of varicose veins and cardiac arrhythmias (Caird *et al.* 1973, Fig. 44.5).

The possibility that orthostatic hypotension without an obvious cause is in fact the result of autonomic dysfunction was reintroduced by the suggestion that there is a defective heart rate response to standing in these subjects (White 1980). Attempts to repeat these observations were, however, unsuccessful (Robinson *et al.*1983), and in these further studies a rapid rise in concentrations of noradrenaline took place in spite of orthostatic hypotension occurring, albeit of a minor degree. Resting catecholamine concentrations were lower than in control elderly subjects even though they had a higher supine diastolic blood pressure. If autonomic failure had been the cause of the orthostatic hypotension in such elderly subjects, raised concentrations of α-adrenoceptors might be expected, but further observations have shown receptor numbers to be depressed rather than exaggerated (Robinson *et al.* 1990; Fig 44.6). It is possible that these patients, instead of having autonomic dysfunction, have increased

Table 44.5. Neurological disorders in which patients of all ages may develop orthostatic hypotension and the parts of the reflex pathway affected.

Afferent pathway IX or X nerves	Central (brainstem integration)	Efferent pathway	
		Spinal cord	Sympathetic chain postganglionic nerves
Acute polyneuropathy	Acute polyneuropathy (?)	Trauma	Acute polyneuropathy
Chronic alcoholism (?)	Acute alcoholism	Transverse myelitis	Pure autonomic neuropathy
Diabetes mellitus (?)	Brainstem lesions	Syringomyelia	Pure autonomic failure
Adie's syndrome	Familial dysautonomia (?)	Intramedullary tumours	Chronic polyneuropathy
Renal failure	Anorexia nervosa (?)	Extramedullary tumours	Chronic alcoholism
Haemodialysis	Drugs	Intermediolateral column degeneration: pure autonomic failure, multiple system atrophy, Parkinson's disease	Diabetes mellitus
			Tumours (non-metastatic complication)
			Rheumatoid arthritis (?)
			Acute intermittent porphyria
			Amyloidosis
			Pernicious anaemia
			Dopamine β_2-hydroxylase deficiency
			Failure of catecholamine release in anorexia nervosa
			Drugs

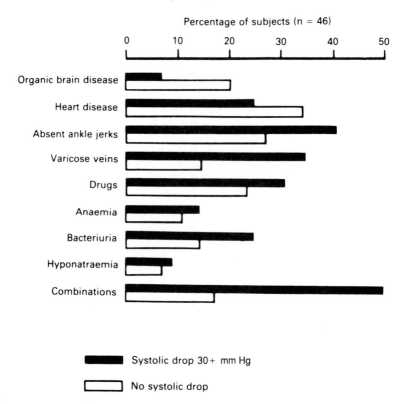

Fig. 44.5. A study of 496 patients, aged 65 years or more, living at home in which a comparison of the frequency of a series of factors was made between subjects with a drop in systolic pressure of 30 mm Hg or more on standing (46 subjects) and a matched group without such a drop. No factor was statistically significant alone, but a combination of factors was significantly more frequent in those with orthostatic hypotension. (Taken with permission from Caird *et al.* (1973).)

rigidity of blood vessels (MacLennan *et al.* 1980). This would be in keeping with the wide pulse pressure frequently observed in elderly subjects. Plasma vasopressin concentrations increased during standing by these patients, which indicated that the afferent part of their baroreflexes was intact. Changes in vessel structure might contribute to loss of baroreflex sensitivity. Loss of elasticity of arterial walls has been demonstrated in post-mortem specimens from elderly people, but there has been no study of vessel elasticity between those patients with, and those without orthostatic hypotension. The abnormality in these patients could also be due to a reduction in vascular α_2-adrenoceptor populations which remains unexplained.

The fall in blood pressure in these patients may lead to symptoms of altered consciousness including dizziness and even loss of consciousness. Another

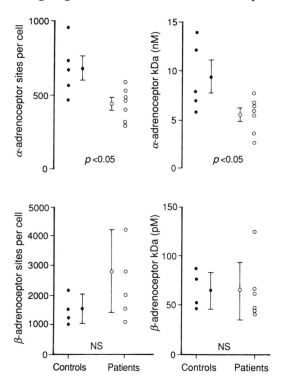

Fig. 44.6. Adrenoceptor sites per cell and binding affinity, (kd) on isolated platelets (α-adrenoceptors) and lymphocytes (β-adrenoceptors) in elderly subjects with (open circle) and without (filled circle) orthostatic hypotension. Results are plotted as individual results and as group means $\pm$ SE. The patients with orthostatic hypotension had lower α-adrenoceptor counts whereas patients with autonomic failure may have raised concentrations. (Taken with permission from Robinson *et al.* (1990).)

possible contributory cause of these symptoms is failure of normal cerebral blood flow regulation in some elderly people. Normally, cerebral blood flow is maintained at a steady level with changes of blood pressure. Maintenance of constant cerebral blood flow occurs within a wide range of arterial blood pressure in normal subjects but in hypertension this range is elevated. This depends on autoregulation of cerebral blood vessel tone as a result of intrinsic mechanisms within the blood vessels themselves. Cerebral autoregulation is generally well maintained, so that it only fails when the mean blood pressure falls below about 60 mm Hg. In patients with orthostatic hypotension the range may be shifted downwards so that lower arterial pressures may be tolerated without symptoms. In some elderly patients, however, failure of cerebral autoregulation has been demonstrated and this may contribute to the development of symptoms (Wollner *et al.* 1979; Fig. 44.7). This finding

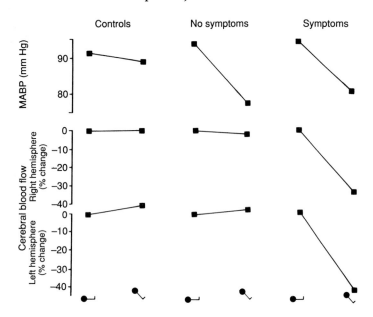

Fig. 44.7. Changes in mean arterial blood pressure (MABP, mm Hg) and cerebral blood flow (percentage change; the method used an inhalation or intravenous xenon 133 technique) with change of posture (75° feet down) in elderly patients with orthostatic hypotension and controls. The patients with symptoms of cerebral ischaemia associated with the minor fall in systemic arterial pressure had bilateral or unilateral failure in cerebral autoregulation. The observations suggest that impaired autoregulation may put some elderly patients at risk of brain damage if they suffer only minor falls of blood pressure. (Data from Wollner *et al.* 1979; graph taken with permission from Johnson *et al.* (1984).)

implies that such patients may be at particular risk of brain damage with only minor falls of blood pressure. Studies in other groups of patients have failed to indicate that cerebral blood vessels need to be normally innervated for cerebral autoregulation to continue, even though the vessels have a substantial sympathetic supply. Cerebral autoregulation is, for example, maintained in patients with cervical cord transection. It is possible that there may be degenerative changes inducing rigidity in the cerebral blood vessels of some elderly people, similar to the changes already suggested in vessels elsewhere.

Postprandial hypotension (see also Chapter 26)

Patients who suffer from orthostatic hypotension due to autonomic failure are prone to develop hypotension after meals—postprandial hypotension.

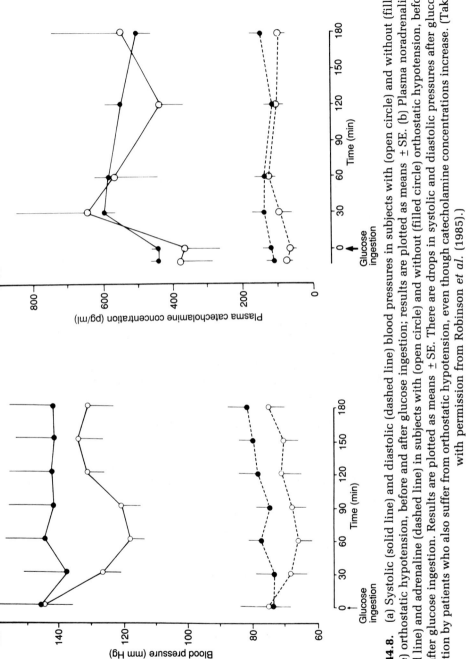

Fig. 44.8. (a) Systolic (solid line) and diastolic (dashed line) blood pressures in subjects with (open circle) and without (filled circle) orthostatic hypotension, before and after glucose ingestion; results are plotted as means ± SE. (b) Plasma noradrenaline (solid line) and adrenaline (dashed line) in subjects with (open circle) and without (filled circle) orthostatic hypotension, before and after glucose ingestion. Results are plotted as means ± SE. There are drops in systolic and diastolic pressures after glucose ingestion by patients who also suffer from orthostatic hypotension, even though catecholamine concentrations increase. (Taken with permission from Robinson *et al.* (1985).)

Patients on drugs causing autonomic dysfunction may also show postprandial hypotension. Cerebrovascular accidents are particularly likely following meals and it has been suggested that this may be due to a hypotensive phase as a result of eating. In patients with orthostatic hypotension without evidence of autonomic failure postprandial hypotension also occurs, even though catecholamine concentrations increase (Robinson *et al.* 1985; Fig. 44.8). It therefore seems likely that the mechanisms involved in postprandial hypotension in the elderly are different from those occurring in the disease of pure autonomic failure or multiple system atrophy and are not primarily related to autonomic dysfunction.

Ingestion of food in normal individuals is not associated with any change of blood pressure, even though there is marked increase in intestinal blood flow. There is also an increase in heart rate and cardiac output and a fall in peripheral blood flow in other regions such as the forearm. These changes compensate for the fall in peripheral resistance in the gut. The overall response to ingestion of food depends upon both sympathetic nervous activity and the release of vasoactive hormones. When patients with pure autonomic failure or multiple system atrophy are studied, a fall of blood pressure may be observed 10–15 min after food ingestion and this may result in dizziness and even mental confusion. In this group of patients there are no changes in plasma adrenaline or noradrenaline, as occurs in normal subjects, but there are still increases in gastrointestinal hormones, such as neurotensin, which has a vasodilatory action. This increases to a greater extent in patients with orthostatic hypotension and may contribute to their problem (Mathias *et al.* 1988). Other hormones may contribute, particularly vasoactive intestinal polypeptide, which may influence splanchnic vasodilatation.

Another hormone that may be important is insulin, as it has been observed that intravenous insulin can lower blood pressure substantially in patients with autonomic failure, independently of changes in blood glucose. Glucose is the most potent of the components of food in the production of hypotension, probably because it is responsible for insulin release. Another feature which may contribute to postprandial hypotension in subjects with autonomic failure is the rapid rate of gastric emptying which may be a concomitant of the condition, analogous to the dumping syndrome which can be a complication of gastric surgery.

As discussed in the previous section, elderly patients without evidence of autonomic failure but with orthostatic hypotension, may develop postprandial hypotension. It is possible that, in this group of patients, a contributory feature to the hypotension is blunting of the baroreflex response, as has been observed in elderly patients after administration of glucose. This may also be secondary to the release of insulin. A dual mechanism therefore, probably contributes to postprandial hypotension in elderly patients with orthostatic hypotension. First, there may be splanchnic vasodilatation resulting from elevation of blood insulin and other vasoactive peptides and, second, baroreflex activity may be depressed as a direct effect of insulin on the baroreflex from the carotid sinus.

The most important aspect of management is to recognize the condition. Advice may then be given about taking small meals and avoiding alcohol, which can contribute to peripheral vasodilatation. Adequate fat and protein content of the diet should be achieved as these have a smaller effect than carbohydrate in producing postprandial hypotension.

Treatment of orthostatic hypotension

Orthostatic hypotension is particularly dangerous if it is unrecognized. Patients may suffer falls and complications including fractures or burns as a result and they may die. It is also possible for susceptible patients to suffer minor orthostatic hypotension when sitting or with the additional contribution of the effect of food and thus to have prolonged periods of cerebral ischaemia with consequent confusion and disorientation and the possibility of developing a stroke. As already described, the condition is frequently multifactorial. A full history of drugs taken is therefore important as many patients have drugs as a major cause of their problem. Clearly defined disorders such as diabetes mellitus should also be excluded. In many elderly patients, however, no clear indication of a major cause is found and it is in this group that the descriptive diagnosis 'orthostatic hypotension in the elderly' is used. Patients with orthostatic hypotension may respond to mechanical procedures such as elastic stockings and a rubber roll-on corset over the abdomen, but they are frequently difficult for elderly people to use and can be uncomfortable in hot weather. Tilting the head of the bed up at night has long been shown to cause improvement in the blood pressure of many patients when standing, probably by stimulating the renin–angiotensin system.

A wide range of drugs has been recommended (Johnson *et al.* 1984) of which the most useful is fludrocortisone (dosage 0.2 mg daily), but it has the disadvantage of increasing both standing and supine blood pressure. The elderly are probably more prone to side-effects from fludrocortisone, especially if higher doses are used. The wide range of drugs implies that the condition is one which is very difficult to treat. In many elderly patients it is not possible to achieve an adequate drug regime. Particular importance should be given to recognition of postprandial hypotension and the consequent avoidance of heavy meals, alcohol, and food with high glucose content.

Patients are likely to require considerable care and assistance and it is important to monitor their blood pressure changes regularly so that they are helped as much as possible over its management; they should also be helped through social work support.

References

Caird, F. I., Andrew, G. R., and Kennedy, R. D. (1973). Effect of posture on blood pressure in the elderly. *Br. Heart J.* **35**, 527–30.

Collins, K. J. (1983). Autonomic failure and the elderly. *In Autonomic failure* (1st edn) (ed. R. Bannister), pp. 489–507. Oxford University Press, Oxford.

Cooper, K. E., Johnson, R. H., and Spalding, J. M. K. (1964). The effects of central body and trunk skin temperatures on reflex vasodilatation in the hand. *J. Physiol.* **174**, 45–54.

Eisenhofer, G., Lambie, D. G., Johnson, R. H., Tan, E. T. H., and Whiteside, E. A. (1982). Deficient catecholamine release as the basis of orthostatic hypotension in pernicious anaemia. *J. Neurosurg. Psychiat.* **45**, 1053–5.

Esler, M., Skews, H., Leonard, P., Jackman, G., Bobik, A., and Korner, P. (1981). Age-dependence of noradrenaline kinetics in normal subjects. *Clin. Sci.* **60**, 217–19.

Foster, K. G., Ellis, F. P., Dore, C., Exton-Smith, A. N., and Weiner, J. S. (1976). Sweat responses in the aged. *Age Ageing* **5**, 91–101.

Horan, M. J., Steinberg, G. M., Dunbar, J. B., and Hadley, E. C. (1986). Summary of NIH workshop on blood pressure regulation and aging. *Hypertension* **8**, 178–80.

Ingall, T. J., McLeod, J. G., and O'Brien, P. C. (1990). The effect of ageing on autonomic nervous system function. *Austral. New Z. J. Med.* **20**, 570–7.

Johnson, R. H. and Park, D. M. (1973). Intermittent hypothermia. *J. Neurol. Neurosurg. Psychiat.* **36**, 411–16.

Johnson, R. H. and Spalding, J. M. K. (1974). *Disorders of the autonomic nervous system*. Blackwell, Oxford.

Johnson, R. H., Smith, A. C., and Spalding, J. M. K. (1965). Effect of posture on blood pressure in elderly patients. *Lancet* **i**, 731–3.

Johnson, R. H., Lambie, D. G., and Spalding, J. M. K. (1984). *Neurocardiology: the interrelationships between dysfunction in the nervous and cardiovascular systems*. W. B. Saunders, London.

Johnson, R. H., Delahunt, J. W., and Robinson, B. J. (1990). Do thermoregulatory reflexes pass through the hypothalamus?—studies of chronic hypothermia due to hypothalamic lesion. *Austral. New Z. J. Med.* **20**, 154–9.

Keatinge, W. R. (1991). Hypothermia: dead or alive? *Br. med. J.* **302**, 3–4.

Keatinge, W. R. and Nadel, J. A. (1965). Immediate respiratory response to sudden cooling of the skin. *J. appl. Physiol.* **20**, 65–9.

MacLennan, W. J., Hall, M. R. P., and Timothy, J. I . (1980). Postural hypotension in old age: is it a disorder of the nervous system or of blood vessels? *Age Ageing* **9**, 25–32.

Macmillan, A. L., Corbett, J. L., Johnson, R. H., Crampton Smith, A., Spalding, J. M. K., and Wollner, L. (1967). Temperature regulation in survivors of accidental hypothermia of the elderly. *Lancet* **ii**, 165–9.

Mankikar, G. D. and Clark, A. N. G. (1975). Cardiac effect of carotid sinus massage in old age. *Age Ageing* **4**, 86–94.

Mathias, C., da Costa, D., and Bannister R. (1988). Postcibal hypotension in autonomic disorders. In *Autonomic failure* (2nd edn) (ed. R. Bannister), pp. 367–80. Oxford University Press, Oxford.

Murphy, A. L., Rowbotham, B. J., Boyle, R. S., Thew, C. M., Farboulys, J. A., and Wilson, K. (1986). Carotid sinus hypersensitivity in elderly nursing home patients. *Austral. New Z. J. Med.* **16**, 24–7.

Robinson, B. J., Johnson, R. H., Lambie, D. G., and Palmer, K. T. (1983). Do elderly patients with an excessive fall in blood pressure on standing have evidence of autonomic failure? *Clin. Sci.* **64**, 587–91.

Robinson, B. J., Johnson, R. H., Lambie, D. G., and Palmer, K. T. (1985). Autonomic responses to glucose ingestion in elderly subjects with orthostatic hypotension. *Age Ageing* **14**, 168–73.

Robinson, B. J., Stowell, L. I., Johnson, R. H., and Palmer, K. T. (1990). Is orthostatic hypotension in the elderly due to autonomic failure? *Age Ageing* **19**, 288–96.

White, N. J. (1980). Heart rate changes on standing in elderly patients with orthostatic hypotension. *Clin. Sci.* **58**, 411–13.

Wollner, L., McCarthy, S. T., Soper, N. D W., and Macy, D. J. (1979). Failure of cerebral autoregulation as a cause of brain dysfunction in the elderly. *Br. Med. J.* **1**, 1117–18.

Young, J. B., Rowe, J. W., Pallotta, J. A., Sparrow, D., and Landsberg, L. (1980). Enhanced plasma norepinephrine response to upright posture and oral glucose administration in elderly human subjects. *Metabolism* **29**, 532–9.

45. Pain and the sympathetic nervous system

G. D. Schott

Introduction

It is by no means established that the sympathetic nervous system is implicated in the generation of painful states. Two clinical features, however, have led to the concept that certain pains may be associated with the sympathetic nervous system. First, blocking the local sympathetic supply relieves some painful conditions. Second, some of these painful conditions are accompanied by features that resemble those encountered in disorders of the sympathetic supply, for instance, vasomotor, sudomotor, and temperature disturbances. As will be considered later, however, caution is required before concluding that the sympathetic nervous system is therefore causing or contributing to the painful state.

The concept that the sympathetic system is concerned with pain developed from the observations of Leriche (1939 pp. 170–201). He noted that patients with causalgia often showed vasomotor changes which were similar to those seen in patients with sympathetically mediated peripheral vascular disorders; he also observed that periarterial sympathectomy could relieve pain. Subsequent workers demonstrated that a variety of procedures on the sympathetic system of a surgical or blocking nature could also result in pain relief. More recently, it was found that peripheral blockade of the sympathetic nervous system using regional sympatholytic drugs, in particular guanethidine, could abolish certain pains.

For a number of reasons, however, the assumption that the sympathetic nervous system is therefore necessarily involved may be too simplistic as exemplified by the following points: (1) some but not other seemingly identical pains respond to sympathetic blockade; (2) effective blockade leading to pain relief, which is transient, may not be achieved again by repeated blocks; (3) one form of blockade, for example, using local anaesthetic, may relieve pain whereas subsequent surgical sympathectomy may not; and (4) sometimes only repeated blocks relieve pain whilst in other instances just a single block proves effective. There also appears to be a striking lack of specificity in what is used for sympathetic blockade. Numerous other techniques ranging from physiotherapy measures to oral and local drugs of many sorts, and from psychological intervention to surgery have all been tried, with very variable and unpredictable results.

Concerning the appearances, which resemble disturbances of peripheral sympathetic control, the vasomotor, sudomotor, thermal, and trophic changes seen in patients with these pains may not be mediated by the sympathetic system at all. Release of vasoactive substances by small-diameter afferents can produce many and possibly all of these features, perhaps mimicking rather than representing sympathetic dysfunction (Cline *et al.* 1989). At present, therefore, the role of the sympathetic nervous system remains possible but not established.

Mechanisms

The mechanisms underlying sympathetically maintained pains are unclear (Jänig 1985). Even whether the mechanisms are peripheral or central is uncertain, and any distinction may be artificial since peripheral lesions give rise to central changes and vice versa.

Clinical evidence that the peripheral nervous system is implicated in some instances seems obvious, since peripheral lesions ranging from injuries to an extremity to nerve damage can give rise to sympathetically maintained pain. Various theories have been proposed for peripheral mechanisms (for reviews, see Richards 1967; Bonica 1979; Schott 1986). These include:

1. Development of abnormal peripheral tissues at the site of damage, both from ischaemia due to sympathetically maintained vasoconstriction and from painful vasodilatation. Although vascular changes can occur in these conditions, their contribution to pain generation is not established.
2. Mechanisms arising from damage to the peripheral nerve itself. Such mechanisms include ephaptic transmission between afferent and sympathetic efferent fibres; selective involvement of large as opposed to small-diameter nerve fibres; and the development of neuromas and other neural abnormalities that result in the nerve showing spontaneous activity, abnormal catecholamine sensitivity, and response to changes in the sympathetic supply. The possibility that in hyperalgesic states, noradrenaline could produce further hyperalgesia by acting on presynaptic receptors on the sympathetic postganglionic neurons, perhaps indirectly via various inflammatory mediators, has also been proposed (Levine *et al.* 1986). There are a number of factors which make each of these possibilities unlikely as complete explanations for sympathetically maintained pains, though a contribution from such mechanisms has not been excluded.

Of major concern is whether the sympathetic nervous system is abnormal in these pain states. Despite the frequently stated or implied belief that the sympathetic system is abnormal, the limited evidence available from microneurographic studies indicates that the sympathetic outflow is normal

(Cline *et al.* 1989; Torebjork 1990) or even reduced (Drummond *et al.* 1991). This accords well with the facts that there is no correlation between the pain and state of temperature and sweating of the affected part and that pain relief after blockade does not correlate with the peripheral state; indeed, pain relief can occur when sympathetic blockade is only partial. If the sympathetic supply is normal and sympathetic blockade alleviates pain, it seems likely that the sympathetic system exerts its effects on the afferent system, and that it is the afferent system which is abnormal.

The way in which the afferent nervous system might become abnormal and sympathetically dependent may be due to a change in the properties of the nerve, either at the terminal receptor or the axon itself. As discussed below, the pain is typically burning and there may be hyperpathia and allodynia. In allodynia, a stimulus such as a light touch or puff of wind produces pain, that is, pain due to a stimulus which does not normally provoke pain. The term allodynia was introduced by the International Association for the Study of Pain (IASP), which also defined hyperpathia as an increased reaction to a stimulus as well as an increased threshold. There is also often hyperalgesia, an increased response to a stimulus which is normally painful, and undue sensitivity to thermal changes. Concerning hyperpathia and allodynia, Loh and Nathan (1978) made an observation of fundamental importance: they observed that those patients with causalgia whose pains were most likely to be relieved by sympathetic blockade were those with allodynia. These authors drew attention to the role of mechanoreceptor fibres in the generation of pain (see Nathan 1983). Concerning thermal sensitivity, in some patients pain is worsened by cold and in others by warming. Both light touch and cold are mediated by large-diameter fibres, and evidence both supports (Campbell *et al.* 1988) and refutes (Cline *et al.* 1989) the possibility that, in patients with causalgia and reflex sympathetic dystrophy, pain and hyperalgesia are subserved by large-diameter, A-beta fibres rather than the expected C and A-delta fibres which typically subserve nociception. The vasodilatation and related phenomena seen in these pain states and referred to above may be attributed to antidromic vasodilatation from substances released at the nerve terminals, rather than due to sympathetic involvement, though some involvement of sympathetic fibres cannot be excluded and could also be an epiphenomenon.

The central nervous system must, at least in some instances, be implicated (for a review, see Schott 1986) because: (1) causalgia can occur both in diseases confined to the central nervous system and in the absence of the part as in phantom states; (2) peripheral pains can spread far outside the territory of the affected nerve or root and can affect a whole quadrant or even more extensively; (3) there may be involvement of non-sensory systems with trophic changes and with weakness, wasting, immobility, and involuntary movements; and (4) sympathetic blockade can abolish pains even when the pains are experienced proximal to the block and are caused by diseases confined to the central nervous system (Loh *et al.* 1981). Many of the mechanisms discussed above could apply to the central nervous system, and the role of mechanoreceptor sensitivity has been considered in relation to the central nervous system.

Roberts (1986) has postulated that, in sympathetically maintained pains, sensitization develops in wide-dynamic-range neurons in the central nervous system that receive afferents from both nociceptor and non-nociceptor inputs. He proposed that these neurons respond abnormally to innocuous input, the non-nociceptive afferents being activated and remaining tonically sensitized by sympathetic activity. Recent clinical evidence not only confirms the importance of A-beta, low-threshold mechanoreceptors in sympathetically maintained pains, but indicates that somatosympathetic interaction may indeed take place centrally (Price *et al.* 1989).

Animal models

Inherent in studying painful conditions is the impossibility of using animal models. The best that can be done is to induce conditions in animals which may resemble the conditions and produce some form of sensory and affective disturbance as seen in man. In sympathetically maintained pains, by definition, improvement of pain or alteration of physiological characteristics by manipulation of the sympathetic supply is required.

The neuroma model has provided important experimental information. Following nerve transection, the fine unmyelinated nerve sprouts which grow out from the cut end show ongoing discharges, mechanical sensitivity, and, of particular importance, increased firing with local application of noradrenaline or sympathetic fibre stimulation, firing which is reduced by sympathetic blockade. The relevance of this model to human causalgia has been questioned, however, since: (1) neuromas in humans are often painless; (2) the animal model shows effects that are very variable in different species; and (3) the specificity of sympathetic sensitivity has not been very fully assessed—indeed other substances such as acetylcholine, anticonvulsants, and axon-transport blockers affect the properties of neuromas.

A more relevant *in vivo* model is that of Bennett and Xie (1988), in which a loosely constrictive ligature is placed around a rat (sciatic) nerve, following which hyperalgesia, allodynia, and perhaps spontaneous pain are produced. Disturbances of temperature of the limb and trophic changes may also be seen, as is autotomy (self-mutilatory behaviour in animals, thought to be related to pain or other sensory disturbances). These phenomena appear to be abolished by sympathetic blockade. A variation of this model has also been reported, in which a partial rather than complete constriction of the nerve is obtained.

Animal models producing trophic changes have also been studied. In rabbits, phenol in paraffin injected into sympathetic ganglia can produce a form of reflex sympathetic dystrophy, with involvement of hair, skin discoloration, oedema, and wound formation. There may be reduction of reflexes and initially functional, then structural changes at the neuromuscular junction, and later skeletal muscle changes. Whether such a technique induces a destructive or irritative lesion of the sympathetic outflow is unclear.

Sympathetically maintained pains

Classification and general characteristics

Painful disorders traditionally associated with the sympathetic nervous system comprise the whole spectrum of 'sympathetically maintained' pains, and those rare, painful diseases associated with damage to the sympathetic system (sympathalgias) which are considered later (for reviews, see Stanton-Hicks 1990; Stanton-Hicks *et al.* 1990).

Sympathetically maintained pains can usefully be separated into their extreme forms: causalgia and reflex sympathetic dystrophy (RSD). The latter is known by numerous other terms (e.g. algodystrophy, minor causalgia) and also includes special forms such as the shoulder–hand syndrome. The nosology of these conditions remains confusing for several reasons: the definitions and terminology are arbitrary; the diseases heterogeneous; the response to treatment unpredictable (and therefore even the concept of 'sympathetically maintained' pain is unreliable); and the mechanisms are unknown.

While it is useful to separate these pains into their extreme forms, they have in common a number of clinical features which may be present in all forms. These include pain, which is typically spontaneous and burning in quality (hence the term causalgia, meaning 'burning pain'). The pain starts in the region of damage but can then spread much more widely and affect areas well beyond the local peripheral nerve or root distribution, and indeed can involve the segment, quadrant, or more widely. Disturbances of sensation over the affected area are often seen. Allodynia and hyperpathia may be seen, and there may also be hyperalgesia. In some instances it may be possible to dissociate the causalgia from the allodynia.

A number of other associated features often occur with 'sympathetically maintained' pains: increased or decreased sweating, excessive warmth or coldness, and swelling or atrophy of the part—changes reminiscent of sympathetic dysfunction. There may also be profound trophic changes, with alterations in the skin (such as loss of wrinkles, glossiness, atrophy), hair (sometimes thin, sometimes coarse) and nails (with thinning, curvature, and even clubbing), thickening of subcutaneous tissues which can resemble Dupuytren's contractures, swelling and contractures of joints, and focal, regional, or sometimes very extensive osteoporotic changes which typically spare the periarticular surfaces. (Sudeck's atrophy strictly refers only to the radiological changes of this osteoporosis.) There may also be changes in the motor system, with weakness and wasting of muscle, tremor, and a variety of involuntary movements such as dystonia and spasms (Schwartzman and Kerrigan 1990). Many of these features will coexist only in a few patients, different patients may show one or more disturbances, and the clinical features may change with time. Finally, patients may or may not show relief of some of their symptoms, in particular pain, following sympathetic blockade.

Predisposing factors

There is controversy as to whether certain individuals are more likely to develop RSD and perhaps causalgia. Patients with underlying diabetes and hyperlipidaemia have been studied, though with indefinite conclusions. The distribution of HLA tissue types is probably no different in patients with sympathetically maintained pains compared with the general population. Age cannot be a significant factor, since RSD has been described on a number of occasions in children.

The possibility that individuals with particular personality traits are susceptible has also been considered and, whilst some authors have commented on the depression, anxiety, and emotional lability of these patients, observations have been made on individuals suffering prolonged and often severe pain, which makes assessment necessarily difficult. Patients may have several injuries, sometimes at the same and sometimes at different times; perhaps just one injury will be associated with RSD, indicating that an underlying personality trait cannot be the sole factor. Noteworthy, however, is the remarkable and perhaps unique prospective study of RSD following surgery for Dupuytren's contracture, in which the development of RSD was generally correctly predicted by a pre-operative psychiatric assessment (Zachariae 1964).

Causalgia

Causalgia means burning pain, and was the term introduced by Weir Mitchell in 1867. He with his colleagues Morehouse and Keen described in 1864 in an unsurpassed account the extremely severe burning pain and nearly all the other features of this condition. Their classical report followed clinical observations made on soldiers who sustained severe nerve injuries during the American Civil War (Mitchell *et al.* 1864).

Nomenclature has subsequently become more complicated, albeit less clear. For example, IASP defines causalgia as 'burning pain, allodynia, and hyperpathia, usually in the hand or foot, after partial injury of a nerve or one of its major branches' and an essential feature is stated to be signs of sympathetic hyperactivity in the distribution of the partially damaged nerve. A number of problems arise with a definition such as this, including the facts that causalgia can occur after complete nerve injuries, burning pain can in some patients be separated from allodynia, and hyperactivity of the sympathetic system is quite possibly incorrect, as discussed below. Indeed, IASP at the same time defines causalgia as 'a syndrome of sustained burning pain, allodynia, and hyperpathia after a traumatic nerve lesion, often combined with vasomotor and sudomotor dysfunction and later trophic changes'. That is a simpler and more useful definition, and closer to the original use of the term first used by Weir Mitchell.

The clinical features have been well summarized by numerous authors, including Richards (1976) and Bonica (1979). The incidence of causalgia is difficult to gauge but probably ranged from 2.5 to 5 per cent of the cases of peripheral nerve injury sustained in the Second World War, compared with less than 1 per cent in the Vietnam War. Nerve injuries can, of course, occur in non-combat situations, such as brachial plexus traction injuries from motor-cycle accidents, and surgical and other iatrogenic nerve injuries.

The onset of the pain is usually immediately after nerve injury, although occasionally some delay occurs, with only around 5 per cent developing pain after more than 1 month. Those injuries particularly likely to be associated with the development of causalgia are lesions of the median or sciatic nerve or brachial plexus; incomplete lesions are more liable to cause causalgia than complete ones. The pain is typically burning, but is often also crushing, throbbing, stabbing, of great severity, and is felt in the periphery of the affected limb. The pain is continuous, poorly localized, and usually spreads outside the affected nerve territory. Not only may the pain spread widely, it can sometimes be experienced in the contralateral, mirror extremity. The pain is worsened by stress of all sorts, and by any additional sensory input, such as bright lights or noise.

The associated sensory, motor, and trophic changes have been referred to earlier, and there is likely to be sensory and motor loss associated with the nerve lesion itself.

The prognosis of causalgia is difficult to gauge and, although there have been reports of spontaneous remission with time (sometimes years), it is more common for pain to persist indefinitely or even worsen. Emphasis therefore has been on trying to institute treatment as rapidly as possible, in particular by sympathetic blockade. There have been reports that early sympathetic blockade, especially if blockade is complete, can result in dramatic relief of causalgia—indeed, some authorities require that causalgia be pain which is relieved by sympathetic blockade.

Reflex sympathetic dystrophy (RSD)

The clinical features are similar to those seen in causalgia, but by definition the cause is not damage to a major peripheral nerve, and often the pain is not so severe (for review, see Doury *et al.* 1981). Indeed,

Evans (1946), who first used the term reflex sympathetic dystrophy, specifically stated that pain could be absent, and he considered the features resembling sympathetic dysfunction to be cardinal.

The causes of RSD are numerous. Probably the most common is virtually any sort of minor peripheral injury, such as a simple sprain, an otherwise unremarkable surgical procedure as for Dupuytren's contracture, a knock or object falling on an extremity or a Colles' fracture. Often the traumatic episode, though comparatively minor and not associated with major nerve damage, appears particularly painful. The pain may or may not disappear and, if it does, it then recurs some days or even weeks later. There are many other causes; these include virtually any damage to the periphery from disease (e.g. herpes zoster) or accident (e.g. electric shock) or immobilization; or damage to the central nervous system, such as from stroke, multiple sclerosis, or cranial or spinal trauma. RSD can be associated with systemic illness, such as pulmonary disease, and can occur after myocardial infarction and cardiac surgery. In the latter situation, as well as following strokes in particular, a focal form of RSD may be encountered, the shoulder–hand syndrome (Steinbrocker and Argyros 1958). Here there is pain and limitation of shoulder movements and an ipsilateral painful, swollen, and immobile hand. An analogous situation can occur in the lower limb. RSD may also occur, not only in association with cerebral tumours and epilepsy, but particularly when there is concurrent use of phenobarbitone. Other drugs, in particular isoniazid, have also been incriminated.

Transient forms of RSD may occur, particularly in pregnancy when it especially affects the hip, and RSD sometimes flits from one area to another (migratory osteoporosis).

The more major forms of RSD, in particular the shoulder–hand syndrome, have been described as going through a process involving three phases, each lasting several weeks or months. These phases are highly variable in their degree and duration, and one phase tends to merge into the next. In the early stages, there are pain and pseudoinflammatory changes with hot, swollen extremities; there is then partial resolution with early atrophic changes and finger contractures; and, finally, there is a third stage of atrophic or dystrophic changes affecting the soft tissues with severe contractures, possibly ankylosis, and immobilization.

The frequency of development of RSD is unknown. The shoulder–hand syndrome following myocardial infarction was estimated to occur in 10–15 per cent of cases some 30 years ago, but the frequency is perhaps around 1–2 per cent at present, possibly due to earlier mobilization and greater awareness of the problem. The incidence of RSD following trauma must be extremely small. Perhaps the largest series is the 14 000 in-patients with limb trauma seen over a 10-year period reported by Poplawski et al. (1983), only 126 of whom developed RSD.

Bilaterality

RSD as well as causalgia affecting one extremity can produce bilateral, mirror involvement, although, unfortunately, clinical descriptions of patients showing this phenomenon often lack detail. It is hardly surprising if patients with conditions, such as cervical spondylosis, that affect midline structures demonstrate bilateral RSD. The clinical involvement not only includes pain and tenderness, but also swelling, weakness, and more complex phenomena such as tremor. Perhaps 25–30 per cent of patients with unilateral disease, particularly the shoulder–hand syndrome, are said to develop bilateral involvement and investigations demonstrate subclinical bilateral involvement even more frequently. Indeed, some authors have reported subclinical bilateral involvement, as determined by isotope scanning, in all the patients they studied, although abnormalities are more marked on the clinically affected side (Kozin *et al.* 1976*a,b*). Successful treatment of the clinical condition results in bilateral improvement. The fact that bilateral involvement can occur following unilateral disease emphasizes the importance of central nervous system mechanisms.

Investigations

The investigation of causalgia and related states is that of the accompanying phenomena. Most emphasis has been on imaging techniques. Plain radiographs show details of bone structure and may demonstrate the focal or more generalized osteoporosis of Sudeck. This is typically periarticular, but spares the joint space itself. Where possible, it is helpful to X-ray the opposite side on the same plate for comparison, though interpretation is, of course, subjective. Isotope scanning techniques demonstrate metabolic activity in the bone and soft tissue and are sometimes useful. The technique may include three phases of imaging: an immediate scan after injection of isotope, an early static phase (3–5 minutes after injection), and a late phase (2–3 h after). There have been reports of different patterns of abnormalities depending on the chronicity of the condition, and increased uptake on delayed images appears to be a sensitive and early finding in patients with RSD.

Whether the abnormalities that may be visualized by various imaging techniques are relevant to pain, its management and underlying mechanisms are unclear. The changes are not specific and other diseases may show abnormalities. Conversely, sympathetically maintained (and other) pains may occur without any radiological or scanning abnormalities. The temporal relationships are imprecise; for example, radiographs and scans may become abnormal before or after RSD develops, can persist long after clinical resolution, and do not correlate with the severity of pain. Perhaps the most useful place for such techniques is in investigating pain for which no cause can be found; an abnormal radiograph or scan indicates some underlying process, though the changes may reflect secondary changes rather than the primary cause.

Various other investigations are of even more uncertain value. These include thermography and other measures of skin temperature; laser–Doppler and other techniques assessing peripheral blood flow; and techniques to measure sweating, joint mobility, and muscle strength. These may be of interest as research techniques in studying patients with pain, but at present provide little diagnostic or therapeutic benefit.

Of particular importance, however, are negative laboratory measurements. In uncomplicated sympathetically maintained pains, the blood count, erythrocyte sedimentation rate (ESR), calcium, phosphorus, alkaline phosphatase, plasma proteins, and electrophoresis, and tests for rheumatological diseases are normal; a small, non-specific increase in urinary hydroxyproline may occur. Increased excretion merely reflects increased bone turnover, is non-specific (for example, can occur in Paget's disease), and indicates increased bone resorption. The latter of course may be seen in RSD and is evident from the osteoporosis seen on X-ray. Abnormal laboratory tests should lead to investigation for an underlying cause if this is not already known. Electromyographic studies are usually unhelpful, except of course where there is underlying nerve damage.

The response of pain to sympathetic blockade cannot be used as a diagnostic tool. Moreover, pain relief after sympathetic blockade does not preclude a serious underlying cause, such a response for instance being reported in the treatment of malignant disease.

Treatment

The mainstay of treatment of causalgia and RSD is sympathetic blockade (for reviews, see Bonica 1979; Gybels and Sweet 1989). Sympathetic nerve blocks using local anaesthetic that produce pain relief may be considered diagnostic procedures; they can be carried out for the upper limb, face, and upper trunk by blocking the stellate ganglion, or for the lower limb by lumbar sympathetic block. The problem then is to achieve a long-term therapeutic effect. Repeated blocks may be tried, although the success rate in causalgia may only be 18–25 per cent (Bonica 1979). In patients in whom repeated blocks are effective, and ideally after negative placebo blocks, permanent pain relief can be attempted either by chemical sympathetic blockade using phenol or by surgical sympathectomy. Unfortunately, effective temporary blocks do not assure a permanent procedure will result in long-term pain relief. The success rate of sympathectomy in patients with causalgia from war-time injuries is said to range from 62–100 per cent, although not all reports are as optimistic. The variability may result from incomplete sympathetic denervation, the persistence of tissue damage from the injuries, and the presence of additional, non-causalgic pains. Other techniques of achieving sympathectomy have also been tried, including temporary blockade of the stellate ganglion using morphine, and more permanent effects using radiofrequency lesioning of the stellate ganglion.

A major advance was achieved when Hannington-Kiff (1974) developed regional intravenous guanethidine infusion to achieve peripheral chemical sympathectomy. Guanethidine is taken up by adrenergic nerve terminals, where it causes release and subsequent depletion of noradrenaline. Guanethidine has other effects, for example, on anticholinesterase activity and histamine-mediated vasodilatation. It is tissue-bound and hence enters the systemic circulation in minimal amounts after regional administration.

In this technique, the previously exsanguinated limb is isolated from the circulation using a blood pressure cuff inflated above arterial blood pressure for 20–30 min. When the cuff has been inflated, guanethidine (in saline, with or without heparin, and often with local anaesthetic) is injected into a small peripheral vein. 10–30 mg guanethidine is used for the upper limb, and up to 30 mg for the lower limb. Some workers use a maximum of 10 mg for the first block, with higher doses for subsequent blocks. Pain relief if it occurs is often dramatic and very rapid; indeed it is observed whilst the cuff is still inflated. Weakness attributable to pain disappears extremely rapidly as well, and the patient is able to use the limb freely.

The injection is often painful, partly because of the application of the cuff, and partly because the noradrenaline released by the guanethidine is painful. Piloerection may be observed in the periphery at the time of noradrenaline release. Side-effects include postural hypotension from systemic effects, especially if the procedure is repeated. Transient headache, mild ptosis, drowsiness, and muscle weakness have also been described and, rarely, an allergic skin reaction may be seen. Temporary impotence and persistent headache have been described as late effects. The affected limb usually becomes warm and vasodilated, sometimes painfully; these sequelae are usually transient, but care is necessary if the patient's pain is worsened by warmth. Resuscitation facilities should be available, particularly for the rare instance of tourniquet failure.

How often blocks need to be repeated, either if the first is ineffective, or if benefit is transient, is not established. Some authors repeat the block two or three times over a fortnight; others give two or three blocks in a week; others have given 20 or more blocks over several weeks. It is difficult to envisage that any effects using the latter regime are due to the same mechanisms that occur when just one or two blocks are effective. As with stellate or lumbar blocks, efficacy is always unpredictable, the duration or benefit uncertain, and there is no correlation between pain relief and the other effects of sympathetic denervation. It is of interest that pain relief can occur even when sympathetic denervation is incomplete. It may be that repeated regional blocks are superior to stellate or lumbar blocks, but this is neither invariably so nor predictable.

Regional blockade using other sympatholytic drugs such as bretylium, phenoxybenzamine and reserpine has been tried, especially in the USA where guanethidine is not available for regional infusion. Systemic sympatholytic drugs have also been used, including oral guanethidine, which tends to cause unacceptable postural hypotension, and oral phenoxybenzamine. Numerous other methods have been described. These include regional intravenous local anaesthetic block with steroids, and ketanserin, and parenteral calcitonin. Oral α- and β-adrenergic blockers, anticonvulsants, analgesics, antidepressants, anti-inflammatory drugs, steroids, calcium-channel blockers, anticholinesterases, and griseofulvin have been tried, as have physical methods including transcutaneous electrical nerve stimulation and acupuncture, in addition to a variety of physiotherapy and psychological techniques. If pain relief is achieved, even in the short term, it is essential that vigorous physiotherapy and mobilization are carried out immediately.

Despite the numerous therapies tried, few studies have involved controlled trials with placebo or comparison with other methods, patients' conditions are often poorly described, groups of patients tend to include heterogeneous conditions, and follow-up is often short. Hence it is often very difficult to assess the value of a specific therapy and, in practice, many patients are treated in a 'trial-and-error' fashion. Nevertheless, sympathetic blockade is the treatment of first choice. There has been a consensus, difficult to prove, that early treatment provides the best outcome; this opinion has, however, also been refuted.

Post-sympathectomy pain (sympathalgia)

There have been a number of reports that damage to the sympathetic nervous system can sometimes cause pain (e.g. Raskin *et al.* 1976). The frequency is difficult to assess, but perhaps over 25 per cent of patients undergoing surgical sympathectomy develop severe pain, typically around rather than within the sympathectomized area. The pain usually occurs 1–2 weeks after surgery, lasts a few weeks, but can persist. There is paradoxically often increased rather than decreased sweating in the painful area. The pain is deep within the muscle, often with aching and hyperaesthesia. After lumbar sympathectomy, the anterior thighs are particularly affected. A similar syndrome has been described after aortic bifurcation surgery, presumably due to involvement of the sympathetic outflow. Occasionally the upper limb can be affected in a similar fashion after cervicothoracic sympathectomy.

The distribution of the pain is not usually that of a peripheral root or nerve, and it approximates to that of the efferent sympathetic outflow and particularly the periphery of this area. The cause is unclear. It may be due to partial peripheral damage to the sympathetic supply and denervation supersensitivity (which would account for the time delay), to partial damage to afferents travelling with the sympathetic efferents, and there may be a compensatory, delayed rise in sensory neuropeptides.

Anticonvulsants, including carbamazepine and phenytoin, may be helpful for the pain and, paradoxically, sympathetic blockade for sympathalgia after aortic bifurcation surgery has been reported as beneficial.

References

Bennett, G. J. and Xie, Y.-K. (1988). A peripheral mononeuropathy in rat that produces disorders of pain sensation like those seen in man. *Pain* **33**, 87–107.

Bonica, J. J. (1979). Causalgia and other reflex sympathetic dystrophies. In *Proceedings of the Second World Congress on Pain, Advances in Pain Research and Therapy*, Vol. 3 (ed. J. J. Bonica, J. C. Liebeskind, and D. G. Albe-Fessard), pp. 141–66. Raven Press, New York.

Campbell, J. N., Raja, S. N., Meyer, R. A., and Mackinnon, S. E. (1988). Myelinated afferents signal the hyperalgesia associated with nerve injury. *Pain* **32**, 89–94.

Cline, M. A., Ochoa, J., and Torebjork, H. E. (1989). Chronic hyperalgesia and skin warming caused by sensitized C nociceptors. *Brain* **112**, 621–47.

Doury, P., Dirheimer, Y., and Pattin, W. (1981). *Algodystrophy*. Springer, Berlin.

Drummond, P. D., Finch, P. M., and Smythe, G. A. (1991). Reflex sympathetic dystrophy: the significance of differing plasma catecholamine concentrations in affected and unaffected limbs. *Brain* **114**, 2025–36.

Evans, J. A. (1946). Reflex sympathetic dystrophy. *Surg. Gynecol. Obstet.* **82**, 36–43.

Gybels, J. M. and Sweet, W. H. (ed.) (1989) *Neurosurgical treatment of persistent pain. Pain and headache*, Vol. 11 pp. 257–81. Karger, Basel.

Hannington-Kiff, J. G. (1974). Intravenous regional sympathetic blockade with guanethidine. *Lancet* **i**, 1091–20.

Jänig, W. (1985). Causalgia and reflex sympathetic dystrophy: in which way is the sympathetic nervous system involved? *Trends Neurosci.* **8**, 471–7.

Kozin, F., Genant, H. K., Bekerman, C., and McCarty, D. J. (1976*a*). The reflex sympathetic dystrophy syndrome. II. Roentgenographic and scintigraphic evidence of bilaterality and of periarticular accentuation. *Am. J. Med.* **60**, 332–8.

Kozin, F., McCarty, D. J., Sims, J., and Genant, H. (1976*b*). The reflex sympathetic dystrophy syndrome. I. Clinical and histologic studies: evidence for bilaterality, response to corticosteroids and articular involvement. *Am. J. Med.* **60**, 321–31.

Leriche, R. (1939). *The surgery of pain*. (English translation) Baillière, Tindall and Cox, London.

Levine, J. D., Taiwo, Y. O., Collins, S. D., and Tam, J. K. (1986). Noradrenaline hyperalgesia is mediated through interaction with sympathetic postganglionic neurone terminals rather than activation of primary afferent nociceptors. *Nature* **323**, 158–60.

Loh, L. and Nathan, P. W. (1978) Painful peripheral states and sympathetic blocks. *J. Neurol. Neurosurg. Psychiat.* **41**, 664–71.

Loh, L., Nathan, P. W., and Schott, G. D. (1981). Pain due to lesions of central nervous system removed by sympathetic block. *Br. med. J.* **282**, 1026–8.

Mitchell, S. W., Morehouse, G. R., and Keen, W. W. (1864) *Gunshot wounds and other injuries of nerves.* Lippincott, Philadelphia.

Nathan, P. W. (1983). Pain and the sympathetic system. *J. autonom. nerv. Syst.* 7, 363-70.

Poplawski, Z. J., Wiley, A. M., and Murray, J. F. (1983). Post traumatic dystrophy of the extremities. A clinical review and trial of treatment. *J. Bone Jt Surg.* **65A**, 642-55.

Price, D. D., Bennett, G. J., and Rafii, A. (1989). Psychophysical observations on patients with neuropathic pain relieved by a sympathetic block. *Pain* **36**, 273-88.

Raskin, N. H., Levinson, S. A., Hoffman, P. M., Pickett, J. B. E., and Fields, H. (1976). Postsympathectomy neuralgia. Amelioration with diphenylhydantoin and carbamazepine. *Am. J. Surg.* **128**, 75-8.

Richards, R. L. (1967). Causalgia. A centennial review. *Arch. Neurol.* **16**, 339-50.

Roberts, W. J. (1986). A hypothesis on the physiological basis for causalgia and related pains. *Pain* **24**, 297-311.

Schott, G. D. (1986). Mechanisms of causalgia and related clinical conditions. The role of the central and the sympathetic nervous systems. *Brain* **109**, 717-38.

Schwartzman, R. J. and Kerrigan, J. (1990). The movement disorder of reflex sympathetic dystrophy. *Neurology, Minneapolis* **40**, 57-61.

Stanton-Hicks, M. (ed.) (1990). *Pain and the sympathetic nervous system.* Kluwer Academic Publishers, Boston.

Stanton-Hicks, M., Jänig, W., and Boas, R. A. (ed.) (1990). *Reflex sympathetic dystrophy.* Kluwer Academic Publishers, Boston.

Steinbrocker, O. and Argyros, T. G. (1958). The shoulder–hand syndrome: present status as a diagnostic and therapeutic entity. *Med. Clinics N. Am.* **42**, 1533-53.

Torebjork, E. (1990). Clinical and neurophysiological observations relating to pathophysiological mechanisms in reflex sympathetic dystrophy. In *Reflex sympathetic dystrophy* (ed. Stanton-Hicks, M., Jänig, W., and Boas, R. A.), pp. 71-9. Kluwer Academic Publishers, Boston.

Zachariae, L. (1964). Incidence and course of posttraumatic dystrophy following operation for Dupuytren's contracture. *Acta chir. scand.* **suppl. 336**, 28-31.

Index

Page numbers in **bold** indicate main discussions. Abbreviations used in sub-headings are: ADH, antidiuretic hormone; ANS, autonomic nervous system; CNS, central nervous system; CSF, cerebrospinal fluid; NANC, non-adrenergic, non-cholinergic; PET, positron emission tomography.